Contents

Introduction to Nutrition and Metabolism

Fourth Edition

David A. Bender

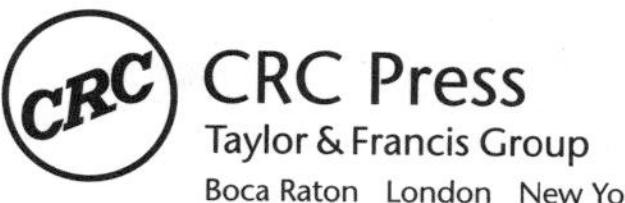

CRC Press
Taylor & Francis Group
Boca Raton London New York

CRC Press is an imprint of the
Taylor & Francis Group, an informa business

CRC Press
Taylor & Francis Group
6000 Broken Sound Parkway NW, Suite 300
Boca Raton, FL 33487-2742

Printed in Canada on acid-free paper
10 9 8 7 6 5 4 3

International Standard Book Number-10: 1-4200-4312-9 (Softcover)
International Standard Book Number-13: 978-1-4200-4312-9 (Softcover)

Library of Congress Cataloging-in-Publication Data

Bender, David A.
Introduction to nutrition and metabolism / by David Allen Bender. -- 4th ed.
p. ; cm.
Includes bibliographical references and index.
ISBN-13: 978-1-4200-4312-9 (hardcover : alk. paper)
ISBN-10: 1-4200-4312-9 (hardcover : alk. paper)
1. Nutrition. 2. Metabolism. I. Title.
[DNLM: 1. Nutrition Physiology. 2. Metabolism--physiology. QU 145 B4582i 2008]

QP141.B38 2008
612.3'9--dc22 2007002481

Visit the Taylor & Francis Web site at
http://www.taylorandfrancis.com

and the CRC Press Web site at
http://www.crcpress.com

Preface

The food we eat has a major effect on our physical health and psychological well-being. An understanding of the way in which nutrients are metabolized, and hence of the principles of biochemistry, is essential for an understanding of the scientific basis of what we would call a prudent or healthy diet.

My aim in the following pages is to explain the conclusions of the many expert committees that have deliberated on the problems of nutritional requirements, diet, and health over the years and also the scientific basis on which these experts have reached their conclusions. Much of what is now presented as "facts" will be proven to be incorrect in years to come. This book is intended to provide a foundation of scientific knowledge and understanding from which to interpret and evaluate future advances in nutrition and health sciences.

Nutrition is one of the basic sciences that underlies a proper understanding of health and human sciences and the ways in which humans and their environment interact. In its turn, the science of nutrition is based on both biochemistry and physiology on the one hand, and the social and behavioral sciences on the other. This book contains such biochemistry as is essential to an understanding of the science of nutrition.

In a book of this kind, which is an introduction to nutrition and metabolism, it is not appropriate to cite the original scientific literature that provides the (sometimes conflicting) evidence for the statements made; in the clinical problems and some of the tables of data, I have acknowledged my sources of data as a simple courtesy to my fellow scientists, and also to guide readers to the original sources of information.

I am grateful to those of my students whose perceptive questions have helped me to formulate and clarify my thoughts, and especially to those who responded to my inquiry as to what they would like to see (for the benefit of future generations of students) in this new edition. At their request, but somewhat against my better judgment, I have included a list of key points at the end of each chapter—against my better judgment because I think that it is the student's task to summarize the key points from reading.

This book is dedicated to those who will use it as a part of their studies, in the hope that they will, in their turn, be able to advance the frontiers of knowledge and help their clients, patients, and students to understand the basis of the advice they offer.

David A. Bender
University College London

Additional resources

The CD that accompanies this book contains a number of additional resources to supplement each chapter. All of these can be run directly from the CD, but it is better to copy the files onto a hard disc. Teachers who adopt the book as a class text are permitted to install the material on the CD onto an institutional server for class use, but this must be password protected and available only to members of the institution.

To access the resources on the CD, you will require an IBM-compatible PC running 32-bit Windows® (95, 98, 2000, XP, or higher), with a minimum screen resolution of 1024 × 768 pixels for the programs; the PowerPoint presentations and html files are not dependent on screen resolution.

Users of Apple Mac® computers will have to install Windows emulation software to run the programs, but should be able to view the PowerPoint presentations and html files without.

All the resources on the CD can be accessed with links from the welcome file, although you may wish to set up shortcuts to specific sections.

If the program on the CD does not autostart when you insert the disc in your CD drive, run the program *welcome.htm*.

The resources on the CD consist of the following:

A review of simple chemistry: The file "chemical basis of life" on the CD provides a very elementary review of the chemistry you may need to know in order to understand some aspects of this book. It is an Adobe Acrobat (.pdf) file, and there is a link to download the Acrobat reader in the welcome file.

PowerPoint presentations: There is a PowerPoint presentation to accompany each chapter, as well as one that provides a tour of the cell. In most cases, the slides build with simple animations as you click the mouse or press the spacebar.

If you have Microsoft PowerPoint installed on your computer, then you can view these presentations immediately. If not, the Microsoft PowerPoint viewer is on the CD and can be installed by running the program *ppviewer.exe* from the CD.

Teachers are welcome to use these PowerPoint presentations, or parts of them, in their lectures, provided that due acknowledgement is made; they are copyright David A. Bender, 2007 and may not be published without written permission.

Self-assessment quizzes: For most chapters, there is a computer-based self-assessment quiz on the CD. This consists of a series of statements to be marked true or false; you assess your confidence in your answer, and gain marks for being correct, or lose marks for being incorrect, scaled according to your confidence in your answer. These quizzes are accessed from the welcome screen, or from the program *Testme.exe* on the CD.

The virtual laboratory: There are a number of simulations of laboratory experiments on the CD; they can be accessed from the welcome file or by going directly to *simulations.htm* in the simulations folder. There are html screens to explain the theory for each program:

- Energy balance
- Enzyme assay
- Enzyme purification
- Mutations in a peptide
- Nitrogen balance

- Oxygen electrode studies
- Peptide sequence
- Radio-immunoassay of steroid hormones
- Urea synthesis

Food composition: This program permits you to analyze the nutrients in more than 2700 foods and display the results in the format of a "food facts" or "nutrition information" label. You can also add each food you analyze to one of four meals, and see the summary of each meal in the same format.

When you start the program, you are offered the choice of using the US/Canadian Daily Value (DV) figures or the EU labeling RDA (RDA), and only this value will be used for on-screen display with the nutrient analysis. However, when you print the results both %DV and %RDA are shown.

You select foods by browsing the aisles of a virtual supermarket; unlike a real supermarket, some aisles appear in more than one place (e.g., cooked meat appears both with other meat and poultry, and also in the food court restaurants). Once you have found the aisle, the foods available appear in a scroll-down box. Just click on the food to select it.

For most foods there is a standard or average serving. You may either use this default portion or enter the weight of the portion in a tick box. You are then shown the analysis of the food, and you are offered the choice of adding it to one of four meals, or ignoring it.

Once more than three foods have been added to a meal, it is possible to see the summary of meals and foods added to date. This screen also offers you the chance to save the results to print out when you end the program.

When you end the program, you are offered the choice of ending without printing or printing out your saved results. The printout consists of the names of foods added to each meal and the summary nutritional analysis of each meal.

The nutrient data come from two sources:

- US Department of Agriculture National Nutrient Database for Standard Reference, Release 17, which is freely available from the USDA Nutrient Data Laboratory website: http://www.nal.usda.gov/fnic/foodcomp.
- Data provided on web sites of fast food restaurants and manufacturers' labels.

Web links: Most people use a search engine to find information on the Internet, but there is a page of links that I have found to be useful sources of reliable information on the CD.

Problems at the end of chapters

At the end of most chapters there are problems to be considered. These are of various kinds:

- Open-ended problems to be thought about.
- Defined calculation problems to which there are correct answers (but the answer is not provided here).
- Problems of data interpretation, in which you are guided through sets of data and prompted to draw conclusions. Again, deliberately, no answers to these problems are provided.

- Clinical problems in which you are given information about a patient and expected to deduce the underlying biochemical basis of the problem, and explain how the defect causes the metabolic disturbances.

Teachers and instructors who adopt this book as a class text can obtain a file containing solutions to the problems from CRC Press.

Review journals

Nutrition Research Reviews, published biannually by Cambridge University Press, for the Nutrition Society.

Nutrition Reviews, published monthly by the International Life Sciences Institute, Washington, DC.

Annual Reviews of Biochemistry and *Annual Review of Nutrition,* published annually by Annual Reviews, Inc.

About the author

David Bender was educated at North Ealing Primary School and Greenford County Grammar School, and then studied biochemistry from 1965 to 1968 at the University of Birmingham. He joined the Courtauld Institute of Biochemistry of the Middlesex Hospital Medical School as a research assistant in 1968, was appointed lecturer in biochemistry in 1970, and received his PhD (on the metabolism of aromatic amino acids) in 1971. The Middlesex Hospital Medical School merged with University College London (UCL) in 1987 and Bender became a member of the Department of Biochemistry and Molecular Biology of UCL. He was appointed senior lecturer in biochemistry in 1994.

Since 1994, David Bender has also been assistant faculty tutor (medical) in the Faculty of Life Sciences and since 1998, subdean (teaching) of the Royal Free and University College Medical School. His research interests have been in the field of amino acid and vitamin nutritional biochemistry, and his main activities now are concerned with teaching and the delivery of the undergraduate medical course; he has also taught a variety of health science courses.

chapter one

Why eat?

An adult eats about a tonne of food a year. This book attempts to answer the question *"why?"* by exploring the need for food and the uses to which that food is put in the body. Some discussion of chemistry and biochemistry is obviously essential in order to understand the fate of food in the body, and why there is a continual need for food throughout life. Therefore, in the following chapters various aspects of biochemistry and metabolism will be discussed. This should provide not only the basis of our present understanding, knowledge, and concepts in nutrition, but also, more importantly, a basis from which to interpret future research findings and evaluate new ideas and hypotheses as they are formulated.

We eat because we are hungry. Why have we evolved complex physiological and psychological mechanisms to control not only hunger, but also our appetite for different types of food? Why do meals form such an important part of our life?

Objectives

After reading this chapter, you should be able to

- Describe the need for metabolic fuels and outline the relationship between food intake, energy expenditure, and body weight
- Outline the importance of an appropriate intake of dietary fat
- Describe the mechanisms involved in short-term and long-term control of food intake
- Outline the mechanisms involved in the sense of taste
- Explain the various factors that influence peoples' choices of foods

1.1 The need for energy

There is an obvious need for energy to perform physical work. Work has to be done to lift a load against the force of gravity, and there must be a source of energy to perform that work. The energy used in various activities can be measured (Section 5.1), as can the metabolic energy yield of the foods that are the fuel for that work (Table 1.1). This means that it is possible to calculate a balance between the intake of energy, as metabolic fuels, and the body's energy expenditure. Obviously, energy intake has to be appropriate for the level of energy expenditure; as discussed in Chapters 7 and 8, neither an excess intake nor a deficiency is desirable.

Figure 1.1 shows the relationship between food intake, physical work, and variations in the body reserves of metabolic fuels, as shown by changes in body weight. This was a study conducted in Germany at the end of the Second World War, when there was a great deal of rubble from bomb-damaged buildings to be cleared, and a large number of people to be fed and employed. Increasing the food intake resulted in an increase in work output—initially with an increase in body weight, indicating that the food supply was greater than was required to meet the (increased) work output. When a financial reward

Table 1.1 The Energy Yield of Metabolic Fuels

	Energy	
	kcal/g	kJ/g
Carbohydrate	4	17
Protein	4	16
Fat	9	37
Alcohol	7	29

Note: 1 kcal = 4.186 kJ or 1 kJ = 0.239 kcal.

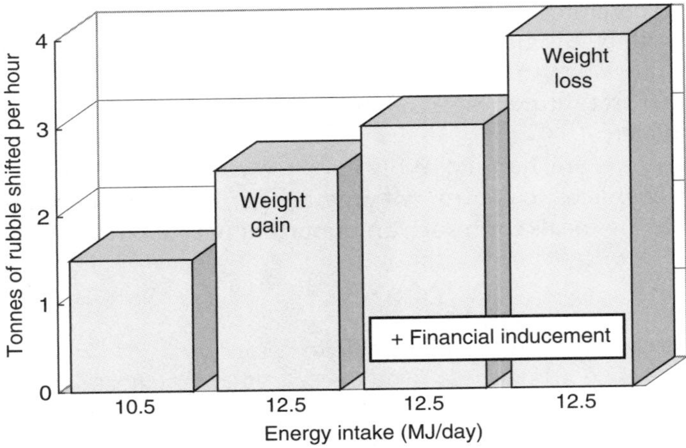

Figure 1.1 The relationship between food intake, work output, and body weight. (From Widdowson, E.M., MRC Special Report series no. 275, London HMSO, 1951.)

was offered as well, the work output increased to such an extent that people now drew on their (sparse) reserves, and there was a loss of body weight.

Quite apart from obvious work output, the body has a considerable requirement for energy, even at rest. Only about one-third of the average person's energy expenditure is for voluntary work (Section 5.1.3). The remaining two-thirds is required for maintenance of the body's functions, homeostasis of the internal environment, and metabolic integrity. This energy requirement at rest, the basal metabolic rate (BMR; Section 5.1.3.1), can be measured by the output of heat or the consumption of oxygen, when the subject is completely at rest. Figure 1.2 shows the proportion of this resting energy expenditure that is accounted for by different organs.

Part of this basal energy requirement is obvious—the heart beats to circulate the blood; respiration continues; and there is considerable electrical activity in nerves and muscles, irrespective of whether they are "working" or not. The brain and nervous system comprise about only 2% of body weight, but account for some 20% of the resting energy expenditure, because of the active transport of ions across nerve membranes to maintain electrical activity. These processes require a metabolic energy source. Less obviously, there is also a requirement for energy for the wide variety of biochemical reactions occurring all the time in the body: laying down reserves of fat and carbohydrate (Section 5.6); turnover of tissue proteins (Section 9.2.3.3); transport of substrates into, and products out of, cells (Section 3.2.2); and the synthesis and secretion of hormones and neurotransmitters.

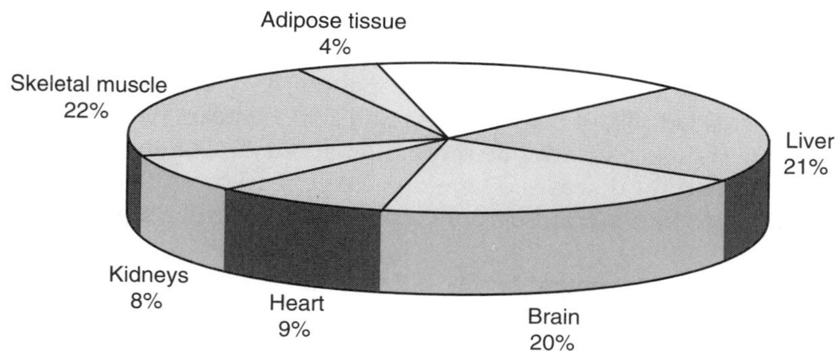

Figure 1.2 Percentage of resting energy expenditure by different organs of the body.

1.1.1 Units of energy

Energy expenditure is measured by the output of heat from the body (Section 5.1.1). The unit of heat used in the early studies was the calorie (cal)—the amount of heat required to raise the temperature of 1 g of water by 1°C. The calorie is still used to some extent in nutrition; in biological systems the kilocalorie (kcal, sometimes written as Calorie with a capital C) is used. One kilocalorie is 1000 calories (10^3 cal), and hence the amount of heat required to raise the temperature of 1 kg of water by 1°C.

Correctly, the joule is used as the unit of energy. Joule is an SI unit, named after James Prescott Joule (1818–1889), who first showed the equivalence of heat, mechanical work, and other forms of energy. In biological systems, the kilojoule (1 kJ = 10^3 J) and megajoule (1 MJ = 10^6 J) are used. To convert between calories and joules:

1 kcal = 4.186 kJ (normally rounded off to 4.2 kJ)
1 kJ = 0.239 kcal (normally rounded off to 0.24 kcal)

The average total daily energy expenditure of adults is between 7.5 and 10 MJ for women and 8 and 12 MJ for men.

1.2 Metabolic fuels

The dietary sources of metabolic energy (the metabolic fuels) are carbohydrates, fats, protein, and alcohol. The metabolism of these fuels results in the production of carbon dioxide and water (and also urea in the case of proteins; Section 9.3.1.4). They can be converted to the same end products chemically by burning in air. Although the process of metabolism in the body is more complex, it is a fundamental law of chemistry that if the starting material and end products are the same, the energy yield is the same, regardless of the route taken. Therefore, the energy yield of foodstuffs can be determined by measuring the heat produced when they are burnt in air, making allowance for the extent to which they are digested and absorbed from foods. The energy yields of the metabolic fuels in the body, allowing for digestion and absorption, are shown in Table 1.1.

1.2.1 The need for carbohydrate and fat

Although there is a requirement for energy sources in the diet, it does not matter unduly how that requirement is met. There is no requirement for a dietary source of carbohydrate; the body can synthesize carbohydrates from the amino acids derived from proteins

(Section 5.7). Similarly, there is no requirement for a dietary source of fat, apart from the essential fatty acids (Section 4.3.1.1), and there is certainly no requirement for a dietary source of alcohol. Diets that provide more than about 35%–40% of energy from fat are associated with increased risk of heart disease and some cancers (Section 6.3.2), and there is some evidence that diets that provide more than about 20% of energy from protein are also associated with chronic diseases. Therefore, the general consensus is that diets should provide about 55% of energy from carbohydrates, 30% from fat, and 15% from protein (Section 6.3).

Although there is no requirement for fat in the diet, fats are nutritionally important and there is a specific mechanism for detecting the taste of fats in foods (Section 1.3.3.1).

- It is difficult to eat enough of a very low-fat diet to meet energy requirements. As shown in Table 1.1, the energy yield per gram of fat is more than twice that of carbohydrate or protein. The problem in many less-developed countries, where undernutrition is a problem (Chapter 8), is that diets provide only 10%–15% of energy from fat and it is difficult to consume a sufficient bulk of food to meet the energy requirements. In contrast, the problem in Western countries is an undesirably high intake of fat, contributing to the development of obesity (Chapter 7) and chronic diseases (Section 6.3.2).
- Four of the vitamins, A, D, E, and K (Chapter 11), are fat- soluble and are found in fatty and oily foods. They are absorbed dissolved in fat; so with a very low-fat diet the absorption of these vitamins may be inadequate to meet requirements, even if the diet provides an adequate amount.
- There is a requirement for small amounts of two essential fatty acids (Section 4.3.1.1) that cannot be synthesized in the body, but must be provided in the diet.
- In many foods, a great deal of the flavor (and hence the pleasure of eating) is carried in the fat.
- Fat lubricates food, making it easier to chew and swallow.

1.2.2 *The need for protein*

Unlike fats and carbohydrates, there is a requirement for protein in the diet. In a growing child this need is obvious. As the child grows, and the size of its body increases, there is an increase in the total amount of protein in the body.

Adults also require protein in their diet (Section 9.1). There is a continual loss of protein from the body, for example, in hair, shed skin cells, enzymes, and other proteins secreted into the gut and not completely digested. More importantly, there is a turnover of tissue proteins, which are continually being broken down and replaced. Although there is no change in the total amount of protein in the body, an adult with an inadequate intake of protein will be unable to replace this loss and will lose tissue protein.

1.2.3 *The need for micronutrients—minerals and vitamins*

In addition to metabolic fuels and protein, the body has a requirement for a variety of mineral salts. If a metal or an ion has a function in the body, it must be provided by the diet, since the different elements cannot be interconverted. Again, the need is obvious for a growing child; as the body grows, the total amounts of minerals in the body will increase. In adults, there is a turnover of minerals in the body and losses must be replaced from the diet (Section 11.15).

There is a requirement for a different group of nutrients in small amounts—vitamins. These are organic compounds that have a variety of functions. They cannot be synthesized in the body and so must be provided by the diet. There is turnover of the vitamins, so there must be replacement of the losses (Sections 11.2 through 11.14).

Other compounds in the diet (especially from fruits and vegetables) are not considered as nutrients, since they are not dietary essentials, but they may have beneficial effects in reducing the risk of developing a variety of chronic diseases (Section 6.6).

1.3 Hunger and appetite

Humans have evolved an elaborate system of physiological and psychological mechanisms, to ensure that the body's needs for metabolic fuels and nutrients are met and also balance energy expenditure with food intake.

1.3.1 Hunger and satiety—short-term control of feeding

There are hunger centers in the brain that stimulate us to begin eating and satiety centers that signal us to stop eating when hunger has been satisfied (Figure 1.3). The hunger centers in the lateral hypothalamus act through neurons that use neuropeptide Y as their transmitter. The satiety centers in the ventro-medial hypothalamus act through neurons that use another peptide, pro-opiomelanocortin (POMC). A number of drugs can modify the responses to hunger and satiety. Although some of these have been used to reduce appetite in the treatment of obesity (Section 7.3.4.11) or stimulate it in people with loss of appetite, or anorexia, none is now legally available because of (sometimes severe) side effects. The synthesis and release of neuropeptide Y is dependent on zinc, and the loss of appetite associated with zinc deficiency is a result of impaired secretion of this neurotransmitter (Section 11.15.2.6).

A variety of factors act on the hunger and the satiety centers to initiate nerve impulses, including the following:

- Direct neuronal input from the gastrointestinal tract.
- The relative concentrations of glucose, triacylglycerols, nonesterified fatty acids, and ketone bodies available as metabolic fuels in the fed and the fasting states (Section 5.3).
- The relative concentrations of the hormones, insulin (secreted by the pancreas in response to increased blood concentrations of glucose and amino acids; Section 5.3.1) and glucagon (secreted by the pancreas in response to a decreased concentration of blood glucose; Section 5.3.2).
- Hormones secreted by the gastrointestinal tract during digestion, including ghrelin, cholecystokinin (secreted by the duodenum), glucagon-like peptide and oxyntomodulin (both derived from the glucagon gene and secreted by gut endocrine cells), and peptide YY (also secreted by gut endocrine cells). Ghrelin is secreted by the stomach. It was originally discovered as the hormone that stimulates growth hormone secretion, but it also acts to increase the synthesis of neuropeptide Y (thus increasing hunger—an orexigenic action) and a peptide that antagonizes the appetite-suppressing action of POMC. The other gut-derived hormones act to suppress appetite.

The hypothalamic centers control food intake remarkably precisely. Without conscious effort, most people regulate their food intake to match energy expenditure very

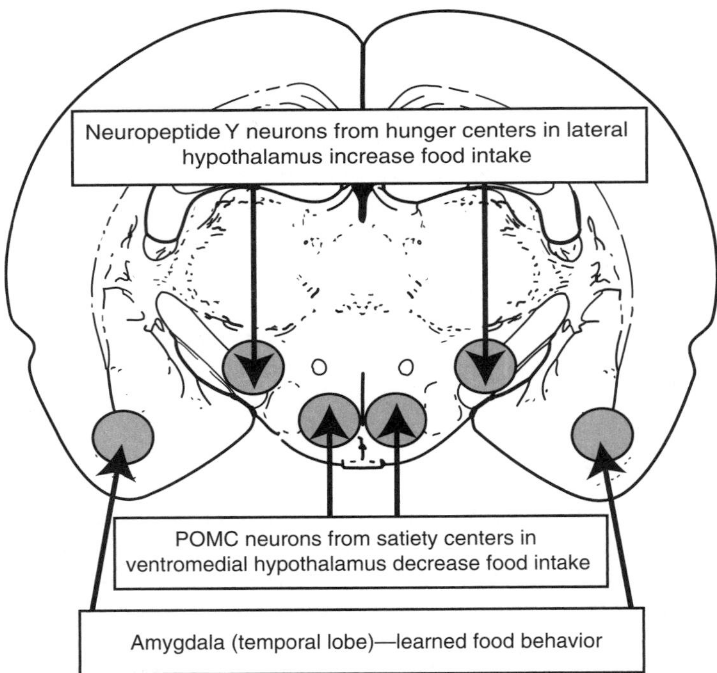

Figure 1.3 Hypothalamic appetite control centers.

closely—they neither waste away from lack of metabolic fuel for physical activity nor lay down excessively large reserves of fat. Even people who have excessive reserves of body fat, and can be considered to be so overweight or obese as to be putting their health at risk (Section 7.2.2), balance their energy intake and expenditure relatively well considering that the average intake of food is a tonne a year, while the record obese people weigh about 250–300 kg (compared with the average weights between 60 and 100 kg) and it takes many years to achieve such a weight. A gain or loss of 5 kg of body weight over 6 months would require only a 1% daily mismatch between food intake and energy expenditure (Section 5.2).

1.3.2 Long-term control of food intake and energy expenditure

In addition to the immediate control of feeding by sensations of hunger and satiety, there is long-term regulation of food intake and energy expenditure in response to the size of the body's fat reserves. This is largely a function of the peptide hormone leptin, which is secreted by adipose tissue. It was discovered as the normal product of the gene that is defective in the homozygous recessive mutant (*ob/ob*) obese mouse; administration of the peptide to the obese mice caused them to lose weight. Further studies showed that the administration of leptin to the genetically obese diabetic (*db/db*) mouse had no effect on body weight; they secreted a normal or a greater than normal amount of leptin. The defect in these animals is in the receptor for leptin in the hypothalamus.

The circulating concentration of leptin is determined largely by the mass of adipose tissue in the body, and leptin signals the size of body fat reserves. Low levels of leptin, reflecting adipose tissue reserves that are inadequate to permit a normal pregnancy, not only increase food intake, but also lead to cessation of ovulation and menstruation (by decreasing the secretion of gonadotrophin-releasing hormone); a loss of weight to below about 45 kg is associated with amenorrhea. In undernourished children, low levels of leptin, reflecting levels of adipose tissue reserves that are inadequate to permit growth, reduce skeletal growth by inhibiting the secretion of the growth hormone.

There is reduced food intake in response to leptin, associated with a decrease in the synthesis of neuropeptide Y (the transmitter for neurons from the hunger centers of the hypothalamus) and increased synthesis of POMC (the transmitter for neurons from the satiety centers). However, the resultant weight loss is greater than can be accounted for by reduced food intake alone, and in response to leptin there is a specific loss of adipose tissue, while in response to reduced food intake there is a loss of both adipose and lean tissue. Leptin receptors are found in a variety of tissues, including muscle and the adipose tissue itself. In addition to its role in appetite control, leptin acts to increase energy expenditure and promote the loss of adipose tissue by several mechanisms, including the following:

- Increased expression of uncoupling proteins (Section 3.3.1.5) in adipose tissue and muscle. This results in relatively uncontrolled oxidation of metabolic fuel, unrelated to requirements for physical and chemical work, and increased heat output from the body (thermogenesis).
- Increased activity of lipase in adipose tissue (Section 10.5.1), resulting in the breakdown of triacylglycerol reserves and release of nonesterified fatty acids that may be either oxidized or be re-esterified in the liver and transported back to adipose tissue. This is metabolically inefficient because of the energy cost of synthesizing triacylglycerol from fatty acids (Section 5.6.1.2); such cycling of lipids is one of the factors involved in the weight loss associated with advanced cancer (Section 8.4.1).
- Decreased expression of acetyl CoA carboxylase in adipose tissue (Section 5.6.1). This results in both decreased synthesis and increased oxidation of fatty acids, as a result of decreased formation of malonyl CoA (Section 10.5.2).
- Increased apoptosis (programmed cell death) in adipose tissue, thus reducing the number of adipocytes available for storage of fat in the body.

The result of these actions of leptin on adipose tissue and muscle is that there is an increase in metabolic rate, and hence energy expenditure, in addition to the reduction in food intake.

Although most leptin is secreted by adipose tissue, it is also secreted by muscles and the gastric mucosa. After a meal there is an increase in circulating leptin, suggesting that apart from its role in long-term control of food intake and energy expenditure, it may also be important in short-term responses to food intake. Some of this leptin comes from the gastric mucosa, but in response to food intake, insulin (Section 5.3.1) stimulates the synthesis and secretion of leptin from adipose tissue. Conversely, leptin increases the synthesis and secretion of insulin but also antagonizes its actions, so that excessively high levels of leptin, associated with obesity, lead to hyperinsulinemia and insulin resistance—part of the metabolic syndrome associated with obesity (Section 7.2.3.1).

There is a circadian variation in leptin secretion, with an increase during the night. This is in response to glucocorticoid hormones, which are secreted in increased amounts during the night. It is likely that the loss of appetite and weight loss associated with chronic stress, when there is increased secretion of glucocorticoids, is mediated by the effect of these hormones on leptin synthesis and secretion.

When leptin was first discovered, there was great excitement that as in the obese mouse, human obesity (Chapter 7) might be due to a failure of leptin synthesis or secretion and that administration of leptin might be a useful treatment for severe obesity. However, most obese people secrete more leptin than lean people (because they have more adipose tissue), and it is likely that the problem is not due to lack of leptin but rather to a loss of sensitivity of the leptin receptors. Only a very small number of people have been found in whom genetically determined obesity is due to a mutation in the gene for leptin, the leptin receptor, or a component of the downstream signaling pathway.

1.3.3 Appetite

In addition to hunger and satiety, which are basic physiological responses, food intake is controlled by appetite, which is related not only to physiological need but also to the pleasure of eating—flavor, texture, and a variety of social and psychological factors.

1.3.3.1 Taste and flavor

Taste buds on the tongue can distinguish five basic tastes: salt, savory, sweet, bitter, and sour, as well as a less well-understood ability to taste fat. The ability to taste salt, sweetness, savoriness, and fat permits detection of nutrients; the ability to taste sourness and bitterness permits avoidance of toxins in foods.

Salt (correctly, the mineral sodium) is essential, to life, and wild animals will travel great distances to a salt lick. Like other animals, humans have evolved a pleasurable response to salty flavors; this ensures that physiological needs are met. There is evidence that sensitivity to salt changes in response to the state of sodium balance in the body, with an increased number of active salt receptors on the tongue at times of sodium depletion. However, there is no shortage of salt in developed countries; indeed average intakes of salt are considerably greater than requirements and pose a hazard to health (Section 6.3.4).

The sensation of savoriness is distinct from that of saltiness and is sometimes called *umami* (Japanese for "savory"). It is largely due to the presence of free amino acids in foods and permits detection of protein-rich foods. Stimulation of the umami receptors of the tongue is the basis of flavor enhancers such as monosodium glutamate, an important constituent of traditional oriental condiments that is widely used in manufactured foods.

The other instinctively pleasurable taste is sweetness, which permits detection of carbohydrates and hence energy sources. While it is only sugars (Section 4.2.1) that have a sweet taste, humans (and a few other animals) secrete the enzyme amylase in saliva, which catalyzes the hydrolysis of starch, the major dietary carbohydrate, to sweet-tasting sugars while the food is being chewed (Section 4.2.2.1).

The tongue is not sensitive to the taste of triacylglycerols, but rather to free fatty acids and especially polyunsaturated fatty acids (Section 4.3.1.1). This suggests that the lipase secreted by the tongue has a role in permitting the detection of fatty foods as an energy source, in addition to a very minor role in fat digestion (Section 4.3.2).

Sourness and bitterness are instinctively unpleasant sensations; many of the toxins that occur in foods have a bitter or a sour flavor. Learnt behavior will overcome the instinctive aversion, but this is a process of learning or acquiring tastes, not an innate or an instinctive response.

The receptors for salt, sourness, and savoriness (umami) all act as ion channels, transporting sodium, hydrogen, and glutamate ions, respectively, into the cells of the taste buds. The receptors for sweetness and bitterness act via cell-surface receptors linked to intracellular formation of second messengers. There is evidence that both cyclic adenosine monophosphate (cAMP, Section 10.3.2) and inositol trisphosphate (Section 10.3.3) mechanisms are involved, and more than one signal transduction pathway may be involved in the responses to sweetness or sourness of different compounds. Some compounds may activate more than one subtype of receptor.

In addition to the sensations of taste provided by the taste buds on the tongue, many flavors can be distinguished by the sense of smell. Some flavors and aromas (fruity flavors, fresh coffee, and, at least to a nonvegetarian, the smell of roasting meat) are pleasurable, tempting people to eat and stimulating appetite. Other flavors and aromas are repulsive, warning us not to eat the food. Again, this can be seen as a warning of possible danger—the smell of decaying meat or fish tells us that it is not safe to eat.

Like the acquisition of a taste for bitter or sour foods, a taste for foods with what would seem at first to be an unpleasant aroma or flavor can also be acquired. Here things become more complex—a pleasant smell to one person may be repulsive to another. Some people enjoy the smell of cooked cabbage and Brussels sprouts, while others can hardly bear to be in the same room. The durian fruit is a highly prized delicacy in southeast Asia, yet to the uninitiated it has the unappetizing aroma of sewage or feces.

1.3.4 *Why do people eat what they do?*

People have different responses to the same taste or flavor. This may be explained in terms of childhood memories, pleasurable or otherwise. An aversion to the smell of a food may protect someone who has a specific allergy or intolerance (although sometimes people have a craving for the foods of which they are intolerant). Most often, we simply cannot explain why some people dislike foods that others eat with great relish. A number of factors influence why people choose to eat particular foods (Table 1.2).

1.3.4.1 *The availability and cost of food*

In developed countries, the simple availability of food is not a constraint on choice. There is a wide variety of foods available, and when fruits and vegetables are out of season at home they are imported; frozen, canned, or dried foods are widespread. In contrast, in developing countries, the availability of food may be a major constraint on what people choose. Little food is imported, and what is available depends on the local soil and climate. In normal times the choice of foods may be limited, while in times of drought there may

Table 1.2 Factors That Influence the Choice of Foods

Availability of foods
Cost of foods
Time for preparation and consumption
Disability and infirmity
Personal likes and dislikes
Intolerance or allergy
Eating alone or in company
Marketing pressure and advertising
Religious and ethical taboos
Perceived or real health benefits and risks
Modified diet for control of disease
Illness or medication

be little or no food available at all, and what little is available will be more expensive than most people can afford. Even in developed countries the cost of food is important, and for the most disadvantaged members of the community, poverty may impose severe constraints on their choice of foods.

1.3.4.2 Religion, habit, and tradition

Religious and ethical considerations are important in determining the choice of foods. Observant Jews and Muslims will only eat meat from animals that have cloven hooves and chew the cud. The terms *kosher* in Jewish law and *halal* in Islamic law both mean clean; the meat of other animals—scavenging animals, birds of prey, and detritus-feeding fish—is regarded as unclean (*traife* or *haram*). We now know that many of these forbidden animals carry parasites that can infect human beings, and the ancient prohibitions are based on food hygiene.

Hindus will not eat beef. The reason for this is that the cow is far too valuable—as a source of milk and dung (as manure and fuel) and as a beast of burden—for it to be killed as a source of meat.

Many people refrain from eating meat as a result of humanitarian concern for the animals involved, or because of real or perceived health benefits. Vegetarians can be divided into various groups according to the strictness of their diet:

- Some avoid red meat, but will eat poultry and fish.
- Some specifically avoid beef because of the potential risk of contracting variant Creutzfeld–Jacob disease from BSE-infected animals.
- Pescetarians eat fish, but not meat or poultry.
- Ovo-lacto-vegetarians will eat eggs and milk, but not meat or fish.
- Lacto-vegetarians will eat milk, but not eggs.
- Vegans will eat only plant-based foods and no foods of animal origin.

Foods that are commonly eaten in one area may be little eaten elsewhere, even though they are available, simply because people have not been accustomed to eating them. To a very great extent, adults continue the eating habits learnt as children.

Haggis and oat cakes travel south from Scotland as specialty items; black pudding is a staple of northern British breakfasts, but is rare in the southeast of England. Until the 1960s yogurt was almost unknown in Britain, apart from a few health food "cranks" and immigrants from eastern Europe. Many British children believe that fish comes as rectangular fish fingers, while children in inland Spain may eat fish and other seafood three or four times a week. The French mock the British habit of eating lamb with mint sauce, and the average British reaction to such French delicacies as frogs' legs and snails in garlic is one of horror. The British eat their cabbage well boiled; the Germans and Dutch ferment it to produce sauerkraut.

This regional and cultural diversity of foods provides one of the pleasures of travel. As people travel more frequently, and become (perhaps grudgingly) more adventurous in their choice of foods, they create a demand for different foods at home and there is an increasing variety of foods available in shops and restaurants.

Another factor that has increased the range of foods available is the immigration of people from a variety of different backgrounds, all of whom have, as they have become established, introduced their traditional foods to their new homes. It is difficult to realize that in the 1960s there was only a handful of tandoori restaurants in the whole of Britain, that pizza was something seen only in southern Italy and a few specialist restaurants, or that Balti cooking and sushi were unknown until the 1990s.

Some people are naturally adventurous and will try a new food just because they have never eaten it before. Others are more conservative and will try a new food only when they see someone else eating it safely and with enjoyment. Others are still more conservative in their food choices; the most conservative eaters "know" that they do not like a new food *because* they have never eaten it before.

1.3.4.3 Luxury status of scarce and expensive foods

Foods that are scarce or expensive have a certain appeal of fashion or style; they are (rightly) regarded as luxuries for special occasions rather than everyday meals. Conversely, foods that are widespread and inexpensive have less appeal.

In the nineteenth century, salmon and oysters were so cheap that the articles of apprentices in London specified that they should not be given salmon more than three times a week, while oysters were eaten by the poor. Through much of the twentieth century, salmon was scarce and a prized luxury food; fish farming has increased the supply of salmon to such an extent that it is again an inexpensive food. Chicken, turkey, guinea fowl, and trout, which were expensive luxury foods in the 1950s, are now widely available as a result of changes in farming practice, and they form the basis of inexpensive meals. In contrast, fish such as cod and skate, once the basis of cheap meals, are now becoming scarce and expensive as a result of depletion of fish stocks by overexploitation.

1.3.4.4 The social functions of food

Humans are social animals, and meals are important social functions. People eating in a group are likely to eat better, or at least have a wider variety of foods and a more lavish and luxurious meal, than people eating alone. Entertaining guests may be an excuse to eat foods that we know to be nutritionally undesirable and perhaps to eat to excess. The greater the variety of dishes offered, the more people are likely to eat. As we reach satiety with one food, another, different flavor is offered to stimulate appetite. A number of studies have shown that when faced with only one food, people tend to reach satiety sooner than when a variety of foods is on offer. This is the difference between hunger and appetite—even when we are satiated, we can still "find room" to try something different.

Conversely, and more importantly, many lonely single people (especially the bereaved elderly) have little incentive to prepare meals and no stimulus to appetite. While poverty may be a factor, apathy (and frequently, in the case of widowed men, ignorance) severely limits the range of foods eaten, possibly leading to undernutrition. When these problems are added to those of ill-fitting dentures (which make eating painful), arthritis (which makes handling many foods difficult), and the difficulty of carrying food home from the shops, it is not surprising that we include the elderly among the vulnerable groups of the population who are at risk of undernutrition (Section 8.2).

In hospitals and other institutions, there is a further problem. People who are unwell may have low physical activity, but they have higher than normal requirements for energy and nutrients as a part of the process of replacing tissue in convalescence (Section 9.2.3.3) or as a result of fever or the metabolic effects of cancer (Section 8.4.1). At the same time, illness impairs appetite and a side effect of many drugs is to distort the sense of taste, depress appetite, or cause nausea. It is difficult to provide a range of exciting and attractive foods under institutional conditions, yet this is what is needed to tempt the patient's appetite.

Key points

- There is a relationship between energy intake from food, energy expenditure in physical activity, and body weight, but two-thirds of the total energy expenditure is required to maintain nerve and muscle tone, circulation and breathing, and metabolic homeostasis.
- The main metabolic fuels are carbohydrate and fat, and there is no absolute requirement for either (apart from small amounts of essential fatty acids). It is difficult to achieve an adequate energy intake on a very low-fat diet, and fat is essential for the absorption of vitamins A, D, E, and K.
- There is a requirement for protein in addition to its role as a metabolic fuel.
- There is a requirement for minerals that have a function in the body and for vitamins.
- Centers in the brain control hunger and satiety.
- Long-term control of food intake and energy expenditure is largely by the hormone leptin, which is secreted by adipose tissue; circulating concentrations of leptin reflect the adequacy (or otherwise) of body fat reserves. Leptin acts on the hypothalamus to regulate food intake, and on muscle and adipose tissue to regulate energy expenditure.
- The sense of taste on the tongue permits detection of nutrients and avoidance of potential toxins.
- Food choices are complex. In addition to the cost and availability of foods, a variety of religious and ethical beliefs and social and individual factors affect what people choose to eat.

chapter two

Enzymes and metabolic pathways

All metabolic processes depend on reactions between molecules, with breaking of some covalent bonds and the formation of others, yielding compounds that are different from the starting materials. Therefore, to understand nutrition and metabolism it is essential to understand how chemical reactions occur, how they are catalyzed by enzymes, and how enzyme activity can be regulated and controlled.

Objectives

After reading this chapter, you should be able to

- Explain how covalent bonds are broken and formed; what is meant by thermoneutral, endothermic, and exothermic reactions, and how reactions come to equilibrium
- Explain how a catalyst increases the rate at which a reaction comes to equilibrium and how enzymes act as catalysts
- Explain how an enzyme exhibits specificity for both the substrates bound and the reaction catalyzed
- Define a unit of enzyme activity
- Explain how pH, temperature, and the concentration of enzyme affect the rate of reaction
- Describe and explain the dependence of the rate of reaction on the concentration of substrate, define the kinetic parameters K_m and V_{max}, and explain how they are determined experimentally
- Explain how enzymes may show cooperative binding of substrate, and how this affects the substrate dependence of activity
- Describe the difference between irreversible and reversible inhibitors of enzymes, their clinical relevance, and how they may be distinguished experimentally
- Describe the difference between competitive, noncompetitive, and uncompetitive reversible inhibitors of enzymes, their clinical relevance, and how they may be distinguished experimentally
- Explain what is meant by the terms coenzyme and prosthetic group, apoenzyme and holoenzyme; describe the roles of coenzymes in oxidation and reduction reactions
- Describe the classification of enzymes on the basis of the reaction catalyzed
- Describe and explain what is meant by a metabolic pathway, and by linear, branched, spiral (looped), and cyclic pathways

2.1 *Chemical reactions: breaking and making covalent bonds*

Breaking covalent bonds requires an initial input of energy in some form—normally as heat, but in some cases also as light or other radiation. This is the activation energy of the reaction. The process of breaking a bond requires activation of the electrons forming the bond—a temporary movement of electrons from orbitals in which they have a stable configuration to orbitals further from the nucleus. Electrons that have been excited in this way have an unstable configuration, and the covalent bonds they contributed to are broken. Electrons cannot remain in this excited state for more than a fraction of a second. Sometimes they simply return to their original unexcited state, emitting the same energy as was taken up to excite them, but usually as a series of small steps, rather than as a single step. Overall, there is no change when this occurs.

More commonly, the excited electrons adopt a different stable configuration by interacting with electrons associated with different atoms and molecules. The result is the formation of new covalent bonds and hence the formation of new compounds. In this case, there are three possibilities (Figure 2.1):

- There may be an output of energy equal to the activation energy of the reaction, so that the energy level of the products is the same as that of the starting materials. Such a reaction is energetically neutral (thermoneutral).
- There may be an output of energy greater than the activation of the reaction, so that the energy level of the products is lower than that of the starting materials. This is an exothermic reaction—it proceeds with the output of heat. An exothermic reaction will proceed spontaneously once the initial activation energy has been provided.
- There may be an output of energy less than the activation energy, so that the energy level of the products is higher than that of the starting materials. The solution will take up heat from its surroundings and will have to be heated for the reaction to proceed. This is an endothermic reaction.

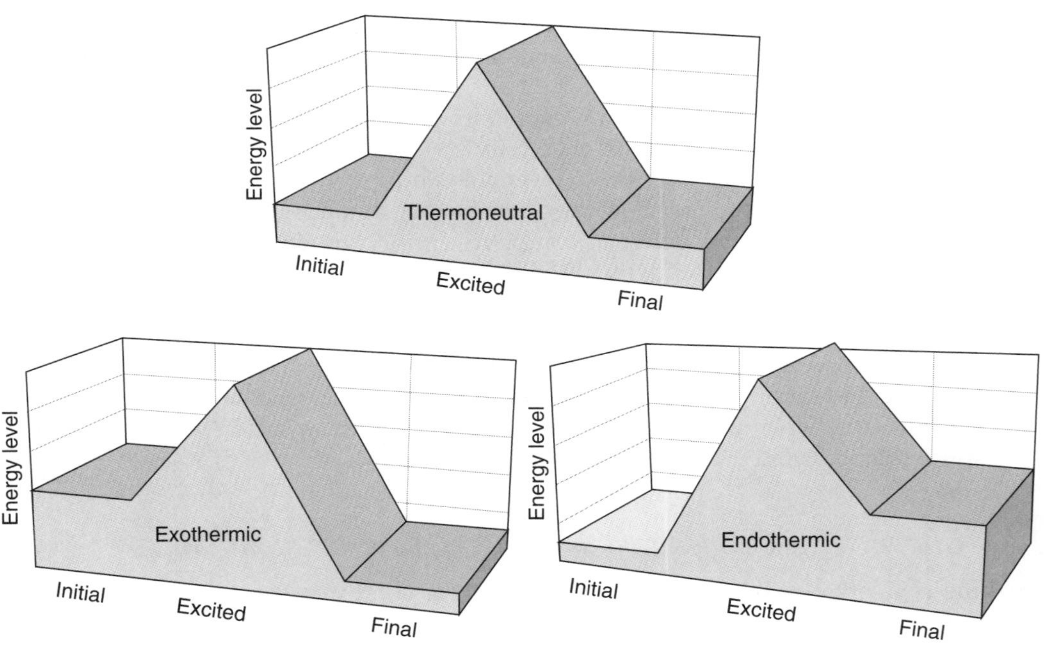

Figure 2.1 Energy changes in chemical reactions: thermoneutral, endothermic, and exothermic reactions.

In general, reactions in which relatively large complex molecules are broken down to smaller molecules are exothermic, while reactions that involve the synthesis of larger molecules from smaller ones are endothermic.

2.1.1 Equilibrium

Some reactions, such as the burning of a hydrocarbon in air to form carbon dioxide and water, are highly exothermic, and the products of the reaction are widely dispersed. Such reactions proceed essentially in one direction only. However, most reactions do not proceed in only one direction. If two compounds A and B can react together to form X and Y, then X and Y can react to form A and B. The reactions can be written as

$$A + B \rightarrow X + Y \tag{2.1}$$

$$X + Y \rightarrow A + B \tag{2.2}$$

Starting with only A and B in the solution, at first only reaction 2.1 will occur, forming X and Y. However, as X and Y accumulate, so they will undergo reaction 2.2, forming A and B. Similarly, starting with X and Y, at first only reaction 2.2 will occur, forming A and B. As A and B accumulate, they will undergo reaction 2.1, forming X and Y.

In both cases, the final result will be a solution containing A, B, X, and Y. The relative amounts of [A + B] and [X + Y] will be the same regardless of whether the starting compounds (substrates) were A and B or X and Y. At this stage, the rate of reaction 2.1 forming X and Y and reaction 2.2 forming A and B will be equal. This is equilibrium, and the reaction can be written as

$$A + B \rightleftharpoons X + Y$$

If there is a large difference in energy level between [A + B] and [X + Y]—i.e., if the reaction is exothermic in one direction (and therefore endothermic in the other)—then the position of the equilibrium will reflect this. If reaction 2.1 above is exothermic, then at equilibrium there will be very little A and B remaining, most will have been converted to X and Y. Conversely, if reaction 2.1 is endothermic, then relatively little of A and B will be converted to X and Y at equilibrium.

At equilibrium, the ratio [A + B]/[X + Y] is a constant for any given reaction. Therefore, if there is a constant addition of substrates, this will disturb the equilibrium and increase the amount of product formed. Similarly, constant removal of the products will increase the rate at which the substrate is utilized.

A metabolic pathway is a sequence of reactions, and *in vivo* very few reactions actually come to equilibrium. The product of one reaction is the substrate for the next, so there is a continual supply of substrate and removal of products for each reaction, and there is a constant flux through the pathway—a dynamic steady state rather than equilibrium.

2.1.2 Catalysts

A catalyst increases the rate at which a reaction comes to equilibrium, without itself being consumed in the reaction, so that a small amount of catalyst can effect the reaction of many thousands of molecules of substrate. While a catalyst increases the rate at which a reaction comes to equilibrium, it does not affect the position of the equilibrium.

Catalysts affect the rate of reaction in three main ways:

- They provide a surface on which the molecules that are to undergo reaction can come together in higher concentrations than would be possible in free solution, thus increasing the probability of them colliding and reacting. Binding also aligns the reactants in the correct orientation to undergo reaction.
- They provide a microenvironment for the reactants that is different from the solution as a whole.
- They participate in the reaction by withdrawing electrons from, or donating electrons to, covalent bonds. This enhances the breaking of bonds that is the essential prerequisite for a chemical reaction, and lowers the activation energy of the reaction.

2.2 Enzymes

Enzymes are proteins that catalyze metabolic reactions. There are also a number of enzymes that are not proteins, but are catalytic molecules of RNA (Section 9.2.2). These are sometimes referred to as ribozymes.

Proteins are linear polymers of amino acids (Section 4.4.2). Any protein adopts a characteristic pattern of folding, determined largely by the amino acids in its sequence. This folding of the protein chain results in reactive groups from amino acids that may be widely separated in the primary sequence coming together at the surface and creating a site that has a defined shape and an array of chemically reactive groups. This is the active site of the enzyme, which can be divided into two distinct domains: the binding site for the compounds that are to undergo reaction (the substrates) and the catalytic site. Figure 2.2 shows how three amino acids that are widely separated in the primary sequence of the enzyme trypsin come together to form a catalytic triad as a result of folding of the protein chain.

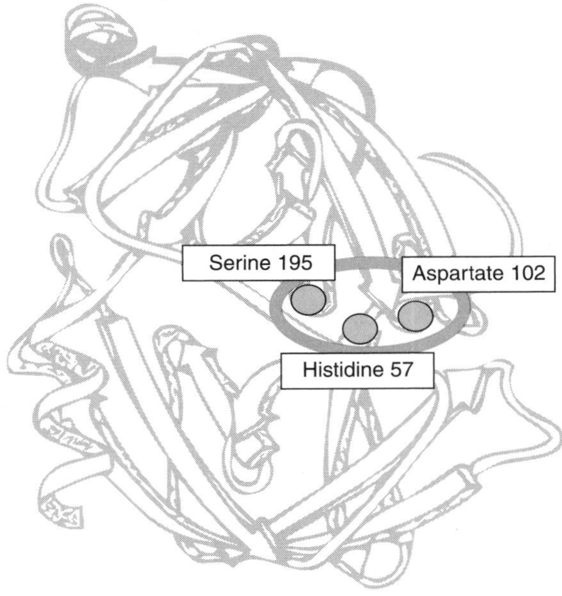

Figure 2.2 The formation of an active site in an enzyme as a result of folding of the protein chain.

Many enzymes also have a nonprotein component of the catalytic site; this may be a metal ion, an organic compound that contains a metal ion (e.g., heme; Section 3.3.1.2), or an organic compound, which may be derived from a vitamin (Table 2.1; Chapter 11) or may be a compound that is readily synthesized in the body. This nonprotein part of the active site may be covalently bound, when it is generally referred to as a prosthetic group, or tightly but not covalently bound, when it is usually referred to as a coenzyme (Section 2.4.1).

Reactive groups in amino acid side chains at the active site (Figure 4.18) facilitate the making or the breaking of specific chemical bonds in the substrate by donating or withdrawing electrons. In this way, the enzyme lowers the activation energy of a chemical reaction (Figure 2.3) and increases the rate at which the reaction attains equilibrium, under much milder conditions than are required for a simple chemical catalyst. To hydrolyze a protein into its constituent amino acids in the laboratory, it is necessary to use concentrated acid as a catalyst and heat the sample at 105°C overnight to provide the activation energy of the hydrolysis. This is the process of digestion of proteins, which occurs under relatively mild acid or alkaline conditions, at 37°C, and is complete within a few hours of eating a meal (Section 4.4.3).

Table 2.1 The Major Coenzymes

		Source	Functions
CoA	Coenzyme A	Pantothenic acid	Acyl transfer reactions
FAD	Flavin adenine dinucleotide	Vitamin B_2	Oxidation reactions
FMN	Flavin mononucleotide	Vitamin B_2	Oxidation reactions
NAD	Nicotinamide adenine dinucleotide	Niacin	Oxidation and reduction reactions
NADP	Nicotinamide adenine dinucleotide phosphate	Niacin	Oxidation and reduction reactions
PLP	Pyridoxal phosphate	Vitamin B_6	Amino acid metabolism

Note: There are a number of other coenzymes, which are discussed as they are relevant to specific metabolic pathways. In addition to those shown in this table, most of the other vitamins also function as coenzymes; see Chapter 11.

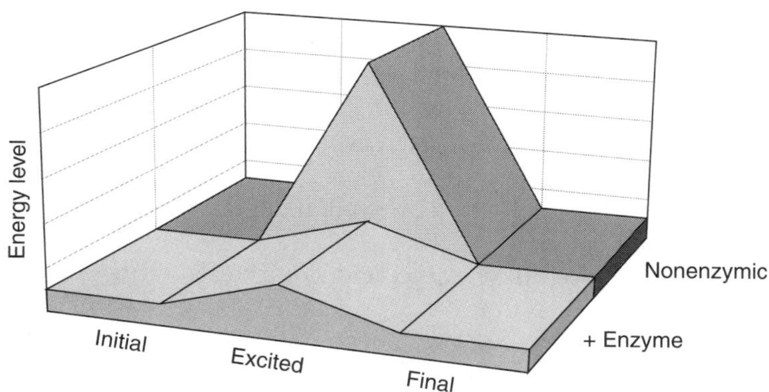

Figure 2.3 The effect of enzyme catalysis on the activation energy of a reaction.

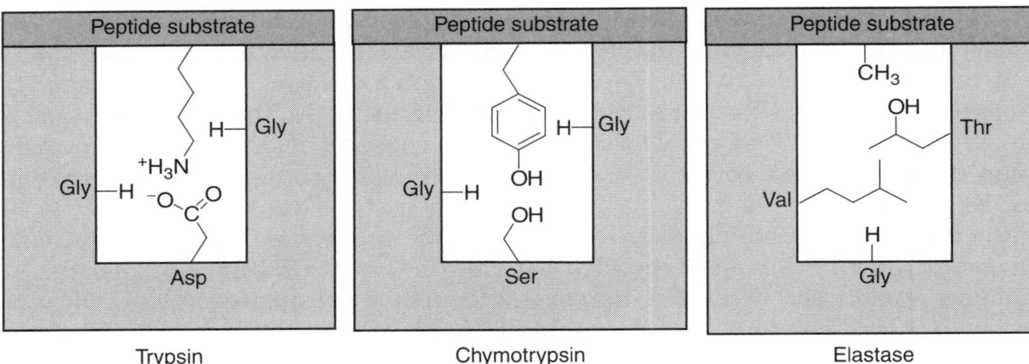

Figure 2.4 Enzyme specificity: the substrate-binding sites of trypsin, chymotrypsin, and elastase.

2.2.1 Specificity of enzymes

The binding of substrates to enzymes involves interactions between the substrates and the reactive groups of the amino acid side chains that make up the active site of the enzyme. This means that enzymes show a considerable specificity for the substrates they bind. Normally, several different interactions must occur before the substrate can bind in the correct orientation to undergo reaction, and binding of the substrate often causes a change in the conformation of the active site, bringing reactive groups closer to the substrate.

Figure 2.4 shows the active sites of three enzymes that catalyze the same reaction: hydrolysis of a peptide bond in a protein (Section 4.4.3); in all three enzymes, the catalytic site is the same as that shown for trypsin in Figure 2.2. The three enzymes show different specificity for the bond that they hydrolyze:

- Trypsin catalyzes hydrolysis of the esters of basic amino acids.
- Chymotrypsin catalyzes hydrolysis of the esters of aromatic amino acids.
- Elastase catalyzes hydrolysis of the esters of small neutral amino acids.

This difference in specificity for the bond to be hydrolyzed is explained by differences in the substrate binding sites of the three enzymes. In all three, the substrate binds in a groove at the surface, in such a way as to bring the bond to be cleaved over the serine residue that initiates the catalysis. The amino acid providing the carboxyl side of the peptide bond to be cleaved sits in a pocket below this groove, and it is the nature of the amino acids that line this pocket that determines the specificity of the enzymes:

- In trypsin, there is an acidic group (from aspartate) at the base of the pocket; this will attract a basic amino acid side chain.
- In chymotrypsin, the pocket is lined by small neutral amino acids, so that a relatively large aromatic group can fit in.
- In elastase, there are two bulky amino acid side chains in the pocket, so that only a small neutral side chain can fit it.

Chemically, D and L isomers (Figure 2.5), and *cis* and *trans* isomers (Figure 2.6) of a compound behave identically, and it can often be difficult to distinguish between isomers. However, the isomers have different shapes, and enzymes readily discriminate between

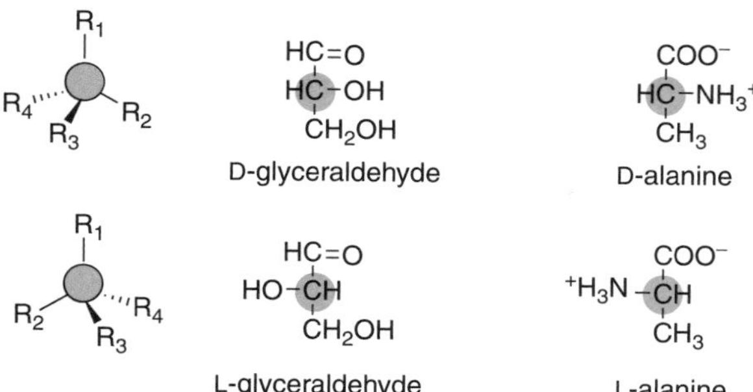

Figure 2.5 DL-Isomerism.

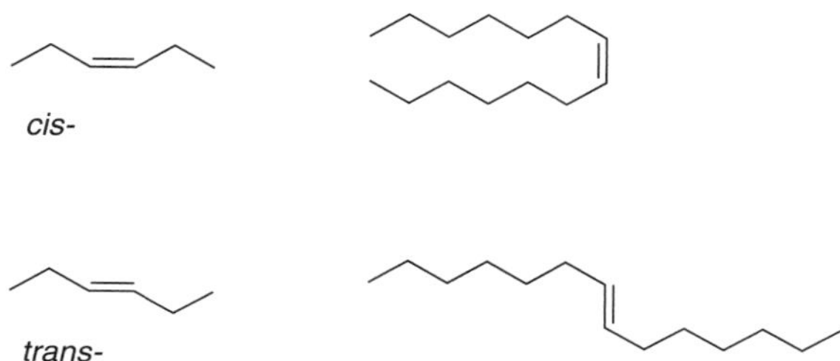

Figure 2.6 *Cis/trans* isomerism.

them—the shape and conformation of the substrate are critically important for binding to an enzyme. (Most of the naturally occurring and physiologically relevant sugars are D isomers, and most amino acids are L isomers; the nutritional and heath importance of *trans* isomers of unsaturated fatty acids is discussed in Section 6.3.2.1.)

The participation of reactive groups at the active site provides not only specificity for the substrates that will bind, but also for the reaction that will be catalyzed. For example, in a nonenzymic model system, an amino acid may undergo α-decarboxylation to yield an amine, transfer of the α-amino group and replacement with an oxo-group (Section 9.3.1.2), isomerization between the D and L isomers, or a variety of reactions involving elimination or replacement of the side chain. In an enzyme-catalyzed reaction, only one of the possible reactions will normally be catalyzed by a given enzyme.

2.2.2 *The stages in an enzyme-catalyzed reaction*

An enzyme-catalyzed reaction can be considered to occur in three distinct steps, each of which is reversible:

- Binding of the substrate (S) to the enzyme (Enz) to form the enzyme–substrate complex: Enz + S $\rightleftharpoons$ Enz-S
- Reaction of the enzyme–substrate complex to form the enzyme–product complex: Enz-S $\rightleftharpoons$ Enz-P
- Breakdown of the enzyme–product complex, with release of the product (P): Enz-P $\rightleftharpoons$ Enz + P

Overall, the process can be written as Enz + S $\rightleftharpoons$ Enz-S $\rightleftharpoons$ Enz-P $\rightleftharpoons$ Enz + P.

2.2.3 Units of enzyme activity

When an enzyme has been purified, it is possible to express the amount of enzyme in tissues or plasma as the number of moles of enzyme protein present, for example, by raising antibodies against the purified protein for use in an immunoassay. However, what is more important is not how much of the enzyme protein is present in the cell, but how much catalytic activity there is—how much substrate can be converted to product in a given time. Therefore, amounts of enzymes are usually expressed in units of activity.

The SI unit of catalysis is the katal—1 mol of substrate converted per second. However, enzyme activity is usually expressed as the number of micromoles (μmol) of substrate converted (or of product formed) per minute. This is the standard unit of enzyme activity, determined under specified optimum conditions for that enzyme, at 30°C. This temperature is a compromise between mammalian biochemists, who would work at body temperature (37°C for humans) and microbiological biochemists, who would normally work at 20°C.

2.3 Factors affecting enzyme activity

Any given enzyme has an innate activity. For many enzymes, the catalytic rate constant is of the order of 1–5000 mol of substrate converted per mole of enzyme per second or higher. However, a number of factors affect the activity of enzymes.

2.3.1 Effect of pH

Both the binding of the substrate to the enzyme and the catalysis of the reaction depend on interactions between the substrates and reactive groups in the amino acid side chains that make up the active site. They have to be in the appropriate ionization state for binding and reaction to occur; this depends on the pH of the medium. Any enzyme will have maximum activity at a specific pH—the optimum pH for that enzyme. When the pH rises or falls away from the optimum, the activity of the enzyme will decrease. Most enzymes have little or no activity 2–3 pH units away from their pH optimum.

Figure 2.7 shows the activity of two enzymes that are found in plasma and catalyze the same reaction: hydrolysis of a phosphate ester: acid phosphatase (released from the prostate gland) has a pH optimum around 3.5, while alkaline phosphatase (released from liver

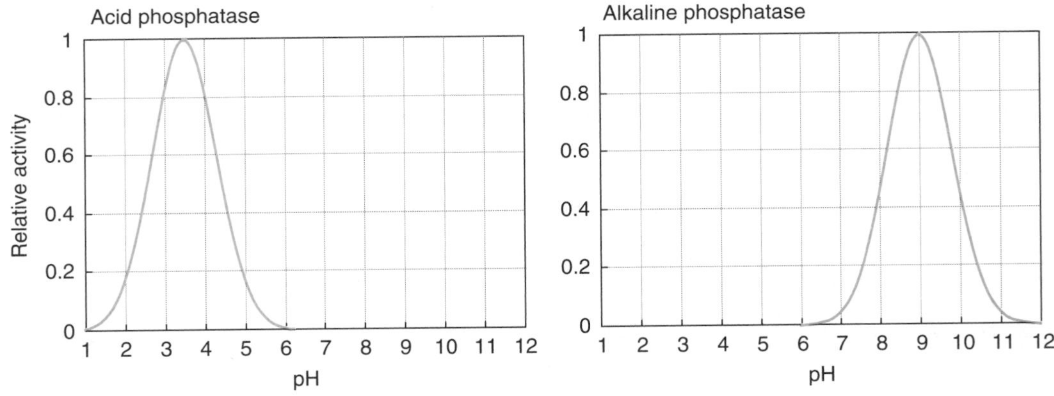

Figure 2.7 The effect of pH on enzyme activity.

and bone) has a pH optimum around 9.0. Neither has any significant activity at pH 7.35–7.45, which is the normal range in plasma. However, alkaline phosphatase is significantly active in the alkaline microenvironment at cell surfaces, and is important, for example, in the hydrolysis of pyridoxal phosphate (the main form of vitamin B_6 in plasma; Section 11.9.1) to free pyridoxal for uptake into tissues.

2.3.2 Effect of temperature

Chemical reactions proceed faster at higher temperatures for two reasons:

- Molecules move faster at higher temperatures and hence have a greater chance of colliding to undergo reaction.
- At a higher temperature, it is easier for electrons to gain activation energy, and hence be excited into unstable orbitals to undergo reaction.

With enzyme-catalyzed reactions, although the rate at which the reaction comes to equilibrium increases with temperature, there is a second effect of temperature—denaturation of the enzyme protein (Section 4.4.2), leading to irreversible loss of activity. As the temperature increases, so does the movement of parts of the protein molecules relative to each other, leading to disruption of the hydrogen bonds that maintain the folded structure of the protein. When this happens, the protein chain unfolds, and the active site is lost. As the temperature increases further, the denatured protein becomes insoluble and precipitates out of solution.

Temperature thus has two opposing effects on enzyme activity (Figure 2.8). At relatively low temperatures (up to about 50°C–55°C), increasing temperature results in an increase in the rate of reaction. However, as the temperature increases further, denaturation of the enzyme protein becomes increasingly important, resulting in a rapid fall in activity at higher temperatures. The rate of increase in the rate of reaction with increasing temperature depends on the activation energy of the reaction being catalyzed; the rate of decrease in activity at higher temperatures is a characteristic of the enzyme itself.

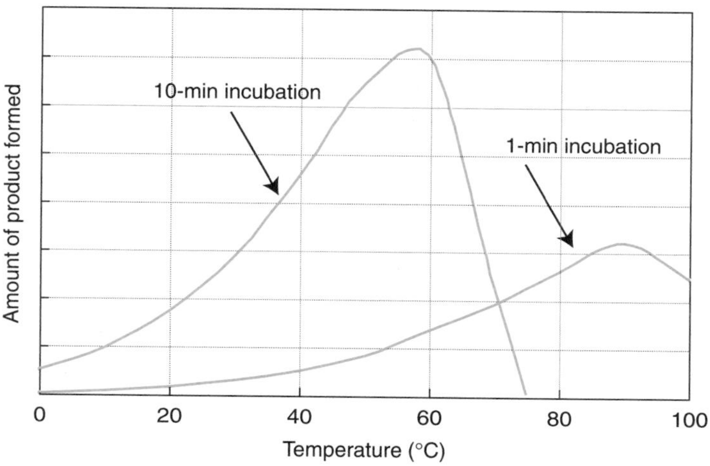

Figure 2.8 The temperature dependence of enzyme activity. In a short (1 min) incubation, the enzyme may have an optimum temperature as high as 90°C, but in longer incubations this falls, so that in a 10-min incubation the optimum temperature is about 55°C.

The apparent temperature optimum of an enzyme-catalyzed reaction depends on the time for which the enzyme is incubated. During a short incubation (e.g., 1 min), there is negligible denaturation, and so the apparent optimum temperature is relatively high, while during a longer incubation denaturation is important, and so the apparent optimum temperature is lower.

The effect of temperature is not normally physiologically important, since body temperature is maintained close to 37°C. However, some of the effects of fever (when body temperature may rise to 40°C) may be due to changes in the rates of enzyme-catalyzed reactions. Because different enzymes respond differently to changes in temperature, there may be a loss of the normal integration between different reactions and metabolic pathways.

2.3.3 *Effect of substrate concentration*

In a simple chemical reaction involving a single substrate, the rate at which product is formed increases linearly as the concentration of the substrate increases. When more substrate is available, more will undergo reaction.

With enzyme-catalyzed reactions, the change in the rate of formation of product with increasing concentration of substrate is not linear, but hyperbolic (Figure 2.9). At relatively low concentrations of substrate (region A in Figure 2.9), the catalytic site of the enzyme will be empty at times, until more substrate binds to undergo reaction. Under these conditions, the rate of product formation is limited by the time taken for another molecule of substrate to bind to the enzyme. A relatively small change in the concentration of substrate has a large effect on the rate at which product is formed in this region of the curve.

At high concentrations of substrate (region B in Figure 2.9), as the product leaves the catalytic site, another molecule of substrate binds more or less immediately, and the enzyme is saturated with substrate. The limiting factor in the formation of product is now the rate at

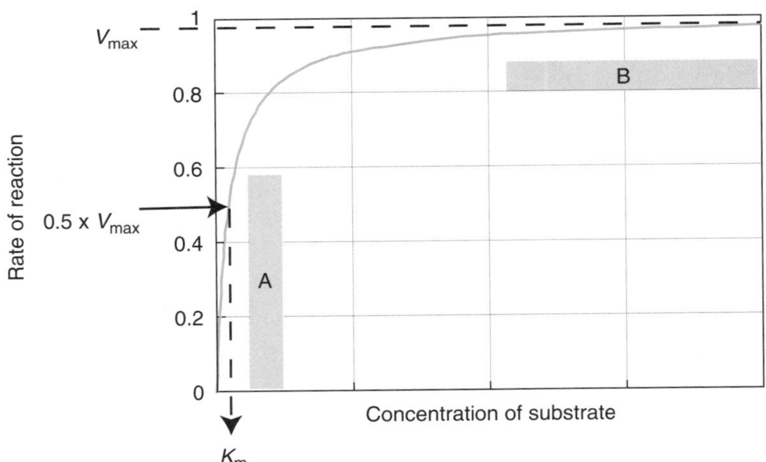

Figure 2.9 The substrate dependence of an enzyme-catalyzed reaction. In region A the enzyme is very unsaturated with substrate, and the rate of reaction increases sharply with increasing concentration of substrate. In region B the enzyme is almost saturated with substrate, and there is little change in the rate of reaction with increasing substrate concentration.

which the enzyme can catalyze the reaction, and not the availability of substrate. The enzyme is acting at or near its maximum rate (or maximum velocity, usually abbreviated to V_{max}). Even a relatively large change in the concentration of substrate has little effect on the rate of formation of product in this region of the curve.

From a graph of the rate of formation of product versus the concentration of substrate (Figure 2.9), it is easy to estimate the maximum rate of reaction that an enzyme can achieve (V_{max}) when it is saturated with substrate. However, it is not possible to determine from this graph the concentration of substrate required to achieve saturation, because the enzyme gradually approaches V_{max} as the concentration of substrate increases, and only really achieves its true V_{max} at an infinite concentration of substrate.

It is easy to estimate the concentration of substrate at which the enzyme has achieved half its maximum rate of reaction. The concentration of substrate to achieve half V_{max} is called the Michaelis constant of the enzyme (abbreviated to K_m), to commemorate Michaelis who, together with Menten, first formulated a mathematical model of the dependence of the rate of enzymic reactions on the concentration of substrate.

The K_m of an enzyme is not affected by the amount of the enzyme protein that is present. It is an (inverse) index of the affinity of the enzyme for its substrate. An enzyme that has a high K_m has a lower affinity for its substrate than an enzyme with a lower K_m. The higher the value of K_m, the greater the concentration of substrate required to achieve half-saturation of the enzyme.

In general, enzymes that have a low K_m compared with the normal concentration of substrate in the cell are likely to be acting at or near their maximum rate, and hence to have a more or less constant rate of reaction despite (modest) changes in the concentration of substrate. In contrast, an enzyme that has a high K_m compared with the normal concentration of substrate in the cell will show a large change in the rate of reaction with relatively small changes in the concentration of substrate.

If two enzymes in a cell can both act on the same substrate, catalyzing different reactions, the enzyme with the lower K_m will be able to bind more substrate, and therefore its reaction will be favored at relatively low concentrations of substrate. Thus, knowing the values of K_m and V_{max} for two enzymes, for example at a branch point in a metabolic pathway (Figure 2.22), it is possible to predict whether one branch or the other will predominate in the presence of different amounts of the substrate. At low concentrations of substrate, the reaction catalyzed by the enzyme with the lower K_m predominates, but as the concentration of substrate increases, this enzyme becomes saturated and acts at a more or less constant rate, while the rate of the reaction catalyzed by the enzyme with the higher K_m continues to increase (Figure 2.10).

2.3.3.1 *Experimental determination of K_m and V_{max}*

Plotting the graph of rate of reaction against substrate concentration, as in Figure 2.9, permits only a very approximate determination of the values of K_m and V_{max}, and a number of methods have been developed to convert this hyperbolic relationship into a linear relationship, to permit more precise fitting of a line to the experimental points, and hence more precise estimation of K_m and V_{max}.

Of such linearization of the data, the most widely used is the Lineweaver–Burk double reciprocal plot of 1/rate of reaction versus 1/[substrate] (Figure 2.11). This has an intercept on the y ($1/v$) axis: $1/V_{max}$ when $1/s = 0$ (i.e., at an infinite concentration of substrate), and an intercept on the x ($1/s$) axis: $-1/K_m$. There are notes on other ways of linearizing the data in the theory screens for the enzyme assay program in the virtual laboratory on the CD.

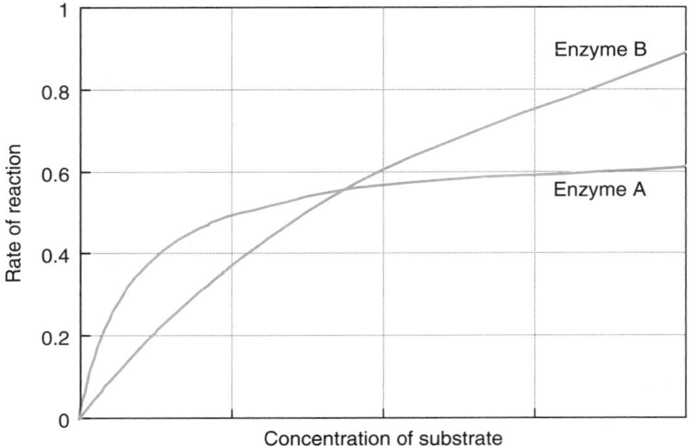

Figure 2.10 Two enzymes competing for the same substrate. Enzyme A has a relatively low K_m and reaches saturation at a low concentration of substrate; enzyme B has a higher K_m and its rate of reaction continues to increase. At low concentrations of substrate, most undergoes the reaction catalyzed by enzyme A; at higher concentrations of substrate, the reaction catalyzed by enzyme B predominates.

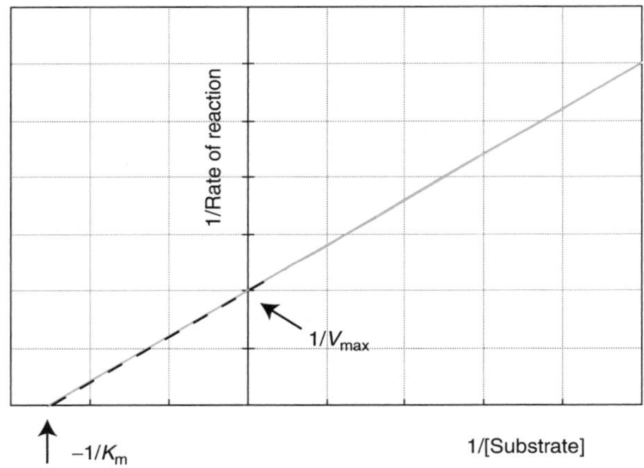

Figure 2.11 The Lineweaver–Burk double reciprocal plot to determine K_m and V_{max}.

Experimentally, the values of K_m and V_{max} are determined by incubating the enzyme (at optimum pH) with different concentrations of substrate, plotting the graph shown in Figure 2.11 and extrapolating back from the experimental points to determine the intercepts.

The Michaelis–Menten equation that describes the dependence of rate of reaction on concentration of substrate is

$$v = \frac{V_{max} \times [S]}{[S] + K_m}$$

One of the underlying assumptions of the Michaelis–Menten model is that there is no change in the concentration of substrate. This means that what should be measured is the initial rate of reaction. This is usually estimated by determining the amount of product formed at a series of short time intervals after the initiation of the reaction, then plotting a rate curve (product formed against time incubated), and estimating the tangent to this curve as the initial rate of reaction.

2.3.3.2 *Enzymes with two substrates*

Most enzyme-catalyzed reactions involve two substrates; it is only enzymes catalyzing lysis of a molecule or an isomerization reaction that have only a single substrate.

For a reaction involving two substrates (and two products)

$$A + B \rightleftharpoons C + D$$

the enzyme may act by

- An ordered mechanism, in which each substrate binds in turn:

$$A + Enz \rightleftharpoons A\text{-}Enz$$
$$A\text{-}Enz + B \rightleftharpoons A\text{-}Enz\text{-}B \rightleftharpoons C\text{-}Enz\text{-}D \rightleftharpoons C\text{-}Enz + D$$
$$C\text{-}Enz \rightleftharpoons Enz + C$$

- A ping-pong mechanism in which one substrate undergoes reaction, modifying the enzyme and releasing product, then the second substrate binds, reacts with the modified enzyme and restores it to the original state:

$$A + Enz \rightleftharpoons A\text{-}Enz \rightleftharpoons C\text{-}Enz^* \rightleftharpoons C + Enz^*$$
$$B + Enz^* \rightleftharpoons B\text{-}Enz^* \rightleftharpoons D\text{-}Enz \rightleftharpoons D + Enz$$

These two different mechanisms can be distinguished by plotting $1/v$ against 1/[substrate A] at several different concentrations of substrate B; as shown in Figure 2.12, the lines converge if the mechanism is ordered, but are parallel for a ping-pong reaction.

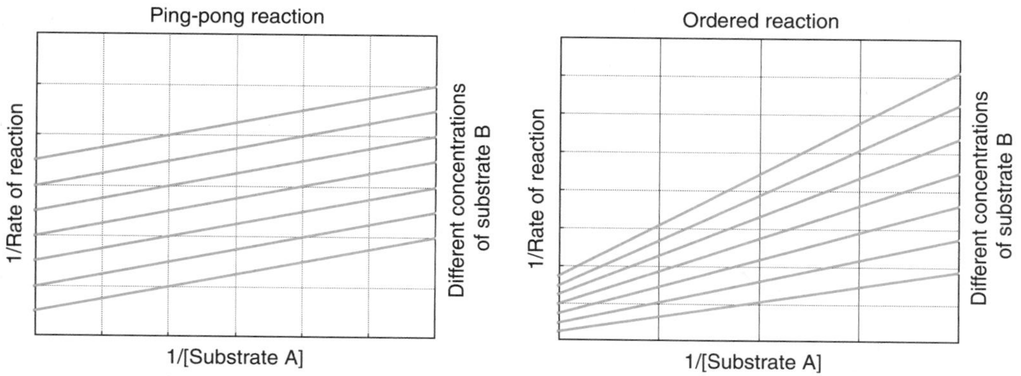

Figure 2.12 The Lineweaver–Burk double reciprocal plots for ordered and ping-pong two-substrate reactions.

2.3.3.3 Cooperative (allosteric) enzymes

Not all enzymes show the simple hyperbolic dependence of the rate of reaction on substrate concentration shown in Figure 2.9. Some enzymes consist of several separate protein chains, each with an active site. In many such enzymes, the binding of the substrate to one active site changes the conformation of not only that active site, but of the whole multi-subunit array. This change in conformation affects the other active sites, altering the ease with which the substrate can bind. This is cooperativity—the different subunits of the complete enzyme cooperate with each other. Because there is a change in the conformation (or shape) of the enzyme molecule, the phenomenon is also called allostericity (from the Greek for *different shape*), and such enzymes are called allosteric enzymes.

Figure 2.13 shows the change in the rate of reaction with increasing concentration of substrate for an enzyme that displays substrate cooperativity. At low concentrations of substrate, the enzyme has little activity. As one of the binding sites is occupied, it causes a conformational change and increases the ease with which the other sites can bind substrate. Therefore, there is a steep increase in the rate of reaction with increasing concentration of substrate. Of course, as all the sites become saturated, the rate of reaction cannot increase any further with increasing concentration of substrate; the enzyme achieves its maximum rate of reaction.

Enzymes that display substrate cooperativity are often important in controlling the overall rate of metabolic pathways (Section 10.2.1). Their rate of reaction is extremely sensitive to the concentration of substrate. Furthermore, this sensitivity can readily be modified by a variety of compounds that bind to specific regulator sites on the enzyme and affect its conformation, thus affecting the conformation of all the active sites of the multi-subunit complex, and either activating the enzyme at low concentrations of substrate by decreasing cooperativity or inhibiting it by increasing cooperativity (Figure 10.2).

2.3.4 Inhibition of enzyme activity

Inhibition of the activity of key enzymes in metabolic pathways by end products or metabolic intermediates is an important part of metabolic integration and control (Section 10.2).

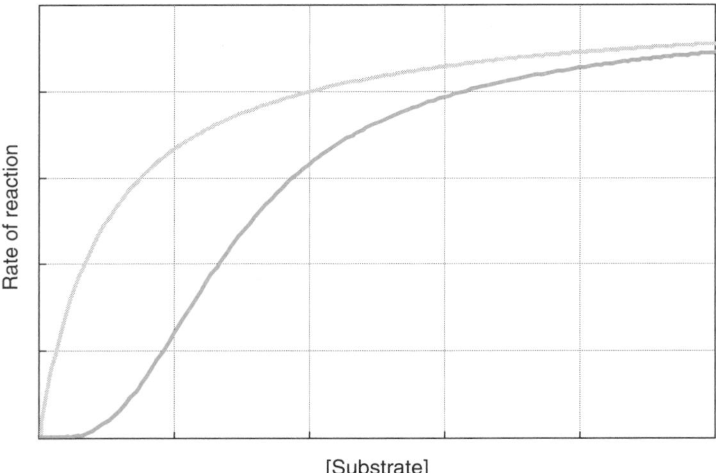

Figure 2.13 The substrate dependence of an enzyme showing subunit cooperativity—a sigmoid curve. For comparison, the hyperbolic substrate dependence of an enzyme not showing substrate cooperativity is shown in gray.

In addition, many of the drugs used to treat diseases act by inhibiting enzymes. Some inhibit the patient's enzyme, thereby altering metabolic regulation; others act by preferentially inhibiting enzymes in the organisms that are causing disease.

Inhibitors may either act reversibly, so that the inhibition wears off as the inhibitor is metabolized, or irreversibly, causing chemical modification of the enzyme protein, so that the effect of the inhibitor is prolonged, and only diminishes gradually as the enzyme protein is catabolized and replaced (Section 9.1.1). It is important when designing drugs to know whether they act as reversible or irreversible inhibitors. An irreversible inhibitor may only need to be administered every few days; however, it is more difficult to adjust its dose to match the patient's needs because of the long duration of action. In contrast, it is easy to adjust the dose of a reversible inhibitor to produce the desired effect, but such a compound may have to be taken several times a day, depending on the rate at which it is metabolized or excreted.

2.3.4.1 Irreversible inhibitors

Irreversible inhibitors are commonly chemical analogs of the substrate and bind to the enzyme in the same way as does the substrate, then undergo part of the normal reaction sequence. However, at some stage, they form a covalent bond to a reactive group in the active site, resulting in inactivation of the enzyme. Such inhibitors are sometimes called mechanism-dependent inhibitors, or suicide inhibitors, because they cause the enzyme to "commit suicide."

Experimentally, it is easy to distinguish between irreversible and reversible inhibitors by dialysis—placing the mixture of enzyme and inhibitor inside a sac of semipermeable membrane with pores that will permit small molecules, such as the inhibitor, to cross, but not large molecules, such as the enzyme (Figure 2.14). A reversible inhibitor is not covalently

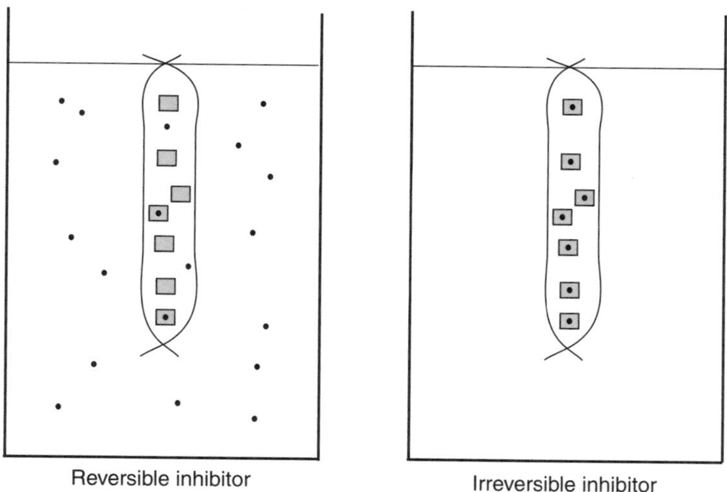

Figure 2.14 Differentiating between reversible and irreversible inhibition by dialysis. The enzyme plus inhibitor is placed in a tube of semipermeable membrane that will allow small molecules (e.g., the inhibitor) but not large ones (e.g., the enzyme) to cross. The reversible inhibitor is not covalently bound to the enzyme, and so can equilibrate across the membrane into the larger volume of buffer outside; as the inhibitor is removed, enzyme activity is restored. The irreversible inhibitor remains covalently bound to the enzyme and cannot be removed.

bound to the enzyme and so can equilibrate across the membrane into the larger volume of buffer outside. Incubation of the enzyme with substrate after a period of dialysis will show that activity has been restored as the inhibitor is removed. In contrast, an irreversible inhibitor is covalently bound to the enzyme and cannot be removed by dialysis, so activity is not restored.

2.3.4.2 Competitive reversible inhibitors

A competitive inhibitor is a compound that binds to the active site of the enzyme in competition with the substrate. Often, but not always, such compounds are chemical analogs of the substrate. Although a competitive inhibitor binds to the active site, it does not undergo reaction, or, if it does, does not yield the product that would have been obtained by reaction of the normal substrate.

A competitive inhibitor reduces the rate of reaction because at any time some molecules of the enzyme have bound the inhibitor and therefore are not free to bind the substrate. However, the binding of the inhibitor to the enzyme is reversible, and therefore there is competition between the substrate and the inhibitor for the enzyme. This means that the sequence of the reaction in the presence of a competitive inhibitor can be shown as

$$\text{Enz} + \text{S} + \text{I} \rightleftharpoons \text{Enz-I}$$

$$\text{Enz} + \text{S} + \text{I} \rightleftharpoons \text{Enz-S} \rightleftharpoons \text{Enz-P} \rightleftharpoons \text{Enz} + \text{P}$$

Figure 2.15 shows the *s/v* and double reciprocal plots for an enzyme incubated with various concentrations of a competitive inhibitor. If the concentration of substrate is increased, it will compete more effectively with the inhibitor for the active site of the enzyme. This means that at high concentrations of substrate, the enzyme will achieve the same maximum rate of reaction (V_{max}) in the presence or absence of inhibitor. It is simply that in the presence of inhibitor the enzyme requires a higher concentration of substrate to achieve saturation; in other words, the K_m of the enzyme is higher in the presence of a competitive inhibitor.

The effect of a competitive inhibitor as a drug is that the final rate at which product is formed is unchanged, but there is an increase in the concentration of the substrate of the inhibited enzyme in the cell. As the inhibitor acts, the concentration of substrate rises, eventually becoming high enough for the enzyme to reach a more or less normal rate of reaction. This means that a competitive inhibitor is appropriate for use as a drug when the

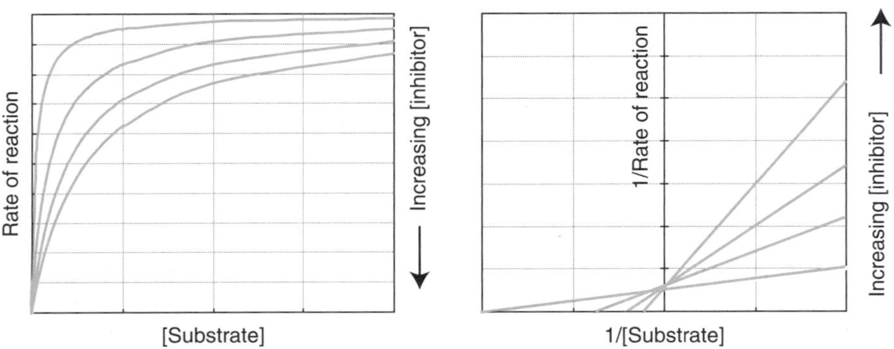

Figure 2.15 Substrate/velocity and Lineweaver–Burk double reciprocal plots for an enzyme incubated with varying concentrations of a competitive inhibitor.

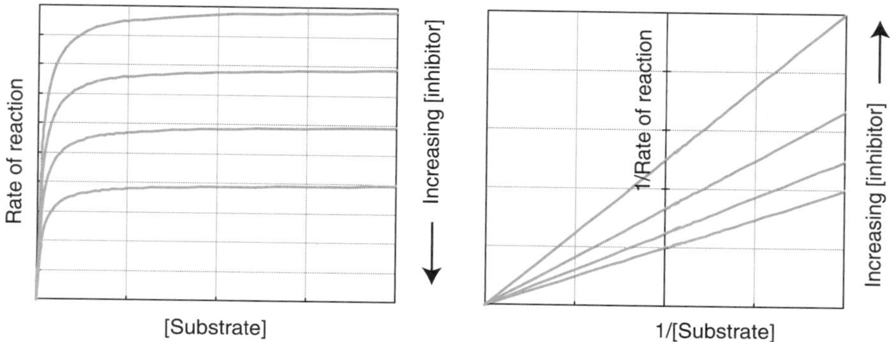

Figure 2.16 Substrate/velocity and Lineweaver–Burk double reciprocal plots for an enzyme incubated with varying concentrations of a noncompetitive inhibitor.

aim is to increase the available pool of substrate (perhaps to allow an alternative reaction to proceed), but inappropriate if the aim is to reduce the amount of product formed.

2.3.4.3 *Noncompetitive reversible inhibitors*

Compounds that are noncompetitive inhibitors bind to the enzyme–substrate complex, rather than to the enzyme itself. The enzyme–substrate–inhibitor complex only reacts slowly to form enzyme–product–inhibitor, so the effect of a noncompetitive inhibitor is to slow down the rate at which the enzyme catalyzes the formation of product. The reaction sequence can be written as

$$\text{Enz} + \text{S} + \text{I} \rightleftharpoons \text{Enz-S} + \text{I} \rightleftharpoons \text{Enz-S-I} (\rightleftharpoons) \text{Enz-P-I} \rightleftharpoons \text{Enz} + \text{P} + \text{I}$$

Because there is no competition between the inhibitor and the substrate for binding to the enzyme, increasing the concentration of substrate has no effect on the activity of the enzyme in the presence of a noncompetitive inhibitor. The K_m of the enzyme is unaffected by a noncompetitive inhibitor, but the V_{max} is reduced. Figure 2.16 shows the s/v and double reciprocal plots for an enzyme incubated with several concentrations of a noncompetitive inhibitor.

A noncompetitive inhibitor would be appropriate for use as a drug when the aim is either to increase the concentration of substrate in the cell or reduce the rate at which the product is formed, since unlike a competitive inhibitor, the accumulation of substrate has no effect on the degree of inhibition.

2.3.4.4 *Uncompetitive reversible inhibitors*

Compounds that are uncompetitive inhibitors bind to the enzyme, but unlike competitive inhibitors (Section 2.3.4.2) enhance the binding of substrate (i.e., they lower K_m). However, as with noncompetitive inhibitors (Section 2.3.4.3), the enzyme–inhibitor–substrate complex undergoes reaction only slowly, so that the V_{max} of the reaction is reduced. The reaction sequence can be written as

$$\text{Enz} + \text{S} + \text{I} \rightleftharpoons \text{Enz-I} + \text{S} \rightleftharpoons \text{Enz-I-S} (\rightleftharpoons) \text{Enz-I-P} \rightleftharpoons \text{Enz} + \text{P} + \text{I}$$

Figure 2.17 shows the s/v and double reciprocal plots for an enzyme incubated with several concentrations of an uncompetitive inhibitor. Because the binding of the inhibitor

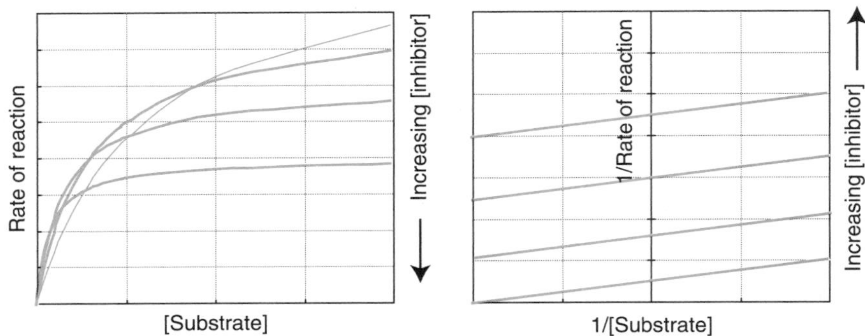

Figure 2.17 Substrate/velocity and Lineweaver–Burk double reciprocal plots for an enzyme incubated with varying concentrations of an uncompetitive inhibitor.

enhances the binding of substrate, addition of more substrate does not overcome the effect of the inhibitor.

Uncompetitive inhibition is rare; like a noncompetitive inhibitor, an uncompetitive inhibitor would be appropriate for use as a drug when the aim is to either increase the concentration of substrate in the cell or reduce the rate at which the product is formed, since the accumulation of substrate has no effect on the degree of inhibition.

2.4 Coenzymes and prosthetic groups

Although most enzymes are proteins, many contain small nonprotein molecules as an integral part of their structure. These may be organic compounds or metal ions. In either case, they are essential to the function of the enzyme, and the enzyme has no activity in the absence of the metal ion or coenzyme.

When an organic compound or a metal ion is covalently bound to the active site of the enzyme, it is referred to as a prosthetic group. Compounds that are tightly, but not covalently, bound are referred to as coenzymes. Like the enzyme itself, the coenzyme or prosthetic group participates in the reaction, but at the end emerges unchanged. Sometimes, the coenzyme is chemically modified in the reaction with the first substrate, then restored to its original state by reaction with the second substrate. This would be a ping-pong reaction (Section 2.3.3.2); transaminases (Section 9.3.1.2) catalyze a ping-pong reaction in which the amino group from the first substrate forms an amino derivative of the coenzyme as an intermediate step in the reaction.

Some compounds that were historically considered to be coenzymes do not remain bound to the active site of the enzyme, but bind and leave in the same way as other substrates. Such compounds include the nicotinamide nucleotide coenzymes (NAD and NADP) and coenzyme A. Although they are not strictly coenzymes, they are present in the cell in very much smaller concentrations than most substrates, and are involved in a relatively large number of reactions, so that they turn over rapidly.

Table 2.1 shows the major coenzymes, the vitamins they are derived from, and their principal metabolic functions.

2.4.1 Coenzymes and metal ions in oxidation and reduction reactions

Oxidation is the process of removing electrons from a molecule, either alone or together with hydrogen ions (protons, H^+). For example, Fe^{3+} is formed by the removal of an electron from Fe^{2+}, while in the oxidation of a hydrocarbon such as ethane (C_2H_6) to ethene (C_2H_4) two hydrogen atoms are transferred onto a carrier: $CH_3{-}CH_3$ + carrier $\rightleftharpoons$ $CH_2{=}CH_2$ + carrier-H_2. In some oxidation reactions, oxygen is reduced to water or hydrogen peroxide by the hydrogen removed from the substrate being oxidized, as in the oxidation of glucose to carbon dioxide:

$$C_6H_{12}O_6 + 6O_2 \rightarrow 6CO_2 + 6H_2O$$

Reduction is the reverse of oxidation—the addition of hydrogen or electrons, or the removal of oxygen, are all reduction reactions. In the reaction above, ethane was oxidized to ethene at the expense of a carrier, which was reduced in the process. The addition of hydrogen to the carrier is a reduction reaction. Similarly, the addition of electrons to a molecule is a reduction, so just as the conversion of Fe^{2+} to Fe^{3+} is an oxidation reaction, the reverse reaction, the conversion of Fe^{3+} to Fe^{2+}, is a reduction.

Most of the reactions involved in energy metabolism involve the oxidation of metabolic fuels, while many of the biosynthetic reactions involved in the formation of metabolic fuel reserves and the synthesis of body components are reductions.

In some metabolic oxidation and reduction reactions, the hydrogen acceptor or donor is a prosthetic group, e.g., heme (Section 2.4.1.1) or riboflavin (Section 2.4.1.2). In other cases, the hydrogen acceptor or donor acts as a substrate of the enzyme (e.g., the nicotinamide nucleotide coenzymes; Section 2.4.1.3).

2.4.1.1 *Metal ions*

The electron acceptor or donor may be a transition metal ion that can have two different stable electron configurations. Commonly iron (which can form Fe^{2+} or Fe^{3+} ions) and copper (which can form Cu^{+} or Cu^{2+} ions) are involved.

In some enzymes, the metal ion is bound to the enzyme protein; in others it is incorporated in an organic molecule, which in turn is attached to the enzyme. For example, heme is an organic compound containing iron, which is the coenzyme for a variety of enzymes collectively known as the cytochromes (Section 3.3.1.2). Heme is also the prosthetic group of hemoglobin, the protein in red blood cells that binds and transports oxygen between the lungs and other tissues, and myoglobin in muscle. However, in hemoglobin and myoglobin, the iron of heme does not undergo oxidation; it binds oxygen but does not react with it.

2.4.1.2 *Riboflavin and flavoproteins*

Vitamin B_2 (riboflavin; Section 11.7) is important in a wide variety of oxidation and reduction reactions. A few enzymes contain riboflavin itself, while others contain a riboflavin derivative: either riboflavin phosphate (sometimes called flavin mononucleotide) or flavin adenine dinucleotide (FAD; Figure 2.18). When an enzyme contains riboflavin, it is usually covalently bound at the active site. Although riboflavin phosphate and FAD are not normally covalently bound to the enzyme, they are very tightly bound and can be regarded as prosthetic groups. The resultant enzymes with attached riboflavin are collectively known as flavoproteins.

The riboflavin moiety of flavoproteins can be reduced in a single step in which two hydrogen atoms are transferred at the same time forming fully reduced flavin-H_2, or in two separate steps in which one hydrogen is transferred, to form the flavin radical (generally

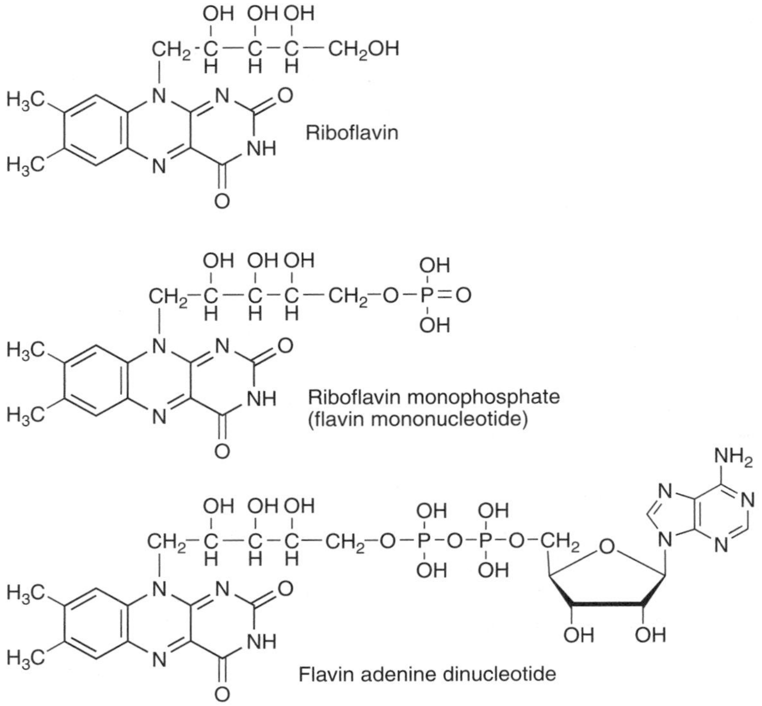

Figure 2.18 Riboflavin and the flavin coenzymes, riboflavin monophosphate, and flavin adenine dinucleotide.

written as flavin-H$^•$), followed by transfer of a second hydrogen to form the fully reduced flavin-H_2 (Figure 2.19).

In some reactions, a single hydrogen is transferred to form flavin-H$^•$, which is then recycled in a separate reaction; in some reactions two molecules of flavin each accept one hydrogen atom from the substrate to be oxidized. Other reactions involve the sequential transfer of two hydrogens onto the flavin, forming first the flavin-H$^•$ radical, then fully reduced flavin-H_2. Flavins can thus act as intermediates between obligatory single-electron reactions, e.g., heme, and obligatory double-electron reactions involving NAD (Section 3.3.1.2).

The reoxidation of reduced flavins in enzymes that react with oxygen is a major source of potentially damaging oxygen radicals (Section 6.5.2.1).

2.4.1.3 The nicotinamide nucleotide coenzymes: NAD and NADP

The vitamin niacin (Section 11.8) is important for the formation of two related compounds, the nicotinamide nucleotide coenzymes—nicotinamide adenine dinucleotide (NAD) and nicotinamide adenine dinucleotide phosphate (NADP; Figure 2.20). They differ only in that NADP has an additional phosphate group attached to the ribose. The whole of the coenzyme molecule is essential for binding to enzymes, and most enzymes can bind and use only one of these two coenzymes, either NAD or NADP, despite the overall similarity in their structures.

The functionally important part of these coenzymes is the nicotinamide ring, which undergoes a two-electron reduction. In the oxidized coenzymes, there is a positive charge associated with the nitrogen atom in the nicotinamide ring, and the oxidized forms of the

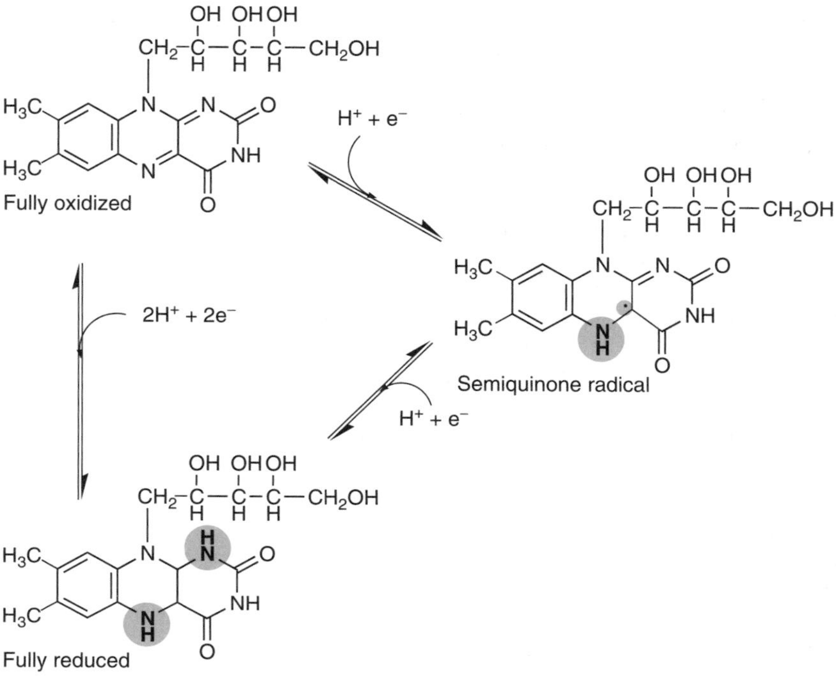

Fully oxidized

$H^+ + e^-$

Semiquinone radical

$2H^+ + 2e^-$

$H^+ + e^-$

Fully reduced

Figure 2.19 Oxidation and reduction of the flavin coenzymes. The reaction may proceed as either a single two-electron reaction or as two single-electron steps with intermediate formation of the riboflavin semiquinone radical.

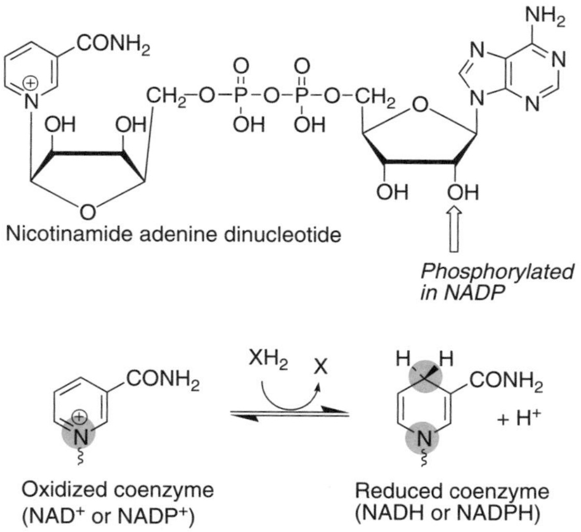

Nicotinamide adenine dinucleotide

Phosphorylated in NADP

XH_2 X

$+ H^+$

Oxidized coenzyme (NAD^+ or $NADP^+$)

Reduced coenzyme (NADH or NADPH)

Figure 2.20 The nicotinamide nucleotide coenzymes, NAD and NADP. In the oxidized coenzyme, there is one hydrogen at carbon-4, but by convention this is not shown when the ring is drawn. In the reduced coenzymes both hydrogens are shown, with a dotted bond to one hydrogen, and a bold bond to the other, to show that the ring as a whole is planar, with one hydrogen at carbon-4 above the plane of the ring, and the other below.

coenzymes are usually shown as NAD^+ and $NADP^+$. Reduction involves the transfer of two electrons and two hydrogen ions (H^+) from the substrate to the coenzyme. One electron neutralizes the positive charge on the nitrogen atom. The other, with its associated H^+ ion, is incorporated into the ring as a second hydrogen at carbon-4.

The second H^+ ion removed from the substrate remains associated with the coenzyme. This means that the reaction can be shown as

$$X\text{-}H_2 + NAD^+ \rightleftharpoons X + NADH + H^+$$

where $X\text{-}H_2$ is the substrate and X is the product (the oxidized form of the substrate).

Note that the reaction is reversible, and NADH can act as a reducing agent:

$$X + NADH + H^+ \rightleftharpoons X\text{-}H_2 + NAD^+$$

where X is now the substrate and $X\text{-}H_2$ is the product (the reduced form of the substrate).

The usual notation is that NAD and NADP are used when the oxidation state is not relevant, and NAD(P) when either NAD or NADP is being discussed. The oxidized coenzymes are shown as $NAD(P)^+$, and the reduced forms as NAD(P)H.

Unlike flavins and metal coenzymes, the nicotinamide nucleotide coenzymes do not remain bound to the enzyme, but act as substrates, binding to the enzyme, undergoing reduction, and then leaving. The reduced coenzyme is then reoxidized either by reaction with another enzyme, for which it acts as a hydrogen donor, or by way of the mitochondrial electron transport chain (Section 3.3.1.2). Cells contain only a small amount of NAD(P) (of the order of 400 nmol/g in liver), which is rapidly cycled between the oxidized and the reduced forms by different enzymes.

In general, NAD^+ is the coenzyme for oxidation reactions, with most of the resultant NADH being reoxidized directly or indirectly via the mitochondrial electron transport chain (Section 3.3.1.2), while NADPH is the main coenzyme for reduction reactions (e.g., the synthesis of fatty acids; Section 5.6.1).

2.5 The classification and naming of enzymes

There is a formal system of enzyme nomenclature, in which each enzyme has a number, and the various enzymes are classified according to the type of reaction catalyzed and the substrates, products, and coenzymes of the reaction. This is used in research publications, when there is a need to identify an enzyme unambiguously, but for general use there is a less formal system of naming enzymes. Almost all enzyme names end in *-ase*, and many are derived simply from the name of the substrate acted on, with the suffix *-ase*. In some cases, the type of reaction catalyzed is also included.

Altogether, there are some 5–10,000 enzymes in human tissues. However, they can be classified into only six groups, depending on the types of chemical reaction they catalyze:

1. Oxidation and reduction reactions
2. Transfer of a reactive group from one substrate onto another
3. Hydrolysis of bonds
4. Addition across carbon–carbon double bonds
5. Rearrangement of groups within a single molecule of substrate
6. Formation of bonds between two substrates, frequently linked to the hydrolysis of ATP → ADP + phosphate

Table 2.2 Classification of Enzyme-Catalyzed Reactions

Oxidoreductases	Oxidation and reduction reactions	
	Dehydrogenases	Addition or removal of H
	Oxidases	Two-electron transfer to O_2 forming H_2O_2
		Two-electron transfer to ½O_2 forming H_2O
	Oxygenases	Incorporate O_2 into product
	Hydroxylases	Incorporate ½O_2 into product as –OH and form H_2O
	Peroxidases	Use as H_2O_2 as oxygen donor, forming H_2O
Transferases	Transfer a chemical group from one substrate to the other kinases	Transfer phosphate from ATP onto substrate
Hydrolases	Hydrolysis of C–O, C–N, O–P, and C–S bonds	For example, esterases, proteases, phosphatases, and deamidases
Lyases	Addition across a carbon–carbon double bond	For example, dehydratases, hydratases, and decarboxylases
Isomerases	Intramolecular rearrangements	
Ligases (synthetases)	Formation of bonds between two substrates	Frequently linked to utilization of ATP, with intermediate formation of phosphorylated enzyme or substrate

This classification of enzymes is expanded in Table 2.2 to give some examples of the types of reactions catalyzed.

Each enzyme has a four-part number indicating the overall class of reaction (1–6 in the list above), then the subclass, sub-subclass, and finally the unique number for that enzyme within its sub-subclass. In formal nomenclature, this is shown as EC (for Enzyme Commission) xx.xx.xx.xx.

2.6 Metabolic pathways

A simple reaction, such as the oxidation of ethanol (alcohol) to carbon dioxide and water, can proceed in a single step, for example, simply by setting fire to the alcohol in air. The reaction is exothermic, and the oxidation of ethanol to carbon dioxide and water has an output of 29 kJ/g.

When alcohol is metabolized in the body, although the overall reaction is the same, it does not proceed in a single step, but as a series of linked reactions, each resulting in a small change in the substrate. In general, any enzyme catalyzes only a single simple change in the substrate, although there are enzymes that catalyze more complex reactions. The metabolic oxidation of ethanol (Figure 2.21) involves 11 enzyme-catalyzed steps, as well as the mitochondrial electron transport chain (Section 3.3.1.2). The energy yield is still

29 kJ/g, since the starting material (ethanol) and the end products (carbon dioxide and water) are the same, and the overall change in energy level is the same, regardless of the route taken. Such a sequence of linked enzyme-catalyzed reactions is a metabolic pathway.

Metabolic pathways can be divided into three broad groups:

- *Catabolic pathways*, involved in the breakdown of relatively large molecules, and oxidation of substrates, ultimately to carbon dioxide and water. These are the main energy-yielding metabolic pathways.
- *Anabolic pathways*, involved in the synthesis of compounds from simpler precursors. These are the main energy-requiring metabolic pathways. Many are reduction reactions, and many involve condensation reactions. Similar reactions are also involved in the metabolism of drugs and other foreign compounds, hormones, and neurotransmitters, to yield products that are excreted in the urine or bile.
- *Central pathways*, involved in interconversions of substrates, that can be regarded as being both catabolic and anabolic, and are sometimes called amphibolic. The principal such pathway is the citric acid cycle (Section 5.4.4).

In some pathways all the enzymes are free in solution, and intermediate products are released from one enzyme, equilibrate with the pool of intermediate in the cell, and then bind to the next enzyme. In other cases, there is channeling of substrates; the product of

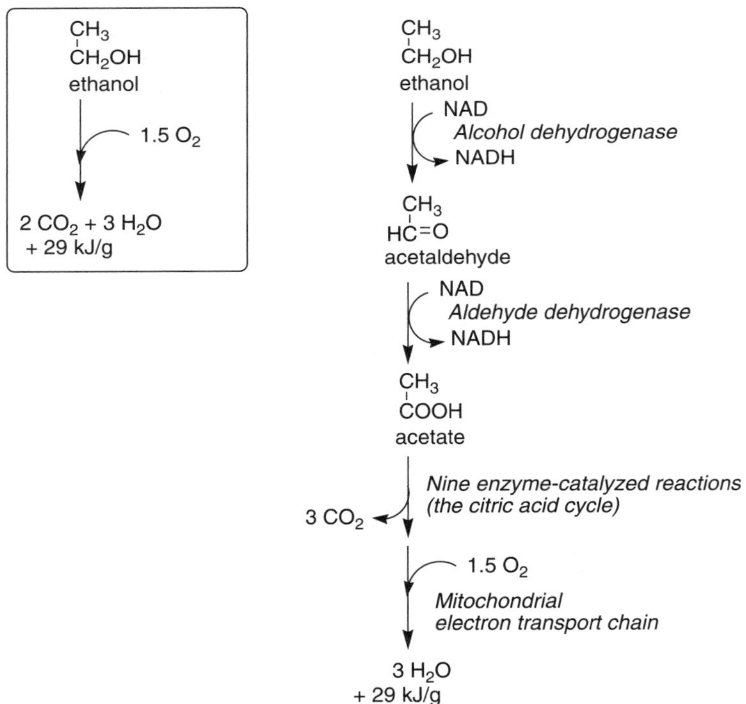

Figure 2.21 The oxidation of ethanol. The box shows the rapid nonenzymic reaction when ethanol is burnt in air; metabolic oxidation of ethanol involves 11 separate enzyme-catalyzed steps, as well as the mitochondrial electron transport chain.

one enzyme is passed directly to the active site of the next, without equilibrating with the pool of intermediate in the cell.

Sometimes, this channeling of substrates is achieved by the assembly of the individual enzymes that catalyze a sequence of reactions into a multienzyme complex that is in free solution in the cytosol; examples of multienzyme complexes include pyruvate dehydrogenase (Section 5.4.3.1) and the very large multienzyme complex that catalyzes the synthesis of fatty acids (Section 5.6.1). In some cases, enzymes that catalyze adjacent steps in a pathway have undergone gene fusion during evolution, so that there is a single protein with two catalytic sites, the first of which passes its product directly onto the next.

In other cases (e.g., the β-oxidation of fatty acids; Section 5.5.2), all the enzymes involved in the pathway are arranged on a membrane in such a way that each passes its product to the next in turn, and none of the intermediates can be detected in solution. Such an array of enzymes is sometimes known as a metabolon.

2.6.1 *Linear and branched pathways*

The simplest type of metabolic pathway is a single sequence of reactions in which the starting material is converted to the end product with no possibility of alternative reactions or branches in the pathway.

Simple linear pathways are rare, since many of the intermediate compounds in metabolism can be used in a variety of pathways, depending on the need for different products. Many metabolic pathways involve branch points (Figure 2.22), where an intermediate may proceed down one branch or another. The fate of an intermediate at a branch point will depend on the relative activities of the two enzymes that are competing for the same substrate. As discussed earlier (Section 2.3.3.1), if the enzymes catalyzing the reactions from D → P and from D → X have different values of K_m, then it is possible to predict which branch will predominate at any given intracellular concentration of D.

Enzymes catalyzing reactions at branch points are usually subject to regulation (Section 10.1), so as to direct substrates through one branch or the other, depending on the body's requirements at the time.

2.6.2 *Spiral or looped reaction sequences*

Sometimes a metabolic pathway involves repeating a series of reactions several times over. For example, the oxidation of fatty acids (Section 5.5.2) proceeds by the sequential removal of two-carbon units. The removal of each two-carbon unit involves a repeated sequence of four reactions, and the end product of each cycle of the pathway is a fatty acid that is two carbons shorter than the one that entered. It then undergoes the same sequence of reactions (Figure 2.23).

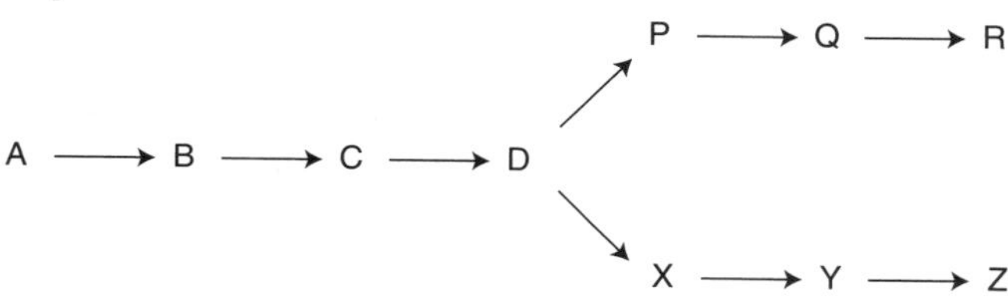

Figure 2.22 Linear and branched metabolic pathways.

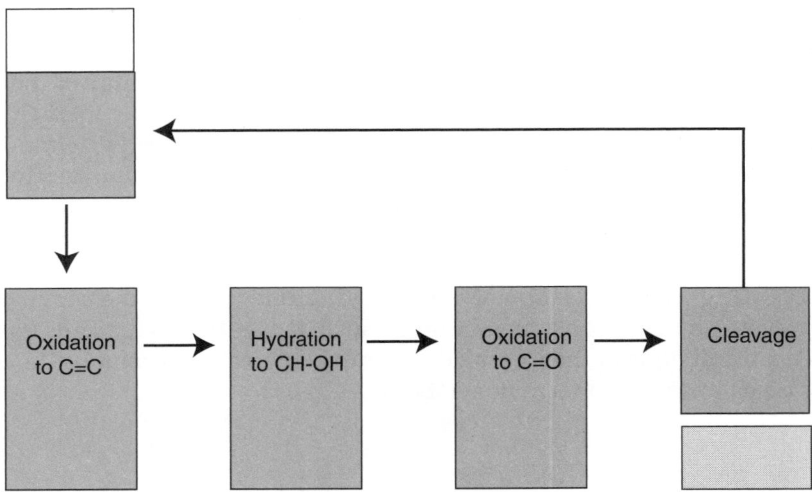

Figure 2.23 A spiral or looped (repeating) metabolic pathway.

Similarly, the synthesis of fatty acids (Section 5.6.1) involves the repeated addition of two-carbon units until the final chain length (commonly, 16 carbon atoms) has been achieved. The addition of each two-carbon unit involves four separate reaction steps, which are repeated in each cycle of the pathway. The enzymes of this pathway form a large multi-enzyme complex in which the enzymes catalyzing each step of the sequence are arranged in a series of concentric rings; the innermost ring catalyzes the reaction sequence until the growing fatty acid chain is long enough to reach to the next ring of enzymes outward from the center.

2.6.3 *Cyclic pathways*

The third type of metabolic pathway is cyclic; a product is assembled, or a substrate is catabolized, attached to a carrier molecule that is unchanged at the end of each cycle of reactions.

Figure 2.24 shows a cyclic biosynthetic pathway in cartoon form; the product is built up in a series of reactions, then released, regenerating the carrier molecule. An example of such a pathway is the urea synthesis cycle (Section 9.3.1.4).

Figure 2.25 shows a cyclic catabolic pathway in cartoon form; the substrate is bound to the carrier molecule, then undergoes a series of reactions in which parts are removed, until at the end of the reaction sequence the original carrier molecule is left. An example of such a pathway is the citric acid cycle (Section 5.4.4).

The intermediates in a cyclic pathway can be considered to be catalysts, in that they participate in the reaction sequence, but at the end they emerge unchanged. Until all the enzymes in a cyclic pathway are saturated (and hence acting at V_{max}), addition of any one of the intermediates will result in an increase in the intracellular concentration of all intermediates, and an increase in the rate at which the cycle runs, and either substrate is catabolized or product is formed (see Problem 5.3 and the urea synthesis experiment in the virtual laboratory on the CD).

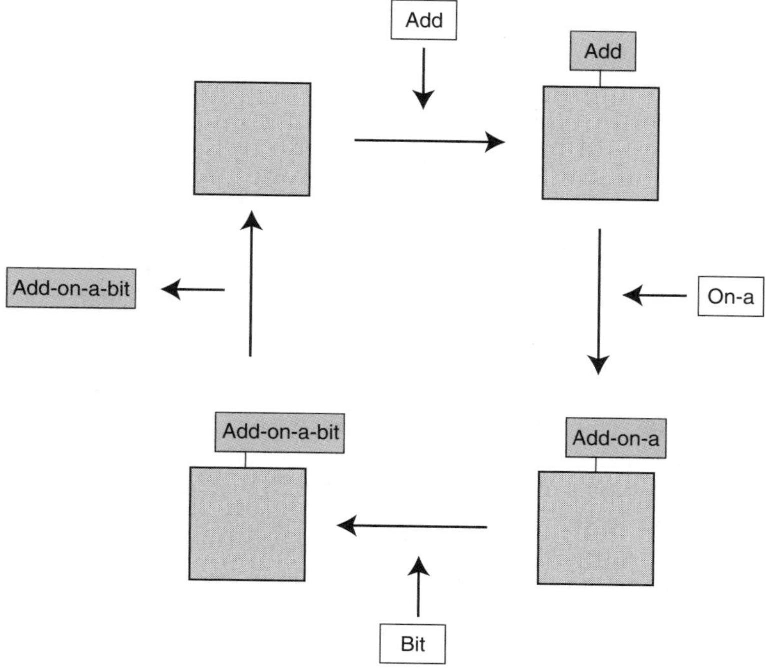

Figure 2.24 A biosynthetic cyclic metabolic pathway.

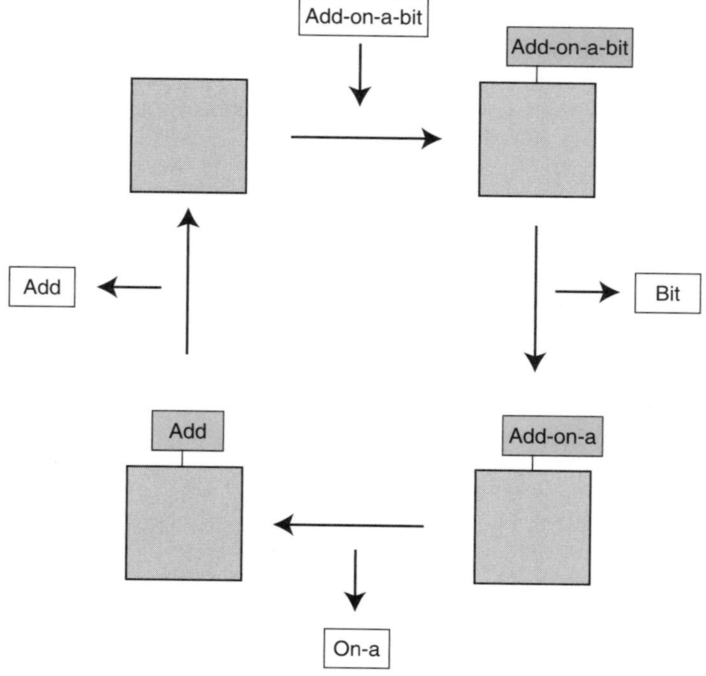

Figure 2.25 A catabolic cyclic metabolic pathway.

2.7 Enzymes in clinical chemistry and medicine

There are three areas in which enzymes can be exploited in clinical chemistry—measurement of metabolites, measurement of enzymes in plasma as a diagnostic tool, and assessment of vitamin nutritional status.

2.7.1 Measurement of metabolites in blood, urine, and tissue samples

Enzyme assays provide two advantages over conventional chemical assays: they have high sensitivity, so that very small amounts of analyte can be detected (and therefore only small amounts of sample are needed); and, because enzymes have a high degree of specificity for their substrates, they are very specific for the substance being measured. For example, the chemical measurement of glucose in urine depends on reduction of Cu^{2+} to Cu^{+} in alkaline solution, and a variety of other compounds that may occur in urine will also reduce copper ions; by contrast, the enzyme glucose oxidase detects only glucose and not other reducing compounds (see Problem 4.1).

Obviously, the limiting factor in the formation of the product must be the concentration of substrate available; the enzyme must be present in excess, and the sample diluted so as to ensure that the concentration of substrate is considerably lower than the K_m of the enzyme—i.e., the reaction conditions are such that the enzyme is operating in region A of Figure 2.9, and a small difference in substrate leads to a large difference in the amount of product formed.

2.7.2 Measurement of enzymes in blood samples

Many enzymes occur in blood plasma as a result of both normal turnover of cells and pathological tissue damage; they are released into the bloodstream by the dying cells. An abnormally high amount of one or more enzymes in a plasma sample is indicative of tissue damage, and the pattern of enzymes released is a useful diagnostic tool (Table 2.3). In a number of cases, there are different forms of the same enzyme in different tissues—isoenzymes that catalyze the same reaction, but differ in their pH optimum, sensitivity to inhibitors, or mild heat treatment, or some other readily measurable property, so that it is possible to differentiate between, for example, alkaline phosphatase from bone or liver,

Table 2.3 Diagnostically Useful Enzymes in Plasma

Enzyme	Elevated in
Acid phosphatase	Prostate cancer
Alanine aminotransferase	Liver disease
Alkaline phosphatase (different tissue-specific isoenzymes in bone and liver)	Cholestatic liver disease, bone disease, rickets, and osteomalacia (see Section 11.3.4)
Amylase	Acute pancreatitis
Aspartate aminotransferase	Liver disease, muscle disease, myocardiac infarction
Creatine kinase	Muscle disease, myocardiac infarction
γ-Glutamyl transpeptidase	Early liver disease
Lactate dehydrogenase (different tissue-specific isoenzymes in liver, skeletal, and cardiac muscle)	Liver disease, muscle disease, myocardiac infarction

which would be useful in determining for example whether bone pain was due to primary bone disease or metastasis of a liver cancer into bone.

Figure 2.26 shows the pattern of enzymes released by damaged cardiac muscle cells after a myocardiac infarction. The extent to which the enzymes are raised above the normal level indicates the severity of the tissue damage. If the activities of the enzymes do not fall in the expected way, this is an indication that the patient has suffered one or more further infarctions, suggesting a poor prognosis.

If the aim is to determine the activity of an enzyme in plasma, then obviously the limiting factor must be the amount of enzyme present, and not the amount of substrate provided in the assay medium. Ideally the enzyme should be saturated with substrate; conventionally the concentration of substrate added is some 10–20 times greater than the K_m of the enzyme, so that it is acting at or near V_{max} (i.e., in region B of Figure 2.9), and a small change in the amount of substrate will have little or no effect on the activity of the enzyme.

2.7.3 Assessment of vitamin nutritional status

For enzymes that have a tightly bound cofactor derived from a vitamin, the extent to which red blood cells can compete with other tissues for the coenzyme provides a sensitive means of assessing nutritional status. Three such coenzymes are:

- Thiamin diphosphate (derived from vitamin B_1; Section 11.6), the coenzyme of transketolase
- Flavin adenine dinucleotide (derived from vitamin B_2; Section 11.7), the coenzyme of glutathione reductase
- Pyridoxal phosphate (derived from vitamin B_6; Section 11.9), the coenzyme of various transaminases

Tissue contains:

- Enzyme protein with coenzyme bound (the holoenzyme)—this is catalytically active
- Enzyme protein without coenzyme (the apoenzyme)—this is catalytically inactive

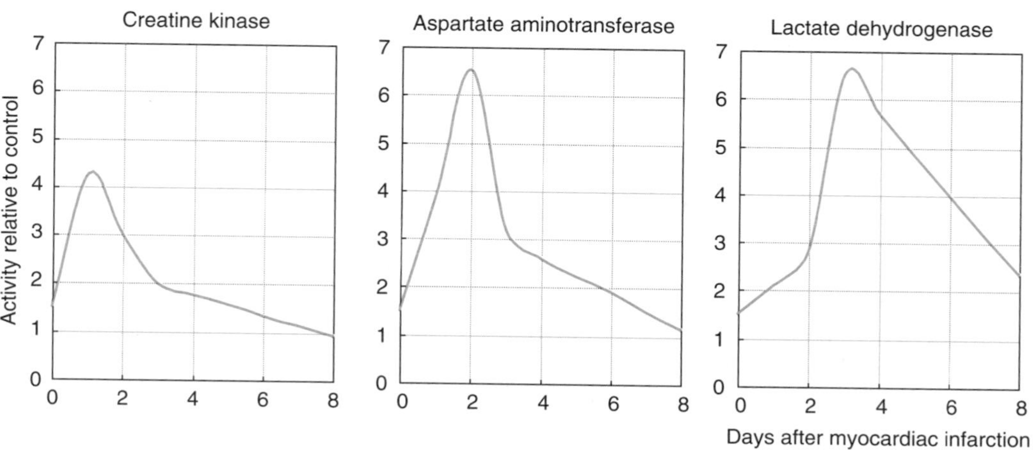

Figure 2.26 Plasma enzymes after myocardiac infarction.

Incubation of a red blood cell lysate *in vitro* without added coenzyme permits measurement of what was initially present as holoenzyme, while incubation after the addition of coenzyme permits activation (and hence measurement) of the apoenzyme as well. The increase in catalytic activity after addition of coenzyme is the activation coefficient; for someone whose vitamin status was good the activation coefficient will be only slightly greater than 1.0; the higher the activation coefficient (meaning that there is more apoenzyme without its coenzyme), the poorer the subject's vitamin status.

Key points

- Breaking covalent bonds involves an input of energy to excite electrons to an unstable configuration (the activation energy).
- Exothermic reactions proceed with output of heat; endothermic reactions require an input of energy.
- Enzymes catalyze reactions by lowering the activation energy; they increase the rate at which equilibrium is reached, but do not affect the position of equilibrium. *In vivo* reactions are not normally at equilibrium because there is constant flux through a pathway.
- The active site of an enzyme comprises a substrate-binding site and a catalytic site; both are formed by reactive groups in the side chains of amino acids that may be some distance apart in the primary sequence of the protein.
- Enzymes show considerable specificity for the substrates bound and the reaction catalyzed.
- Enzymes may have nonprotein components; coenzymes that may be covalently or noncovalently bound to the protein and are essential for activity.
- Most enzymes show a hyperbolic relation between the concentration of substrate and the rate of reaction; V_{max} is the maximum rate of reaction when the enzyme is saturated with substrate.
- K_m is an inverse measure of the affinity of an enzyme for its substrate; it is the concentration of substrate at which the enzyme achieves half V_{max}.
- A variety of compounds inhibit enzymes; irreversible inhibitors bind covalently to the active site, permanently inactivating a molecule of enzyme. Reversible inhibitors may be competitive with respect to substrate, noncompetitive, or uncompetitive.
- A metabolic pathway is a sequence of enzyme-catalyzed reactions; pathways may be linear, branched, looped, or cyclic.
- Enzymes can be used to measure metabolites in blood, urine, and tissue samples; measurement of enzymes in plasma samples is useful diagnostically.

Problem 2.1: An unusual cause of diabetes

This problem concerns a *small* number of families with a clear pattern of dominant inheritance of an *unusual* form of diabetes (Section 10.7), which can be classified as non-insulin-dependent since they secrete significant amounts of insulin (although less than normal subjects), but which develops in early childhood. It is generally referred to as maturity-onset diabetes of the young (MODY). There are a number of different types of MODY, each caused by mutations in a different gene; this problem concerns just one type.

The β-islet cells of the pancreas secrete insulin in response to an increase in blood glucose. This problem is concerned with the way in which the β-cells detect the increased blood concentration of glucose. One hypothesis was that there is a glucose receptor on the outer surface of the β-cell membrane, and when this binds glucose it initiates a series of intracellular events that lead to secretion of insulin.

Coore and Randle (1964) measured the secretion of insulin by rabbit pancreas incubated *in vitro* with two concentrations of glucose, with and without the addition of the seven-carbon sugar mannoheptulose, which they had previously shown to be an inhibitor of phosphorylation of glucose to glucose 6-phosphate. Their results are shown in Table 2.4.

What conclusions can you draw from these observations?

Glucose enters the cells of tissues such as skeletal muscle and adipose tissue by means of an active transport mechanism, which is stimulated in response to the hormone insulin. This means that insulin promotes the uptake and utilization of glucose in these tissues. In contrast, glucose enters liver cells by facilitated diffusion and is then trapped intracellularly by phosphorylation to glucose 6-phosphate, which cannot cross cell membranes. Glucose 6-phosphate is then either metabolized as a metabolic fuel (Section 5.4.1) or used to synthesize the storage carbohydrate glycogen (Section 5.6.3).

Two enzymes catalyze the formation of glucose 6-phosphate from glucose:

- Hexokinase is expressed in all tissues; it has a K_m for glucose of ~0.15 mmol/L.
- Glucokinase is expressed only in liver and the β-cells of the pancreas; it has a K_m for glucose of ~20 mmol/L.

The normal range of plasma glucose is between 3.5 and 5 mmol/L, rising in peripheral blood to 8–10 mmol/L after a moderately high intake of glucose. After a meal, the concentration of glucose in the portal blood, coming from the small intestine to the liver, may be considerably higher than this.

- What effect do you think changes in the plasma concentration of glucose will have on the rate of formation of glucose 6-phosphate catalyzed by hexokinase?

Table 2.4 Secretion of Insulin (μg/min/incubation) by Rabbit Pancreas *In Vitro*

Glucose (mmol/L)	Control	+ Mannoheptulose
3.3	3.5	3.5
16.6	12.5	3.5

Source: Data reported by Coore, H.G. and Randle, P.J., *Biochem. J.*, 93, 66–77, 1964.

- What effect do you think changes in the plasma concentration of glucose will have on the rate of formation of glucose 6-phosphate catalyzed by glucokinase?
- What do you think is the importance of glucokinase in the liver?

Froguel and coworkers (1993) reported studies of the glucokinase gene in a number of families affected by MODY, and also in unaffected families. They published a list of 16 variants of the glucokinase gene, shown in Table 2.5. All their patients with MODY had an abnormality of the gene.

- Using the genetic code shown in Table 9.8, fill in the amino acid changes associated with each mutation in the gene.
- Why do you think the mutations affecting codons 4, 10, and 116 had no effect on the people involved?
- What conclusions can you draw from this information?

The same authors also studied the secretion of insulin in response to glucose infusion in patients with MODY and normal control subjects. They were given an intravenous infusion of glucose; the rate of infusion was varied so as to maintain a constant plasma concentration of glucose of 10 mmol/L. Their plasma concentrations of glucose and insulin were measured before and after 60 min of glucose infusion (Table 2.6).

- What conclusions can you draw from this information about the probable role of glucokinase in the β-cells of the pancreas?

Table 2.5 Mutations in the Glucokinase Gene

Codon	Nucleotide Change	Amino Acid Change	Effect
4	GAC ⇨ AAC	?	None
10	GCC ⇨ GCT	?	None
70	GAA ⇨ AAA	?	MODY
98	CAG ⇨ TAG	?	MODY
116	ACC ⇨ ACT	?	None
175	GGA ⇨ AGA	?	MODY
182	GTG ⇨ ATG	?	MODY
186	CGA ⇨ TGA	?	MODY
203	GTG ⇨ GCG	?	MODY
228	ACG ⇨ ATG	?	MODY
261	GGG ⇨ AGG	?	MODY
279	GAG ⇨ TAG	?	MODY
300	GAG ⇨ AAG	?	MODY
300	GAG ⇨ CAG	?	MODY
309	CTC ⇨ CCC	?	MODY
414	AAG ⇨ GAG	?	MODY

Source: Data reported by Froguel, P. et al., *New Engl. J. Med.*, 328, 697–702, 1993.

Table 2.6 Plasma Concentrations of Glucose and Insulin before and after 60 min of Glucose Infusion

	Plasma Glucose (mmol/L)		Insulin (mU/L)	
	Patients	Controls	Patients	Controls
Fasting	7.0 ± 0.4	5.1 ± 0.3	5 ± 2	6 ± 2
60 min infusion	Maintained at 10 mmol/L by varying rate of infusion		12 ± 7	40 ± 11

Source: Data reported by Froguel, P. et al., *New Engl. J. Med.*, 328, 697–702, 1993.

Table 2.7 Substrate Dependence of a Novel Endopeptidase

Concentration of *p*-Nitrophenyl Acetate Added (mol/L)	Nitrophenol Formed (μmol/10 min)
1.4×10^{-4}	2.22
2.0×10^{-4}	2.94
3.3×10^{-4}	4.44
5.0×10^{-4}	5.88
1.0×10^{-3}	9.08

- Can you deduce the way in which the β-cells of the pancreas sense an increase in plasma glucose and signal the secretion of insulin?

Problem 2.2: Studies of a novel endopeptidase

A new enzyme, of bacterial origin, is being studied for its potential use in a washing powder preparation. The enzyme is an endopeptidase and has been purified by a variety of chromatographic techniques. The activity of the enzyme has been determined using an assay based on the hydrolysis of a synthetic substrate, *p*-nitrophenyl acetate. On hydrolysis, this (colorless) substrate yields 1 mol of *p*-nitrophenol (which is yellow) for each mole of substrate hydrolyzed.

0.1 mL of a solution containing 1 mg of the purified protein per liter was used in each incubation. The enzyme was incubated at 30°C and pH 7.5 for 10 min; the formation of *p*-nitrophenol was followed spectrophotometrically. The results are shown in Table 2.7.

- Using these results, determine the V_{max} of the enzyme under these incubation conditions.
- Given the relative molecular mass of the enzyme (50,000), calculate the catalytic rate constant, k_{cat} (the maximum rate of reaction expressed in moles of product formed per mole of enzyme per second).

Table 2.8 Results of Measuring Alkaline Phosphatase in Serum Samples

Subject	Absorbance at 405 nm	Enzyme Activity (units/L)
1	0.610	
2	0.302	
3	1.407	
4	1.016	
5	0.871	
6	0.573	
7	0.511	
8	0.497	

Note: A standard solution of 0.1 mmol/L *p*-nitrophenylate in buffer at pH 12 in the same cuvette had an absorbance at 405 nm of 1.83.

Problem 2.3: Determination of serum alkaline phosphatase activity

The activity of alkaline phosphatase in serum is elevated above normal in a variety of different bone diseases, as well as biliary obstruction and some other liver diseases. Measurement of alkaline phosphatase activity in serum can thus give useful information about these conditions. It is especially useful for diagnosis of preclinical rickets and osteomalacia (Section 11.3.4).

The range of alkaline phosphatase activity in serum from healthy adults is (mean ± SD) 75 ± 12 units/L. The reference range (that which is considered "normal") is ± 2 × SD around the mean; values outside this range are considered abnormal.

The activity of alkaline phosphatase is measured by hydrolysis of *p*-nitrophenyl phosphate to yield *p*-nitrophenol and free phosphate. At alkaline pH, *p*-nitrophenol dissociates; the *p*-nitrophenylate ion has a strong yellow color, with maximum absorbance at 405 nm.

The activity of alkaline phosphatase in serum samples was determined by incubating 0.1 mL serum with 0.2 mL *p*-nitrophenyl phosphate at 14 mmol/L in 2.7 mL buffer at pH 10.4 at 30°C for 10 min. The reaction was stopped by addition of 3 mL of 0.2 mol/L sodium hydroxide, which both denatures the enzyme and also raises the pH of the incubation mixture to 12. The absorbance of the final reaction mixture was then determined at 405 nm using a cuvette with a 1 cm light path. The results are shown in Table 2.8. A standard solution of 0.1 mmol/L *p*-nitrophenylate in buffer at pH 12 in the same cuvette had an absorbance at 405 nm of 1.83.

Were the results from the samples within the reference range?

chapter three

The role of ATP in metabolism

Adenosine triphosphate (ATP) acts as the central link between energy-yielding metabolic pathways and energy expenditure in physical and chemical work. The oxidation of metabolic fuels is linked to the phosphorylation of adenosine diphosphate (ADP) to ATP, while the expenditure of metabolic energy for the synthesis of body constituents, transport of compounds across cell membranes, and the contraction of muscle result in the hydrolysis of ATP to yield ADP and phosphate ions. The total body content of ATP plus ADP is under 350 mmol (about 10 g), but the amount of ATP synthesized and used each day is about 100 mol—about 70 kg, an amount equal to the body weight.

Objectives

After reading this chapter, you should be able to

- Explain how endothermic reactions can be linked to the overall hydrolysis of ATP to ADP and phosphate
- Describe how compounds can be transported across cell membranes against a concentration gradient and explain the roles of ATP and proton gradients in active transport
- Describe the role of ATP in muscle contraction and the role of creatine phosphate as a phosphagen
- Describe the structure and functions of the mitochondrion and explain the processes involved in the mitochondrial electron transport chain and oxidative phosphorylation, explain how substrate oxidation is regulated by the availability of ADP and how respiratory poisons and uncouplers act

3.1 The adenine nucleotides

Nucleotides consist of a purine or a pyrimidine base linked to the five-carbon sugar ribose. The base plus sugar is a nucleoside; in a nucleotide the sugar is phosphorylated. Nucleotides may be mono-, di-, or triphosphates.

Figure 3.1 shows the nucleotides formed from the purine adenine—the adenine nucleotides, adenosine monophosphate (AMP), ADP, and ATP. Similar families of nucleotides that are important in metabolism are formed from guanine and uracil. See also Section 10.3.2 for a discussion of the role of cyclic AMP in metabolic regulation and hormone action, and Section 10.3.1 for the role of guanine nucleotides in response to hormone action.

In nucleic acids (DNA and RNA; Sections 9.2.1 and 9.2.2, respectively), it is the purine or the pyrimidine that is important, carrying the genetic information. However, in the link between energy-yielding metabolism and the performance of physical and chemical work, what is important is the phosphorylation of the ribose. Although most enzymic reactions are linked to the utilization of ATP, a small number are linked to guanosine triphosphate (GTP; e.g., Section 5.7) or uridine triphosphate (UTP; Section 5.6.3).

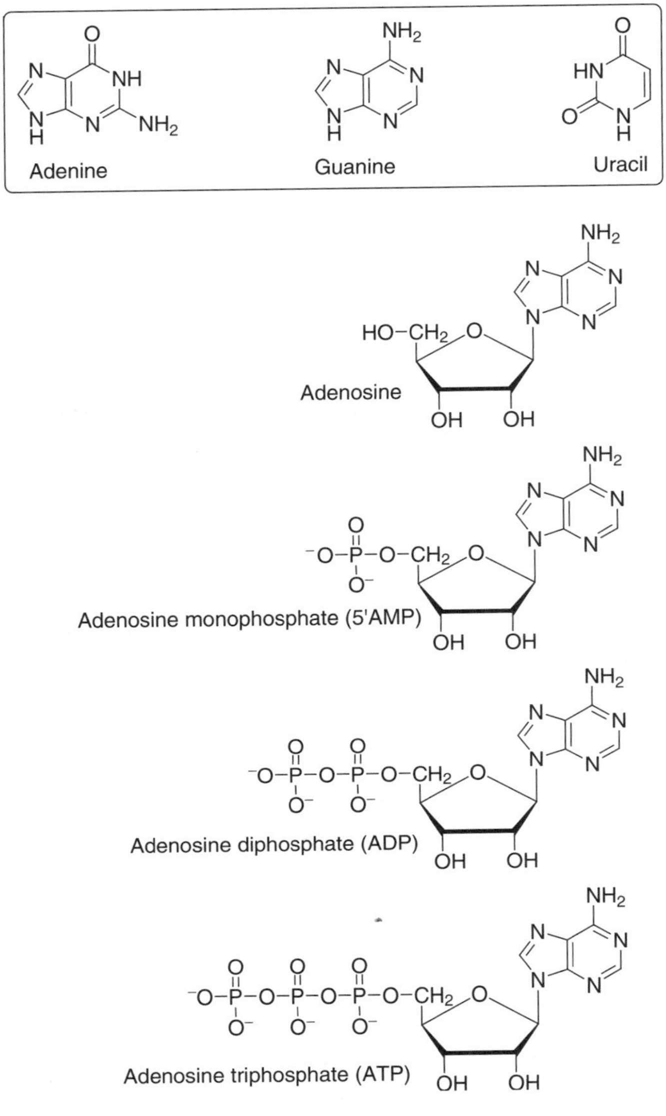

Figure 3.1 The adenine nucleotides (the box shows the structures of adenine, guanine, and uracil; guanine and uracil form a similar series of nucleotides).

3.2 Functions of ATP

Under normal conditions, the processes shown in Figure 3.2 are tightly coupled, so that the oxidation of metabolic fuels is controlled by the availability of ADP, which in turn is controlled by the rate at which ATP is utilized in performing physical and chemical work. Work output, or energy expenditure, thus controls the rate at which metabolic fuels are oxidized and hence the amount of food that must be eaten to meet energy requirements. Metabolic fuels in excess of immediate requirements are stored as reserves of glycogen in muscle and liver (Section 5.6.3), and as fat in adipose tissue (Section 5.6.1).

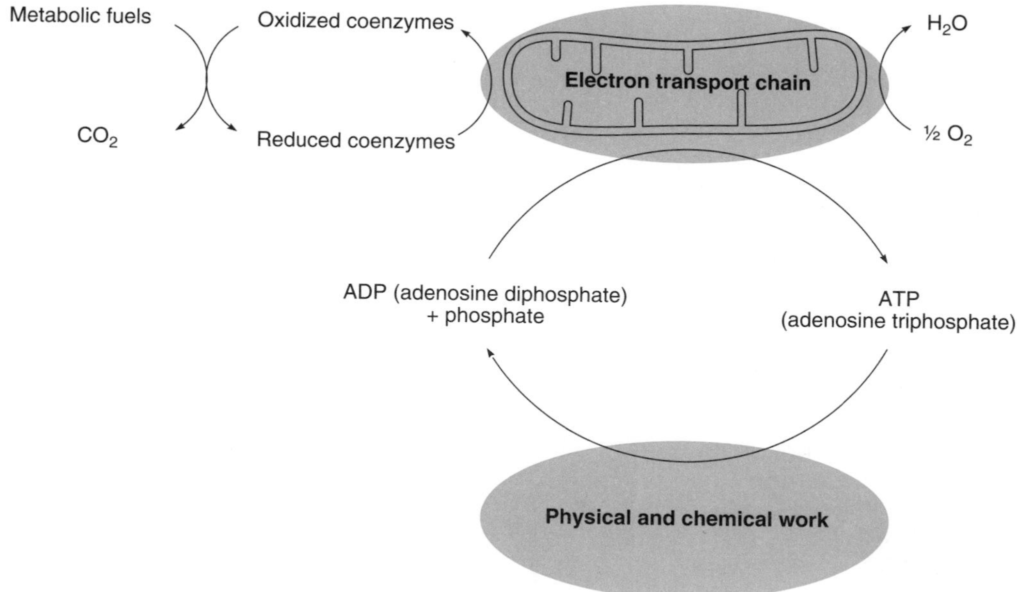

Figure 3.2 Linkage between ATP utilization in physical and chemical work, and the oxidation of metabolic fuels.

In all the reactions in which ATP is utilized, what is observed overall is the hydrolysis of ATP to ADP and phosphate. However, although this is the overall reaction, simple hydrolysis of ATP does not achieve any useful result; it is the intermediate steps in the reaction of ATP + $H_2O \rightarrow$ ADP + phosphate that are important.

3.2.1 *The role of ATP in endothermic reactions*

The equilibrium of an endothermic reaction A + B $\rightleftharpoons$ C + D lies well to the left unless there is an input of energy (Section 2.1.1). The hydrolysis of ATP is exothermic and the equilibrium of the reaction ATP + $H_2O \rightleftharpoons$ ADP + phosphate lies well to the right. Linkage between the two reactions could thus ensure that the (unfavorable) endothermic reaction could proceed together with overall hydrolysis of ATP $\rightarrow$ ADP + phosphate.

Such linkage between two apparently unrelated reactions can easily be achieved in enzyme-catalyzed reactions; there are three possible mechanisms:

1. Phosphorylation of the hydroxyl group of a serine, threonine, or tyrosine residue in the enzyme (Figure 3.3), thereby altering the chemical nature of its catalytic site. Phosphorylation of the enzyme is also important in regulating metabolic pathways, especially in response to hormone action (Section 10.3).
2. Phosphorylation of one of the substrates; the synthesis of glutamine from glutamate and ammonia (Figure 3.4; Section 9.3.1.3) involves the formation of a phosphorylated intermediate.
3. Transfer of the adenosyl group of ATP onto one of the substrates (Figure 3.5); the activation of the methyl group of the amino acid methionine in methyl transfer reactions involves the formation of *S*-adenosyl methionine (Figure 11.21).

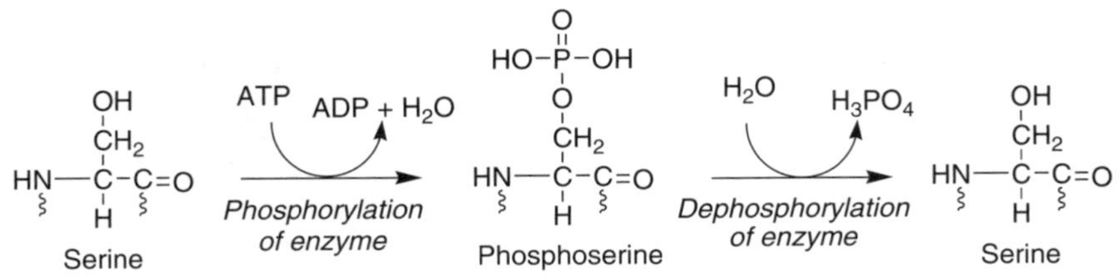

Figure 3.3 The role of ATP in endothermic reactions—phosphorylation of the enzyme.

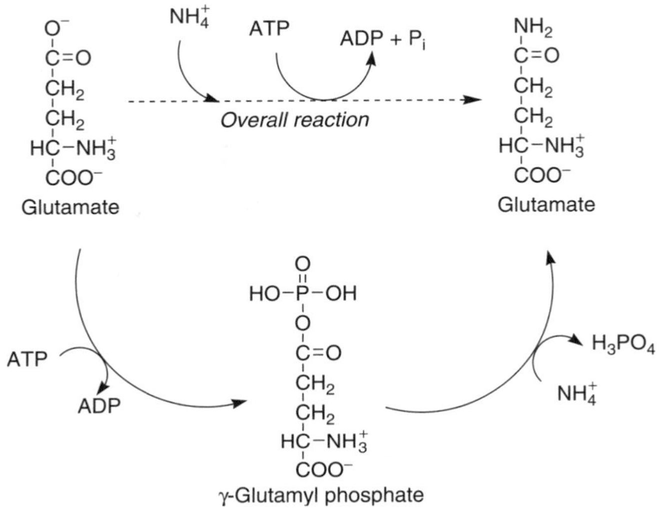

Figure 3.4 The role of ATP in endothermic reactions—phosphorylation of the substrate.

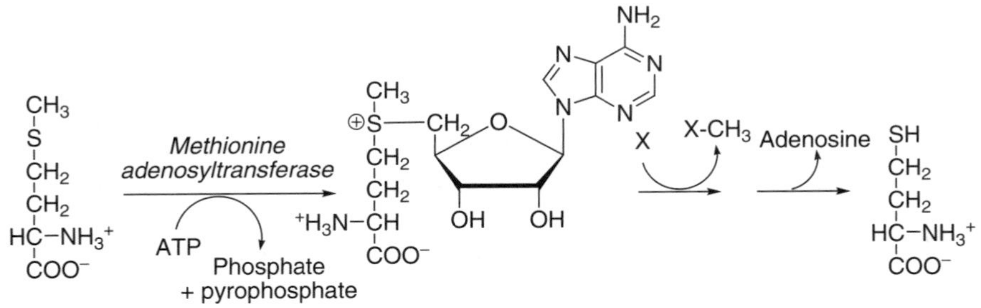

Figure 3.5 The role of ATP in endothermic reactions—adenylation of the substrate. (See also Figure 11.21.)

Not only is the hydrolysis of ATP to ADP and phosphate an exothermic reaction, but the concentration of ATP in cells is always very much higher than that of ADP (a ratio of about 500:1), which again ensures that the reaction will proceed in the direction of ATP hydrolysis. The concentration of ADP in the cell is kept low in two ways:

- ADP is normally rapidly phosphorylated to ATP, linked to the oxidation of metabolic fuels (Section 3.3.1).

- If ADP begins to accumulate, adenylate kinase catalyzes the reaction 2 ADP → AMP + ATP. This not only removes ADP but also provides (a small amount of) ATP; AMP acts as a signal of the energy state of the cell and is a potent activator or inhibitor of a number of key enzymes that regulate metabolic pathways (Section 10.2).

In a number of cases, there is a further mechanism to ensure that the equilibrium of an ATP-linked reaction lies to the right, to such an extent that the reaction is essentially irreversible. The reaction shown in Figure 3.6 results in the hydrolysis of ATP to AMP and pyrophosphate. There is an active pyrophosphatase in cells, which catalyzes the hydrolysis of pyrophosphate to yield 2 mol of phosphate, thereby removing one of the products of the reaction so that the substrate for the reverse reaction is not available.

3.2.2 *Transport of materials across cell membranes*

Lipid-soluble compounds will diffuse freely across cell membranes since they can dissolve in the membrane—this is passive diffusion. Hydrophilic compounds require a transport protein to cross the lipid membrane—this is facilitated or carrier-mediated diffusion. Neither passive nor facilitated diffusion alone can lead to a greater concentration of the material being transported inside the cell than that present outside.

Concentrative uptake of the material being transported may be achieved in three main ways: protein binding, metabolic trapping, and active transport. The latter two mechanisms are ATP dependent.

3.2.2.1 *Protein binding for concentrative uptake*

Hydrophobic compounds are transported in plasma bound to transport proteins (e.g., the plasma retinol binding protein, Section 11.2.2.2, and steroid hormone binding

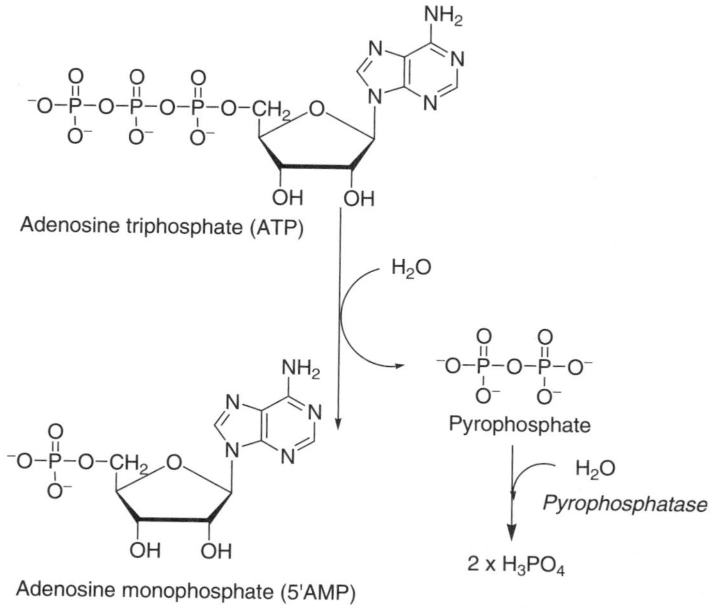

Adenosine triphosphate (ATP)

H_2O

Pyrophosphate

H_2O

Pyrophosphatase

2 x H_3PO_4

Adenosine monophosphate (5'AMP)

Figure 3.6 Hydrolysis of ATP to AMP and pyrophosphate.

proteins, Section 10.4) or dissolved in the lipid core of plasma lipoproteins (Section 5.6.2). Accumulation to a concentration higher than that in plasma depends on an intracellular binding protein that has a greater affinity for the ligand than does the plasma transport protein. The different isomers of vitamin E (Section 11.4.1) have very different biological activity (or potency); at least part of this is explained by the specificity of the intracellular vitamin E binding proteins for the different vitamers.

For a hydrophilic compound that enters the cell by carrier-mediated diffusion, a net increase in concentration inside the cell can sometimes be achieved by binding it to an intracellular protein. Binding proteins are important in the intestinal absorption of calcium (Section 4.5.3) and iron (Section 4.5.3.1).

3.2.2.2 *Metabolic trapping*

Glucose enters and leaves liver cells by carrier-mediated diffusion. In the fed state, when there is a great deal of glucose to be stored as glycogen, it diffuses into the liver cells and is phosphorylated to glucose 6-phosphate, a reaction catalyzed by the enzymes hexokinase and glucokinase using ATP as the phosphate donor (Section 5.4.1 and see Problem 2.1). Glucose 6-phosphate does not cross cell membranes, and therefore there is a net accumulation of glucose as glucose 6-phosphate inside the cell, at the expense of 1 mol of ATP per mole of glucose trapped in this way. Vitamins B_2 (riboflavin; Section 11.7.1) and B_6 (Section 11.9.1) are similarly accumulated inside cells by phosphorylation at the expense of ATP.

3.2.2.3 *Active transport*

Active transport is the accumulation of a higher concentration of a compound on one side of a cell membrane than the other, without chemical modification such as phosphorylation. The process is dependent on the hydrolysis of ATP to ADP and phosphate, either directly, in the case of ion pumps, or indirectly, when metabolites are transported by proton- or sodium-dependent transporters.

3.2.2.4 *P-type transporters*

In P-type transporters, which transport cations, the transport protein is phosphorylated as part of the cycle of activity. Figure 3.7 shows the role of ATP in the sodium–potassium transporter. When the protein has bound ATP, it has a high affinity for Na^+ ions inside the cell. Phosphorylation of the protein causes a conformational change, so that the Na^+ ions are expelled from the cell and the transport now binds K^+ ions at the outer surface of the membrane. Binding of K^+ ions causes a further conformational change, with dephosphorylation of the protein, which now binds ATP again, expels K^+ ions into the cytosol, and is ready to bind more Na^+ ions.

3.2.2.5 *ABC-transporters*

Figure 3.8 shows the role of ATP in transport proteins that bind and hydrolyze ATP, but are not phosphorylated. These proteins all have a similar ATP-binding motif and are known as ATP-binding cassette proteins (ABC transporters). The transporter with the bound ligand binds ATP. Hydrolysis of the bound ATP causes a conformational change in the protein so that the ligand is transported to the opposite face of the membrane and expelled. Expulsion of the ligand causes the reverse conformational change, so that the transporter is open at the opposite side of the membrane, ready to bind more ligand. The intestinal transport proteins that expel sterols into the lumen (Section 4.3.1.3) are ABC transporters, as is the chloride transport protein that is defective in cystic fibrosis.

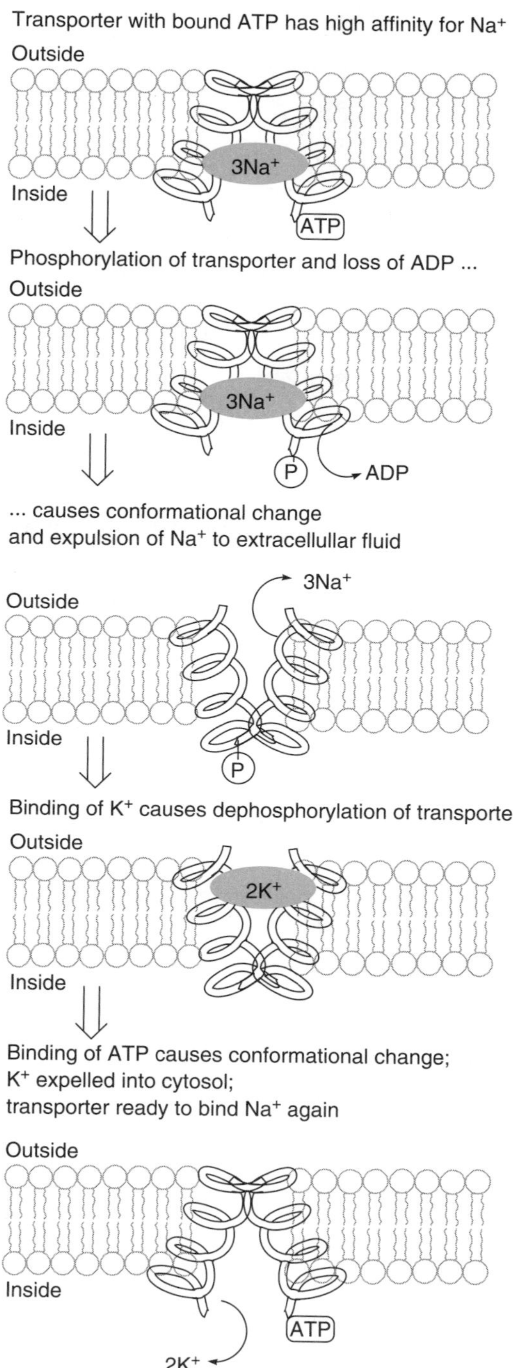

Figure 3.7 The role of ATP in active transport: P-type transporters that have to be phosphorylated to permit transport across the cell membrane.

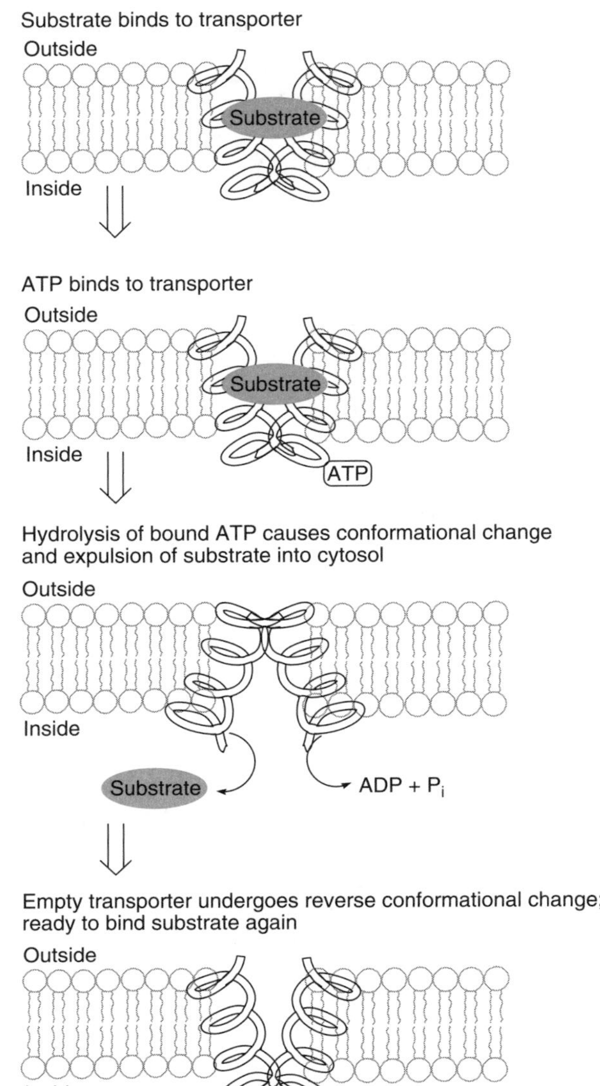

Figure 3.8 The role of ATP in active transport: ATP-binding cassette (ABC) transporters that bind and hydrolyze ATP, but are not phosphorylated.

3.2.2.6 The sodium pump

Figure 3.9 shows the sodium pump, which generates a Na^+ gradient across the membrane that can then be used for transport of other materials against their concentration gradient. The key to understanding the role of ATP in the sodium pump lies in the fact that the hydrolysis is effected not by H_2O, but by H^+ and OH^- ions. The ATPase that catalyzes the hydrolysis of ATP to ADP and phosphate is within the membrane and takes an H^+ ion from inside the cell and an OH^- ion from the extracellular fluid, thus creating a pH gradient across the membrane.

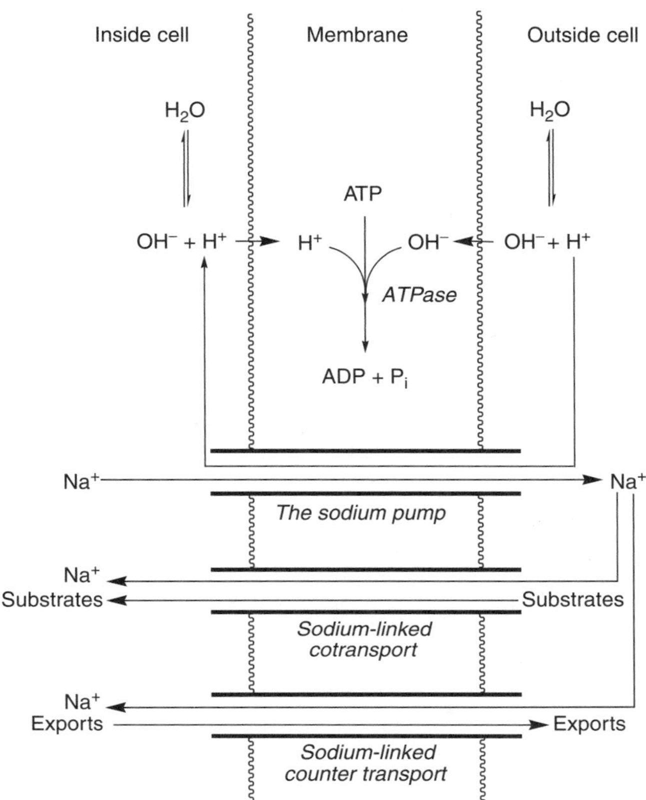

Figure 3.9 The role of ATP in active transport: generation of a proton gradient linked to the sodium pump and sodium-dependent transporters.

The protons in the extracellular fluid then reenter the cell on a transmembrane carrier protein and react with the hydroxyl ions within the cell, thereby discharging the pH gradient. The carrier protein that transports the protons across the cell membrane does so only in exchange for sodium ions. The sodium ions in turn reenter the cell in either of the following ways:

- Together with substrates such as glucose and amino acids, thus providing a mechanism for net accumulation of these substrates, driven by the sodium gradient, which in turn has been created by the proton gradient produced by the hydrolysis of ATP. This is a cotransport mechanism since the sodium ions and substrates travel in the same direction across the cell membrane.
- In exchange for compounds being exported or excreted from the cell. This is a countertransport mechanism, since the sodium ions and the compounds being transported move in opposite directions across the membrane.

3.2.3 The role of ATP in muscle contraction

The important proteins for muscle contraction are actin and myosin (Figure 3.10). Myosin is a filamentous protein, consisting of several subunits, with ATPase activity in the head region.

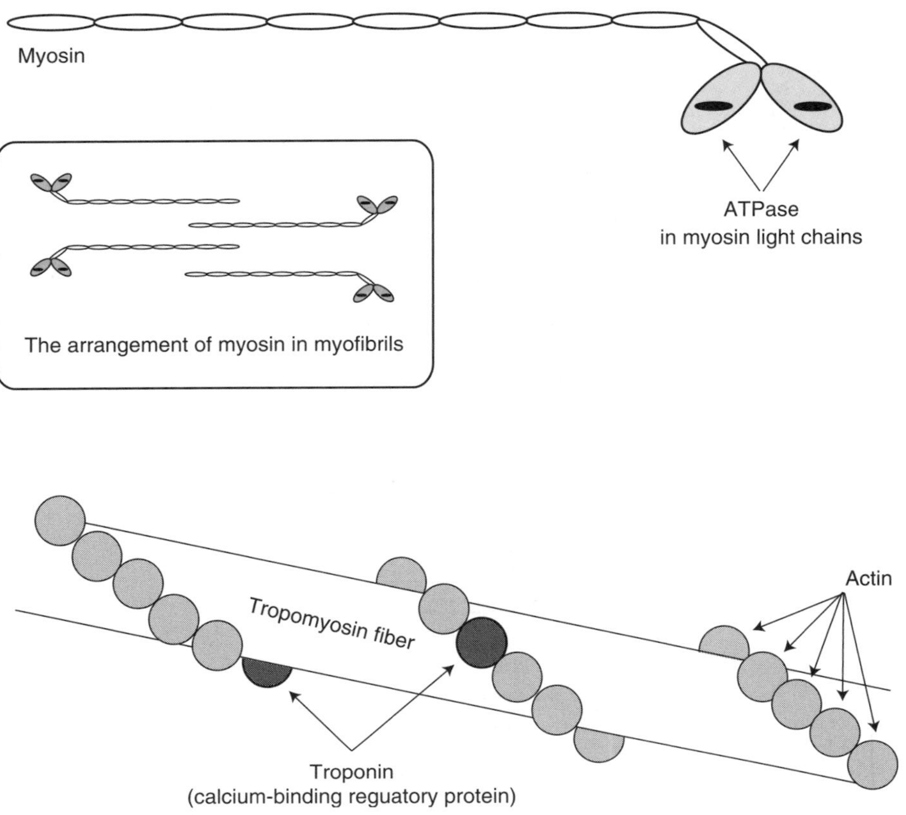

Figure 3.10 The contractile proteins of muscle.

In myofibrils, myosin molecules are arranged in clusters with the tail regions overlapping. Actin is a smaller, globular protein and actin molecules are arranged along a fibrous protein, tropomyosin, thus creating a chain of actin molecules interspersed with molecules of a calcium-binding regulatory protein, troponin.

In resting muscle, each myosin head unit binds ADP and is tightly bound to an actin molecule (Figure 3.11). The binding of ATP to myosin displaces the bound ADP and causes a conformational change in the molecule such that while it remains associated with the actin molecule, it is no longer tightly bound. Hydrolysis of the bound ATP to ADP and phosphate causes a further conformational change in the myosin molecule, so that it is only loosely associated with the actin molecule. Release of the phosphate causes a conformational change affecting the tail region, so that the head region becomes associated with an actin molecule further along. This is the power stroke that causes the actin and myosin filaments to slide over one another, contracting the muscle filament. With ADP bound, the myosin molecule is again tightly bound to actin, but to a molecule further along the actin chain.

3.2.3.1 Creatine phosphate in muscle

The small amount of ATP in cells turns over rapidly and ADP is rapidly rephosphorylated to ATP. However, neither the small amount of ATP in muscle nor the speed with

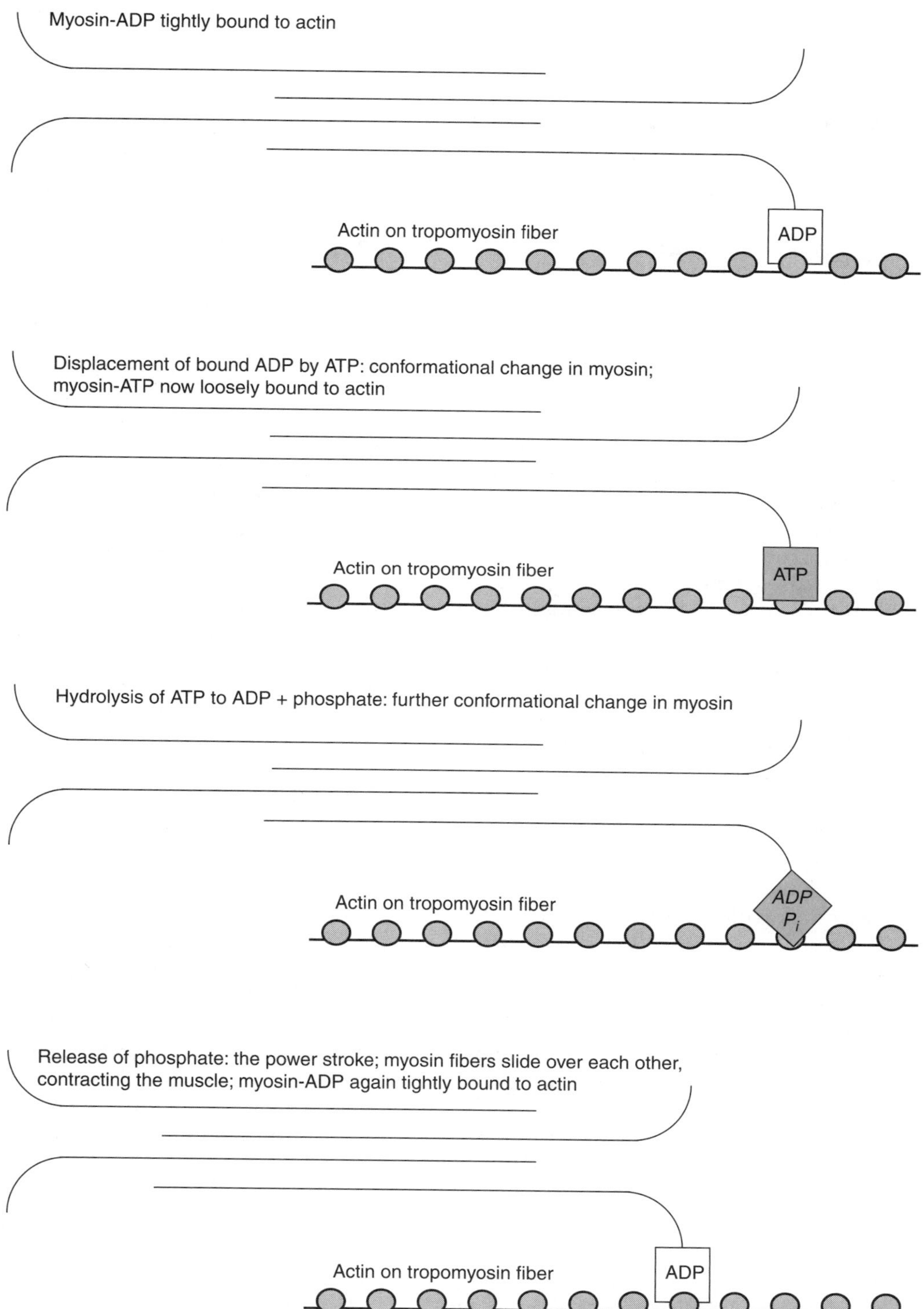

Figure 3.11 The role of ATP in muscle contraction.

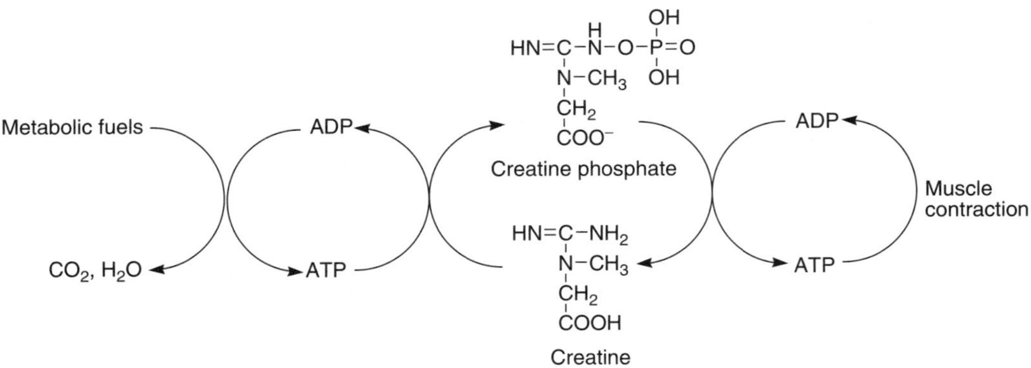

Figure 3.12 The role of creatine phosphate in muscle.

which metabolic activity can be increased, and hence ADP rephosphorylation, matches the demand for ATP for rapid muscle contraction. Muscle contains about four times more creatine phosphate than it does ATP. ADP formed in muscle contraction is rephosphorylated to ATP at the expense of creatine phosphate, which thus acts as a phosphagen—a reservoir or a buffer to maintain a supply of ATP for muscle contraction for the short time until metabolic activity increases (Figure 3.12).

Creatine is not a dietary essential; it is synthesized from the amino acids glycine, arginine, and methionine (Figure 3.13). However, a single serving of meat will provide about 1 g of preformed creatine, compared with *de novo* synthesis of 1–2 g/day. Both creatine and creatine phosphate undergo a nonenzymic reaction to yield creatinine, which is metabolically useless and is excreted in the urine. Since the formation of creatinine is a nonenzymic reaction, the rate at which it is formed, and hence the amount excreted each day, depends mainly on muscle mass and is therefore relatively constant from day to day in any individual. This is useful in clinical chemistry; urinary metabolites are commonly expressed per mole of creatinine and the excretion of creatinine is measured to assess the completeness of a 24 h urine collection; obviously, simple concentration of urinary metabolites is not a useful measurement since the concentration will depend on the volume of urine excreted, which in turn depends on fluid intake and fluid losses from the body. The rate at which creatinine is cleared from the bloodstream (creatinine clearance) provides an index of renal function. There is normally little or no excretion of creatine; significant amounts occur in the urine only when there is breakdown of muscle tissue.

Because of its role as a phosphagen in muscle, creatine supplements are often used as an ergogenic aid to enhance athletic performance and muscle work output. In people who have an initially low muscle concentration of creatine, supplements of 2–5 g/day do increase muscle creatine; however, in people whose muscle creatine is within the normal range, additional creatine has little or no effect, because there is control over the uptake and retention of creatine in muscle cells.

3.3 Phosphorylation of ADP to ATP

A small number of metabolic reactions involve direct transfer of phosphate from a phosphorylated substrate onto ADP, forming ATP—substrate-level phosphorylation. Two such reactions are shown in Figure 3.14; both are reactions in the glycolytic pathway of glucose metabolism (Section 5.4.1). Substrate-level phosphorylation is usually of relatively

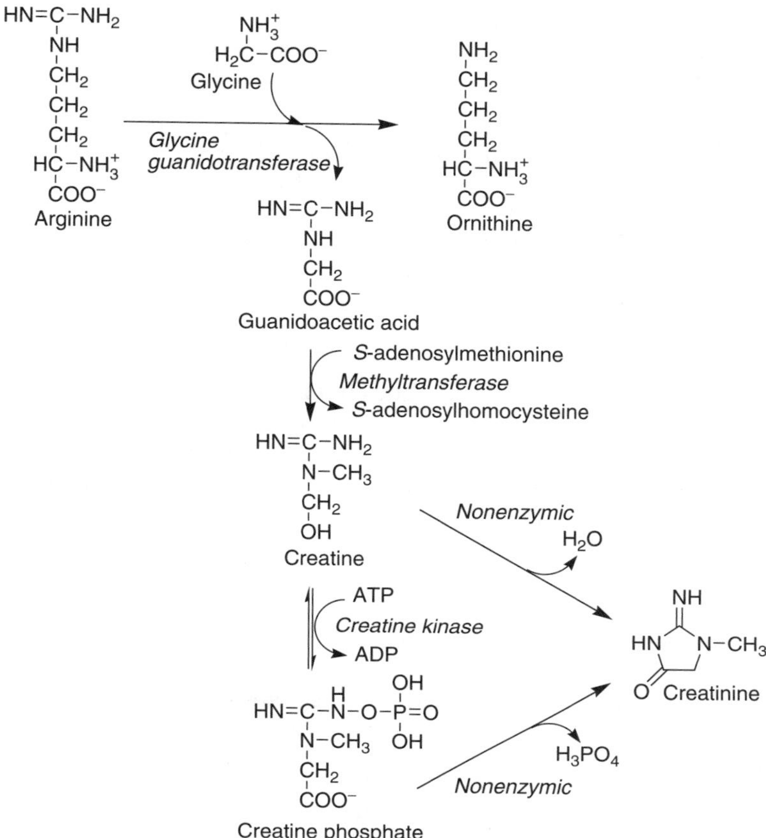

Figure 3.13 The synthesis of creatine and nonenzymic formation of creatinine.

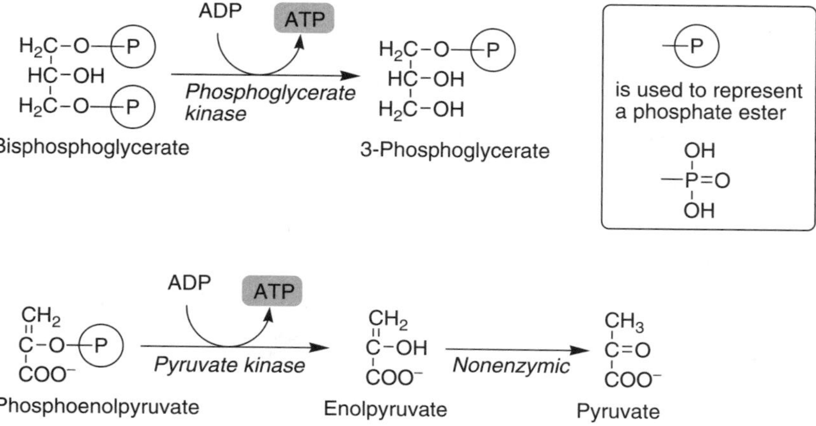

Figure 3.14 Formation of ATP by substrate-level phosphorylation. (See also Figure 5.10.)

minor importance in ensuring a supply of ATP, although it is important in muscle under conditions of maximum exertion (Section 5.4.1.2). Normally, almost all the phosphorylation of ADP to ATP occurs in the mitochondria by the process of oxidative phosphorylation.

3.3.1 Oxidative phosphorylation: the phosphorylation of ADP to ATP linked to the oxidation of metabolic fuels

With the exception of glycolysis (Section 5.4.1), which is a cytosolic pathway, most reactions in the oxidation of metabolic fuels occur inside the mitochondria and lead to the reduction of nicotinamide nucleotide and flavin coenzymes (Section 2.4.1). The reduced coenzymes are then reoxidized, ultimately leading to the reduction of oxygen to water. Within the crista membrane of the mitochondrion, there is a series of coenzymes that undergo reduction and oxidation (Section 3.3.1.2). The first coenzyme in the chain is reduced by reaction with NADH and is then reoxidized by reducing the next coenzyme. In turn, each coenzyme in the chain is reduced by the preceding coenzyme and then reoxidized by reducing the next one. The final step is the oxidation of a reduced coenzyme by oxygen, resulting in the formation of water.

Experimentally, mitochondrial metabolism is measured using the oxygen electrode, in which the percentage saturation of the buffer with oxygen is measured electrochemically as the mitochondria oxidize substrates and reduce oxygen to water.

Figure 3.15 shows the oxygen electrode traces for mitochondria incubated with varying amounts of ADP and a superabundant amount of malate. As more ADP is provided, oxidation of the substrate increases and hence consumption of oxygen is more. This illustrates the tight coupling between the oxidation of metabolic fuels and the availability of ADP (Figure 3.2).

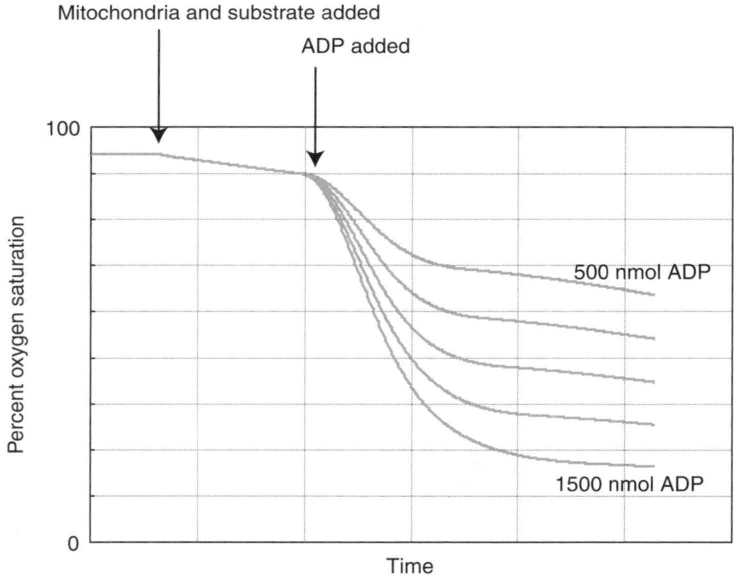

Figure 3.15 Oxygen consumption by mitochondria incubated with malate and varying amounts of ADP.

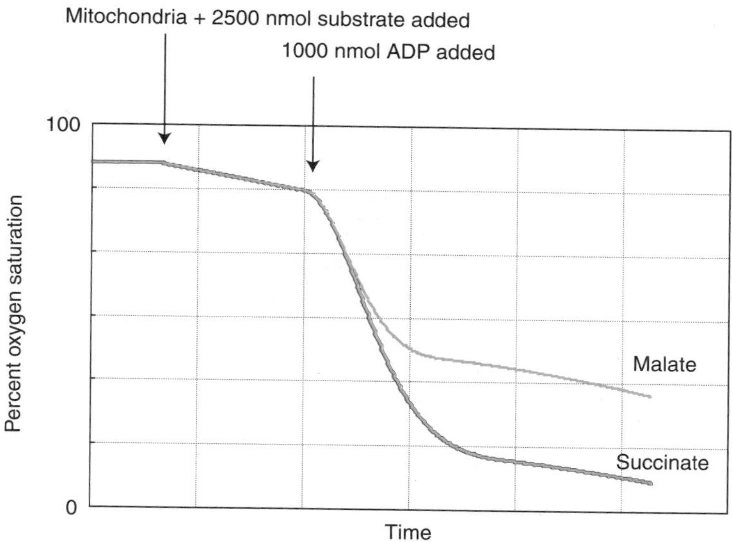

Figure 3.16 Oxygen consumption by mitochondria incubated with malate or succinate and a constant amount of ADP.

Figure 3.16 shows the oxygen electrode traces for incubation of mitochondria with a limiting amount of ADP and:

(a) malate, which reduces NAD^+ to NADH;
(b) succinate, which reduces a flavin coenzyme, then ubiquinone.

The stepwise oxidation of NADH and reduction of oxygen to water is obligatorily linked to the phosphorylation of ADP to ATP. Approximately 2.5 mol of ATP is formed for each mole of NADH that is oxidized. Flavoproteins reduce ubiquinone, which is an intermediate coenzyme in the chain, and approximately 1.5 mol of ADP are phosphorylated to ATP for each mole of reduced flavoprotein that is oxidized.

This means that 1.5 mol of ADP are required for the oxidation of a substrate such as succinate, but 2.5 mol of ADP are required for the oxidation of malate. Therefore, the oxidation of succinate will consume more oxygen when ADP is limiting than does the oxidation of malate. This is usually expressed as the ratio of phosphate to oxygen consumed in the reaction; the P:O ratio is approximately 2.5 for malate and 1.5 for succinate, respectively.

3.3.1.1 The mitochondrion

Mitochondria are intracellular organelles with a double-membrane structure. Both the number and the size of mitochondria vary in different cells; for example, a liver cell contains some 800 mitochondria, a renal tubule cell some 300, and a sperm about 20. The outer mitochondrial membrane is permeable to a great many substrates, while the inner membrane provides a barrier to regulate the uptake of substrates and output of products (e.g., the regulation of palmitoyl CoA uptake into the mitochondrion for oxidation; Section 5.5.1).

The inner mitochondrial membrane forms the cristae, which are paddle-shaped double-membrane structures that protrude from the inner membrane into the matrix (Figure 3.17). The crista membrane is continuous with the inner mitochondrial

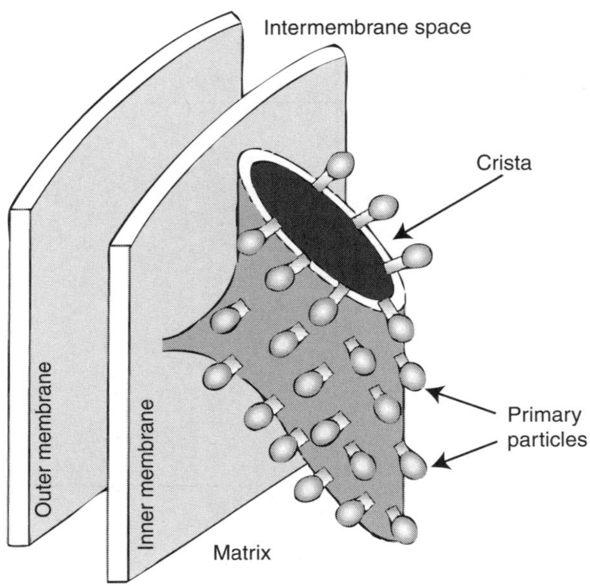

Figure 3.17 The structure of the mitochondrial cristae.

membrane, and the internal space of the cristae is contiguous with the intermembrane space. However, there is only a relatively narrow stalk connecting the crista to the intermembrane space, so that the crista space is effectively separate from, albeit communicating with, the intermembrane space.

The five compartments of the mitochondrion have a range of specialized functions:

1. The outer membrane contains enzymes that are responsible for the desaturation and elongation of fatty acids synthesized in the cytosol (Section 5.6.1.1), enzymes for triacylglycerol synthesis from fatty acids (Section 5.6.1.2), and phospholipases that catalyze the hydrolysis of phospholipids (Section 4.3.1.2).
2. The intermembrane space contains enzymes involved in nucleotide metabolism, transamination of amino acids (Section 9.3.1.2), and a variety of kinases.
3. The inner membrane regulates the uptake of substrates into the matrix for oxidation. There is also a transport protein in the mitochondrial inner membrane that transports ADP into the matrix to undergo phosphorylation, only in exchange for ATP being transported out to the cytosol.
4. The membrane of the cristae contains the coenzymes associated with electron transport; the oxidation of reduced coenzymes, and the reduction of oxygen to water occur here (Section 3.3.1.2). The primary particles on the matrix surface of the cristae are ATP synthase, the enzyme that catalyzes the phosphorylation of ADP to ATP (Section 3.3.1.3).
5. The mitochondrial matrix contains enzymes concerned with the β-oxidation of fatty acids (Section 5.5.2), the citric acid cycle (Section 5.4.4), a variety of other oxidases and dehydrogenases, the enzymes for mitochondrial replication, and the DNA that codes for some of the mitochondrial proteins.

The overall process of oxidation of reduced coenzymes, reduction of oxygen to water, and phosphorylation of ADP to ATP requires intact mitochondria or intact sealed vesicles of mitochondrial inner membrane prepared by disruption of mitochondria; it will not occur with solubilized preparations from mitochondria or open fragments of mitochondrial inner membrane. Under normal conditions, these three processes are linked and none can occur in the absence of the others.

3.3.1.2 The mitochondrial electron transport chain

The mitochondrial electron transport chain is a series of enzymes and coenzymes in the crista membrane, each of which is reduced by the preceding coenzyme and in turn reduces the next, until finally the protons and electrons that have entered the chain from either NADH or reduced flavin reduce oxygen to water. The sequence of the electron carriers (Figure 3.18) has been determined in two ways:

- By considering their electrochemical redox potential, which permits determination of which carrier is likely to reduce another and which is likely to be reduced. There is a steady fall in redox potential between the enzyme that oxidizes NADH and that which reduces oxygen to water.
- By incubating mitochondria with substrates, in the absence of oxygen, when all the carriers become reduced, then introducing a limited amount of oxygen, and following the sequence in which the carriers become oxidized, shown by changes in their absorption spectra.

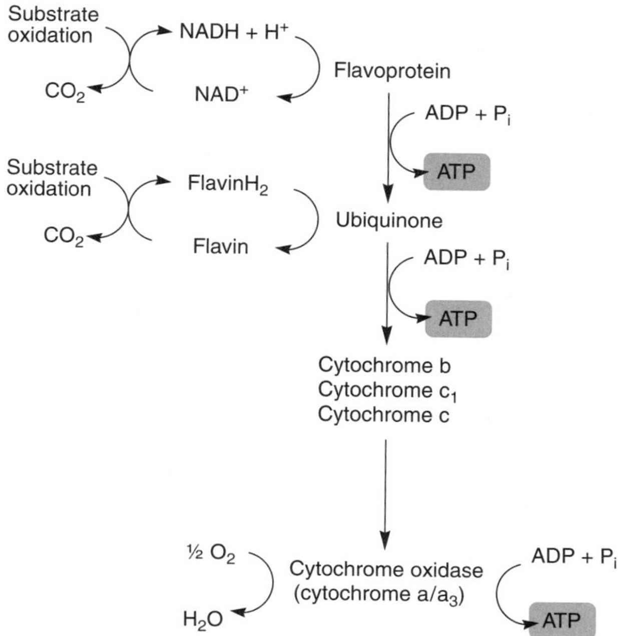

Figure 3.18 An overview of the mitochondrial electron transport chain.

Studies with inhibitors of specific electron carriers, and with artificial substrates that oxidize or reduce one specific carrier, permit dissection of the electron transport chain into four complexes of electron carriers.

- Complex I catalyzes the oxidation of NADH and the reduction of ubiquinone, and is associated with the phosphorylation of ADP to ATP.
- Complex II catalyzes the oxidation of reduced flavins and the reduction of ubiquinone. This complex is not associated with the phosphorylation of ADP to ATP.
- Complex III catalyzes the oxidation of reduced ubiquinone and the reduction of cytochrome c, and is associated with the phosphorylation of ADP to ATP.
- Complex IV catalyzes the oxidation of reduced cytochrome c and the reduction of oxygen to water, and is associated with the phosphorylation of ADP to ATP.

In order to understand how the transfer of electrons through the electron transport chain is linked to the phosphorylation of ADP to ATP, it is necessary to consider the chemistry of the various electron carriers. They can be classified into two groups, hydrogen carriers and electron carriers.

Hydrogen carriers (NAD, flavins, and ubiquinone) undergo reduction and oxidation reactions involving both protons and electrons. NAD undergoes a two-electron oxidation/reduction reaction (Figure 2.20), while the flavins (Figure 2.19) may undergo a two-electron or a two single-electron reaction to form a half-reduced radical and then the fully reduced coenzyme. Ubiquinone (Figure 3.19) undergoes only two single-electron reactions to form a half-reduced radical and then the fully reduced coenzyme.

Electron carriers (the cytochromes and nonheme iron proteins; Figure 3.20) contain iron (and in the case of cytochrome oxidase also copper); they undergo oxidation and reduction by electron transfer alone. In the cytochromes, the iron is present in a heme molecule while in the nonheme iron proteins the iron is bound to the protein through the sulfur of the amino acid cysteine—these are sometimes called iron–sulfur proteins.

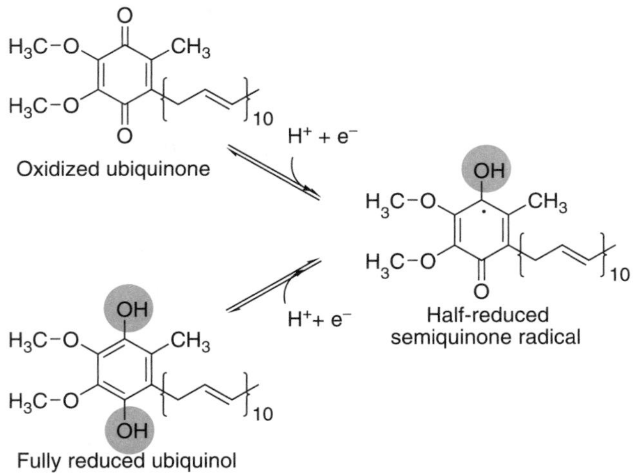

Figure 3.19 Oxidation and reduction of ubiquinone (coenzyme Q).

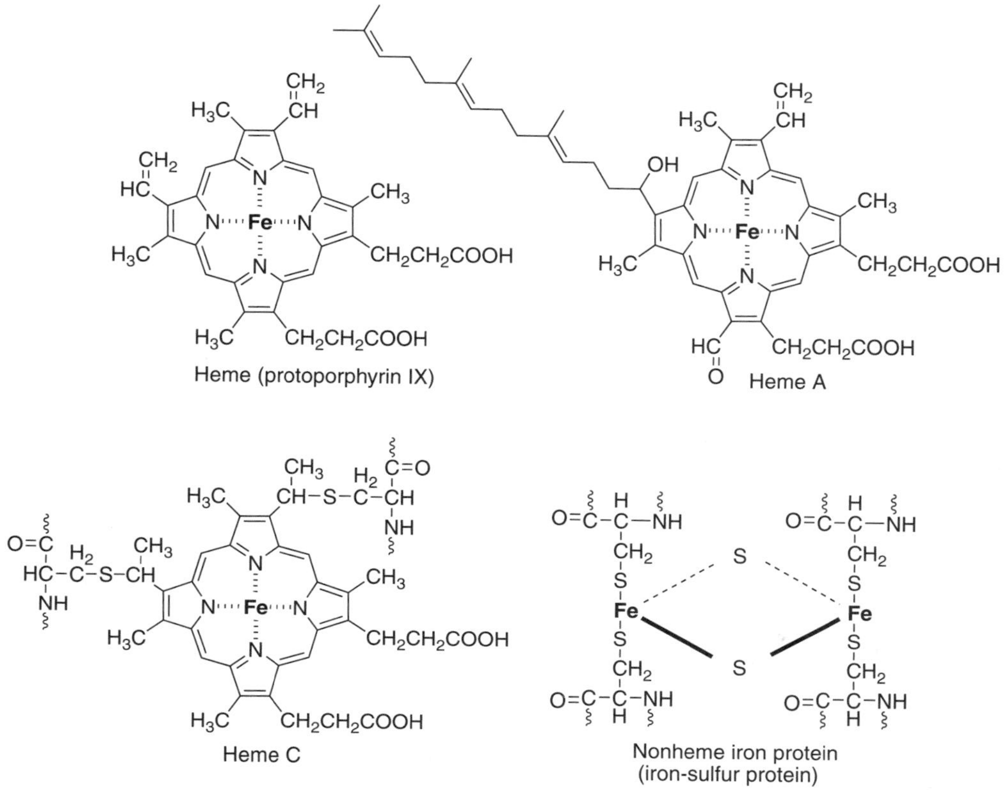

Figure 3.20 Iron-containing carriers of the electron transport chain: heme and nonheme iron proteins.

Three different types of heme occur in cytochromes:

- Heme (protoporphyrin IX) is tightly but noncovalently bound to proteins, including cytochromes b and b_1, as well as enzymes such as catalase, and the oxygen transport proteins hemoglobin and myoglobin.
- Heme C is covalently bound to protein in cytochromes c and c_1.
- Heme A is anchored in the membrane by its hydrophobic side chain in cytochromes a and a_3 (which together form cytochrome oxidase).

The hydrogen and electron carriers of the electron transport chain are arranged in sequence in the crista membrane (Figure 3.21). Some carriers are located entirely within the membrane, while others are at the inner or outer surface of the membrane.

There are two steps in which a hydrogen carrier reduces an electron carrier: the reaction between the flavin and nonheme iron protein in complex I, and the reaction between ubiquinol and cytochrome b plus a nonheme iron protein in complex II. The reaction between nonheme iron protein and ubiquinone in complex I is the reverse—a hydrogen carrier is reduced by an electron carrier.

When a hydrogen carrier reduces an electron carrier, there is a proton that is not transferred onto the electron carrier, but is extruded from the membrane into the crista space (Figure 3.22). When an electron carrier reduces a hydrogen carrier, there is a need

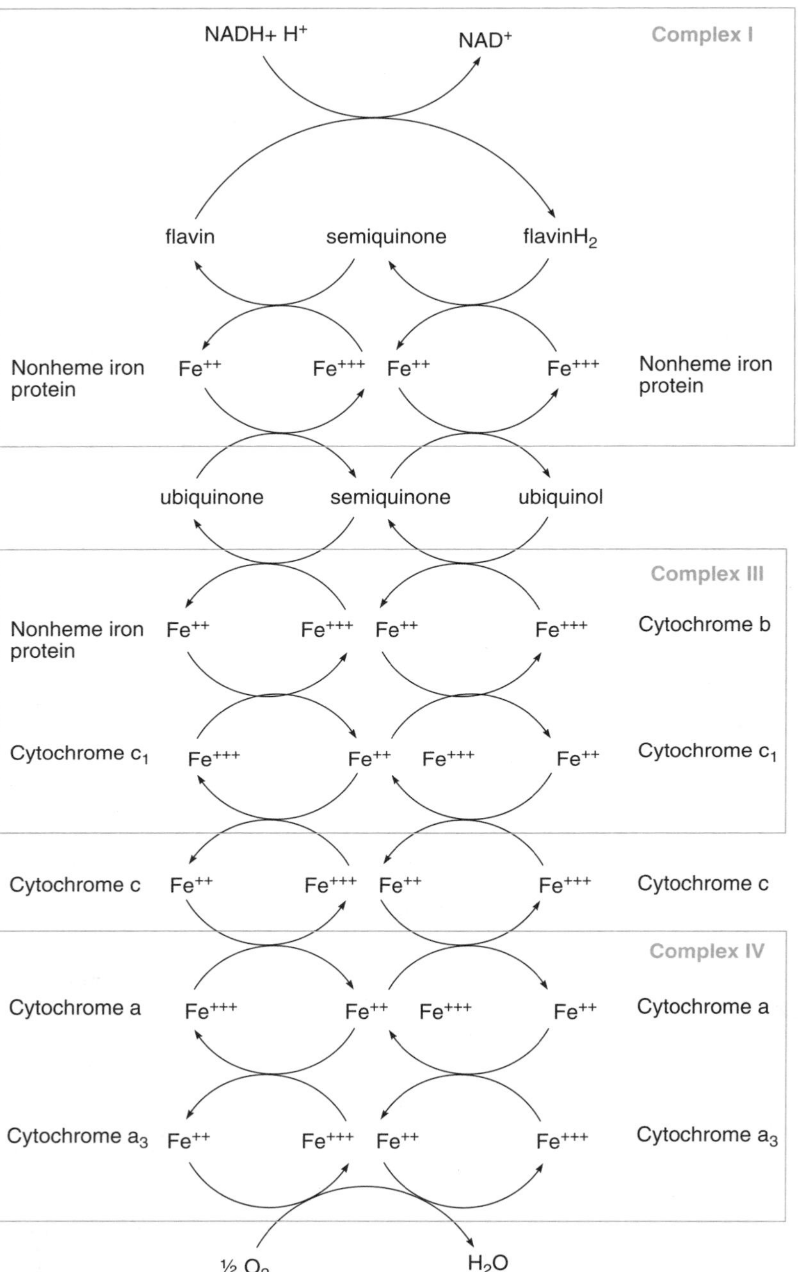

Figure 3.21 Complexes of the mitochondrial electron transport chain.

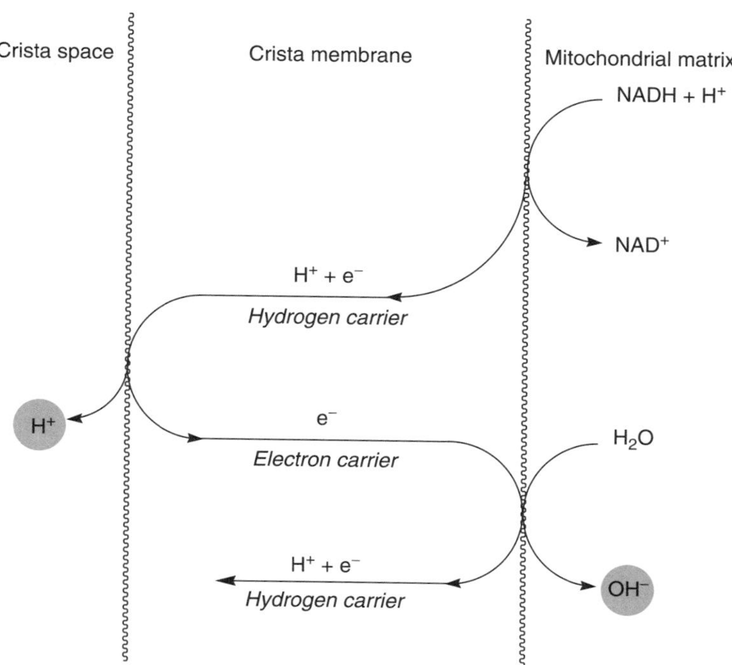

Figure 3.22 Hydrogen and electron carriers in the mitochondrial electron transport chain—generation of a transmembrane proton gradient.

for a proton to accompany the electron that is transferred. This is acquired from the mitochondrial matrix, thus shifting the equilibrium between $H_2O \rightleftharpoons H^+ + OH^-$, resulting in an accumulation of hydroxyl ions in the matrix.

3.3.1.3 Phosphorylation of ADP linked to electron transport

The result of electron transport through the electron transport chain and the alternation between hydrogen carriers and electron carriers is a separation of protons and hydroxyl ions across the crista membrane, with an accumulation of protons in the crista space and an accumulation of hydroxyl ions in the matrix, i.e., creation of a pH gradient across the inner membrane. Overall, approximately ten protons are expelled into the intermembrane space when NADH is oxidized and seven when reduced flavin is oxidized. These protons reenter the mitochondrial matrix through a proton transport pore that forms the stalk of ATP synthase (Figure 3.23), and the proton gradient provides the driving force for the highly endothermic phosphorylation of ADP to ATP (Figure 3.24).

ATP synthase acts as a molecular motor, driven by the flow of protons down the concentration gradient from the crista space into the matrix, through the transmembrane stalk of the primary particle. As protons flow through the stalk, they cause rotation of the core of the multienzyme complex that makes up ATP synthase.

There are three equivalent catalytic sites in ATP synthase, and each one-third turn of the central core causes a conformational change at each active site (Figure 3.25). At one site the conformational change permits binding of ADP and phosphate, while at the next site the conformational change brings ADP and phosphate close enough to undergo condensation

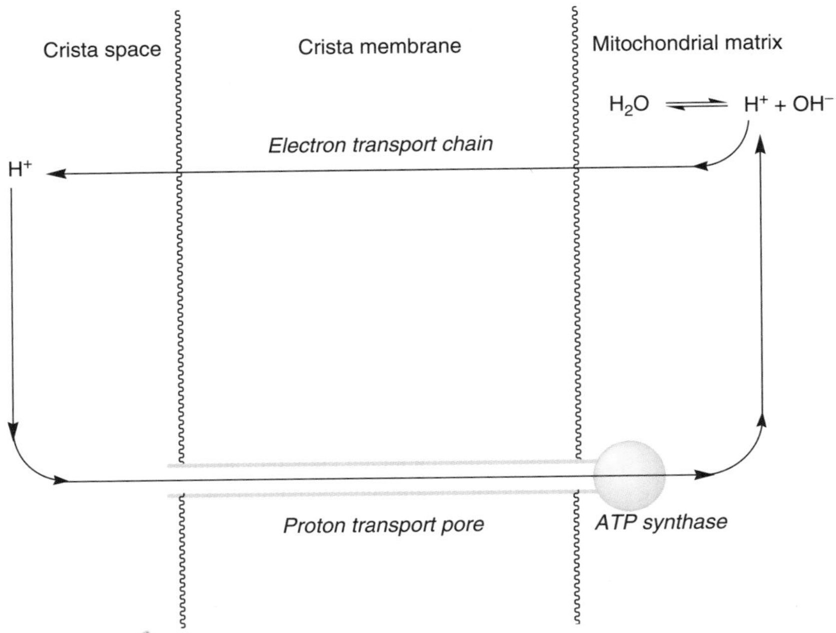

Figure 3.23 The reentry of protons into the mitochondrial matrix through the stalk of ATP synthase.

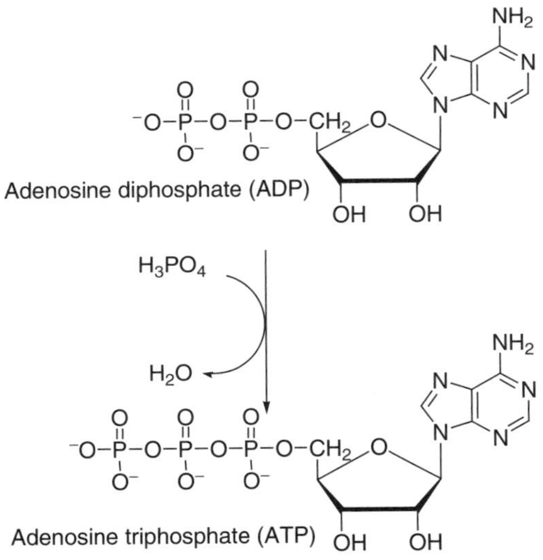

Adenosine diphosphate (ADP)

H_3PO_4

H_2O

Adenosine triphosphate (ATP)

Figure 3.24 Condensation of ADP + phosphate → ATP.

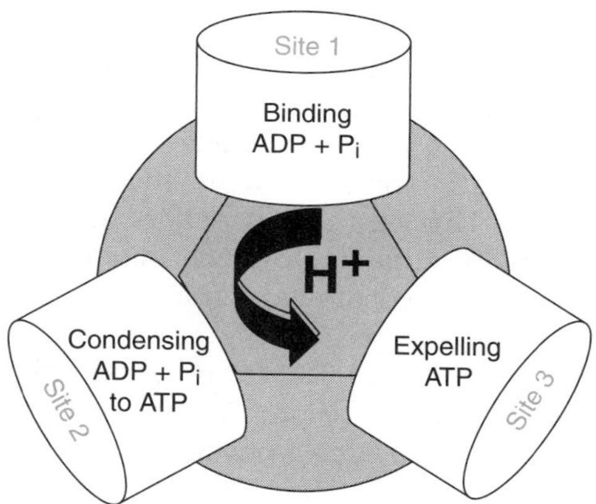

Figure 3.25 Mitochondrial ATP synthase—a molecular motor. As the central core rotates, each site in turn undergoes a conformational change, site 1 becoming equivalent to 2, 2 to 3, and 3 to 1.

and expel water. At the third site, the conformational change causes expulsion of ATP from the site, leaving it free to accept ADP and phosphate at the next turn.

At any time, one site is binding ADP and phosphate, one is undergoing condensation, and the third is expelling ATP. If ADP is not available to bind at the empty site, then rotation cannot occur, and if rotation cannot occur, then protons cannot flow through the stalk from the crista space into the matrix.

3.3.1.4 Coupling of electron transport, oxidative phosphorylation, and fuel oxidation

The processes of oxidation of reduced coenzymes and phosphorylation of ADP to ATP are normally tightly coupled:

- ADP phosphorylation cannot occur unless there is a proton gradient across the crista membrane, resulting from the oxidation of NADH or reduced flavins.
- If there is no ADP available, the oxidation of NADH and reduced flavins cannot occur, because the protons cannot reenter through the stalk of ATP synthase, and so the proton gradient becomes large enough to inhibit further transport of protons into the crista space. Indeed, experimentally it is possible to force reverse electron transport and reduction of NAD^+ and flavins by creating a proton gradient across the crista membrane.

Metabolic fuels can only be oxidized when NAD^+ and oxidized flavoproteins are available. Therefore, if there is little or no ADP available in the mitochondria (i.e., it has all been phosphorylated to ATP), there will be an accumulation of reduced coenzymes and hence a slowing of the rate of oxidation of metabolic fuels. This means that substrates are only oxidized when ADP is available and there is a need for the formation of ATP. The availability of ADP is dependent on the utilization of ATP in performing physical and chemical work (Figure 3.2). The rate of oxidation of metabolic fuels, and hence utilization of oxygen, is controlled by energy expenditure in physical and chemical work.

3.3.1.5 Uncouplers

It is possible to uncouple electron transport and ADP phosphorylation by adding a weak acid such as dinitrophenol that transports protons across the crista membrane. In the presence of such an uncoupler, the protons expelled during electron transport do not accumulate in the crista space, but are transported into the mitochondrial matrix, bypassing the ATP synthase (Figure 3.26). This means that ADP is not phosphorylated to ATP, and the oxidation of NADH and reduced flavins can continue unimpeded until all the available oxygen (or substrate) has been consumed. Figure 3.27 shows the oxygen electrode trace in the presence of an uncoupler.

The result of uncoupling electron transport from the phosphorylation of ADP is that a great deal of substrate is oxidized, with little production of ATP, although heat is produced. A moderate degree of uncoupling provides a physiological mechanism for nonshivering thermogenesis (heat production to maintain body temperature without performing physical work) by activating uncoupling proteins in mitochondria.

The first such uncoupling protein to be identified was in brown adipose tissue and was called thermogenin because of its role in thermogenesis. Brown adipose tissue is anatomically and functionally distinct from the white adipose tissue that is the main site of fat storage in the body. It has a red-brown color because of the large number of mitochondria that it contains. Brown adipose tissue is especially important in the maintenance of body temperature in infants, but it remains active in adults, although its importance compared with uncoupling proteins in muscle and other tissues is unclear.

In addition to the maintenance of body temperature, uncoupling proteins are important in overall energy balance and maintenance of body weight. One of the actions of the hormone leptin secreted by white adipose tissue (Section 1.3.2) is to increase the expression

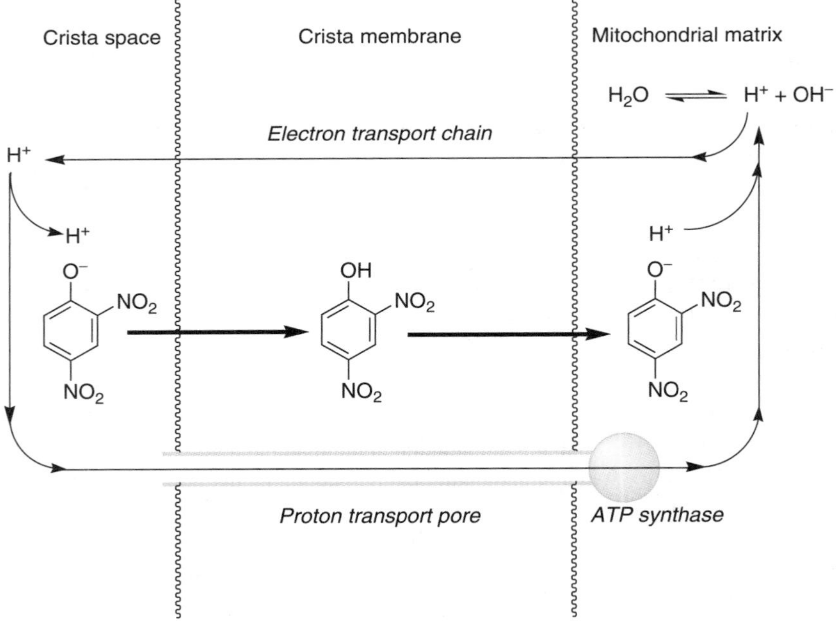

Figure 3.26 Uncoupling of electron transport and oxidative phosphorylation by a weak acid such as 2,4-dinitrophenol.

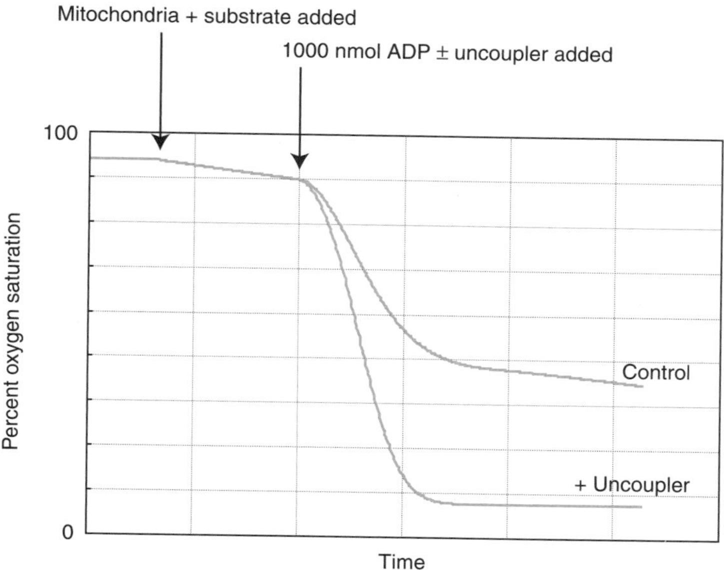

Figure 3.27 Oxygen consumption by mitochondria incubated with malate and ADP, with and without an uncoupler.

of uncoupling proteins in muscle and adipose tissue, thereby increasing energy expenditure and the utilization of adipose tissue fat reserves.

3.3.1.6 *Respiratory poisons*

Much of our knowledge of the processes involved in electron transport and oxidative phosphorylation has come from studies using inhibitors. Figure 3.28 shows the oxygen electrode traces from mitochondria incubated with malate and an inhibitor of electron transport, with or without the addition of dinitrophenol as an uncoupler. Inhibitors of electron transport include:

(a) Rotenone, the active ingredient of derris powder, an insecticide prepared from the roots of the leguminous plant *Lonchocarpus nicou*. It is an inhibitor of complex I (NADH → ubiquinone reduction). The same effect is seen in the presence of amytal (amobarbital), a barbiturate sedative drug, which again inhibits complex I. These two compounds inhibit oxidation of malate, which requires complex I, but not succinate, which reduces ubiquinone directly. The addition of the uncoupler has no effect on malate oxidation in the presence of these two inhibitors of electron transport, but leads to uncontrolled oxidation of succinate.

(b) Antimycin A, an antibiotic produced by *Streptomyces* spp., which is used as a fungicide against fungi that are parasitic on rice. It inhibits complex III (ubiquinone → cytochrome c reduction), and so inhibits the oxidation of both malate and succinate, because both require complex III and the addition of the uncoupler has no effect.

(c) Cyanide, azide, and carbon monoxide, all of which bind irreversibly to the iron of cytochrome a_3 and thus inhibit complex IV. Again, these compounds inhibit oxidation of malate and succinate, since both rely on cytochrome oxidase, and again the addition of the uncoupler has no effect.

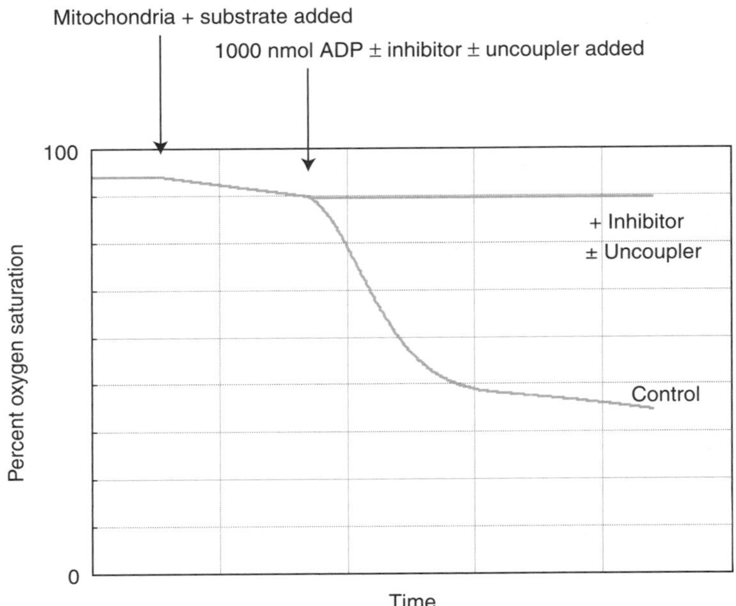

Figure 3.28 Oxygen consumption by mitochondria incubated with malate and ADP, plus an inhibitor of electron transport, with and without an uncoupler.

Figure 3.29 shows the oxygen electrode traces from mitochondria incubated with malate and an inhibitor of ATP synthesis, with or without the addition of dinitrophenol as an uncoupler. Oligomycin is a toxic, and therefore a clinically useless, antibiotic produced by *Streptomyces* spp.; it inhibits the transport of protons across the stalk of ATP synthase. This results in inhibition of oxidation of both malate and succinate, since if the protons cannot be transported back into the matrix, they will accumulate and inhibit further electron transport. In this case, addition of the uncoupler permits reentry of protons across the crista membrane, and hence uncontrolled oxidation of substrates.

Two further compounds also inhibit ATP synthesis, not by inhibiting the ATP synthase, but by inhibiting the transport of ADP into, and ATP out of, the mitochondria:

- Atractyloside is a toxic glycoside from the rhizomes of the Mediterranean thistle *Atractylis gummifera*; it competes with ADP for binding to the carrier protein at the outer face of the membrane and so prevents the entry of ADP into the matrix.
- Bongkrekic acid is a toxic antibiotic formed by *Pseudomonas cocovenenans* growing on coconut; it is named after bongkrek, an Indonesian mold-fermented coconut product that becomes highly toxic when *Pseudomonas* outgrows the mold. It fixes the carrier protein at the inner face of the membrane, so that ATP cannot be transported out nor ADP in.

Both compounds thus inhibit ATP synthesis and therefore the oxidation of substrates. However, as with oligomycin (Figure 3.29), addition of an uncoupler permits rapid and complete utilization of oxygen, since electron transport can now continue uncontrolled by the availability of ADP.

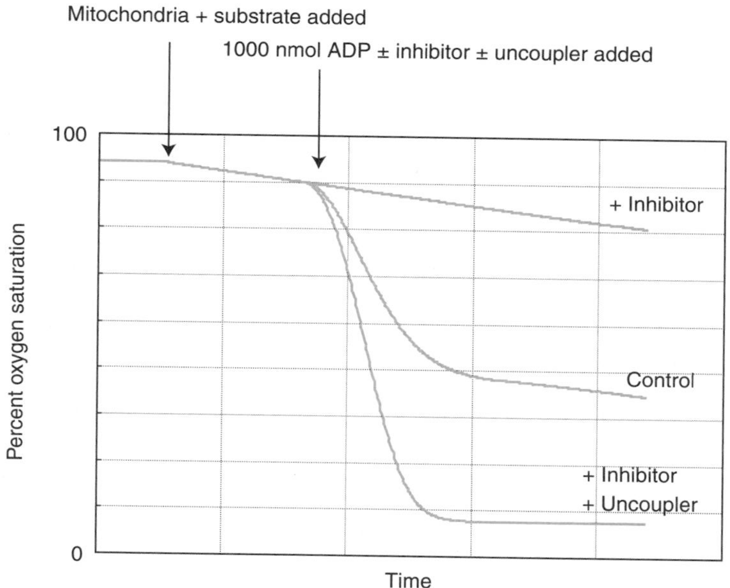

Figure 3.29 Oxygen consumption by mitochondria incubated with malate and ADP, plus an inhibitor of ATP synthesis such as oligomycin, with and without an uncoupler.

Key points

- Endothermic reactions are coupled to the (exothermic) hydrolysis of ATP → ADP + phosphate. This may involve intermediate phosphorylation of the enzyme or substrate, or, in some cases, adenylation of the substrate.
- Compounds that enter cells by passive or carrier-mediated diffusion may be accumulated to a higher concentration than in the extracellular fluid by binding to proteins or by phosphorylation at the expense of ATP (metabolic trapping).
- Active transport is the accumulation of a substance against a concentration gradient, linked to the utilization of ATP in one of three ways:
  - The carrier may be phosphorylated, leading to a conformational change.
  - The carrier may bind and hydrolyze ATP, again leading to a conformational change.
  - ATPase action in a membrane leads to formation of a proton gradient; protons reenter the cell in exchange for Na^+ ions, which then reenter the cell together with, or in exchange for, substrates and metabolites.
- Muscle contraction involves conformational changes in myosin due to the displacement of ADP by ATP, hydrolysis of ATP → ADP + phosphate, and expulsion of phosphate from the active site of the protein.
- A relatively small amount of ATP is formed by substrate-level phosphorylation of ADP; most is formed in the mitochondria, linked to electron transport and the oxidation of reduced coenzymes and reduction of oxygen to water.
- The oxidation of NADH yields approximately 2.5 mol of ATP and that of reduced flavins 1.5.

- Transfer of electrons along the electron transport chain from reduced coenzymes to oxygen results in the pumping of protons across the crista membrane and formation of a pH gradient across the membrane.
- Protons reenter the mitochondrial matrix through a proton transport pore that forms the stalk of ATP synthase. This causes rotation of the central core of the enzyme and provides the driving force for the synthesis of ATP from ADP and phosphate.
- Electron transport and ATP synthesis are tightly coupled, so that the oxidation of metabolic fuels and utilization of oxygen are controlled by the availability of ADP, and hence by the utilization of ATP in physical and chemical work.
- Uncouplers permit uncontrolled oxidation of substrates (and hence generation of heat) by providing an alternative route for protons to reenter the mitochondrial matrix, bypassing ATP synthase.

Problem 3.1: Dinitrophenol as a slimming agent

Dinitrophenol was at one time used as a slimming agent. Explain how it acted and describe what you would expect to observe in a person who had consumed a modest (nontoxic) amount of dinitrophenol.

Problem 3.2: ATP in working muscle

Table 3.1 shows the concentrations of ATP, ADP, creatine phosphate, and creatine in rat gastrocnemius muscle (1) at rest, and (2) after electrical stimulation (causing contraction) for 3 min. What conclusions can you draw from these results?

Table 3.1 ATP, ADP, and Creatine Phosphate in Muscle

	At Rest µmol/g Muscle	After Stimulation µmol/g Muscle
ATP	5.0	4.9
ADP	0.01	0.11
Creatine phosphate	17.0	1.0
Creatine	0.1	16.1

chapter four

Digestion and absorption

The major components of the diet are starches, sugars, fats, and proteins. These have to be hydrolyzed to their constituent smaller molecules for absorption and metabolism. Starches and sugars are absorbed as monosaccharides, fats as free fatty acids and glycerol (plus a small amount of intact triacylglycerol), and proteins as their constituent amino acids and small peptides.

The fat-soluble vitamins (A, D, E, and K) are absorbed dissolved in dietary lipids; there are active transport systems (Section 3.2.2) in the small intestinal mucosa for the absorption of the water-soluble vitamins. The absorption of vitamin B_{12} (Section 4.5.2.1) requires a specific binding protein that is secreted in the gastric juice in order to bind to the mucosal transport system.

Minerals generally enter the intestinal mucosal cells by carrier-mediated diffusion and are accumulated intracellularly by binding to specific binding proteins (Section 3.2.2.1). They are then transferred into the bloodstream by active transport mechanisms (P-type transport proteins; Section 3.2.2.4) at the serosal side of the epithelial cells, usually onto plasma-binding proteins.

Objectives

After reading this chapter you should be able to

- Describe the major functions of each region of the gastrointestinal tract
- Describe and explain the classification of carbohydrates according to their chemical and nutritional properties; explain what is meant by glycemic index
- Describe and explain the digestion and absorption of carbohydrates
- Describe and explain the classification of dietary lipids and the different types of fatty acid
- Describe and explain the digestion and absorption of lipids, the role of bile salts, and the formation of lipid micelles and chylomicrons
- Describe and explain the classification of amino acids according to their chemical and nutritional properties
- Describe the levels of protein structure and explain what is meant by denaturation;
- Describe and explain the digestion and absorption of proteins
- Describe the absorption of vitamins and minerals, especially vitamin B_{12}, iron, and calcium

4.1 The gastrointestinal tract

The gastrointestinal tract is shown in Figure 4.1. The major functions of each region are:
Mouth:

- Hydrolysis of a small amount of starch catalyzed by amylase, secreted by the salivary glands

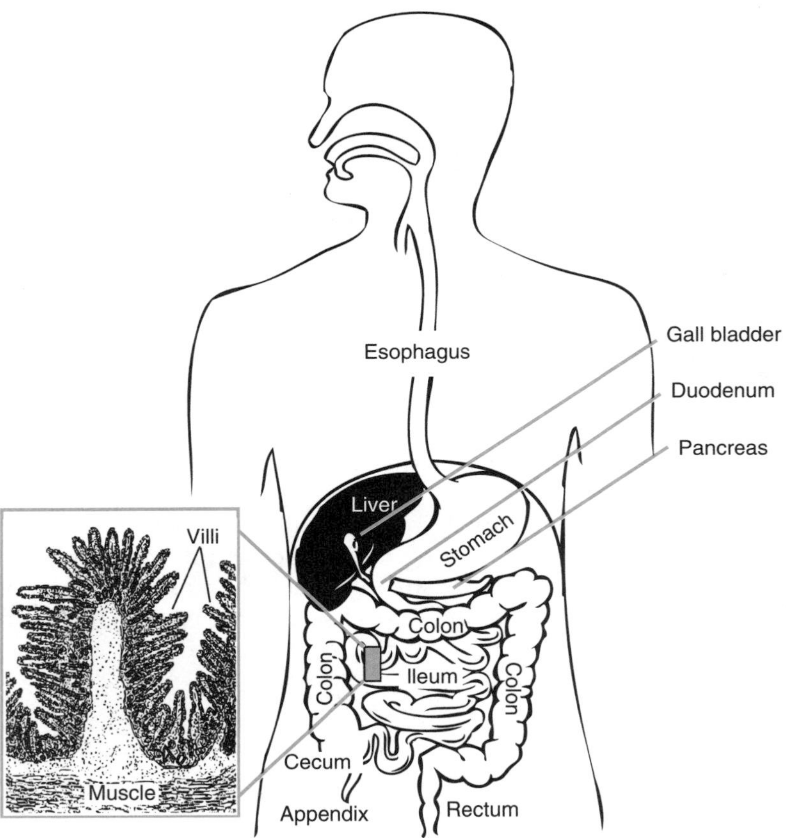

Figure 4.1 The gastrointestinal tract.

- Hydrolysis of a small amount of fat, catalyzed by lingual lipase, secreted by the tongue
- Absorption of small amounts of vitamin C and a variety of nonnutrients (including nicotine)

Stomach:

- Denaturation of dietary proteins (Section 4.4.2.3) and the release of vitamin B_{12}, iron, and other minerals from protein binding, for which gastric acid is important
- Hydrolysis of protein catalyzed by pepsin
- Hydrolysis of fat catalyzed by lipase
- Secretion of intrinsic factor for the absorption of vitamin B_{12}

Small intestine (duodenum, jejunum, and ileum):

- Hydrolysis of starch catalyzed by amylase secreted by the pancreas
- Hydrolysis of disaccharides within the brush border of the intestinal mucosa
- Hydrolysis of fat catalyzed by lipase, phospholipase, and esterase secreted by the pancreas

- Hydrolysis of protein catalyzed by a variety of exo- and endopeptidases (Section 4.4.3) secreted by the pancreas and small-intestinal mucosa
- Hydrolysis of di- and tripeptides within the brush border of the intestinal mucosa
- Absorption of the products of digestion
- Absorption of water (failure of water absorption, as in diarrhea, can lead to serious dehydration)

Large intestine (cecum and colon):

- Bacterial metabolism of undigested carbohydrates, proteins, and shed intestinal mucosal cells
- Absorption of some of the products of bacterial metabolism
- Absorption of water

Rectum:

- Storage of undigested gut contents prior to evacuation as feces

Throughout the gastrointestinal tract, and especially in the small intestine, the surface area of the mucosa is considerably greater than would appear from its superficial appearance. As shown in the inset in Figure 4.1, the intestinal mucosa is folded into the lumen. The surface of these folds is covered with villi, fingerlike projections into the lumen, some 0.5–1.5 mm long. There are some 20–40 villi/mm^2, giving a total absorptive surface area of some 300 m^2 in the small intestine.

Each villus has both blood capillaries, which drain into the hepatic portal vein, and a lacteal, which drains into the lymphatic system (Figure 4.2). Water-soluble products of digestion (carbohydrates and amino acids) are absorbed into the blood capillaries, and the

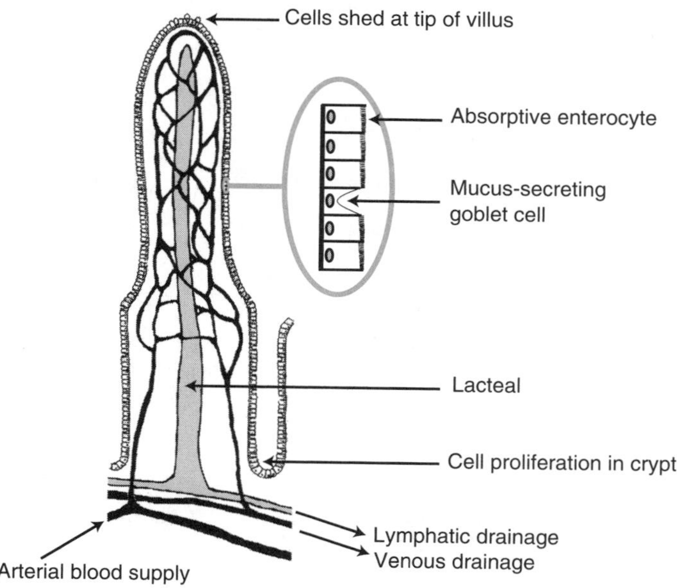

Figure 4.2 An intestinal villus.

liver has a major role in controlling the availability of the products of carbohydrate and protein digestion to other tissues in the body. Lipids are absorbed into the lacteals; the lymphatic system joins the bloodstream at the thoracic duct; and extrahepatic tissues are exposed to the products of lipid digestion uncontrolled by the liver, which functions to clear the remnants from the circulation.

There is rapid turnover of the cells of the intestinal mucosa; epithelial cells proliferate in the crypts, alongside the cells that secrete digestive enzymes and mucus, and migrate to the tip of the villus, where they are shed into the lumen. The average life of an intestinal mucosal epithelial cell is about 48 h. This rapid turnover of epithelial cells is important in controlling the absorption of iron and possibly other minerals (Section 4.5.3.1).

The rapid turnover of intestinal mucosal cells is also important for protection against the digestive enzymes secreted into the lumen. Further protection is afforded by the secretion of mucus, a solution of mucin and other proteins that are resistant to enzymic hydrolysis, which coats the intestinal mucosa. The secretion of intestinal mucus explains a considerable part of an adult's continuing requirement for dietary protein (Section 9.1.2).

4.2 Digestion and absorption of carbohydrates

Carbohydrates are compounds of carbon, hydrogen, and oxygen in the ratio C_n:H_{2n}:O_n. The basic unit of the carbohydrates is the sugar molecule or monosaccharide. Note that sugar is used here in a chemical sense and includes a variety of simple carbohydrates, which are collectively known as sugars. Ordinary table sugar (cane sugar or beet sugar) is correctly known as sucrose—it is a disaccharide (Section 4.2.1.3). It is only one of a number of different sugars found in the diet.

4.2.1 The classification of carbohydrates

Dietary carbohydrates can be considered in two main groups: sugars and polysaccharides; the polysaccharides can be further subdivided into starches and nonstarch polysaccharides (Figure 4.3).

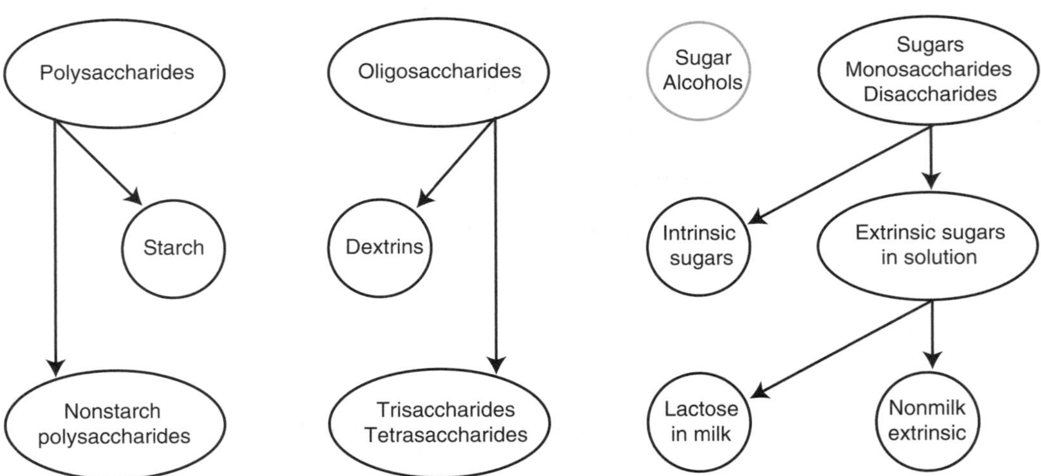

Figure 4.3 Nutritional classification of carbohydrates.

The simplest type of sugar is a monosaccharide—a single sugar unit (Section 4.2.1.1). Monosaccharides consist of between three and seven carbon atoms (and the corresponding number of hydrogen and oxygen atoms). A few larger monosaccharides also occur, although they are not important in nutrition and metabolism.

Disaccharides (Section 4.2.1.3) are formed by condensation between two monosaccharides to form a glycoside bond. The reverse reaction, cleavage of the glycoside bond to release the individual monosaccharides, is a hydrolysis.

Oligosaccharides consist of three or four monosaccharide units (trisaccharides and tetrasaccharides), and occasionally more, linked by glycoside bonds. Most are not digested, but are fermented by intestinal bacteria, yielding short-chain fatty acids that provide a metabolic fuel to intestinal mucosal cells, and may be protective against colorectal cancer (Section 6.3.3.2). The oligosaccharides also make a significant contribution to the production of intestinal gas.

Nutritionally, it is useful to consider sugars (both monosaccharides and disaccharides) in two groups:

- Intrinsic sugars that are contained within plant cell walls in foods.
- Sugars that are in free solution in foods, and therefore provide a substrate for oral bacteria, leading to the formation of dental plaque and caries. These are known as extrinsic sugars; it is considered desirable to reduce the consumption of extrinsic sugars (Section 6.3.3.1), both because of their role in dental decay and also because of the ease with which excessive amounts of sweet foods can be consumed, thus leading to obesity (Chapter 7).

A complication in the classification of sugars as intrinsic (which are considered desirable in the diet) and extrinsic (which are considered undesirable in the diet) is that lactose (Section 4.2.1.3) is in free solution in milk, and hence is an extrinsic sugar. However, lactose is not a cause of dental decay, and milk is an important source of calcium (Section 11.15.1), protein (Chapter 9), and vitamin B_2 (Section 11.7). It is not considered desirable to reduce intakes of milk, which is the only significant source of lactose, and extrinsic sugars are further subdivided into milk sugar and nonmilk extrinsic sugars.

Polysaccharides are polymers of many hundreds of monosaccharide units, again linked by glycoside bonds. The most important are starch and glycogen (Section 4.2.1.5), both of which are polymers of glucose. There are a number of other polysaccharides, composed of other monosaccharides, or of glucose units linked differently from the linkages in starch and glycogen. Collectively these are known as nonstarch polysaccharides. They are generally not digested but have important roles in nutrition (Section 4.2.1.6).

4.2.1.1 Monosaccharides

The classes of monosaccharides are named by the number of carbon atoms in the ring, using the Greek names for the numbers, with the ending "-ose" to show that they are sugars. The names of all sugars end in "-ose" are provided.

- Three-carbon monosaccharides are trioses.
- Four-carbon monosaccharides are tetroses.
- Five-carbon monosaccharides are pentoses.
- Six-carbon monosaccharides are hexoses.
- Seven-carbon monosaccharides are heptoses.

In general, trioses, tetroses, and heptoses are important as intermediate compounds in the metabolism of pentoses and hexoses. Hexoses are the nutritionally important sugars.

The pentoses and hexoses can exist as either straight-chain compounds or can form heterocyclic rings (Figure 4.4). By convention, the ring of sugars is drawn with the bonds of one side thicker than the other. This is to show that the rings are planar and can be considered to lie at right angles to the plane of the paper. The boldly drawn part of the molecule comes forward out of the paper, and the lightly drawn part goes behind the paper. The hydroxyl groups lie above or below the plane of the ring in the plane of the paper. Each carbon has a hydrogen atom attached as well as a hydroxyl group; this is generally omitted when the structures are drawn as rings.

The nutritionally important hexoses are glucose, galactose, and fructose. Glucose and galactose differ from each other only in the arrangement of one hydroxyl group above or below the plane of the ring. Fructose differs from glucose and galactose in that it has a C=O (keto) group at carbon 2, while the other two have an H–C=O (aldehyde) group at carbon 1.

There are two important pentose sugars, ribose and deoxyribose. Deoxyribose is unusual, in that it has lost one of its hydroxyl groups. The main role of ribose and deoxyribose is in the nucleotides (Figure 3.1) and the nucleic acids—ribonucleic acid (RNA)—in which the sugar is ribose (Section 9.2.2), and DNA, in which the sugar is deoxyribose

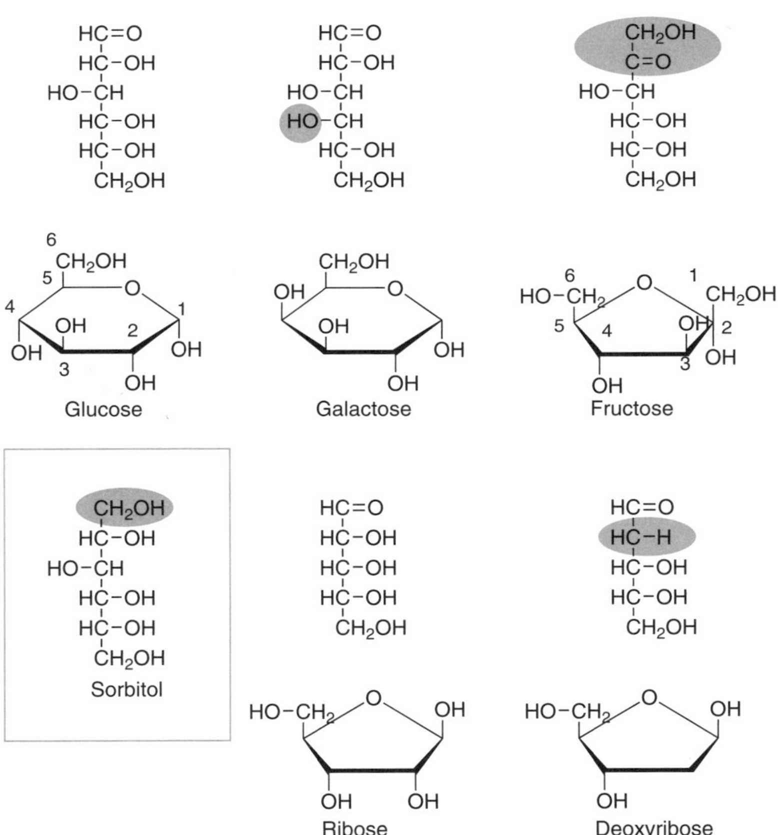

Figure 4.4 The nutritionally important monosaccharides.

(Section 9.2.1). Although pentoses do occur in the diet, they are also readily synthesized from glucose (Section 5.4.2).

4.2.1.2 Sugar alcohols

Sugar alcohols (or polyols) are formed by the reduction of the aldehyde group of a monosaccharide to a hydroxyl (–OH) group. Quantitatively, the most important is sorbitol, formed by the reduction of glucose. It is poorly absorbed from the intestinal tract, so that it has very much less effect on blood glucose than other carbohydrates. Because of this, it is widely used in preparation of foods suitable for use by diabetics, since it tastes sweet, and can replace sucrose and other sugars in food manufacture. However, it is metabolized as a metabolic fuel, although because of its poor absorption, it has an energy yield approximately half that of glucose, so that it is not suitable for the replacement of sugar in weight-reducing diets.

Sugar alcohols are poor substrates for metabolism by the plaque-forming bacteria that are associated with dental caries and are used in the manufacture of "tooth-friendly" sweets and chewing gum. There is some evidence that xylitol, the sugar alcohol formed by reduction of the 5-carbon sugar xylose (an isomer of ribose), may have a positive effect in preventing dental caries.

4.2.1.3 Disaccharides

The major dietary disaccharides (Figure 4.5) are the following:

- Sucrose, cane or beet sugar, which is glucosyl-fructose
- Lactose, the sugar of milk, which is galactosyl-glucose
- Maltose, the sugar originally isolated from malt, and a product of starch digestion, which is glucosyl-glucose
- Isomaltose, a product of starch digestion, which is glucosyl-glucose linked 1→6
- Trehalose, found especially in mushrooms, but also as the blood sugar of some insects, which is glucosyl-glucoside

4.2.1.4 Reducing and nonreducing sugars

Chemically, the aldehyde group of glucose is a reducing agent. This provides a simple test for glucose in urine (Figure 4.6). Glucose reacts with copper (Cu^{2+}) ions in alkaline solution, reducing them to Cu^{+} oxide and itself being oxidized. The original solution of Cu^{2+} ions has a blue color; the copper oxide forms a red-brown precipitate. This reaction is not specific for glucose. Other sugars with a free aldehyde group at carbon-1, including vitamin C (Section 11.14), and a number of pentose sugars that occur in foods can undergo the same reaction, giving a false-positive result.

While alkaline copper reagents are sometimes used to measure urine glucose in monitoring diabetic control (Section 10.7), a test using the enzyme glucose oxidase measures only glucose. Glucose oxidase reduces oxygen to hydrogen peroxide, which, in the presence of catalase, can be reduced to water by oxidation of the colorless compound ABTS to yield a blue color that can readily be measured. High concentrations of vitamin C (Section 11.14), as may occur in the urine of people taking supplements of the vitamin, can react with hydrogen peroxide before it oxidizes the colorless precursor or can reduce the dyestuff back to its colorless form. This means that tests using glucose oxidase can yield a false-negative result in the presence of high concentrations of vitamin C (see Problem 4.1).

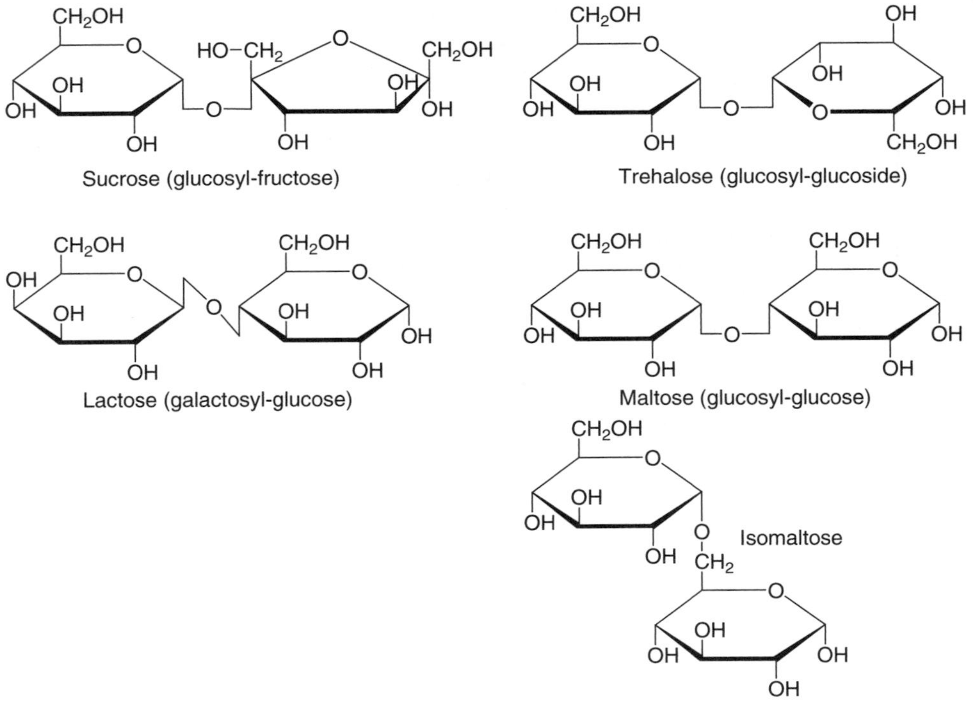

Sucrose (glucosyl-fructose)

Trehalose (glucosyl-glucoside)

Lactose (galactosyl-glucose)

Maltose (glucosyl-glucose)

Isomaltose

Figure 4.5 The nutritionally important disaccharides.

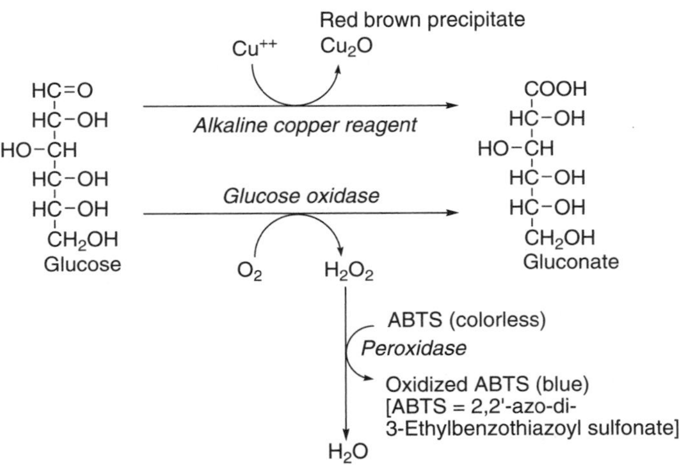

Figure 4.6 Measurement of glucose using alkaline copper reagent and glucose oxidase.

The term *reducing sugars* reflects a chemical reaction of the sugars—the ability to reduce a suitable acceptor such as copper ions. It has nothing to do with weight reduction and slimming, although some people erroneously believe that reducing sugars somehow help one to reduce excessive weight. This is not correct—the energy yield from reducing sugars and nonreducing sugars is exactly the same, and excess of either will contribute to obesity.

4.2.1.5 Polysaccharides: starches and glycogen

Starch is a polymer of glucose containing a large but variable number of glucose units. It is thus impossible to quote a relative molecular mass for starch or discuss amounts of starch in terms of moles. It can, however, be hydrolyzed to glucose, and the results expressed as moles of glucose.

The simplest type of starch is amylose, a straight chain of glucose molecules, with glycoside links between carbon-1 of one glucose unit and carbon-4 of the next. Amylopectin has a branched structure, where every thirtieth glucose molecule has glycoside links to three others instead of just two. The branch is formed by linkage between carbon-1 of one glucose unit and carbon-6 of the next (Figure 4.7).

Starches are the storage carbohydrates of plants, and the relative amounts of amylose and amylopectin differ in starches from different sources, as indeed does the size of the overall starch molecule. On average, about 20%–25% of dietary starch is amylose and the remaining 75%– 80%, amylopectin.

Glycogen is the storage carbohydrate of mammalian muscle and liver. It is synthesized from glucose in the fed state (Section 5.6.3), and its constituent glucose units are used as a metabolic fuel in the fasting state. Glycogen is a branched polymer with a similar structure to amylopectin, but more highly branched with a 1→6 bond about every tenth glucose. Because of its highly branched structure, glycogen traps a great deal of water in the cell; as glycogen stores are depleted during a period of fasting or reduced food intake, this water is released, leading to a considerable loss of body weight during the early stages of food restriction (Section 5.2).

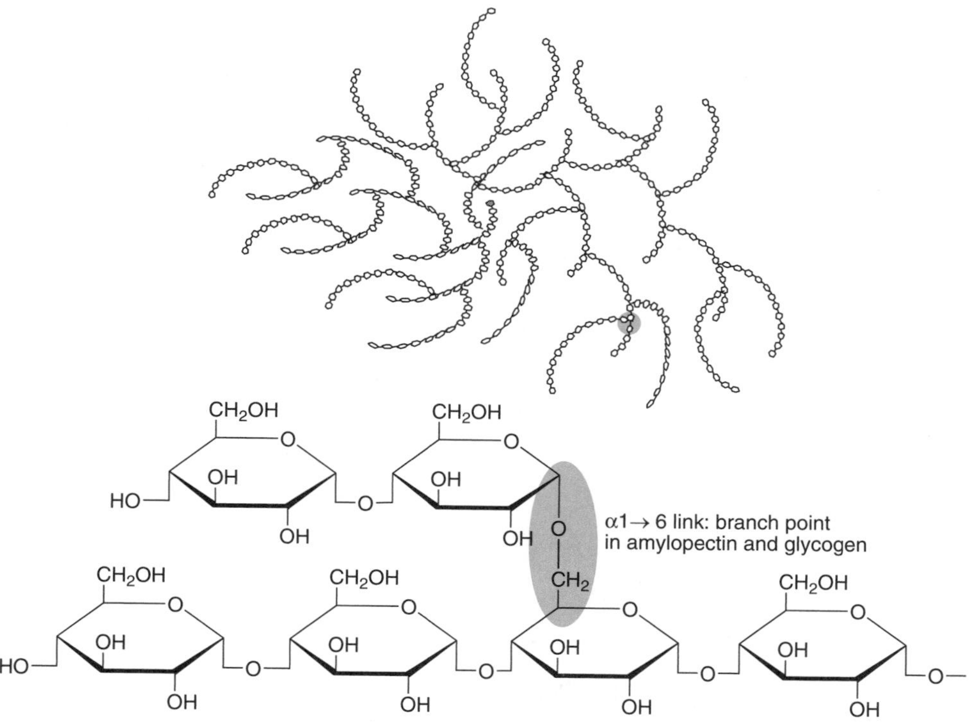

Figure 4.7 The branched structure of starch and glycogen.

4.2.1.6 Nonstarch polysaccharides (dietary fiber)

There are a number of other polysaccharides in foods. Collectively they are known as nonstarch polysaccharides and are the major components of dietary fiber (Section 6.3.3.2). Nonstarch polysaccharides are not digested by human enzymes, although all can be fermented to some extent by intestinal bacteria, and the products of bacterial fermentation may be absorbed and metabolized as metabolic fuels. The major nonstarch polysaccharides (Figure 4.8) are:

- Cellulose, a polymer of glucose in which the configuration of the glycoside bond between the glucose units is in the opposite configuration (β1→4) from that in starch (α1→4) and cannot be hydrolyzed by human enzymes
- Hemicelluloses, branched polymers of pentose (5-carbon) and hexose (6-carbon) sugars
- Inulin, a polymer of fructose, which is the storage carbohydrate of Jerusalem artichoke and some other root vegetables
- Pectin, a complex polymer of a variety of monosaccharides, including some methylated sugars
- Plant gums such as gum arabic, gum tragacanth, acacia, carob, and guar gums—complex polymers of mixed monosaccharides
- Mucilages such as alginates, agar, and carrageen; complex polymers of mixed monosaccharides found in seaweeds and other algae

Cellulose, hemicelluloses, and inulin are insoluble nonstarch polysaccharides, while pectin and the plant gums and mucilages are soluble. The other major constituent of dietary fiber, lignin, is not a carbohydrate at all, but a complex polymer of a variety of aromatic alcohols.

Soluble nonstarch polysaccharides increase the viscosity of the intestinal contents and so slow the absorption of the products of digestion. This can be valuable in the treatment

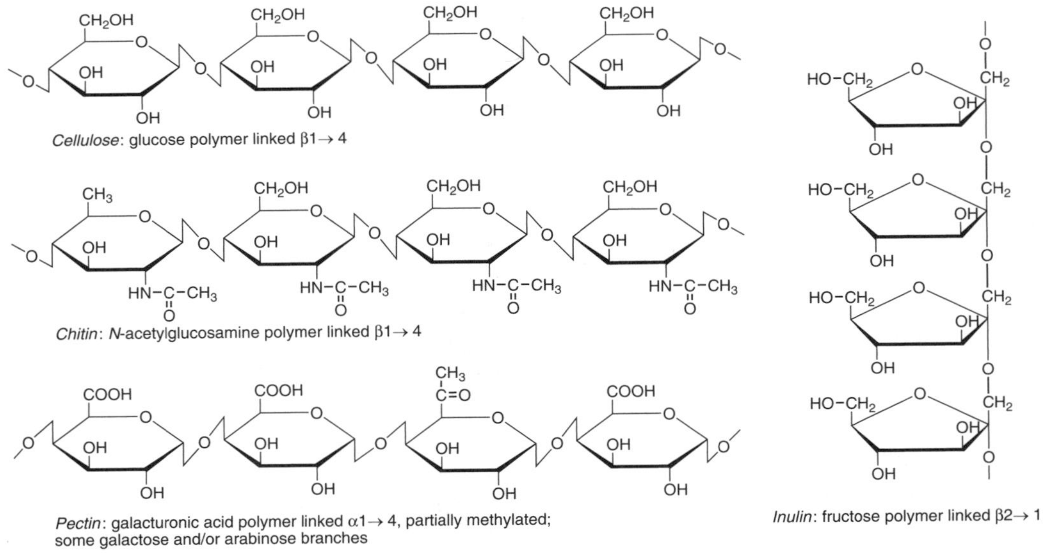

Cellulose: glucose polymer linked β1→ 4

Chitin: *N*-acetylglucosamine polymer linked β1→ 4

Pectin: galacturonic acid polymer linked α1→ 4, partially methylated; some galactose and/or arabinose branches

Inulin: fructose polymer linked β2→ 1

Figure 4.8 The major types of dietary nonstarch polysaccharide.

of diabetes mellitus (Section 10.7), and a number of studies have shown that consuming a relatively large amount of soluble nonstarch polysaccharide before a meal lowers the postprandial rise of blood glucose, thus enhancing glycemic control. Insoluble nonstarch polysaccharides increase the bulk of the intestinal contents, thus aiding peristalsis; they may also adsorb the bile salts and potential carcinogens in the diet, thus reducing their absorption (Section 6.3.3.2).

Both soluble and insoluble nonstarch polysaccharides, as well as oligosaccharides and starch that is resistant to digestion (Section 4.2.2.1), are substrates for bacterial fermentation in the large intestine, yielding short-chain fatty acids (especially butyrate) that are absorbed and provide a significant metabolic fuel for intestinal enterocytes, and may provide protection against the development of colorectal cancer (Section 6.3.3.2). Provision of a substrate for bacterial fermentation in the form of oligosaccharides, resistant starch, and nonstarch polysaccharides alters the composition of the intestinal flora, enhancing the growth of beneficial bacteria at the expense of potential pathogens. Carbohydrates that occur in, or are added to, foods for this purpose are known as prebiotics. Foods that contain the bacteria (mainly *Lactobacillus* and *Bifidobacterium* spp.) themselves are known as probiotics. One of the advantages of breast-feeding over infant formula is that human milk is rich in prebiotic oligosaccharides that enhance the infant's ability to develop a desirable intestinal bacterial flora.

4.2.2 Carbohydrate digestion and absorption

The digestion of carbohydrates is by hydrolysis to liberate small oligosaccharides, then free mono- and disaccharides. The extent and speed with which a carbohydrate is hydrolyzed and the resultant monosaccharides absorbed is measured as the glycemic index—the increase in blood glucose after a test dose of the carbohydrate compared with that after an equivalent amount of glucose, either as a glucose solution or a reference source of carbohydrate such as white bread or boiled rice.

Glucose and galactose have a glycemic index of 1, as do lactose, maltose, isomaltose, and trehalose, which give rise to these monosaccharides on hydrolysis. However, because plant cell walls are largely cellulose, which is not digested, intrinsic sugars in fruits and vegetables have a lower glycemic index. Other monosaccharides (e.g., fructose) and the sugar alcohols are absorbed less rapidly (Section 4.2.2.3) and have a lower glycemic index, as does sucrose, which yields glucose and fructose on hydrolysis. The glycemic index of starch is variable (Section 4.2.2.1), and that of nonstarch polysaccharides is zero.

Carbohydrates with a high glycemic index lead to a greater secretion of insulin after a meal than do those with a lower glycemic index; this results in increased synthesis of fatty acids and triacylglycerol (Section 5.6.1), and may therefore be a factor in the development of obesity (Chapter 7) and diabetes mellitus (Sections 7.2.3.1 and 10.7).

4.2.2.1 Starch digestion

The enzymes that catalyze the hydrolysis of starch are amylases, which are secreted both in the saliva and the pancreatic juice. (Salivary amylase is sometimes known by its old name of ptyalin.) Both salivary and pancreatic amylases catalyze random hydrolysis of glycoside bonds, initially yielding dextrins and other oligosaccharides, then a mixture of glucose, maltose, and isomaltose (from the branch points in amylopectin).

The digestion of starch begins when food is chewed and continues for a time in the stomach. Hydrolysis of starch to sweet sugars in the mouth may be a factor in determining food and nutrient intake (Section 1.3.3.1).

The gastric juice is very acidic (about pH 1.5–2), and amylase is inactive at this pH; as the food bolus is mixed with gastric juice, starch digestion ceases. When the food leaves the stomach and enters the small intestine, it is neutralized by the alkaline pancreatic juice (pH 8.8) and bile (pH 8). Amylase secreted by the pancreas continues the digestion of starch begun by salivary amylase.

Starches can be classified as:

- Rapidly hydrolyzed, with a glycemic index near 1; these are more or less completely hydrolyzed in the small intestine.
- Slowly hydrolyzed, with a glycemic index significantly <1, so that a proportion remains in the gut lumen and is a substrate for bacterial fermentation in the colon.
- Resistant to hydrolysis, with a glycemic index near to zero, so that most remains in the gut lumen and is a substrate for bacterial fermentation in the colon.

A proportion of the starch in foods is still enclosed by plant cell walls, which are mainly composed of cellulose. Cellulose is not digested by human enzymes, and therefore this starch is protected against digestion. Similarly, intrinsic sugars (Section 4.2.1) have a lower glycemic index than would be expected, because they are within intact cells.

Uncooked starch is resistant to amylase action, because it is present as small insoluble granules. The process of cooking swells the starch granules, resulting in a gel on which amylase can act. However, as cooked starch cools, a proportion undergoes crystallization to a form that is again resistant to amylase action—this is part of the process of staling of starchy foods.

Like nonstarch polysaccharides, much of the resistant and slowly hydrolyzed starch is fermented by bacteria in the colon, and a proportion of the products of bacterial metabolism, including short-chain fatty acids, may be absorbed and metabolized.

4.2.2.2 *Digestion of disaccharides*

The enzymes that catalyze the hydrolysis of disaccharides (the disaccharidases) are located on the brush border of the intestinal mucosal cells; the resultant monosaccharides are absorbed together with dietary monosaccharides and glucose arising from the digestion of starch (Section 4.2.2.1). There are four disaccharidases:

- Maltase catalyzes the hydrolysis of maltose to two molecules of glucose.
- Sucrase-isomaltase is a bifunctional enzyme that catalyzes the hydrolysis of sucrose to glucose and fructose, and of isomaltose to two molecules of glucose.
- Lactase catalyzes the hydrolysis of lactose to glucose and galactose.
- Trehalase catalyzes the hydrolysis of trehalose to two molecules of glucose.

Deficiency of the enzyme lactase is common. Indeed, it is mainly in people of north European origin that lactase persists after adolescence. In most other people, and in a number of Europeans, lactase is gradually lost through early adult life—alactasia (see Problem 4.2). In the absence of lactase, lactose cannot be absorbed, but remains in the intestinal lumen, where it is a substrate for bacterial fermentation to lactate (Section 5.4.1.2). This results in a considerable increase in the osmolality of the intestinal contents, since 1 mol of lactose yields 4 mol of lactate and 4 mol of protons. In addition, bacterial fermentation produces carbon dioxide, methane, and hydrogen, and the result of consuming a moderate amount of lactose is an explosive watery diarrhea with severe abdominal pain. Even the relatively small amounts of lactose in milk may upset people with a complete deficiency of lactase. Such people can normally tolerate yogurt and other fermented milk products, since much of the lactose has been converted to lactic acid. Fortunately, for people who suffer from alactasia, milk is the only significant source of lactose in the diet, so it is relatively easy to avoid consuming it. Lactose is widely used in manufacture of pharmaceuticals, but the small amounts consumed seem to be tolerated by people who are alactasic.

Rarely, people may lack sucrase-isomaltase, maltase, or trehalase. This may either be a genetic lack of the enzyme, or an acquired loss as a result of intestinal infection, when all four disaccharidases are lost. These people are intolerant of the sugar(s) that cannot be hydrolyzed and suffer in the same way as alactasic subjects given lactose. It is relatively easy to avoid maltose and trehalose, since there are few sources in the diet. People who lack sucrase have a more serious problem, since as well as the obvious sugar in cakes, biscuits, and jams, many manufactured foods contain added sucrose.

Genetic lack of sucrase-isomaltase is very common among the Inuit of North America. This caused no problems on their traditional diet, since they had no significant sources of sucrose or isomaltose. With the adoption of a more Western diet, sucrose-induced diarrhea has become a significant cause of undernutrition among infants and children.

4.2.2.3 The absorption of monosaccharides

There are two separate mechanisms for the absorption of monosaccharides in the small intestine (Figure 4.9).

Glucose and galactose are absorbed by a sodium-dependent active process (Section 3.2.2.3). The sodium pump (Section 3.2.2.6) and the sodium/potassium ATPase (Section 3.2.2.4), as well as sodium secreted in the alkaline pancreatic juice, create a sodium gradient across the membrane. The sodium ions then enter the cell together with glucose or galactose. These two monosaccharides are carried by the same transport protein and compete with each other for intestinal absorption.

Other monosaccharides are absorbed by carrier-mediated diffusion; there are at least three distinct carrier proteins, one for fructose, one for other monosaccharides, and one for sugar alcohols. Because they are not actively transported, fructose and sugar alcohols are only absorbed to a limited extent, and after a moderately high intake, a significant amount will avoid absorption, and remain in the intestinal lumen, acting as a substrate for colon bacteria and, like unabsorbed disaccharides in people with disaccharidase deficiency, causing abdominal pain and diarrhea.

4.3 Digestion and absorption of fats

The major fats in the diet are triacylglycerols and, to a lesser extent, phospholipids. Lipids are hydrophobic and have to be emulsified to very small droplets (micelles; Section 4.3.2.2) before they can be absorbed. This emulsification is achieved by hydrolysis of triacylglycerols to mono- and diacylglycerols and free fatty acids, and also by the action of the bile salts (Section 4.3.2.1).

4.3.1 The classification of dietary lipids

Four groups of metabolically important compounds can be considered under the heading of lipids:

- Triacylglycerols (sometimes also known as triglycerides), in which glycerol is esterified to three fatty acids (Figure 4.10). These are the oils and fats of the diet, which provide

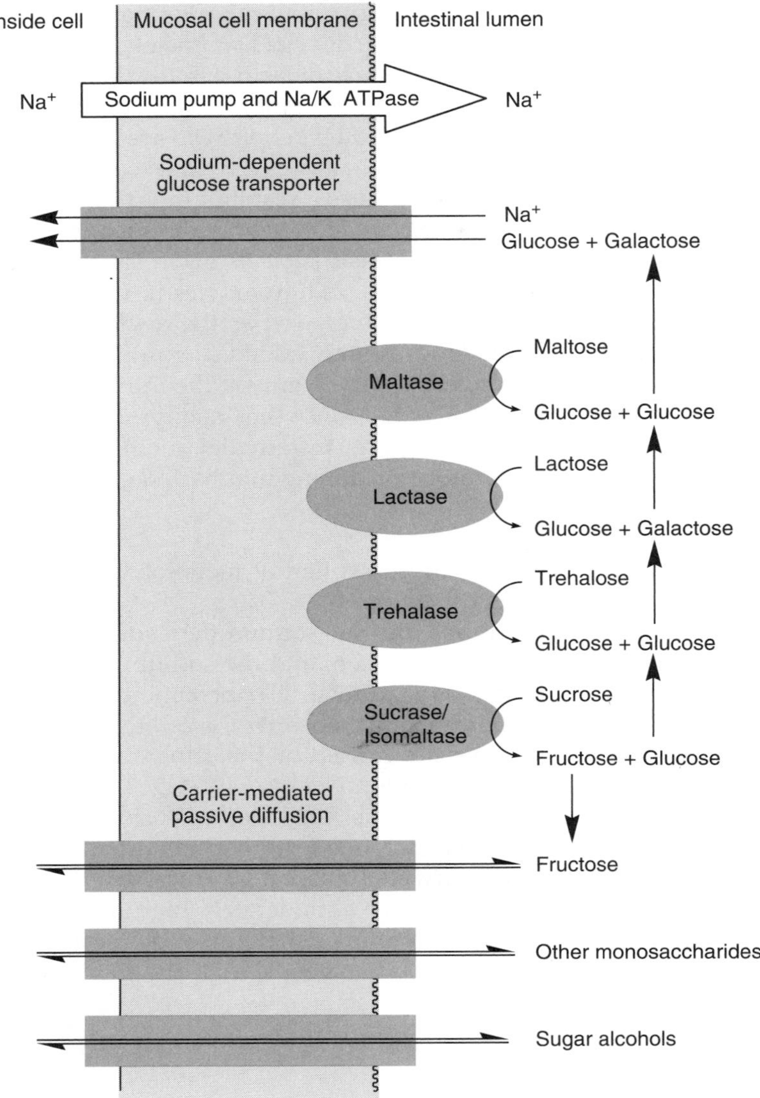

Figure 4.9 The hydrolysis of disaccharides and absorption of monosaccharides.

between 30% and 45% of average energy intake. The difference between oils and fats is that oils are liquid at room temperature, whereas fats are solid.

- Phospholipids, in which glycerol is esterified to two fatty acids, with a hydrophilic group esterified to carbon-3 by a phosphate diester bond (Section 4.3.1.2). Phospholipids are major constituents of cell membranes.
- Steroids, including cholesterol, a variety of plant sterols and stanols (Section 4.3.1.3), and extremely small amounts of steroid hormones (Section 10.4). Chemically, these are completely different from triacylglycerols and phospholipids, and are not a significant source of metabolic fuel.

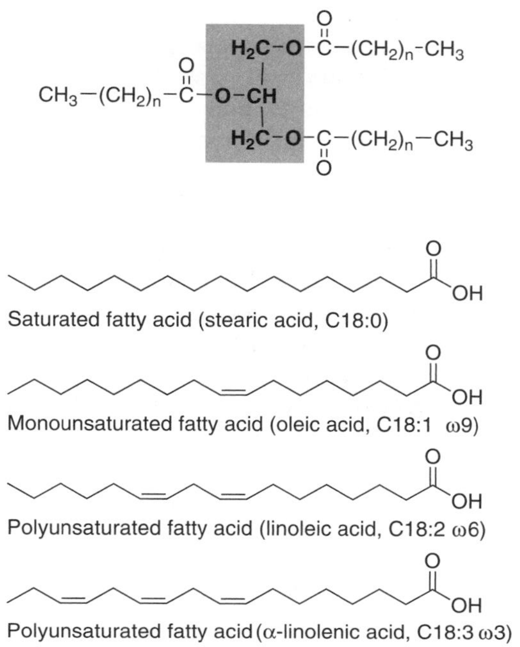

Saturated fatty acid (stearic acid, C18:0)

Monounsaturated fatty acid (oleic acid, C18:1 ω9)

Polyunsaturated fatty acid (linoleic acid, C18:2 ω6)

Polyunsaturated fatty acid (α-linolenic acid, C18:3 ω3)

Figure 4.10 The structure of triacylglycerol and classes of fatty acids.

- A variety of other compounds, including vitamin A and carotenes (Section 11.2), vitamin D (Section 11.3), vitamin E (Section 11.4), and vitamin K (Section 11.5). They are absorbed in lipid micelles (Section 4.3.2.2), and their absorption depends on an adequate intake of fat.

4.3.1.1 Fatty acids

There are a number of different fatty acids, differing in both the length of the carbon chain and whether or not they have one or more double bonds (–CH=CH–) in the chain (Figure 4.10). Those with no double bonds are saturated fatty acids—the carbon chain is completely saturated with hydrogen. Those with double bonds are unsaturated fatty acids—the carbon chain is not completely saturated with hydrogen. Fatty acids with one double bond are known as monounsaturated, while those with two or more double bonds are known as polyunsaturated.

While it is the fatty acids that are saturated or unsaturated, it is common to discuss saturated and unsaturated fats. Although not really correct, it is a useful shorthand, reflecting the fact that fats from different sources contain a greater or lesser proportion of saturated and unsaturated fatty acids.

There are three different ways of naming the fatty acids (Table 4.1):

- Many have trivial names, often derived from the source from which they were originally isolated—thus oleic acid was first isolated from olive oil, stearic acid from beef tallow, palmitic acid from palm oil, linoleic and linolenic acids from linseed oil.
- All have systematic chemical names based on the number of carbon atoms in the chain and the number and position of double bonds (if any).

- A shorthand notation to show the number of carbon atoms in the molecule followed by a colon and the number of double bonds. The position of the first double bond from the methyl group of the fatty acid is shown by n- or ω- (the ω-carbon is the furthest from the α-carbon, which is the one to which the carboxyl group is attached; ω [omega] is the last letter of the Greek alphabet).

In the nutritionally important unsaturated fatty acids, the carbon–carbon double bonds are in the *cis* configuration (Figure 2.6). The *trans* isomers of unsaturated fatty acids occur in foods to some extent, both as a result of hydrogenation of unsaturated oils to more solid fats for food manufacture and also naturally occurring in fat from ruminants, as a result of rumen bacterial fermentation. They do not have the desirable biological actions of the *cis* isomers, and indeed there is evidence that *trans* fatty acids have adverse effects. It is recommended that *trans* unsaturated fatty acids should not exceed 1% of energy intake (Section 6.3.2.1).

Table 4.1 Fatty Acid Nomenclature

		Double Bonds		
	C Atoms	Number	First	Shorthand
Saturated				
Butyric	4	0	–	C4:0
Caproic	6	0	–	C6:0
Caprylic	8	0	–	C8:0
Capric	10	0	–	C10:0
Lauric	12	0	–	C12:0
Myristic	14	0	–	C14:0
Palmitic	16	0	–	C16:0
Stearic	18	0	–	C18:0
Arachidic	20	0	–	C20:0
Behenic	22	0	–	C22:0
Lignoceric	24	0	–	C24:0
Monounsaturated				
Palmitoleic	16	1	7	C16:1 ω7
Oleic	18	1	9	C18:1 ω9
Cetoleic	22	1	11	C22:1 ω11
Nervonic	24	1	9	C24:1 ω9
Polyunsaturated				
Linoleic	18	2	6	C18:2 ω6
α-Linolenic	18	3	3	C18:3 ω3
γ-Linolenic	18	3	6	C18:3 ω6
Arachidonic	20	4	6	C20:4 ω6
Eicosapentaenoic	20	5	3	C20:5 ω3
Docosatetraenoic	22	4	6	C22:4 ω6
Docosapentaenoic	22	5	3	C22:5 ω3
Docosapentaenoic	22	5	6	C22:5 ω6
Docosahexaenoic	22	6	3	C22:6 ω3

Polyunsaturated fatty acids have two main functions in the body:

- As major constituents of the phospholipids in cell membranes, where they are important in maintaining membrane fluidity (Figure 4.12).
- As precursors for the synthesis of a group of compounds known as eicosanoids, including prostaglandins, prostacyclins, and thromboxanes. These function as local hormones (paracrine agents), being secreted into the extracellular fluid and acting on nearby cells.

The polyunsaturated fatty acids can be interconverted to a limited extent in the body, but there is a requirement for a dietary intake of linoleic acid (C18:2 ω6) and linolenic acid (C18:3 ω3), since these two, which can each be considered to be the precursor of a family of related fatty acids and eicosanoids, cannot be synthesized in the body.

An intake of polyunsaturated fatty acids greater than needed to meet physiological requirements may confer benefits in terms of lowering the plasma concentration of cholesterol and reducing the risk of atherosclerosis and ischemic heart disease. The requirement is less than 1% of energy intake, but it is recommended that 6% of energy intake should come from polyunsaturated fatty acids (Section 6.3.2.1).

High intakes of the long-chain ω3 polyunsaturated fatty acids (as found in fish oils) may additionally provide protection against thrombosis, since they form the ω3-series eicosanoids, which inhibit platelet cohesiveness. However, the same enzymes are involved in the metabolism of both ω3 and ω6 polyunsaturated fatty acids to form eicosanoids, and the two families of fatty acids compete with each other for metabolism. This means that the balance between ω3 and ω6 polyunsaturated fatty acids in the diet is important; excessive intakes of one group will lead to reduced formation of the other group of eicosanoids.

4.3.1.2 *Phospholipids*

As their name suggests, phospholipids are lipids that contain a phosphate group (Figure 4.11). They consist of glycerol esterified to two fatty acids, one of which (esterified to carbon-2 of glycerol) is polyunsaturated. The third hydroxyl group of glycerol is esterified to phosphate, which in turn is esterified to one of a variety of compounds, including the amino acid serine (Section 4.4.1), ethanolamine (which is formed from serine), choline (which is formed from ethanolamine), and inositol (Section 10.3.3). A phospholipid lacking the group esterified to the phosphate is known as a phosphatidic acid, and the complete phospholipids are called phosphatidyl serine, phosphatidyl ethanolamine, phosphatidyl choline (also called lecithin), phosphatidyl inositol, etc.

Phospholipids in cell membranes form a lipid bilayer, with the hydrophobic fatty acid chains inside, and the hydrophilic groups outside (Figure 4.12). Various proteins may be embedded in the membrane at one surface or the other, or may span the membrane (transmembrane proteins) as either transport proteins (Section 3.2.2) or receptors for hormones and neurotransmitters (Section 10.3.1). The polyunsaturated fatty acids esterified at carbon-2 of glycerol in phospholipids are essential for membrane fluidity; neither saturated fatty acids nor the *trans* isomers of polyunsaturated fatty acids will pack to form an adequately fluid membrane. Other lipids, including cholesterol (Section 4.3.1.3) and vitamin E (Section 11.4), are dissolved in the hydrophobic interior of the membrane and are essential to its function.

In addition to its structural role, phosphatidyl inositol has a specialized function in membranes, acting as the source of inositol trisphosphate and diacylglycerol that are

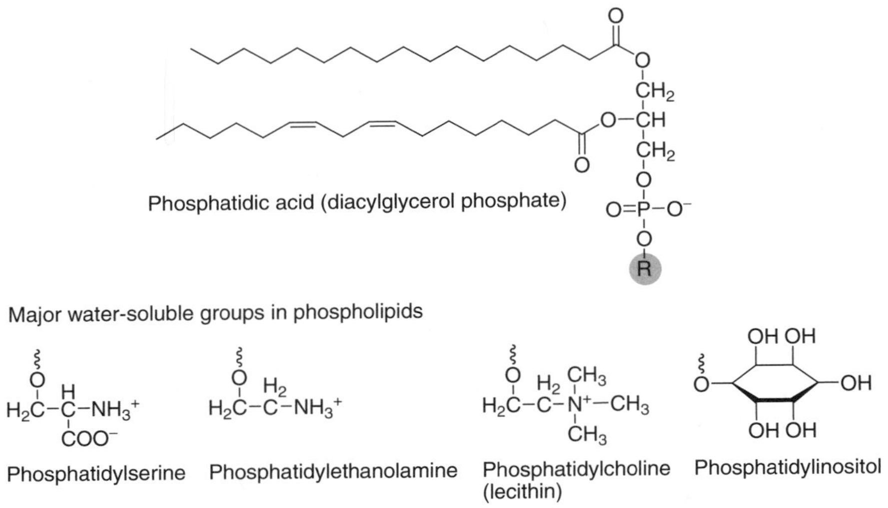

Phosphatidic acid (diacylglycerol phosphate)

Major water-soluble groups in phospholipids

Phosphatidylserine Phosphatidylethanolamine Phosphatidylcholine (lecithin) Phosphatidylinositol

Figure 4.11 The structure of phospholipids.

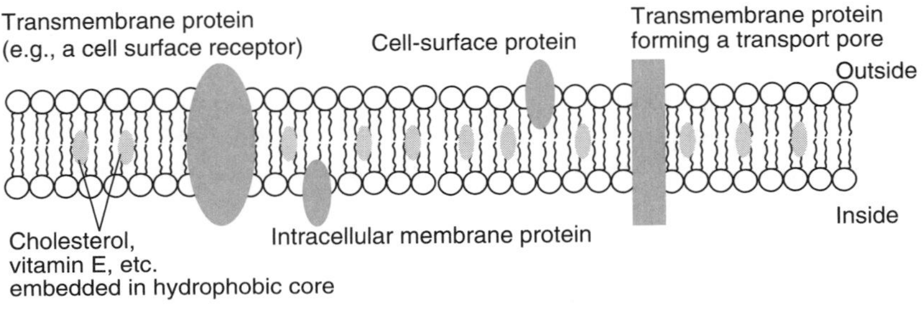

Figure 4.12 The arrangement of phospholipids in cell membranes.

produced as intracellular second messengers in response to fast-acting hormones and neurotransmitters (Section 10.3.3).

4.3.1.3 *Cholesterol and the steroids*

Steroids are chemically completely different from triacylglycerols or phospholipids (Figure 4.13). The parent compound of all the steroids in the body is cholesterol; different steroids are then formed by replacing one or more of the hydrogens with hydroxyl groups or oxo-groups, and in some cases by modifying the side chain.

Apart from cholesterol, which is important in membrane structure and the synthesis of bile salts (Section 4.3.2.1) steroids are slow-acting hormones (Section 10.4). Vitamin D (Section 11.3) is a derivative of cholesterol, and can also be considered to be a steroid hormone.

The cholesterol that is required for membrane synthesis, and the very much smaller amount required for the synthesis of steroid hormones, may either be synthesized in the body or provided by the diet; average intakes are of the order of 200–500 mg/day.

An elevated plasma concentration of cholesterol (in low density lipoproteins; Section 5.6.2.2) is a risk factor for atherosclerosis and ischemic heart disease. The dietary intake of cholesterol is less important as a determinant of plasma cholesterol than is the intake

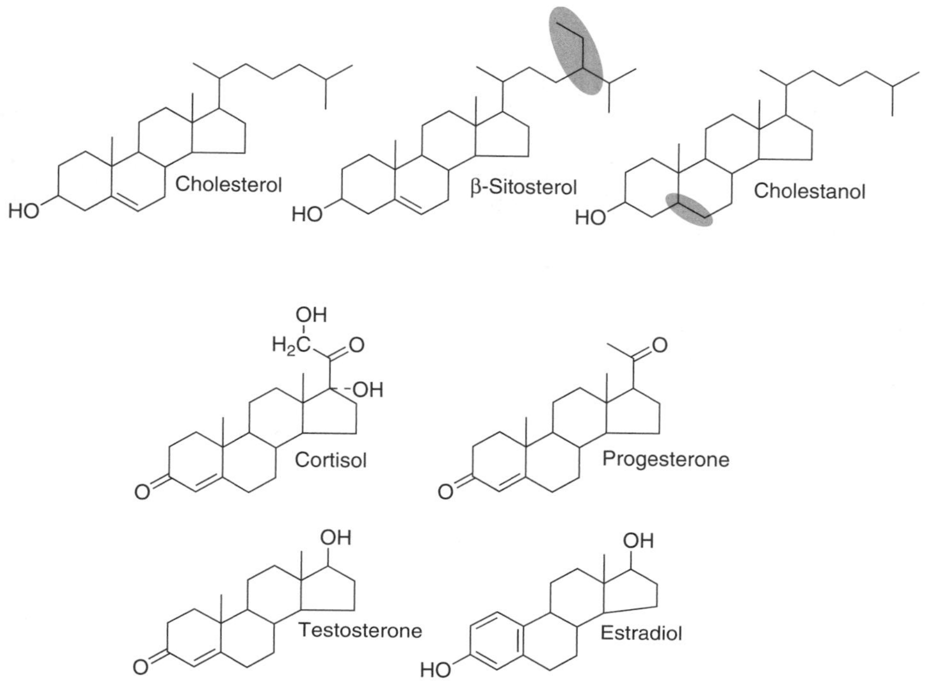

Figure 4.13 Cholesterol, plant sterols and stanols, and some steroid hormones.

of total and saturated fat (Section 6.3.2.1), the intake of compounds such as sitosterol and cholestanol that inhibit the absorption of dietary cholesterol and the reabsorption of cholesterol secreted in bile, or the reabsorption of bile salts themselves (Section 4.3.2.1).

4.3.2 Digestion and absorption of triacylglycerols

The digestion of triacylglycerols begins with lipase secreted by the tongue; lingual lipase may be important in permitting the detection of fat in the diet, and hence in determining food choices (Section 1.3.3.1). However, it makes only a marginal contribution to overall triacylglycerol hydrolysis, which continues in the stomach, where gastric lipase is secreted. Hydrolysis of the fatty acids esterified to carbons 1 and 3 of the triacylglycerol results in the liberation of free fatty acids and 2-mono-acylglycerol (Figure 4.14). These have both hydrophobic and hydrophilic regions, and will therefore emulsify the lipid into increasingly small droplets. Triacylglycerol hydrolysis continues in the small intestine, catalyzed by pancreatic lipase, which requires a further pancreatic protein, colipase, for activity. Monoacylglycerols are hydrolyzed to glycerol and free fatty acids by pancreatic esterase in the intestinal lumen and intracellular lipase within intestinal mucosal cells. The drug orlistat (Xenical®) used in the treatment of severe obesity acts by inhibiting pancreatic lipase, and so reducing the digestion and absorption of dietary triacylglycerol.

4.3.2.1 Bile salts

The final emulsification of dietary lipids into micelles (droplets that are small enough to be absorbed across the intestinal mucosa) is achieved by the action of the bile salts. They are synthesized from cholesterol in the liver, and secreted, together with phospholipids and cholesterol, by the gall bladder. Some 2 g of cholesterol and 30 g of bile salts are secreted by the gall bladder each day, almost all of which is reabsorbed, so that the total fecal output of steroids and bile salts is 0.2–1 g/day (Figure 4.15).

The primary bile salts (those synthesized in the liver) are conjugates of chenodeoxycholic acid and cholic acid with taurine or glycine (Figure 4.16). Intestinal bacteria catalyze deconjugation and further metabolism to yield the secondary bile salts, lithocholic and deoxycholic acids. These are also absorbed from the gut, and are reconjugated in the liver and secreted in the bile.

The bile salts can be bound physically by insoluble nonstarch polysaccharide (Section 4.2.1.6) in the intestinal lumen, so that they cannot be reabsorbed. This is the basis of the cholesterol-lowering effect of moderately high intakes of nonstarch polysaccharide

Triacylglycerol: $H_2C-O-C(=O)-(CH_2)_n-CH_3$ / $CH_3-(CH_2)_n-C(=O)-O-CH$ / $H_2C-O-C(=O)-(CH_2)_n-CH_3$

↓ H_2O, *Lipase* → $CH_3-(CH_2)_n-C(=O)-O^-$

Diacylglycerol: H_2C-OH / $CH_3-(CH_2)_n-C(=O)-O-CH$ / $H_2C-O-C(=O)-(CH_2)_n-CH_3$

↓ H_2O, *Lipase* → $CH_3-(CH_2)_n-C(=O)-O^-$

Monoacylglycerol: H_2C-OH / $CH_3-(CH_2)_n-C(=O)-O-CH$ / H_2C-OH

↓ H_2O, *Pancreatic esterases and intracellular lipase* → $CH_3-(CH_2)_n-C(=O)-O^-$

Glycerol: H_2C-OH / $HO-CH$ / H_2C-OH

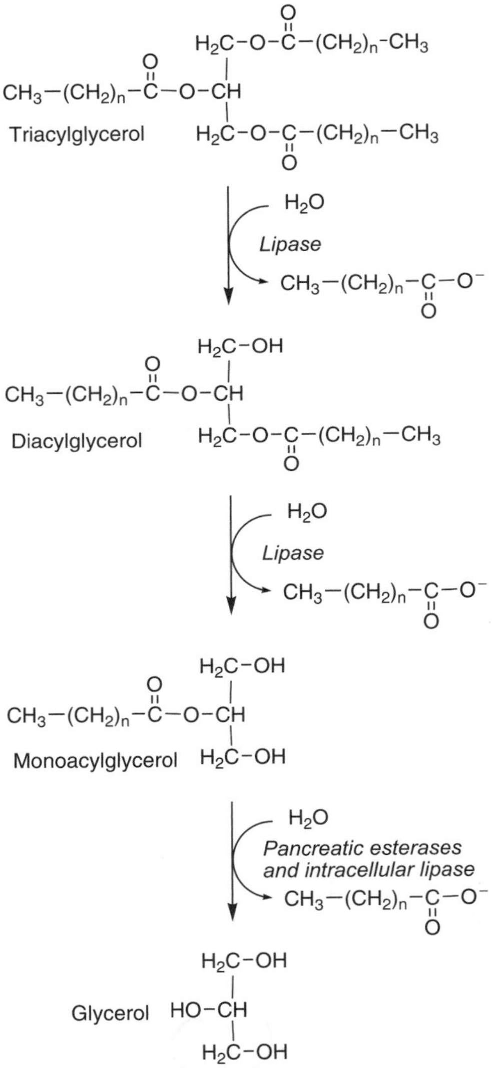

Figure 4.14 Lipase and the hydrolysis of triacylglycerol.

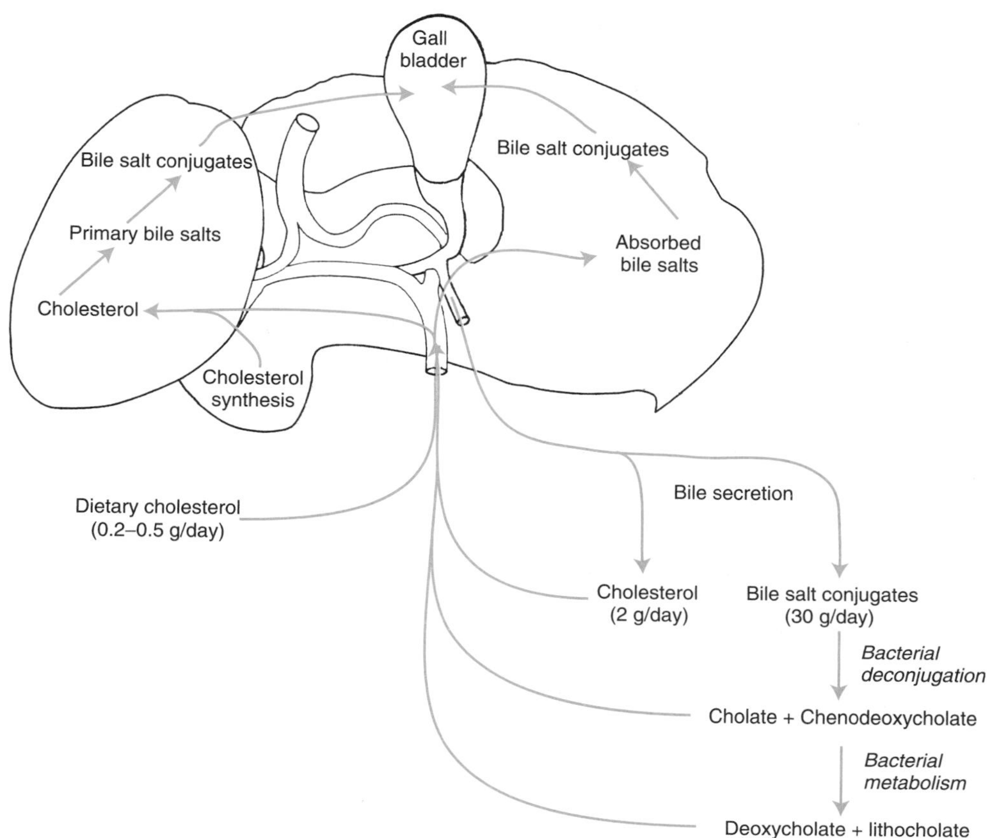

Figure 4.15 Enterohepatic cycling of cholesterol and bile salts.

(Section 6.3.3.2)—if the bile salts are not reabsorbed and reutilized, then there must be further synthesis from cholesterol in the liver, thus depleting body cholesterol.

Under normal conditions, the concentration of cholesterol in bile, relative to that of bile salts and phospholipids, is such that cholesterol is at or near its limit of solubility. It only requires a relatively small increase in the concentration of cholesterol in bile for it to crystallize out, resulting in the formation of gallstones. Obesity (Section 7.2.2) and high-fat diets (especially diets high in saturated fat, which increase the synthesis of cholesterol in the liver) are associated with a considerably increased incidence of gallstones (Figure 4.17).

4.3.2.2 Lipid absorption and chylomicron formation

The finely emulsified lipid micelles, containing free fatty acids, monoacylglycerol, phospholipids, cholesterol, and fat-soluble vitamins, together with a small amount of intact triacylglycerol, are absorbed across the intestinal wall into the mucosal cells. There are membrane transport proteins for fatty acids and cholesterol.

Inside the enterocyte, fatty acids are reesterified to form triacylglycerol (Figure 5.29), and cholesterol is esterified. Newly esterified triacylglycerol, cholesterol esters, and lipid-soluble vitamins are packaged with proteins synthesized in the enterocyte to form chylomicrons, which are secreted into the lacteal in the center of the villus (Figure 4.2), and enter the lymphatic system, which drains into the bloodstream at the thoracic duct. In response to the action of insulin (Section 10.5), lipoprotein lipase at the surface of blood vessel endothelial

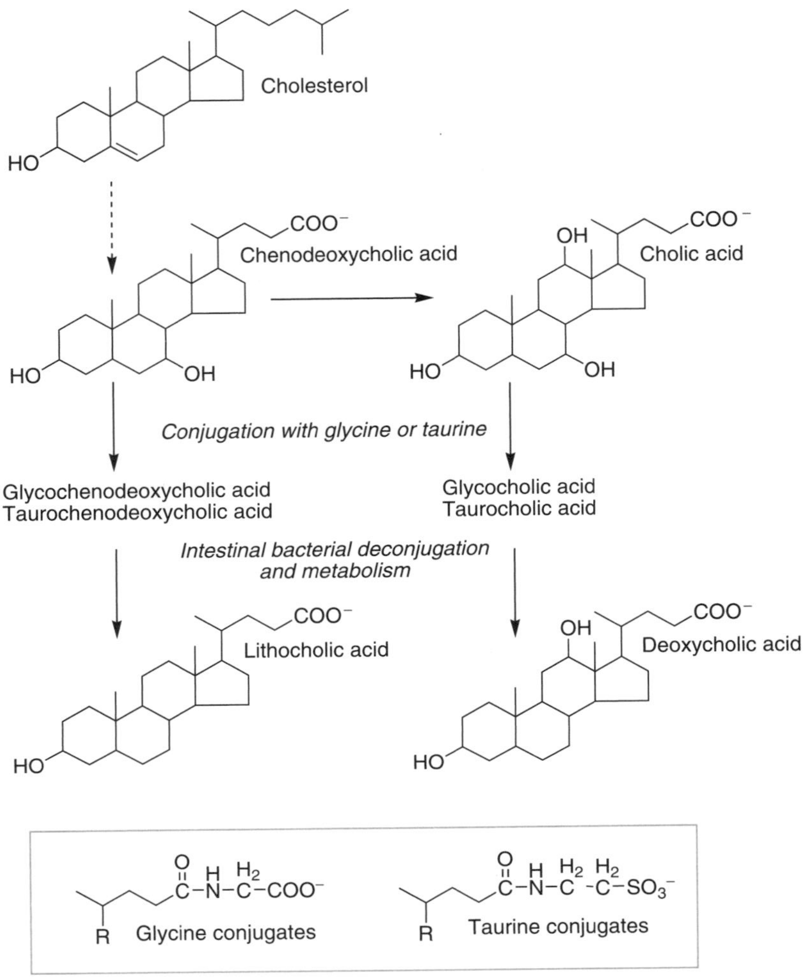

Figure 4.16 The metabolism of bile salts.

cells in adipose tissue and muscle is activated and catalyzes the hydrolysis of chylomicron triacylglycerol. The resultant fatty acids are taken up by adipose tissue and reesterified for storage; in muscle the fatty acids may either be used as a metabolic fuel or be reesterified for storage between muscle fibers. A proportion of the fatty acid released by lipoprotein lipase remains in the bloodstream and is taken up by the liver, where it is reesterified and incorporated into very low density lipoprotein (Section 5.6.2.2).

The triacylglycerol-depleted chylomicron remnants are taken up by the liver through receptor-mediated endocytosis, and most of the residual lipid is secreted in very low-density lipoprotein, together with triacylglycerol synthesized in the liver. See Section 5.6.2 for a discussion of the metabolism of chylomicrons and other plasma lipoproteins.

4.4 Digestion and absorption of proteins

Proteins are polypeptides—polymers of amino acids linked by peptide bonds. Unlike starch and glycogen, which are polymers of only a single type of monomer unit

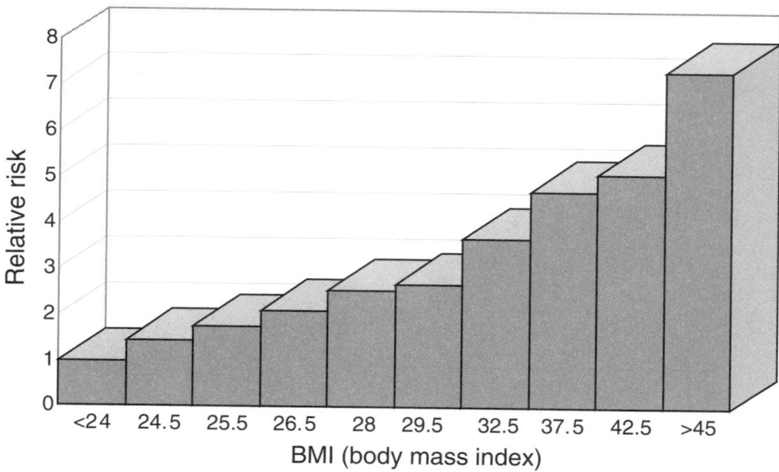

Figure 4.17 The incidence of gallstones with obesity (body mass index = weight [kg]/height [m^2]; the desirable range is 20–25. (From data reported by Stampfer, M.J. et al., *Am. J. Clin. Nutr.*, 55, 652–628, 1992.)

(glucose), proteins contain 21 different amino acids that are incorporated during synthesis (Section 9.2) as well as a number of others that are formed as a result of postsynthetic modification. Since any individual polypeptide chain may contain 50–1000 amino acids, there is an almost infinite possible variety of proteins. There are some 30,000–40,000 different proteins and polypeptides in the human body; each has a specific sequence of amino acids.

Small proteins have a molecular mass of about $50–100 \times 10^3$, while some of the large complex proteins have a molecular mass of up to 10^4 or more. Smaller polypep-tides (containing between 3 and 50 amino acids) are important in the regulation of metabolism.

4.4.1 The amino acids

Chemically, all the amino acids all have the same basic structure—an amino group ($-NH_3^+$) and a carboxylic acid group ($-COO^-$) attached to the same carbon atom (the α-carbon); what differs between the amino acids is the nature of the other group that is attached to the α-carbon. In the simplest amino acid, glycine, there are two hydrogen atoms, while in all other amino acids there is one hydrogen atom and a side chain, varying in chemical complexity from the simple methyl group ($-CH_3$) of alanine to the aromatic ring structures of phenylalanine, tyrosine, and tryptophan. The twenty-first amino acid is selenocysteine, the selenium analogue of cysteine.

Nine of the amino acids are dietary essentials that cannot be synthesized in the body (Section 9.1.3); these are starred in Figure 4.18. The amino acids can be classified according to the chemical nature of the side chain: whether it is hydrophobic (on the left-hand side of Figure 4.18) or hydrophilic (on the right-hand side of Figure 4.18) and the nature of the group:

- Small hydrophobic amino acids: glycine, alanine, proline
- Large hydrophobic, branched-chain amino acids: leucine, isoleucine, valine
- Aromatic amino acids: phenylalanine, tyrosine, tryptophan
- Sulfur-containing amino acids: cysteine and methionine
- Neutral hydrophilic amino acids: serine and threonine

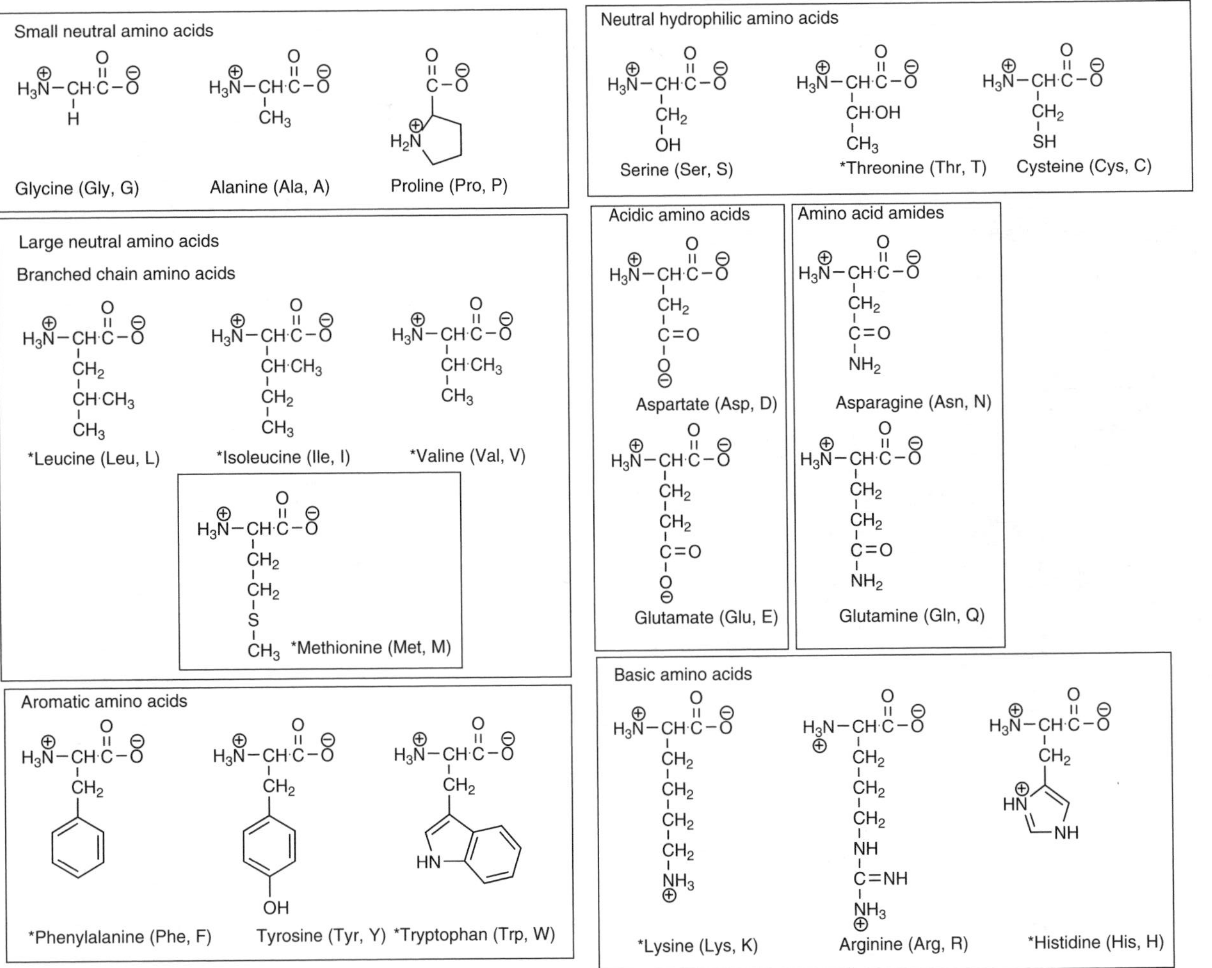

Figure 4.18 The amino acids, showing their three-letter and single-letter codes. *Starred amino acids are dietary essentials that cannot be synthesized in the body.

- Acidic amino acids: glutamic and aspartic acids (the salts of these acids are glutamate and aspartate, respectively)
- Amides of the acidic amino acids: glutamine and asparagine
- Basic amino acids: lysine, arginine, histidine

In addition to the three-letter abbreviations that are commonly used for the amino acids, there is a single-letter code for each that is generally used for showing protein sequences.

4.4.2 Protein structure and denaturation of proteins

Proteins are composed of linear chains of amino acids, joined by condensation of the carboxyl group of one with the amino group of another, to form a peptide bond (Figure 4.19). The sequence of amino acids in a protein is its primary structure. It is different for each protein, although proteins that are closely related to each other often have very similar primary structures. The primary structure of a protein is determined by the gene containing the information for that protein (Section 9.2).

4.4.2.1 Secondary structure of proteins

Polypeptide chains fold up in a variety of ways, stabilized by hydrogen bonds between the oxygen of one peptide bond and the nitrogen of another (Figure 4.20). Interactions between the side chains of the amino acids determine which of the following patterns of secondary structure any given region of a protein adopts:

- α-Helix, in which the peptide backbone of the protein adopts a spiral (helix) form. The hydrogen bonds are formed between peptide bonds that are near each other in the primary sequence.
- β–Pleated sheet, in which regions of the polypeptide chain lie alongside one another, forming a "corrugated" or pleated surface. The hydrogen bonds are between peptide bonds in different parts of the primary sequence, and the regions of polypeptide chain forming a pleated sheet may run parallel or antiparallel.
- Hairpins and loops, in which small regions of the polypeptide chain form very tight bends.
- Random coil, in which there is no recognizable organized structure. Although this appears to be random, for any one protein the shape of a random coil region will always be the same.

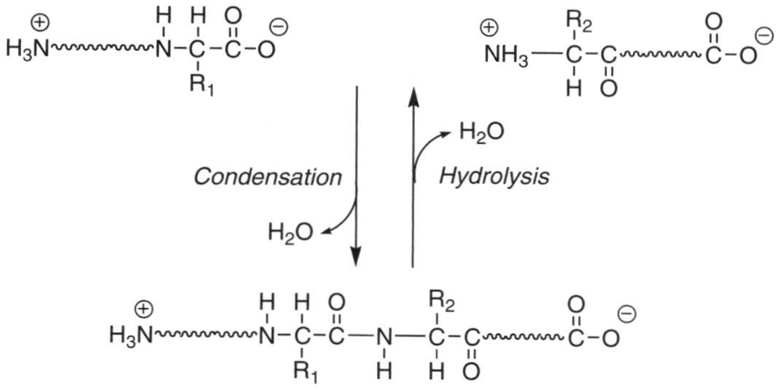

Condensation

H_2O

Hydrolysis

H_2O

Figure 4.19 Condensation of amino acids to form a peptide bond.

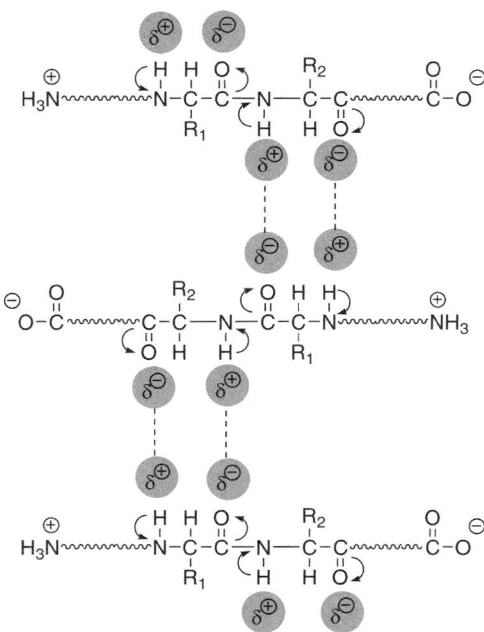

Figure 4.20 Hydrogen bonds in peptide chains.

A protein may have several regions of α-helix, β-pleated sheet (with the peptide chains running parallel or antiparallel), hairpins, and random coil, all in the same molecule.

4.4.2.2 Tertiary and quaternary structures of proteins

Having formed regions of secondary structure, the whole protein molecule then folds up into a compact shape. This is the third (tertiary) level of structure and is largely the result of interactions of the side chains of the amino acids with each other and their environment. Proteins in an aqueous medium in the cell generally adopt a tertiary structure in which hydrophobic side chains are inside the molecule and can interact with each other, while hydrophilic side chains are exposed to interact with water. In contrast, proteins that are embedded in membranes (Figure 4.12) have a hydrophobic region on the outside to interact with the membrane lipids.

Two further interactions between amino acid side chains may be involved in the tertiary structure, in this case forming covalent bonds between regions of the peptide chain (Figure 4.21):

- The ε-amino group on the side chain of lysine can form a peptide bond with the carboxyl group on the side chain of aspartate or glutamate. This is nutritionally important, since the side chain peptide bond is not hydrolyzed by digestive enzymes, and the lysine, which is an essential amino acid, is not available for absorption (Section 9.1.3.2).
- The sulfydryl (–SH) groups of two cysteine molecules may be oxidized to form a disulfide bridge between two parts of the protein chain.

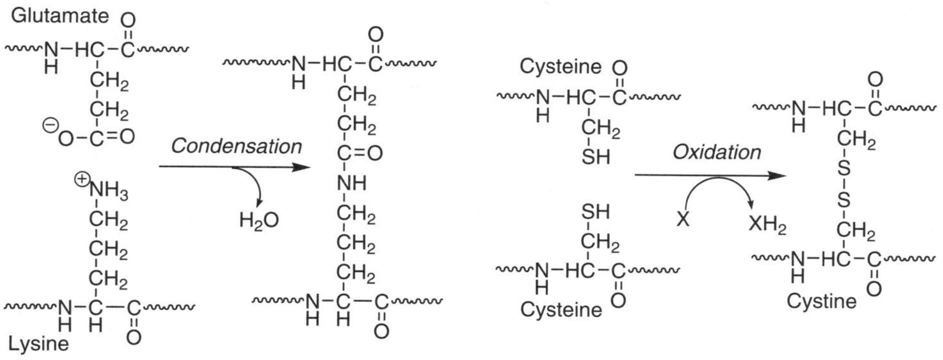

Figure 4.21 Covalent links between peptide chains—on the left-hand side, a side chain peptide between the ε-amino group of lysine and the γ-carboxyl group of glutamate, on the right-hand side, a disulfide bridge formed by oxidation of two cysteine residues.

Some proteins consist of more than one polypeptide chain; the way in which the chains interact with each other, after each has formed its secondary and tertiary structures, is the quaternary structure of the protein. Interactions between the subunits of multi-subunit proteins, involving changes in quaternary structure and the conformation of the protein, are important in a number of regulatory enzymes (Sections 2.3.3.3 and 10.2.1).

4.4.2.3 Denaturation of proteins

Because of their compact secondary and tertiary structures, most proteins are resistant to digestive enzymes—few bonds are accessible to the proteolytic enzymes that catalyze hydrolysis of peptide bonds. However, apart from covalent links formed by reaction between the side chains of lysine and aspartate or glutamate, and disulfide bridges, the native structure of proteins is maintained by relatively weak noncovalent forces: ionic interactions, hydrogen bonding, and van der Waals forces.

Denaturation of a protein is the loss of its compact secondary and tertiary structures, opening out the molecule so that it becomes insoluble (and in the case of an enzyme, loses its catalytic activity, Section 2.3.2). Denatured proteins are susceptible to the action of digestive enzymes, so that denaturation is an important precursor to protein digestion. The relatively weak bonds that maintain the native structure of proteins can be disrupted by heat and extremes of pH, so that both cooking and gastric acid are important in protein digestion.

4.4.3 Protein digestion

Protein digestion occurs by hydrolysis of the peptide bonds between amino acids. There are two main classes of protein digestive enzymes (proteases) with different specificities for the amino acids forming the peptide bond to be hydrolyzed (Table 4.2):

- *Endopeptidases* cleave proteins by hydrolyzing peptide bonds between specific amino acids throughout the molecule.
- *Exopeptidases* remove amino acids one at a time from either the amino or carboxyl end of the molecule, again by the hydrolysis of the peptide bond.

Table 4.2 Protein Digestive Enzymes

	Secreted by	Specificity
Endopeptidases		
Pepsin	Gastric mucosa	Adjacent to aromatic amino acid, leucine, or methionine
Trypsin	Pancreas	Lysine or arginine esters
Chymotrypsin	Pancreas	Aromatic esters
Elastase	Pancreas	Neutral aliphatic esters
Enteropeptidase	Intestinal mucosa	Trypsinogen → trypsin
Exopeptidases		
Carboxypeptidases	Pancreas	Carboxy-terminal amino acids
Aminopeptidases	Intestinal mucosa	Amino-terminal amino acids
Tripeptidases	Mucosal brush border	Tripeptides
Dipeptidases	Mucosal brush border	Dipeptides

The first enzymes to act on dietary proteins are the endopeptidases: pepsin in the gastric juice and trypsin, chymotrypsin, and elastase in the small intestine. (The different specificities of trypsin, chymotrypsin, and elastase are discussed in Section 2.2.1.) The result of the combined action of the endopeptidases is that the large protein molecules are broken down into smaller polypeptides with a large number of amino and carboxyl terminals for the exopeptidases to act on. There are two classes of exopeptidase:

- *Carboxypeptidases,* secreted in the pancreatic juice, release amino acids from the free carboxyl terminal of peptides.
- *Aminopeptidases,* secreted by the intestinal mucosal cells, release amino acids from the amino terminal of peptides.

Both amino- and carboxypeptidases continue to act until the final product is a di- or tripeptide, which is hydrolyzed by di- and tripeptidases inside the mucosal cell.

4.4.3.1 *Activation of zymogens of proteolytic enzymes*

The proteases are secreted as inactive precursors (zymogens)—this is essential if they are not to digest themselves and tissue proteins before they are secreted. In each case, the active site of the enzyme is masked by a small region of the peptide chain that has to be removed for the enzyme to have activity. This is achieved by hydrolysis of a specific peptide bond in the precursor molecule, releasing the blocking peptide and revealing the active site of the enzyme.

Pepsin is secreted in the gastric juice as pepsinogen, which is activated by the action of gastric acid, and also by the action of already activated pepsin. In the small intestine, trypsinogen, the precursor of trypsin, is activated by the action of a specific enzyme, enteropeptidase (sometimes known by its obsolete name of enterokinase), which is secreted by the duodenal epithelial cells; trypsin can then activate chymotrypsinogen to chymotrypsin, proelastase to elastase, procarboxypeptidase to carboxypeptidase, and proaminopeptidase to aminopeptidase.

4.4.3.2 Absorption of the products of protein digestion

The end product of the action of endopeptidases and exopeptidases is a mixture of free amino acids, di- and tripeptides, and oligopeptides.

Free amino acids are absorbed across the intestinal mucosa by sodium-dependent active transport, as occurs in the absorption of glucose and galactose (Figure 4.9). There are a number of different amino acid transport systems, with specificity for the chemical nature of the side chain (large or small neutral, acidic, or basic). Similar group-specific amino acid transporters occur in the renal tubules (for reabsorption of amino acids filtered at the glomerulus) and for uptake of amino acids into tissues. The various amino acids carried by any one transporter compete with each other for absorption and tissue uptake.

Dipeptides and tripeptides enter the brush border of the intestinal mucosal cells, where they are hydrolyzed to free amino acids, which are then transported into the bloodstream. Patients with (rare) genetic defects of one or other of the amino acid transporters can still absorb dipeptides and so have a (limited) dietary source of all the amino acids (see Problem 4.3).

Relatively large peptides can be absorbed intact, either by uptake into mucosal epithelial cells (the transcellular route) or by passing between epithelial cells (the paracellular route). These peptides may be large enough to stimulate antibody production; this is the basis of allergic reactions to foods. In infants, there is greater absorption of intact small proteins and oligopeptides than in adults; this permits the infant to gain passive immunity by absorbing immunoglobulins in breast milk. However, it also means that early exposure to foreign proteins can result in the development of food allergy; cow's milk, egg, and peanut proteins are common food allergens.

4.5 The absorption of vitamins and minerals

In addition to compounds that enter the small intestine from the diet, a number of vitamins and other compounds are secreted in the bile, then reabsorbed from the small intestine—a process of enterohepatic circulation. For example, the total amount of cholesterol entering the gut is some four-to fivefold higher than the dietary intake, so that inhibition of cholesterol absorption has a considerably greater effect than might be expected (Figure 4.15). Folate and vitamin B_{12} undergo similar enterohepatic circulation. In the case of vitamin B_{12}, this serves to remove degradation products and metabolites that have antivitamin activity, since the intestinal binding protein that is required for vitamin B_{12} absorption (intrinsic factor; Section 4.5.2.1) binds only biologically active vitamin B_{12} and none of its analogs.

4.5.1 Absorption of lipid-soluble vitamins and cholesterol

Absorption of the lipid-soluble vitamins (A, D, E, and K) depends on an adequate total amount of fat in the diet, because they are absorbed dissolved in the core of lipid micelles and then incorporated into chylomicrons together with reesterified fatty acids (Section 4.3.2.2). Vitamins D and E and carotenes are absorbed passively by diffusion. Vitamin A enters enterocytes by carrier-mediated transport followed by esterification to permit accumulation; when the carrier is saturated, there is also passive uptake of the vitamin. Vitamin K is transported into enterocytes by an ATP-dependent transporter.

Cholesterol enters enterocytes by carrier-mediated transport. Plant sterols and stanols (Figure 4.13) compete with cholesterol for the transport protein, thus reducing the absorption of both dietary cholesterol and that secreted in the bile. They also inhibit the esterification of cholesterol; any unesterified cholesterol in the enterocyte, as well as unesterified plant sterols and stanols, is actively transported out of the enterocyte back into the intestinal lumen by an ATP-binding transport protein (Section 3.2.2.5).

4.5.2 Absorption of water-soluble vitamins

The absorption of water-soluble vitamins requires a transport protein at the luminal surface of the mucosal cell; this may involve active or passive transport, and may be followed by metabolic trapping (Section 3.2.2.2) to permit accumulation. In some cases, active transport is involved in the efflux of the vitamin from the enterocyte into the bloodstream.

Thiamin (vitamin B_1; Section 11.6) enters the enterocyte by active transport via a proton-pumping ATPase. Some is phosphorylated intracellularly, and there is Na^+-dependent active transport into the bloodstream. The active transport of thiamin out of the enterocyte into the bloodstream is inhibited by alcohol, which, together with a poor diet, explains the relatively common occurrence of thiamin deficiency in alcoholics and heavy drinkers (see Problem 5.2).

Riboflavin (vitamin B_2; Section 11.7) enters the enterocyte by Na^+-dependent active transport, followed by metabolic trapping as riboflavin monophosphate.

The niacin vitamers, nicotinic acid and nicotinamide (Section 11.8), enter the enterocyte by Na^+-dependent active transport.

Vitamin B_6 (Section 11.9) enters the enterocyte by carrier-mediated passive transport, followed by metabolic trapping as pyridoxal phosphate. However, much is dephosphorylated by alkaline phosphatase at the serosal surface of the cell, so that it is mainly pyridoxal rather than pyridoxal phosphate that enters the bloodstream.

Dietary folate (Section 11.11) is a mixture of derivatives with different lengths of a poly-γ-glutamyl side chain. In the intestinal lumen, the side chain is removed by conjugase (a zinc-dependent enzyme), and folate monoglutamate enters the enterocyte by carrier-mediated passive uptake, followed by reduction and methylation, so that what enters the bloodstream is mainly methyl-tetrahydrofolate.

Despite their very different structures, biotin (Section 11.12) and pantothenic acid (Section 11.13) enter the enterocyte using the same Na^+-dependent active transport protein.

Vitamin C (Section 11.14) enters the enterocyte by Na^+-dependent active transport. This transport protein is found elsewhere in the gastrointestinal tract, and a modest amount of vitamin C can be absorbed in the mouth.

4.5.2.1 Absorption of vitamin B_{12}

Very small amounts of vitamin B_{12} (Section 11.10) can be absorbed by passive diffusion across the intestinal mucosa, but under normal conditions this is insignificant, accounting for less than 1% of a large oral dose; the major route of vitamin B_{12} absorption is by way of attachment to a specific binding protein in the intestinal lumen. This binding protein is "intrinsic factor," so called because in the early studies of pernicious anemia (Section 11.10.2), it was found that two curative factors were involved—an extrinsic or dietary factor, which we now know to be vitamin B_{12}, and an intrinsic or endogenously produced factor. Intrinsic factor is a small glycoprotein secreted by the parietal cells of the gastric mucosa, which also secrete hydrochloric acid.

Both gastric acid and pepsin have a role in vitamin B_{12} absorption, serving to release the vitamin from the proteins it is bound to in foods. Atrophic gastritis is a relatively common problem of advancing age; in the early stages there is impaired acid secretion but more or less normal secretion of intrinsic factor. This can result in vitamin B_{12} depletion due to failure to release the vitamin from dietary proteins, but the absorption of free vitamin B_{12} (as in nutritional supplements) is unaffected. Inhibition of gastric acid secretion to treat gastric ulcers and hiatus hernia will also impair the release of vitamin B_{12} from dietary proteins, but there is no evidence that even prolonged use of the proton pump inhibiting drugs results in vitamin B_{12} deficiency.

In the stomach, vitamin B_{12} binds to cobalophilin, a binding protein secreted in the saliva. Cobalophilin is hydrolyzed in the duodenum, releasing the vitamin B_{12} for binding to intrinsic factor. Pancreatic insufficiency can therefore be a factor in the development of vitamin B_{12} deficiency, since failure to hydrolyze cobalophilin will result in the excretion of cobalophilin-bound vitamin B_{12} rather than transfer to intrinsic factor. Intrinsic factor binds biologically active vitamin B_{12}, but not analogs that have no biological activity. Considerably more intrinsic factor is normally secreted than is needed for the binding and absorption of dietary vitamin B_{12}, which requires only about 1% of the total intrinsic factor available.

Vitamin B_{12} is absorbed from the distal third of the ileum by receptor-mediated endocytosis. There are intrinsic factor–vitamin B_{12} binding sites on the brush border of the mucosal cells in this region; free intrinsic factor does not interact with these receptors. The absorption of vitamin B_{12} is limited by the number of binding sites in the ileal mucosa, so that not more than about 1–1.5 μg of a single oral dose of the vitamin is absorbed.

Within the mucosal cell, the vitamin is released by lysosomal proteolysis of intrinsic factor, and is bound to transcobalamin II, a binding protein synthesized in the enterocytes, and stored in vesicles destined for export from the cell. In plasma, vitamin B_{12} circulates bound to transcobalamin I, which is required for tissue uptake of the vitamin, and transcobalamin II, which seems to be a storage form of the vitamin.

There is a considerable enterohepatic circulation of vitamin B_{12}. Vitamin B_{12} and its metabolites (some of which are biologically inactive) are transferred from peripheral tissues to the liver bound to transcobalamin III. They are then secreted into the bile, bound to cobalophilins; 3–8 μg of vitamin B_{12} may be secreted in the bile each day, about the same as the average dietary intake. Like dietary vitamin B_{12} bound to salivary cobalophilin, the biliary cobalophilins are hydrolyzed in the duodenum, and the vitamin binds to intrinsic factor, thereby permitting reabsorption in the ileum. While cobalophilins and transcorrin III have low specificity, and will bind a variety of vitamin B_{12} analogs, intrinsic factor binds only cobalamins, and thus only the biologically active vitamin will be reabsorbed to any significant extent.

4.5.3 Absorption of minerals

Mineral ions require a transport protein at the luminal surface of the mucosal cell and are accumulated inside the mucosal cell by binding to intracellular proteins. Transfer from mucosal cells into the bloodstream is usually by ATP-dependent active transport (Section 3.2.2.4), commonly onto a plasma-binding protein. Genetic defects of the intracellular binding proteins or the active transport systems at the basal membrane of the mucosal cell can result in deficiency despite an apparently adequate intake of the mineral (see Problem 4.4).

The absorption of calcium is dependent on vitamin D (Section 11.3). Synthesis of calbindin, the intracellular binding protein that is required for accumulation of calcium, requires the nuclear action of vitamin D, so that when vitamin D-deficient animals are repleted with the vitamin there is a significant time lag before calcium absorption increases.

The calcium transport protein only migrates from intracellular vesicles to the cell surface, to permit uptake of calcium, in response to rapid (cell-surface receptor-mediated) actions of vitamin D.

The absorption of many minerals is affected by other compounds present in the intestinal lumen. Reducing compounds can enhance the absorption of iron (Section 4.5.3.1), and chelating compounds enhance the absorption of other minerals. For example, zinc absorption is dependent on the secretion by the pancreas of a zinc-binding ligand (tentatively identified as the tryptophan metabolite picolinic acid). Failure to synthesize and secrete this zinc-binding ligand as a result of a genetic disease leads to the condition of acrodermatitis enteropathica—functional zinc deficiency despite an apparently adequate intake.

Diets based on unleavened wheat bread contain a relatively large amount of phytic acid (inositol hexaphosphate), which can bind calcium, iron, and zinc to form insoluble complexes that are not absorbed. Phytases in yeast catalyze dephosphorylation of phytate to products that do not chelate the minerals. Polyphenols (Section 6.6.2.3), especially tannic acid in tea, can also chelate iron and other minerals, reducing their absorption, and large amounts of free fatty acids in the gut lumen (associated with defects of fat absorption, Section 4.3.2) can impair the absorption of calcium and magnesium, by forming insoluble soaps.

4.5.3.1 Iron absorption

Only about 10%–15% of total dietary iron is absorbed, depending on the state of body iron reserves, and as little as 1%–5% of the inorganic iron in plant foods. Heme iron in meat is better absorbed by a separate transport system (Figure 4.22).

Inorganic iron is absorbed only in the Fe^{2+} (reduced) form. This means that a variety of reducing agents present in the intestinal lumen together with dietary iron will enhance its absorption. The most effective of such compounds is vitamin C (Section 11.14.4.1); while

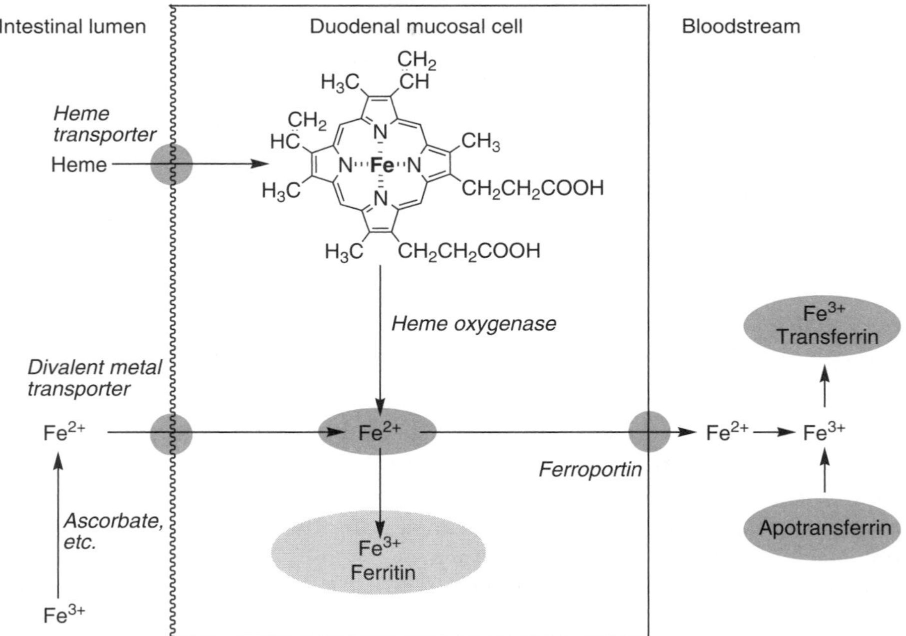

Figure 4.22 Iron absorption.

intakes of 40–100 mg/day of vitamin C are more than adequate to meet requirements, an intake of 25–50 mg/meal is sometimes recommended to enhance iron absorption. Alcohol, fructose, and a number of organic acids also enhance iron absorption.

Inorganic iron enters the mucosal cells by a proton-linked active transport mechanism, while there is a separate transporter for the uptake of heme. Heme iron is released as Fe^{2+} by the action of heme oxygenase. Iron can only leave the mucosal cell via the transport protein ferroportin, and only if there is free apotransferrin in the bloodstream to oxidize it to Fe^{3+} and bind it. The activity of ferroportin (and possibly also that of the divalent metal transporter) is downregulated by hepcidin, a peptide secreted by the liver. In response to anemia, hypoxia, or hemorrhage, hepcidin secretion is reduced and the activity of ferroportin increases, so that more iron can enter the bloodstream from the mucosal cells. Iron in the mucosal cell that is not transported out by ferroportin is oxidized to Fe^{3+} and bound to ferritin. It is then lost into the intestinal lumen when the cells are shed at the tip of the villus (section 4.1).

This mucosal barrier to the absorption of iron has a protective function. There is no pathway for excretion of iron from the body, although there are obligatory losses in shed skin and intestinal cells; thus iron reserves are controlled by regulation of intestinal absorption. About 10% of the population are genetically susceptible to iron overload (hemochromatosis). This is a serious condition, with deposition of inappropriately large amounts of iron in hemosiderin in tissues, and the accumulation of free iron ions, which generate tissue-damaging oxygen radicals (Section 6.5). The consequences of hemochromatosis include enlargement of the liver; diabetes mellitus, as a result of radical damage to pancreatic β-islet cells (because of the skin pigmentation associated with hemochromatosis, the condition is sometimes called bronze diabetes); painful inflammation of joints; heart disease; and depletion of vitamin C, leading to scurvy.

One of the reasons why women are less at risk of atherosclerosis than are men may be that women generally have a lower iron status than men, because of menstrual blood losses. This raises the interesting problem of whether or not it is desirable to recommend high intakes of iron for women of child-bearing age in order to raise their iron reserves to the same level as seen in men. This would prevent the development of iron deficiency, but might also put them at risk of iron overload and increased risk of atherosclerosis.

Key points

- Carbohydrates provide the main source of metabolic fuel. They can be classified into three main groups: sugars (mono- and disaccharides), oligosaccharides, and polysaccharides. Starch is a nutritionally important polysaccharide; a variety of non-starch polysaccharides occur in foods, but are not digested, although they provide a substrate for intestinal bacterial fermentation.
- Dietary carbohydrates can be classified according to their glycemic index—the extent to which they raise blood glucose compared with an equivalent amount of glucose or a reference carbohydrate.
- Starch digestion begins with amylase secreted in saliva and then continues with pancreatic amylase, yielding a mixture of glucose, maltose, and isomaltose.
- Dietary disaccharides are hydrolyzed by disaccharidases in the brush border of the intestinal mucosa. Glucose and galactose are absorbed by Na^+-linked active transport; other sugars are absorbed by facilitated (passive) diffusion.

- Disaccharides that cannot be hydrolyzed because of lack of the disaccharidase, and unabsorbed monosaccharides and sugar alcohols provide a substrate for bacterial fermentation, leading to osmotic diarrhea and intestinal pain.
- Triacylglycerols contain saturated or unsaturated fatty acids esterified to glycerol; the amount of saturated, monounsaturated, and polyunsaturated fatty acids in the diet has significant health effects. *Trans* isomers of unsaturated fatty acids have adverse health effects.
- Triacylglycerols are hydrolyzed by lipase secreted by the tongue, in gastric juice, and by the pancreas, leading to liberation of free fatty acids and 2-mono-acylglycerol; this latter is hydrolyzed by pancreatic and intracellular esterases.
- The bile salts are required to complete the emulsification of dietary lipids to micelles that are small enough to be absorbed into intestinal mucosal cells.
- Within the mucosal cell, fatty acids are reesterified to triacylglycerol and packaged with proteins to form chylomicrons, which enter the lymphatic system. Peripheral tissues take up fatty acids from chylomicrons by the action of extracellular lipoprotein lipase; the liver clears chylomicron remnants.
- Proteins are polymers of amino acids; 21 amino acids are involved in protein synthesis, and others are formed by postsynthetic modification of proteins. Nine of the amino acids are dietary essentials that cannot be synthesized in the body.
- Protein digestion involves denaturation of dietary proteins by heat and the action of gastric acid, followed by the action of endopeptidases that cleave the proteins into smaller peptides, and then the action of exopeptidases that sequentially remove amino and carboxyl terminal amino acids.
- Free amino acids are absorbed by Na^+-linked active transport; di- and tripeptides are hydrolyzed inside the mucosal cell. Significant amounts of relatively large peptides can be absorbed intact; this may result in allergic reactions to foods.
- Absorption of the lipid-soluble vitamins requires an adequate amount of dietary fat.
- Water-soluble vitamins are absorbed in various ways, generally involving active transport into or out of the mucosal cell, sometimes with metabolic trapping to achieve intracellular accumulation.
- Vitamin B_{12} absorption requires gastric acid to release the vitamin from binding to dietary proteins, and specific binding proteins secreted in saliva and by the gastric mucosa. There is considerable enterohepatic cycling of vitamin B_{12}.
- The absorption of minerals generally involves active transport into and out of the mucosal cell, as well as intracellular protein binding. A variety of nonnutrient compounds present in foods (especially phytate and polyphenols) can impair the absorption of minerals.
- The absorption of iron is limited and controlled by the state of body iron reserves.

Problem 4.1: Measurement of urine glucose

Glucose in plasma and urine can be determined in two ways—using an alkaline copper reagent or using glucose oxidase linked to a dyestuff (Section 4.2.1.3). Both methods were used to determine urine glucose in six people:

A. A person with hitherto undiagnosed diabetes mellitus (Section 10.7)
B. A known diabetic, with poor glycemic control, taking supplements of 500 mg of vitamin C per day

C. A nondiabetic subject taking supplements of 500 mg of vitamin C per day
D. A person with idiopathic pentosuria (excretion of five-carbon sugars in the urine)
E. A person with idiopathic pentosuria taking supplements of 500 mg of vitamin C per day
F. A nondiabetic subject taking no supplements

Which subjects would be expected to give the following results for urine glucose tests?

- Positive using glucose oxidase, positive using alkaline copper reagent
- Positive using glucose oxidase, negative using alkaline copper reagent
- Negative using glucose oxidase, positive using alkaline copper reagent
- Negative using glucose oxidase, negative using alkaline copper reagent

Problem 4.2: Tina C

Figure 4.23 shows the results of measuring blood glucose in a group of people after a test dose of 50 g of lactose taken at 08:30, before they had eaten breakfast. The shaded area shows the range of results obtained for 10 of the subjects; the solid line marked with squares shows the results for one subject, Tina C.

Can you explain why Tina C's results were so different from the others?

About 15 min after the test dose of lactose, Tina C's developed severe abdominal pain and had frequent bouts of explosive watery diarrhea, which persisted for about 2 h. Can you account for this?

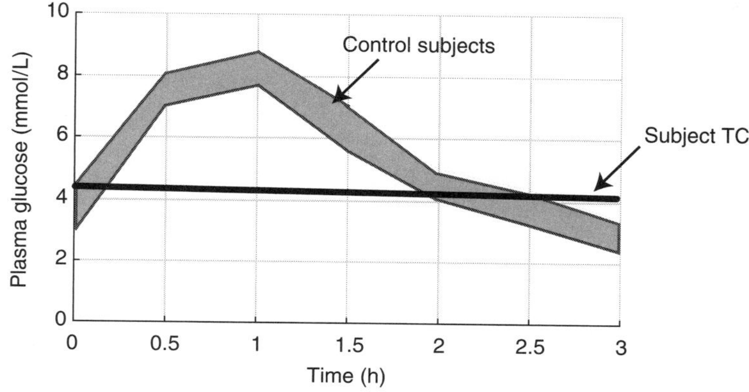

Figure 4.23 The effect on plasma glucose of a 50-g test dose of lactose.

A number of papers in gastroenterology journals have reported fatal explosions during endoscopic removal of colorectal polyps using a heated wire when the gut had been prepared for surgery using an oral dose of the sugar alcohol mannitol (Section 4.2.1.2) and it was insufflated with air. How does mannitol prepare the gut for surgery? What caused the explosions?

Very rarely, infants lack lactase, as a result of a genetic defect, and therefore are severely lactose intolerant. They cannot tolerate breast milk or normal infant formula, and have to be fed on special lactose-free formula.

Relatively commonly, people lose intestinal lactase in late adolescence or early adulthood, and become progressively lactose intolerant. Frequently, they present a history of abdominal discomfort and diarrhea. Careful questioning may reveal that this occurs especially after drinking milk, but commonly it is necessary to test their response to a test dose of lactose. As noted above, the classical method was to give a 50 g dose of lactose and measure the glycemic response—Tina C suffered considerable discomfort during this test.

A number of workers have used measurement of hydrogen in exhaled air after a small test dose of lactose, as a less unpleasant way of detecting lactose intolerance. Can you explain how measuring breath hydrogen can give information about lactose digestion?

A number of studies have been performed to determine lactose tolerance in adults from different populations; some of the results are shown in Table 4.3. What conclusions can you draw from these results?

Table 4.3 Lactose Intolerance in Different Population Groups

Population Group or Country of Study	Lactose Intolerant (%)
UK white	4.7
Northern Germany[a]	7.5
Tuareg (nomads of the central Sahara)	12.7
Western Austria[a]	15.0
Southern Germany[a]	23.0
Eastern Austria[a]	25.0
U.S. black	26.2
Turkey	71.2
Sri Lankan	72.5
Italy	75.0
Greece	75.0
South African black	78.0
Japan	89.0
Singapore-born Chinese	92.4
Canadian-born Chinese	97.9
Papua New Guinea	98.0

[a] The populations of eastern and western Austria are of different origin, as are the populations of northern and southern Germany.

Problem 4.3: Eddie H

At the age of 12, Eddie H was referred to the pediatric outpatient clinic at the Middlesex Hospital in early June, suffering from a severe sunburn-like red scaly rash on exposed areas of his skin. His mother said that she thought he was suffering from pellagra (Section 11.8.4). His older sister, now aged 20, had been treated for pellagra some 10 years ago.

At the time, he had a number of neurological signs that are not characteristic of pellagra, including unsteady gait, jerky arm movements, and intention tremor. He also showed nystagmus and complained of double vision. His mother stated that several times during childhood he had suffered similar attacks, usually associated with the common winter illnesses such as flu, measles, and mumps. He had always made a complete recovery after such attacks, which had not been associated with the pellagra-like rash.

A diet history showed that Eddie had a normal, and apparently adequate, intake of tryptophan and niacin. Therefore, dietary deficiency seemed improbable.

Chromatography revealed excretion of a number of amino acids in his urine, with abnormally high concentrations of tryptophan, phenylalanine, tyrosine, leucine, isoleucine, and valine. His urine also contained relatively high concentrations of a number of indolic compounds, including indoxyl sulfate (indican), indolyllactate, indolylacetate, indolylacetamide, and indolylacetylglutamine, which are not detectable in the urine of normal subjects.

Figure 4.24 shows the effect on Eddie's plasma tryptophan of giving him an oral or intravenous dose of 0.5 mmol tryptophan per kilogram body weight, or an equivalent amount of tryptophanyl-glycine by mouth. What conclusions can you draw from this information?

Problem 4.4: Michael M

Michael is the second child of unrelated parents who are farmers in Sussex. His older sister, now aged 6, is fit and well, with no history of anything other than the usual childhood infections.

After an uneventful pregnancy, Michael weighed 2.8 kg at birth (just above the 5th centile; median birth weight is 3.5 kg). He was a slow developer, achieving the usual milestones considerably later than his sister did, and later than most of his mother's friends' children.

Since the age of 4 months he has suffered occasional convulsive seizures. He has been seen three times at his local hospital's Accident and Emergency Department with broken limbs (twice an arm and once a leg). The frequency of these broken limbs raised a suspicion that they may not be accidental, and his family was investigated by a social worker for possible physical abuse, although at no time was there any evidence of widespread bruising or other injuries. There is no evidence that his parents are other than loving and caring, and no evidence that his injuries were not indeed accidental.

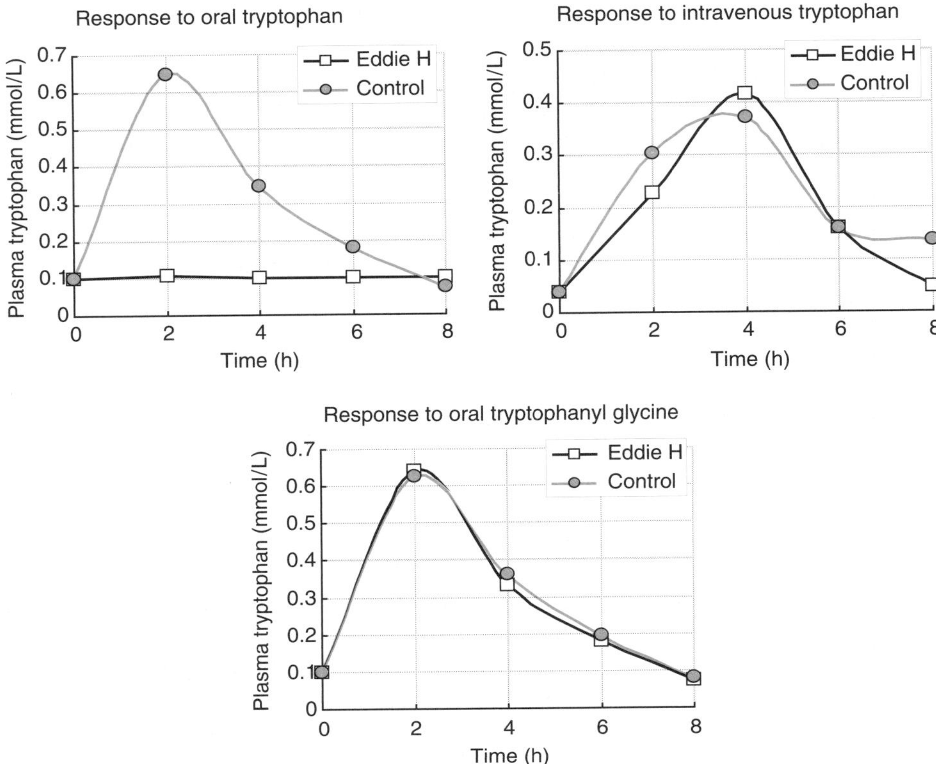

Figure 4.24 The response of plasma tryptophan to 0.5 mmol oral or intravenous tryptophan/kg body weight, and to an oral dose of 0.5 mmol/kg body weight tryptophanyl-glycine dipeptide. (From data reported by Baron, D.N. et al., *Lancet*, ii, 421–428, 1956.)

Michael's father is the youngest of five; both of his brothers and both sisters are married with families. Altogether he has 8 nieces and 9 nephews, aged between 5 and 17, all of whom are fit and healthy. Michael's mother has three sisters, but her two brothers died before they were 3 years old; both death certificates recorded aortic rupture as the cause of death. She remembers that she had three elderly aunts on her mother's side, but no surviving uncles; there had been two brothers, but they had died as infants. On her father's side she had four uncles and one aunt. One of his mother's sisters is married with two healthy daughters.

The most striking feature about Michael was his hair, which was short, tangled, grey, and fragile. His mother said that it could not be grown long as it always broke when she brushed it, and his hairbrush was regularly clogged with broken hairs.

As a young man, Michael's father spent some years on a sheep farm in Tasmania. He remembered that they had had a problem with their wool, which was unsaleable because it was matted and brittle; eventually the problem was traced down to copper deficiency, and use of copper-containing fertilizers on the pasture cured the problem. Therefore, he had tried giving Michael a copper supplement, bought from a health food store, when he was about 18 months old. After 3 months, when the condition of his hair had not improved, the copper supplements were discontinued.

At 2½ years of age, Michael suffered from another convulsive seizure and was admitted to UCL Hospital. Preliminary examination showed a sickly child, obviously mentally retarded. He was 85 cm tall (median height at age 2½ = 90 cm, 5th centile = 87 cm, 95th centile = 97 cm) and weighed 10.5 kg (median = 13.3 kg, 5th centile = 11.4 kg, 95th centile = 16 kg).

Routine clinical chemistry and hematology revealed:

- No abnormalities of plasma enzymes
- Normal plasma electrolytes
- Normal blood clotting (i.e., a normal prothrombin time)
- No evidence of anemia
- A normal differential leukocyte count

Amino acid analysis of a sample of Michael's hair after acid hydrolysis showed that cysteine made up 7.4% of the total (in control subjects the range was 0.86 ± 0.11), while cystine was only 11.4% of the total (compared with a control range of 17.3 ± 1.7). There were no significant differences in any of the other amino acids that were measured.

Because Michael's father referred to the similarity between the appearance of his son's hair and the wool of copper-deficient sheep, his plasma copper was also determined and was found to be 3 μmol/L (95% reference range for infants is 11–24 μmol/L).

Although it seemed unlikely, since it is extremely rare, nutritional copper deficiency was suspected. Therefore, copper was determined on a finger-prick blood sample taken daily over the next week; during which he received an oral dose of 2 mg copper sulfate each day (the reference nutrient intake for copper for a child of 2–4 years is 0.6 mg/day). There was no increase in his plasma concentration of copper.

Unfortunately, while still a patient in UCL Hospital, Michael died; *postmortem* examination revealed that he had died from rupture of the aorta.

What conclusions can you draw from these results?

Problem 4.5: Andrew S

Andrew is 13 years old and has xanthomas (deposits of cholesterol and other lipids) on the tendons of his hands, Achilles tendon, and in various parts of his body under the skin. He also suffers from angina on moderate exercise. His older brother was similarly affected and died at the age of 18 from a heart attack; *postmortem* examination showed that he had very severe atherosclerosis.

Gas–liquid chromatography of serum sterols showed that his total serum cholesterol was at the lower end of the normal range (4 mmol/L). However, his serum also contained 0.7 mmol/L β-sitosterol (Figure 4.13) and 0.2 mmol/L campesterol (another plant sterol), neither of which is normally found in more than trace amounts in serum. About 60% of the β-sitosterol and campesterol was esterified, and 80% of the plant sterols were found in low density lipoprotein.

Analysis of the lipids in red cell membranes showed that about 13% of the total sterols were plant sterols; normally these would not be present in cell membranes to any significant extent. Biopsy of one of the subcutaneous xanthomas showed that in addition to a normal amount of cholesterol, it contained a large amount of unesterified β-sitosterol and campesterol.

After a test dose of β-sitosterol his serum concentration rose sharply; cannulation of his bile duct showed that his bile contained very much less cholesterol than normal, and almost no β-sitosterol or other plant sterols. In normal subjects given a test dose of β-sitosterol little appears in plasma, and what is absorbed is rapidly excreted in bile.

Studies of whole-body cholesterol turnover suggested that his rate of cholesterol synthesis was about 60% of normal, and the rate of cholesterol synthesis from [^{14}C]acetate in freshly isolated mononuclear leukocytes was about half that seen in control subjects. This was due to low activity of hydroxymethylglutaryl CoA (HMG CoA) reductase (the rate-limiting enzyme of cholesterol synthesis). Immunoassay showed that there was less of the enzyme protein present than normal, and northern blotting showed that there was only about half the normal amount of HMG CoA mRNA present in the cells.

What conclusions can you draw from these results?

chapter five

Energy nutrition—the metabolism of carbohydrates and fats

If the intake of metabolic fuels is equivalent to energy expenditure, there is a state of energy balance. Overall, there will be equal periods of fed state metabolism (during which nutrient reserves are accumulated as liver and muscle glycogen, adipose tissue triacylglycerols, and labile protein stores), and fasting state metabolism, during which these reserves are utilized. Averaged out over several days, there will be no change in body weight or body composition.

By contrast, if the intake of metabolic fuels is greater than is required to meet energy expenditure, the body will spend more time in the fed state than the fasting state; there will be more accumulation of nutrient reserves than utilization. The result of this is an increase in body size, and especially an increase in adipose tissue stores. If continued for long enough, this will result in overweight or obesity, with potentially serious health consequences (Chapter 7).

The opposite state of affairs is when the intake of metabolic fuels is lower than is required to meet energy expenditure. Now the body has to mobilize its nutrient reserves and overall spends more time in the fasting state than in the fed state. The result of this is undernutrition, starvation, and eventually death (Chapter 8).

Objectives

After reading this chapter you should be able to

- Define the terms used in energy metabolism and explain how energy expenditure is measured
- Describe the sources of metabolic fuels in the fed and fasting states
- Describe and explain the relationship between energy intake, energy expenditure, and body weight
- Describe the pathway of glycolysis and explain how anaerobic glycolysis under conditions of maximum exertion leads to oxygen debt
- Describe the pentose phosphate pathway and explain how deficiency of glucose 6-phosphate dehydrogenase results in hemolytic crisis
- Describe the metabolic fates of pyruvate arising from glycolysis
- Describe the citric acid cycle and explain how it acts both as a central energy-yielding pathway and also for interconversion of metabolites
- Explain the importance of carnitine in fatty acid uptake into mitochondria and describe the β-oxidation of fatty acids
- Describe the formation and utilization of ketone bodies and explain their importance in fasting and starvation
- Describe the synthesis of fatty acids and triacylglycerol as a major energy reserve
- Describe the roles of plasma lipoproteins in transport of lipids
- Describe the synthesis and utilization of glycogen and the pathways for gluconeogenesis in the fasting state

5.1 Estimation of energy expenditure

Energy expenditure can be determined directly by measuring heat output from the body. This requires a thermally insulated chamber, in which the temperature can be controlled so as to maintain the subject's comfort, and in which it is possible to measure the amount of heat produced, for example, by the increase in temperature of the water used to cool the chamber. Calorimeters of this sort are relatively small, so that it is possible for measurements of direct heat production to be made only for subjects performing a limited range of tasks, and only for a relatively short time. Most estimates of energy expenditure are based on indirect measurements—either measurement of oxygen consumption and carbon dioxide production (indirect calorimetry; Section 5.1.1) or indirect assessment of carbon dioxide production by use of dual isotopically labeled water (Section 5.1.2). From the results of a number of studies in which energy expenditure in different activities has been measured, it is possible to calculate total energy expenditure from the time spent in each type of activity (Section 5.1.3.2).

5.1.1 Indirect calorimetry and the respiratory quotient

Energy expenditure can be determined from the rate of consumption of oxygen. This is known as indirect calorimetry since there is no direct measurement of the heat produced. There is an output or expenditure of approximately 20 kJ for each liter of oxygen consumed, regardless of whether the fuel being metabolized is carbohydrate, fat, or protein (Table 5.1). Measurement of oxygen consumption is quite simple using a spirometer. Such instruments are portable, and so people can carry on more or less normal activities for several hours at a time, while their energy expenditure is being estimated.

Measurement of both oxygen consumption and carbon dioxide production at the same time provides information on the mixture of metabolic fuels being metabolized. In the metabolism of carbohydrates, the same amount of carbon dioxide is produced as the amount of oxygen consumed, that is, the ratio of carbon dioxide produced to oxygen consumed (the respiratory quotient, RQ) is 1.0. This is because the overall reaction is $C_6H_{12}O_6 + 6O_2 \rightarrow 6CO_2 + 6H_2O$.

Proportionally more oxygen is required for the oxidation of fat. The major process involved is the oxidation of $-CH_2-$ units: $-CH_2 + 1\frac{1}{2}O_2 \rightarrow CO_2 + H_2O$. Allowing for the fact that in triacylglycerols there are also the glycerol and three carboxyl groups to be considered, overall the RQ for the oxidation of fat is 0.7.

The oxidation of amino acids arising from proteins gives an RQ of 0.8. The amount of protein being oxidized can be determined separately by measuring the excretion of urea, the end product of amino acid metabolism (Section 9.3.1.4).

Measurement of the respiratory quotient and urinary excretion of urea thus permits calculation of the relative amounts of fat, carbohydrate, and protein being metabolized. In the fasting state (Section 5.3.2), when a relatively large amount of fat is being used as fuel, the RQ is around 0.8–0.85; after a meal, when there is more carbohydrate available to be

Table 5.1 Oxygen Consumption and Carbon Dioxide Production in Oxidation of Metabolic Fuels

	Energy Yield (kJ/g)	Oxygen Consumed (L/g)	Carbon Dioxide Produced (L/g)	Respiratory Quotient (CO_2/O_2)	Energy/Oxygen Consumption (kJ/L Oxygen)
Carbohydrate	16	0.829	0.829	1.0	
Protein	17	0.966	0.782	0.809	~20
Fat	37	2.016	1.427	0.707	

metabolized (Section 5.3.1), the RQ rises to about 0.9–1.0. If there is a significant amount of lipid being synthesized from carbohydrate (Section 5.6.1), then the RQ may rise above 1.0.

5.1.2 Long-term measurement of energy expenditure—the dual isotopically labeled water method

Measurement of oxygen consumption only permits measurement of energy expenditure over a period of a few hours. An alternative technique permits estimation of total energy expenditure over a period of 1–2 weeks, by giving a dose of dual isotopically labeled water, $^{2}H_2{}^{18}O$, and determining the rate of loss of the isotopes from body water.

The deuterium (^{2}H) is lost from the body only in water. However, the labeled oxygen (^{18}O) can be lost in either water or carbon dioxide because of the rapid equilibrium between carbon dioxide and bicarbonate: $H_2O + CO_2 \rightleftharpoons H^+ + HCO_3^-$. This means that the rate of loss of ^{18}O is faster than that of ^{2}H (Figure 5.1). The difference between the rates of loss of the two isotopes from body water (plasma, saliva, or urine) thus reflects the total amount of carbon dioxide that has been produced:

$$CO_2 \text{ production} = (0.5 \times \text{total body water}) \times (k_O - k_H)$$

where k_O is the rate constant for loss of label from ^{18}O, and k_H the rate constant for loss of label from ^{2}H.

Estimating the average RQ over the period from the proportions of fat, carbohydrate, and protein in the diet, and allowing for any changes in body fat, permit calculation of the total amount of oxygen that has been consumed, and hence the total energy expenditure over a period of 2–3 weeks. This technique thus provides a noninvasive way of estimating energy expenditure over several days in normal activities.

5.1.3 Calculation of energy expenditure

Key terms in energy metabolism are defined in Table 5.2. Energy expenditure depends on the following:

- The requirement for maintenance of normal body structure, function, and metabolic integrity—the basal metabolic rate (BMR) (Section 5.1.3.1)

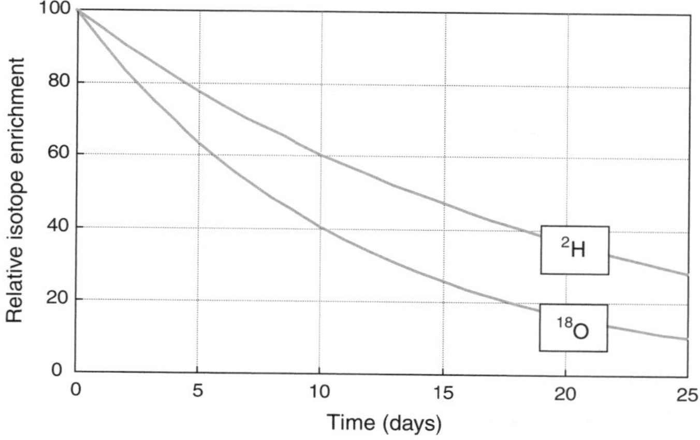

Figure 5.1 The estimation of energy expenditure using dual isotopically labeled water ($^{2}H_2{}^{18}O$).

Table 5.2 Definitions in Energy Metabolism

BMR	Basal metabolic rate	Energy expenditure in the postabsorptive state; measured under standardized conditions of thermal neutrality (environmental temperature 26°C–30°C), awake but completely at rest
RMR	Resting metabolic rate	Energy expenditure at rest, not measured under strictly standardized conditions
PAR	Physical activity ratio	Energy cost of physical activity, on a minute-by-minute basis, expressed as ratio of BMR
IEI	Integrated energy index	Energy cost of an activity over a period of time, including time spent pausing or resting, expressed as the average (integrated) value over the time, as a ratio of BMR
PAL	Physical activity level	Sum of PAR or IEI multiplied by time spent in each activity over 24 h, expressed as ratio of BMR
DIT	Diet-induced thermogenesis	Increased energy expenditure after a meal
TEE	Total energy expenditure	PAL × BMR (+ DIT)

- The energy required for work and physical activity (Section 5.1.3.2)
- The energy cost of synthesizing reserves of fat and glycogen as well as the increase in protein synthesis in the fed state (Section 5.1.3.3)

5.1.3.1 Basal metabolic rate

BMR is the energy expenditure by the body when at rest, but not asleep, under controlled conditions of thermal neutrality, and about 12 h after the last meal. It is the energy requirement for the maintenance of metabolic integrity, nerve and muscle tone, circulation, and respiration (see Figure 1.2 for the contribution of different organs to resting energy expenditure). It is important that the subject is awake, since some people show an increased metabolic rate (and hence increased heat output) when they are asleep, while others have a reduced metabolic rate and a slight fall in body temperature. Where the measurement of metabolic rate has been made under less strictly controlled conditions, the result is more correctly called the resting metabolic rate.

BMR depends on body weight, age, and gender (Figure 5.2):

- Body weight affects BMR because there is a greater amount of metabolically active tissue in a larger body.
- The decrease in BMR with increasing age is due to changes in body composition. With increasing age, even if body weight remains constant, there is loss of muscle and replacement by adipose tissue, which is metabolically less active since 80% of the weight of adipose tissue consists of reserves of triacylglycerol.
- Women have a significantly lower BMR than men of the same weight, because the proportion of body weight that is adipose tissue reserves in lean women is higher than in men (Figure 5.3 and Section 7.1.2).

5.1.3.2 Energy costs of physical activity

The most useful way of expressing the energy cost of physical activities is as a multiple of BMR. The physical activity ratio (PAR) for an activity is the ratio of the energy expended while performing the activity to that expended at rest (= BMR). Very gentle, sedentary

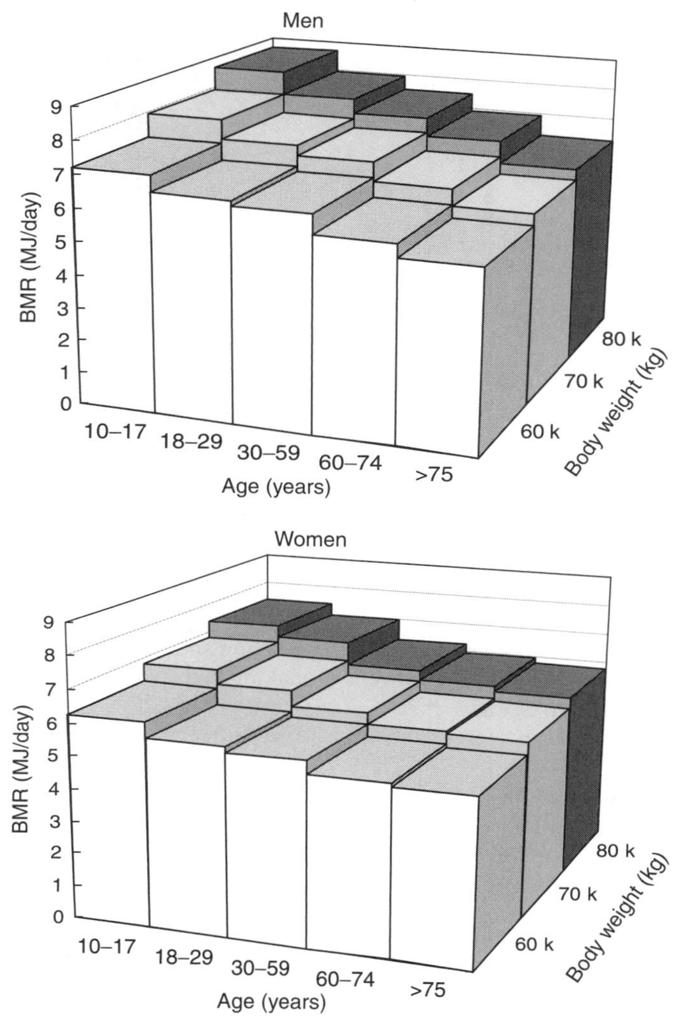

Figure 5.2 The effects of age and gender on basal metabolic rate.

activities use only about 1.1–1.2 × BMR. By contrast, vigorous exertion, such as climbing stairs or walking uphill, may use 6–8 × BMR.

Using data such as those in Table 5.3 and allowing for the time spent during each type of activity through the day permits calculation of an individual's physical activity level (PAL)—the sum of the PAR of each activity performed multiplied by the time spent in that activity. A desirable level of physical activity, in terms of cardiovascular and respiratory health, is a PAL of 1.7.

Table 5.4 shows the classification of different types of occupational work by PAR. This is the average PAR during the 8 h working day and makes no allowance for leisure activities. From these figures, it might seem that there would be no problem in achieving the desirable PAL of 1.7. However, in Britain the average PAL is only 1.4, and the desirable level of 1.7 is achieved by only 22% of men and 13% of women.

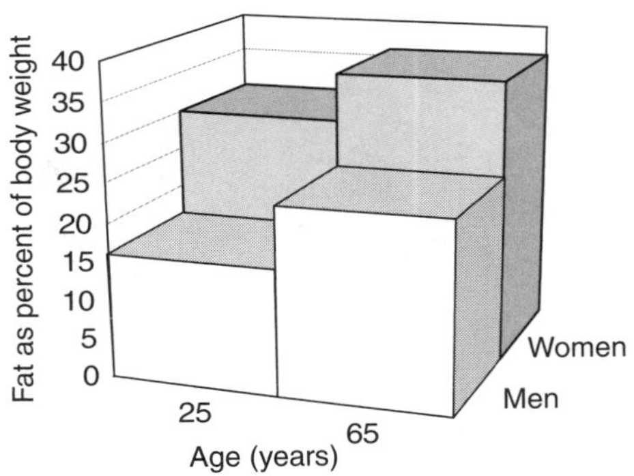

Figure 5.3 Body fat as a percentage of weight with age and gender.

Table 5.3 Physical Activity Ratios in Different Types of Activity

PAR	
1.0–1.4	Lying, standing, or sitting at rest, e.g., watching TV, reading, writing, eating, playing cards, board games
1.5–1.8	*Sitting*: sewing, knitting, playing piano, driving *Standing*: preparing vegetables, washing dishes, ironing, general office, laboratory work
1.9–2.4	*Standing*: mixed household chores, cooking, playing snooker or bowls
2.5–3.3	*Standing*: dressing, undressing, showering, making beds, vacuum cleaning *Walking*: 3–4 km/h, playing cricket *Occupational*: tailoring, shoemaking, electrical and machine tool industry, painting, decorating
3.4 – 4.4	*Standing*: mopping floors, gardening, cleaning windows, table tennis, sailing *Walking*: 4–6 km/h, playing golf *Occupational*: motor vehicle repairs, carpentry and joinery, chemical industry, bricklaying
4.5–5.9	*Standing*: polishing furniture, chopping wood, heavy gardening, volley ball *Walking*: 6–7 km/h *Exercise*: dancing, moderate swimming, gentle cycling, slow jogging *Occupational*: laboring, hoeing, road construction, digging and shoveling, felling trees
6.0–7.9	*Walking*: uphill with load or cross-country, climbing stairs *Exercise*: jogging, cycling, energetic swimming, skiing, tennis, football

The energy cost of physical activity is obviously affected by body weight, because more energy is required to move a heavier body. Figure 5.4 shows the effects of body weight on BMR and total energy expenditure at different levels of physical activity. Table 5.5 shows estimated average energy requirements at different ages, assuming average body weight and, for adults, the average PAL of 1.4 × BMR.

5.1.3.3 *Diet-induced thermogenesis*

There is a considerable increase in metabolic rate after a meal. A small part of this is the energy cost of secreting digestive enzymes and the active transport of the products of digestion (Section 3.2.2). The major part is the energy cost of synthesizing reserves of glycogen (Section 5.6.3) and triacylglycerol (Section 5.6.1), as well as the increased protein synthesis that occurs in the fed state (Section 9.2.3.3).

The cost of synthesizing glycogen from glucose is about 5% of the ingested energy, while the cost of synthesizing triacylglycerol from glucose is about 20% of the ingested

Table 5.4 Classification of Types of Occupational Work by Physical Activity Ratio

Work Intensity	PAR[a]	
Light	1.7	Professional, clerical and technical workers, administrative and managerial staff, sales representatives, housewives
Moderate	2.2–2.7	Sales staff, domestic service, students, transport workers, joiners, roofing workers
Moderately heavy	2.3–3.0	Machine operators, laborers, agricultural workers, bricklaying, masonry
Heavy	2.8–3.8	Laborers, agricultural workers, bricklaying, masonry where there is little or no mechanization

Note: Figures show the average PAR through 8 h working day, excluding leisure activities.
[a]Where a range of PAR is shown, the lower figure is for women and the higher for men.

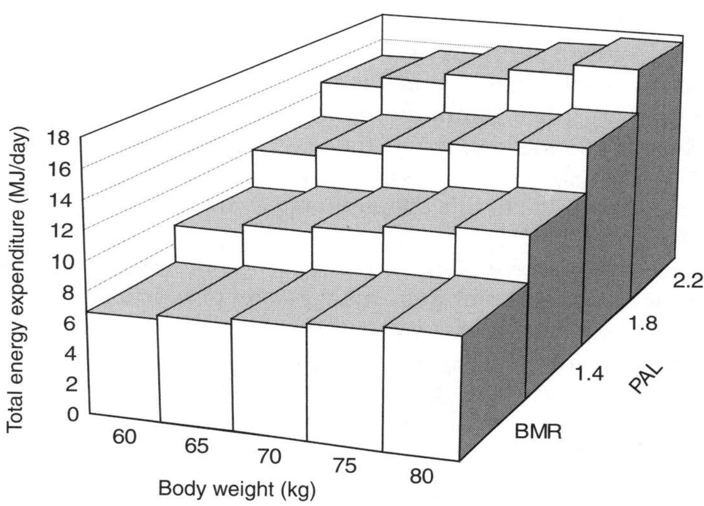

Figure 5.4 The effects of weight and physical activity on total energy expenditure.

Table 5.5 Average Requirements for Energy Based on Average Weights

Age (years)	Males (MJ/day)	Females (MJ/day)
1–3	5.2	4.9
4–6	7.2	6.5
7–10	8.2	7.3
11–14	9.3	7.9
15–18	11.5	8.8
Adults	10.6	8.0

Note: Assuming PAL = 1.4 for adults.

energy. Depending on the relative amounts of fat and carbohydrate in the diet, and the amounts of triacylglycerol and glycogen being synthesized, diet-induced thermogenesis may account for 10% or more of the total energy yield of a meal.

5.2 Energy balance and changes in body weight

When energy intake is greater than expenditure (positive energy balance), there is increased storage of surplus metabolic fuel, largely as triacylglycerol in adipose tissue; similarly, if energy intake is inadequate to meet expenditure (negative energy balance), adipose tissue triacylglycerol reserves are utilized.

Adipose tissue contains 80% triacylglycerol (with an energy yield of 37 kJ/g) and 5% protein (energy yield of 17 kJ/g); the remaining 15% is water. Hence, adipose tissue reserves are equivalent to approximately 30 kJ/g or 30 MJ/kg. This means that the theoretical change in body weight is 33 g/MJ energy imbalance per day, or 230 g/MJ energy imbalance per week. On this basis, it is possible to calculate that even during total starvation, a person with an energy expenditure of 10 MJ/day would lose only 330 g body weight per day or 2.3 kg/week.

This calculation suggests that there will be a constant change of body weight with a constant excessive or deficient energy intake, but this is not observed in practice. The rate of weight gain in positive energy balance is never as great as would be predicted and gradually slows down, so that after a time the subject regains energy balance, albeit with a higher body weight (Figure 5.5). Similarly, in negative energy balance, weight is not lost at a constant rate; the rate of loss slows down and (assuming that the energy deficit is not too severe) levels off, and the subject regains energy balance at a lower body weight.
A number of factors contribute to this adaptation to changing energy balance:

- As more food is eaten, there is an increased energy cost of digestion and absorption.
- When intake is in excess of requirements, a greater proportion is used for synthesis of adipose tissue triacylglycerol reserves, so there is more diet-induced thermogenesis. Conversely, in negative energy balance there is less synthesis of adipose tissue reserves and so less diet-induced thermogenesis.
- The rate of protein turnover increases with greater food intake (Section 9.2.3.3) and decreases with lower food intake.

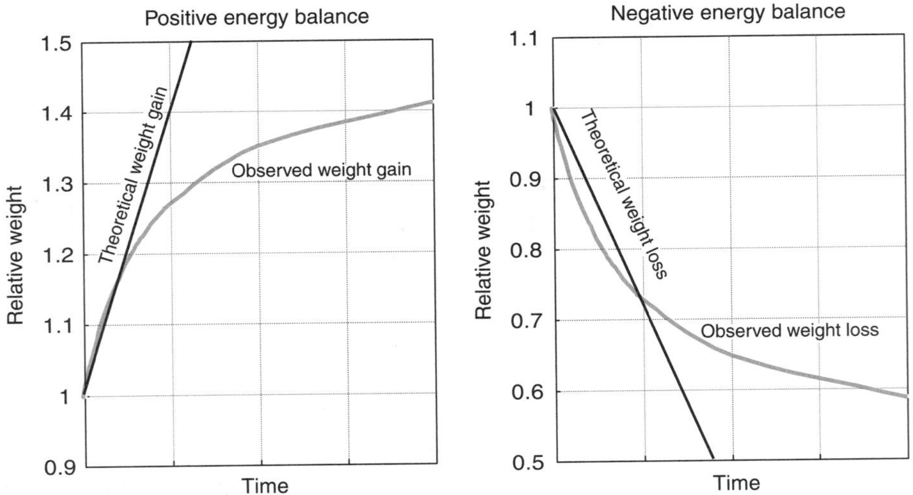

Figure 5.5 Predicted and observed changes in body weight with energy imbalance.

- Although adipose tissue is less metabolically active than muscle, 5% of its weight is metabolically active, and therefore the BMR increases as body weight rises and decreases as it falls.
- The energy cost of physical activity is markedly affected by body weight, so even with a constant level of physical activity, total energy expenditure will increase with increasing body weight (Figure 5.4). There is some evidence that people with habitually low energy intakes are more efficient in their movements, and thus have a lower cost of activity.

Figure 5.5 shows that in the early stages of negative energy balance, the rate of weight loss may be greater than the theoretical rate calculated from the energy yield of adipose tissue. This is because of the loss of relatively large amounts of water associated with liver and muscle glycogen reserves (Section 4.2.1.5), which are considerably depleted during energy restriction.

5.3 *Metabolic fuels in the fed and fasting states*

Energy expenditure is relatively constant throughout the day, but food intake normally occurs in two or three meals. There is therefore a need to ensure that there is a constant supply of metabolic fuel, regardless of the variation in intake. See Section 10.5 for a more detailed discussion of the hormonal control of metabolism in the fed and fasting states.

5.3.1 *The fed state*

During 3–4 h after a meal, there is an ample supply of metabolic fuel entering the circulation from the gut (Figure 5.6). Glucose from carbohydrate digestion (Section 4.2.2) and amino acids from protein digestion (Section 4.4.3) are absorbed into the portal circulation, and to a considerable extent the liver controls the amounts that enter the peripheral circulation. By contrast, the products of fat digestion are absorbed into the lymphatic system as chylomicrons (Sections 4.3.2.2 and 5.6.2.1) and are available to peripheral tissues first; the liver clears chylomicron remnants. Much of the triacylglycerol in chylomicrons goes directly to adipose tissue for storage; when there is a plentiful supply of glucose, it is the main metabolic fuel for most tissues.

The increased concentration of glucose and amino acids in the portal blood stimulates the β-cells of the pancreas to secrete insulin and suppresses the secretion of glucagon by the α-cells of the pancreas. In response to insulin, there is

- Increased uptake of glucose into muscle and adipose tissue, as a result of migration to the cell surface of glucose transporters that are in intracellular vesicles in the fasting state
- Increased synthesis of glycogen (Section 5.6.3) from glucose in both liver and muscle, as a result of activation of glycogen synthetase
- Increased synthesis of fatty acids in adipose tissue (Section 5.6.1) by activation of acetyl CoA carboxylase and inhibition of fatty acid release by inactivation of hormone-sensitive lipase
- Increased uptake of fatty acids from chylomicrons and very low density lipoprotein (Section 5.6.2) by increasing the synthesis of lipoprotein lipase and stimulating its migration into blood capillaries
- Increased amino acid uptake into tissues and stimulation of protein synthesis

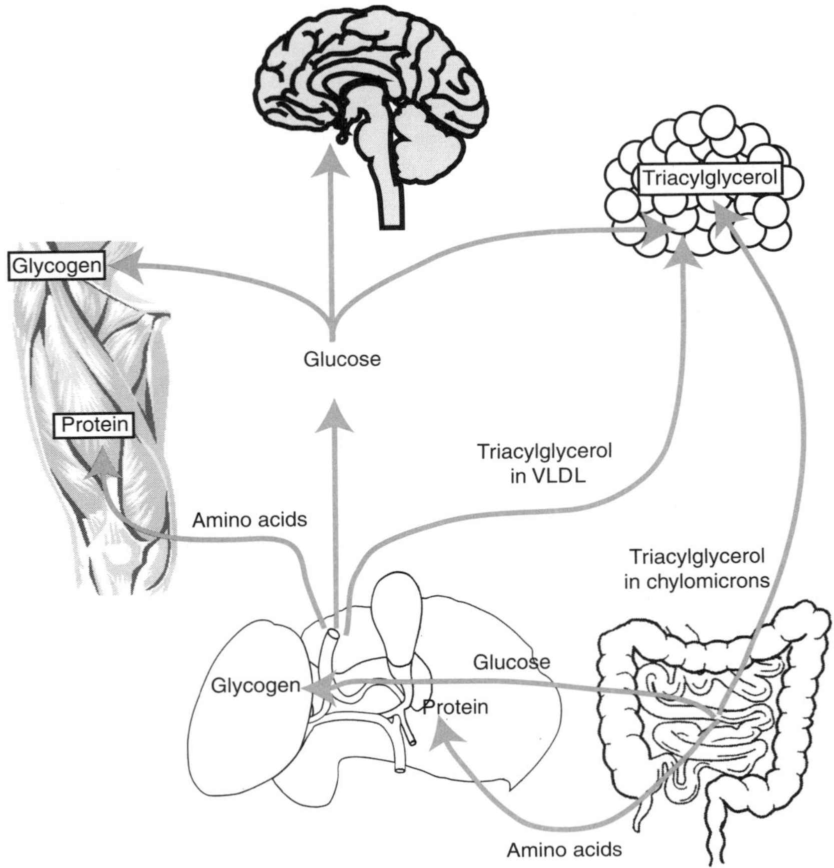

Figure 5.6 An overview of metabolism in the fed state.

In the liver, glucose uptake is by carrier-mediated diffusion and metabolic trapping as glucose 6-phosphate (Section 3.2.2.2) and is independent of insulin. The uptake of glucose into the liver increases very significantly as the concentration of glucose in the portal vein increases, and the liver has a major role in controlling the amount of glucose that reaches peripheral tissues after a meal. There are two isoenzymes that catalyze the formation of glucose 6-phosphate in liver:

- *Hexokinase* has a K_m of approximately 0.15 mmol/L, is saturated, and therefore acting at its V_{max} under all conditions. It acts mainly to ensure an adequate uptake of glucose into the liver to meet the demands for liver metabolism.
- *Glucokinase* has a K_m of approximately 20 mmol/L and will have very low activity in the fasting state when the concentration of glucose in the portal blood is between 3 and 5 mmol/L. However, after a meal the portal concentration of glucose may well reach 20 mmol/L or higher, and under these conditions glucokinase has significant activity and there is increased formation of glucose 6-phosphate. Most of this will be used for synthesis of glycogen (Section 5.6.3), although some will also be used for synthesis of fatty acids that will be exported in very low density lipoprotein (Section 5.6.2.2; see also Problem 2.1).

5.3.2 The fasting state

In the fasting or postabsorptive state (beginning about 4–5 h after a meal, when the products of digestion have been absorbed), metabolic fuels enter the circulation from the reserves of glycogen, triacylglycerol, and protein laid down in the fed state (Figure 5.7).

As the concentration of glucose and amino acids in the portal blood falls, the secretion of insulin by the β-cells of the pancreas decreases and the secretion of glucagon by the α-cells increases. In response to glucagon, there is

- Increased breakdown of liver glycogen to glucose 1-phosphate to release glucose into the circulation (muscle glycogen cannot be used directly as a source of free glucose)
- Increased synthesis of glucose from amino acids in liver and kidney (gluconeogenesis; Section 5.7)

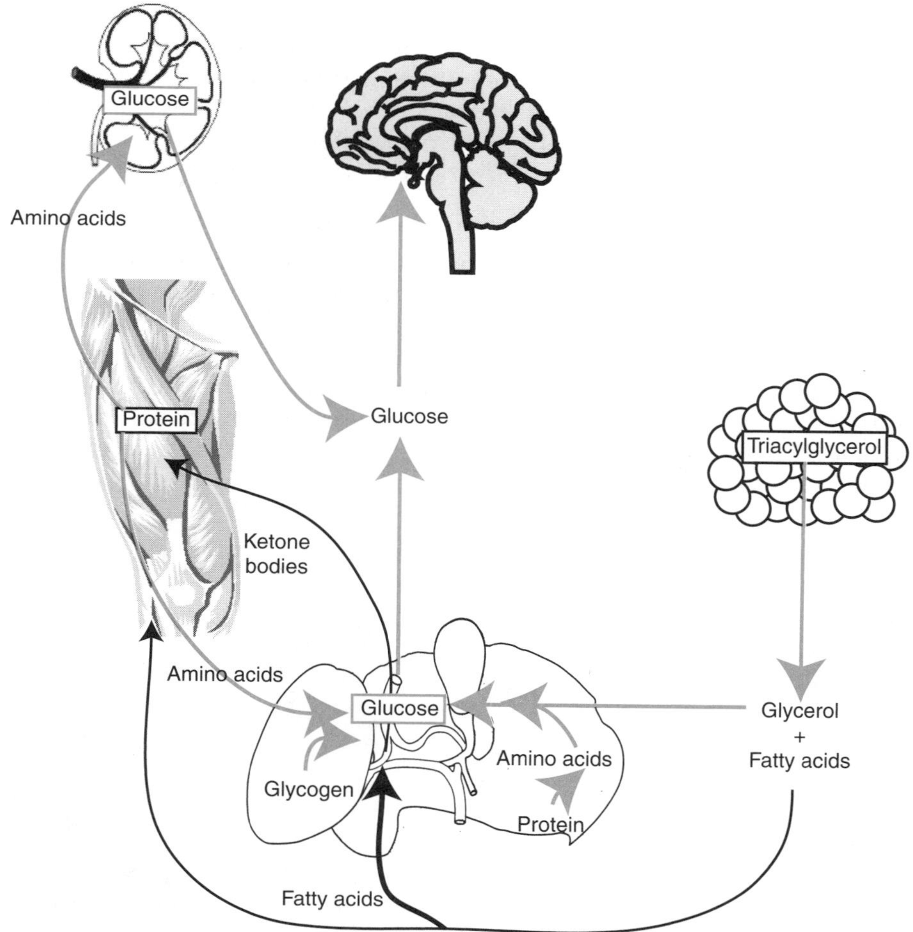

Figure 5.7 An overview of metabolism in the fasting state.

At the same time, in response to the reduced secretion of insulin there is

- Decreased uptake of glucose into muscle and adipose tissue because the glucose transporter is internalized in the absence of insulin
- Decreased protein synthesis, so that the amino acids arising from protein catabolism (Section 9.1.1) are available for gluconeogenesis (Section 5.7)
- Release of nonesterified fatty acids from adipose tissue, as a result of relief of the inhibition of hormone-sensitive lipase

The metabolic imperative in the fasting state is that the brain is largely dependent on glucose as its metabolic fuel, and red blood cells (which lack mitochondria) and the renal medulla can only utilize glucose. Therefore, those tissues that can utilize other fuels do so, to spare glucose for the brain, red blood cells, and renal medulla. Any metabolites that can be used for gluconeogenesis will be used to supplement the relatively small amount of glucose that is available from glycogen reserves; the total liver and muscle glycogen reserves would only meet requirements for 12–18 h. The main substrates for gluconeogenesis are amino acids (Sections 5.7 and 9.3.2) and the glycerol of triacylglycerol. Fatty acids can never be substrates for gluconeogenesis.

Muscle and other tissues can utilize fatty acids as a metabolic fuel, but only to a limited extent, and not enough to meet energy requirements completely. By contrast, the liver has a greater capacity for the oxidation of fatty acids than is required to meet its own energy needs. Therefore, in the fasting state the liver synthesizes ketone bodies (acetoacetate and β-hydroxybutyrate; Section 5.5.3), which it exports to other tissues for use as a metabolic fuel.

The result of these metabolic changes is shown in Figure 5.8. The plasma concentration of glucose falls somewhat, but is maintained through fasting into starvation, as a result of gluconeogenesis. The concentration of free fatty acids in plasma increases in fasting, but does not increase any further in starvation, while the concentration of ketone bodies increases continually through fasting into starvation. After about 2–3 weeks of starvation, the plasma concentration of ketone bodies is high enough for them to be a significant fuel for the brain, providing about 20% of its energy requirement. This means that in prolonged starvation, there is a decrease in the amount of tissue protein that needs to be catabolized for gluconeogenesis.

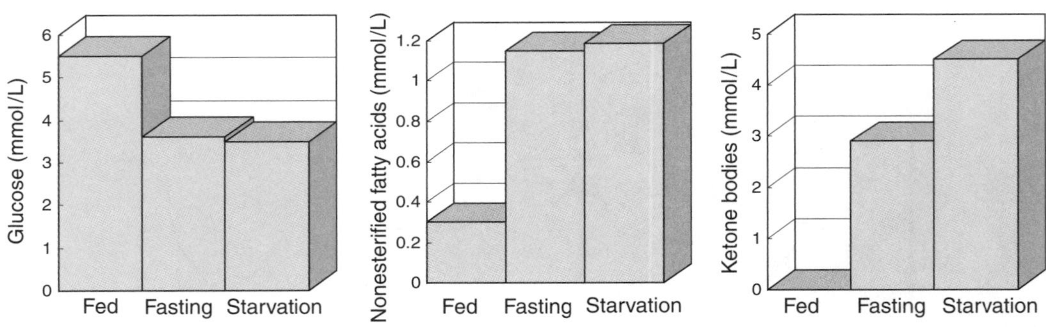

Figure 5.8 Plasma concentrations of metabolic fuels in the fed and fasting states and in starvation.

5.4 Energy-yielding metabolism

5.4.1 Glycolysis—the (anaerobic) metabolism of glucose

Overall, the pathway of glycolysis is cleavage of the six-carbon glucose molecule into two three-carbon units. The key steps in the pathway are the following:

- Two phosphorylation reactions to form fructose-bisphosphate
- Cleavage of fructose-bisphosphate to yield two molecules of triose (three-carbon sugar) phosphate
- Two steps in which phosphate is transferred from a substrate onto ADP forming ATP (and hence a yield of 4 mol of ATP per mole of glucose metabolized)
- One step in which NAD^+ is reduced to NADH (equivalent to 2.5 mol of ATP per mole of triose phosphate metabolized, or 5 mol of ATP per mole of glucose metabolized when the NADH is reoxidized in the mitochondrial electron transport chain [Section 3.3.1.2])
- Formation of 2 mol of pyruvate per mole of glucose metabolized

The immediate substrate for glycolysis is glucose 6-phosphate (Figure 5.9), which may arise by:

- Phosphorylation of glucose, catalyzed by hexokinase (and also by glucokinase in the liver in the fed state) at the expense of ATP.
- Phosphorolysis of glycogen in liver and muscle to yield glucose 1-phosphate, catalyzed by glycogen phosphorylase, using inorganic phosphate. Glucose 1-phosphate is readily isomerized to glucose 6-phosphate.

The pathway of glycolysis is shown in Figure 5.10. Although the aim of glucose oxidation is to phosphorylate ADP to ATP, the pathway involves two steps in which ATP is used, one to form glucose 6-phosphate when glucose is the substrate, and the other to form

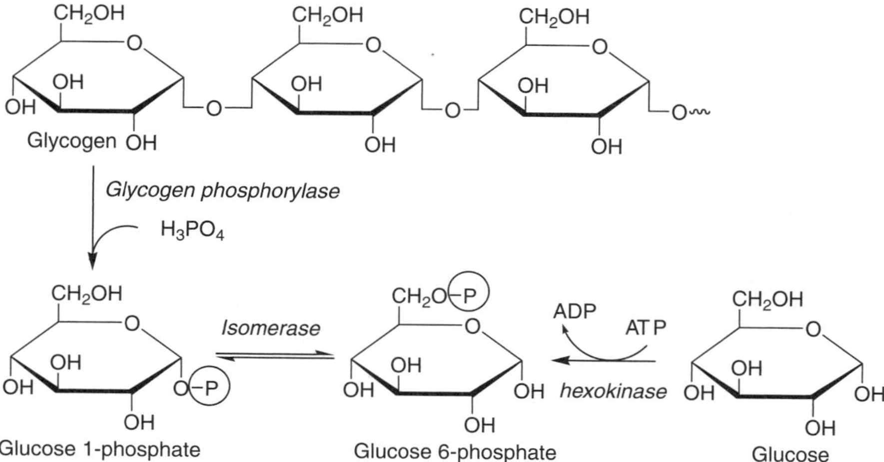

Figure 5.9 Sources of glucose 6-phosphate for glycolysis.

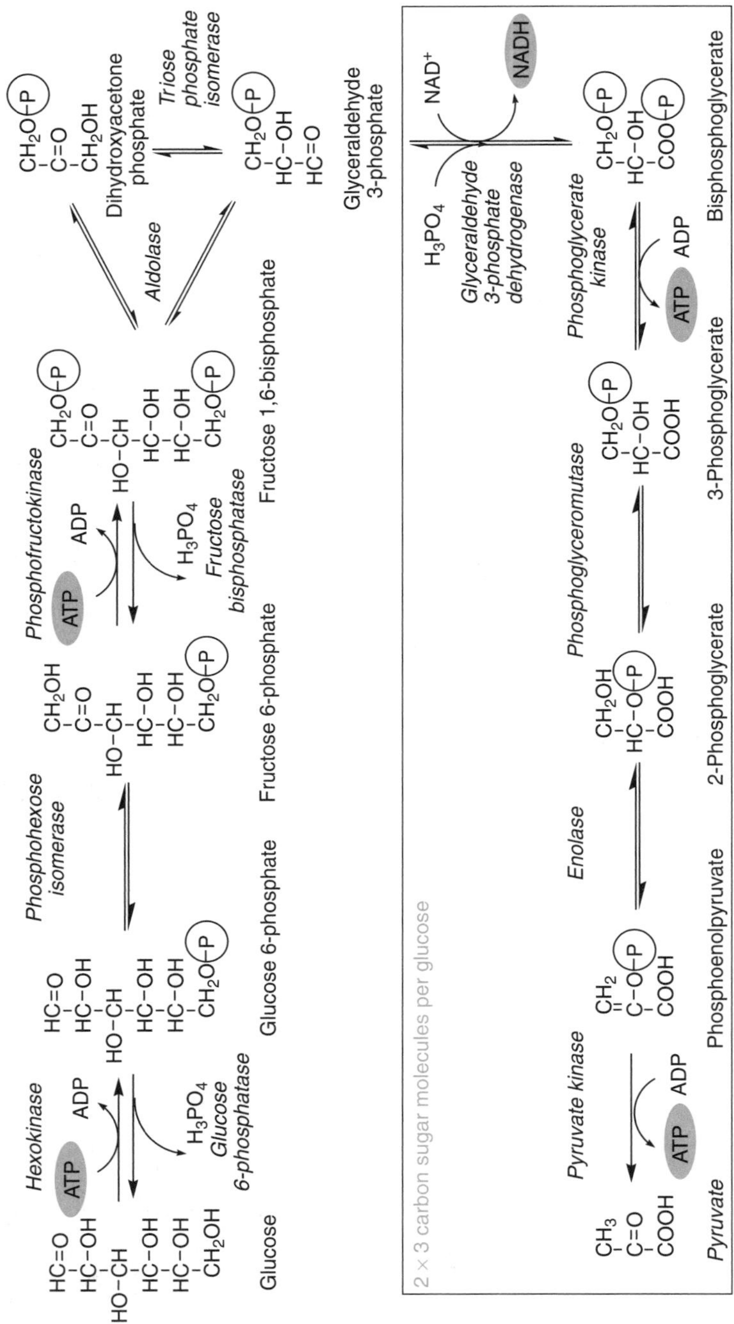

Figure 5.10 Glycolysis.

fructose bisphosphate. In other words, there is a modest cost of ATP to initiate the metabolism of glucose. When glycogen is the source of glucose 6-phosphate there is a cost of only 1 × ATP for glycolysis, but there is a cost of 2 × ATP equivalents for each mole of glucose added in glycogen synthesis (Section 5.6.3).

The formation of fructose bisphosphate, catalyzed by phosphofructokinase, is an important step for the regulation of glucose metabolism (Section 10.2.2). Once it has been formed, fructose bisphosphate is cleaved to yield two interconvertible three-carbon compounds. The metabolism of these three-carbon sugars is linked to both the reduction of NAD^+ to NADH, and direct (substrate level) phosphorylation of ADP to ATP (Section 3.3). The result is the formation of 2 mol of pyruvate from each mole of glucose.

Glycolysis thus requires the utilization of 2 mol of ATP (giving ADP) per mole of glucose metabolized, and yields 4 × ATP by substrate level phosphorylation, and 2 × NADH (formed from NAD^+), equivalent to a further 5 × ATP when oxidized in the electron transport chain (Section 3.3.1.2). There is thus a net yield of 7 × ADP + phosphate → ATP from the oxidation of 1 mol of glucose to 2 mol of pyruvate.

The reverse of glycolysis is important as a means of glucose synthesis—the process of gluconeogenesis (Section 5.7). Most of the reactions of glycolysis are readily reversible, but at three points (the reactions catalyzed by hexokinase, phosphofructokinase, and pyruvate kinase), there are separate enzymes involved in glycolysis and gluconeogenesis.

For two of these reactions, hexokinase and phosphofructokinase, the equilibrium is in the direction of glycolysis because of the utilization of ATP in the reaction and the high ratio of ATP to ADP in the cell. The reactions of phosphofructokinase and hexokinase are reversed in gluconeogenesis by hydrolysis of fructose bisphosphate to fructose 6-phosphate and phosphate (catalyzed by fructose bisphosphatase) and of glucose 6-phosphate to glucose and phosphate (catalyzed by glucose 6-phosphatase).

The equilibrium of pyruvate kinase is also strongly in the direction of glycolysis, because the immediate product of the reaction is enolpyruvate, which is chemically unstable, and undergoes a nonenzymic reaction to yield pyruvate (Figure 5.32). This means that little of the product is available to undergo the reverse reaction in the direction of gluconeogenesis. The conversion of pyruvate to phosphoenolpyruvate for gluconeogenesis is discussed in Section 5.7.

The glycolytic pathway also provides a route for the metabolism of fructose, galactose (which undergoes phosphorylation to galactose 1-phosphate and isomerization to glucose 1-phosphate), and glycerol. Some fructose is phosphorylated directly to fructose 6-phosphate by hexokinase, but most is phosphorylated to fructose 1-phosphate by a specific enzyme, fructokinase. Fructose 1-phosphate is then cleaved to yield dihydroxyacetone phosphate and glyceraldehyde; the glyceraldehyde can be phosphorylated to glyceraldehyde 3-phosphate by triose kinase. This means that fructose enters glycolysis after the main regulatory step is catalyzed by phosphofructokinase (Section 10.2.2), and its utilization is not controlled by the need for ATP formation. There is excessive formation of acetyl CoA, which is used for fatty acid synthesis, so that a high intake of fructose may be a significant factor in the development of obesity.

Glycerol arising from the hydrolysis of triacylglycerols can be phosphorylated and oxidized to dihydroxyacetone phosphate. In triacylglycerol synthesis (Section 5.6.1.2), most glycerol phosphate is formed from dihydroxyacetone phosphate.

5.4.1.1 *Transfer of NADH from glycolysis into the mitochondria*

The mitochondrial inner membrane is impermeable to NAD, and therefore the NADH produced in the cytosol in glycolysis cannot enter the mitochondria for reoxidation.

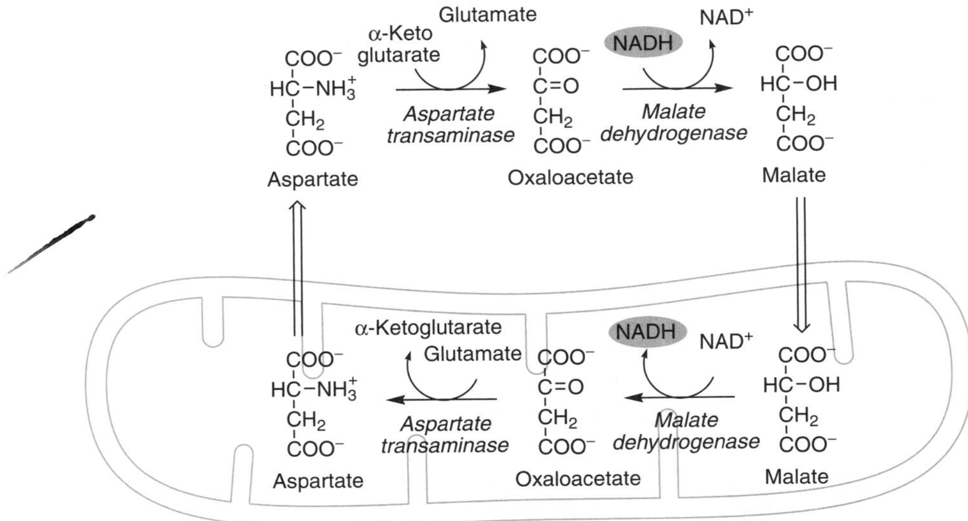

Figure 5.11 The malate-aspartate shuttle for transfer of reducing equivalents from the cytosol into the mitochondrion.

To transfer the reducing equivalents from cytosolic NADH into the mitochondria, two substrate shuttles are used.

The malate-aspartate shuttle (Figure 5.11) involves reduction of oxaloacetate in the cytosol to malate (with the oxidation of cytosolic NADH to NAD^+). Malate enters the mitochondria and is reduced back to oxaloacetate, with the reduction of intramitochondrial NAD^+ to NADH. Oxaloacetate cannot cross the mitochondrial inner membrane but undergoes transamination to aspartate (Section 9.3.1.2), with glutamate acting as amino donor, yielding α-ketoglutarate. α-Ketoglutarate then leaves the mitochondria using an antiporter, which transports malate inward. Aspartate leaves the mitochondria in exchange for glutamate entering; in the cytosol the reverse transamination reaction occurs, forming oxaloacetate (for reduction to malate) from aspartate, and glutamate (for transport back into the mitochondria) from α-ketoglutarate.

The glycerophosphate shuttle (Figure 5.12) involves reduction of dihydroxyacetone phosphate to glycerol 3-phosphate in the cytosol (with oxidation of NADH to NAD^+), and oxidation of glycerol 3-phosphate to dihydroxyacetone phosphate inside the mitochondrion. Dihydroxyacetone phosphate and glycerol 3-phosphate are transported in opposite directions by an antiporter in the mitochondrial membrane.

The cytosolic glycerol 3-phosphate dehydrogenase uses NADH to reduce dihydroxyacetone phosphate to glycerol 3-phosphate, but the mitochondrial enzyme uses flavin adenine dinucleotide (FAD) to reduce glycerol 3-phosphate to dihydroxyacetone phosphate. This means that when this shuttle is used there is a yield of 1.5 mol of ATP rather than the 2.5 mol of ATP that would be expected from reoxidation of NADH.

The malate-aspartate shuttle is sensitive to the relative amounts of NADH and NAD^+ in the cytosol and mitochondria, and cannot operate if the mitochondrial NADH:NAD^+ ratio is higher than that in the cytosol. However, because it does not use NAD^+ in the mitochondrion, the glycerophosphate shuttle can operate even when the mitochondrial NADH:NAD^+ ratio is higher than that in the cytosol.

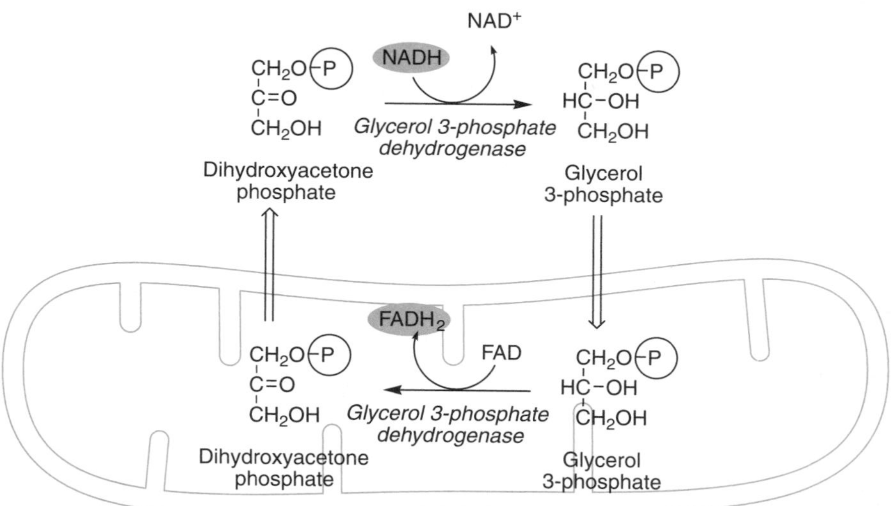

Figure 5.12 The glycerophosphate shuttle for transfer of reducing equivalents from the cytosol into the mitochondrion.

The glycerophosphate shuttle is important in muscle where there is a very high rate of glycolysis (especially insect flight muscle); the malate–aspartate shuttle is especially important in heart and liver.

5.4.1.2 The reduction of pyruvate to lactate: anaerobic glycolysis

Under conditions of maximum exertion, for example, in sprinting, the rate at which oxygen can be transported into the muscle is not great enough to allow for the reoxidation of all the NADH formed in glycolysis. To maintain the oxidation of glucose and the net yield of 2 × ATP per mole of glucose oxidized (or 3 × ATP if the source is muscle glycogen), NADH is oxidized to NAD^+ by the reduction of pyruvate to lactate, catalyzed by lactate dehydrogenase (Figure 5.13). In red blood cells, which lack mitochondria, formation of lactate is the only way to reoxidize NADH.

The resultant lactate is exported from the muscle and red blood cells, and is taken up by the liver, where it is used for the resynthesis of glucose. As shown on the right-hand side of Figure 5.13, synthesis of glucose from lactate is an ATP (and GTP) requiring process. The oxygen debt after strenuous physical activity is due to an increased rate of energy-yielding metabolism to provide the ATP and GTP that are required for gluconeogenesis from lactate. Although most of the lactate will be used for gluconeogenesis, a proportion will undergo oxidation to pyruvate and be oxidized further in the citric acid cycle (Sections 5.4.3 and 5.4.4) to provide the ATP and GTP needed (see Problem 5.1).

Lactate may also be taken up by tissues such as the heart, where oxygen availability is not a limiting factor. Here it is oxidized to pyruvate, and the resultant NADH is oxidized in the mitochondrial electron transport chain, yielding 2.5 × ATP. The pyruvate is then a substrate for complete oxidation through the citric acid cycle. The isoenzyme of lactate dehydrogenase in heart muscle acts preferentially in the direction of lactate oxidation to pyruvate, while the skeletal muscle isoenzyme acts preferentially in the direction of pyruvate reduction to lactate.

Many tumors have a low capacity for oxidative metabolism and metabolize glucose anaerobically to lactate, which is exported to the liver for gluconeogenesis. This cycling of

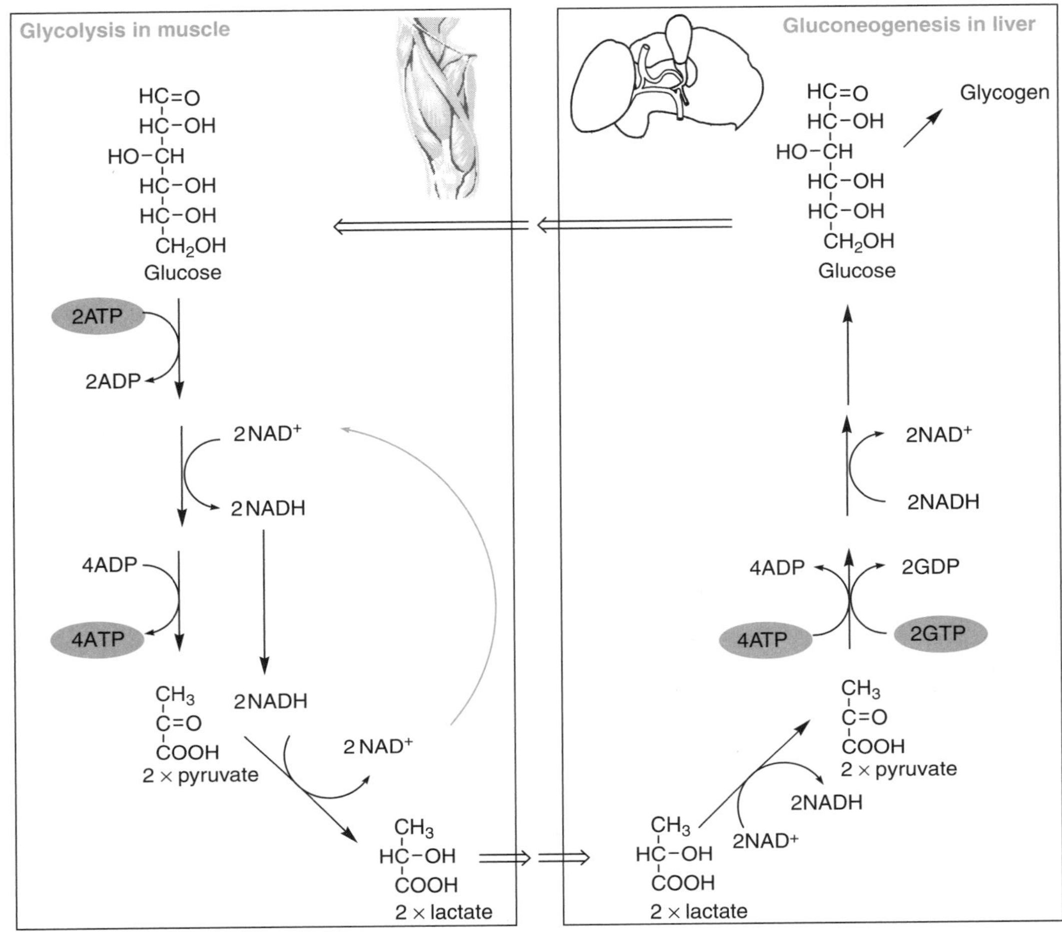

Figure 5.13 The Cori cycle—anaerobic glycolysis in muscle and gluconeogenesis in the liver.

glucose between anaerobic glycolysis in the tumor and gluconeogenesis in the liver may account for much of the increased metabolism and consequent weight loss (cachexia) that is seen in patients with advanced cancer (Section 8.4).

Anaerobic glycolysis is the main pathway in microorganisms that are capable of living in the absence of oxygen. Here there are two possible fates for the pyruvate formed from glucose, both of which involve the oxidation of NADH to NAD^+:

- Reduction to lactate as occurs in human muscle. This is the pathway in lactic acid bacteria, which are responsible for both the fermentation of lactose in milk for manufacture of yogurt and cheese, and also the gastrointestinal discomfort after consumption of lactose in people who lack intestinal lactase (Section 4.2.2.2).
- Decarboxylation and reduction to ethanol. This is the pathway of fermentation in yeast, which is exploited to produce alcoholic beverages. Human gastrointestinal bacteria normally produce lactate rather than ethanol, although there have been reports of people with a high intestinal population of yeasts that produce significant amounts of ethanol after consumption of resistant starch (Section 4.2.2.1).

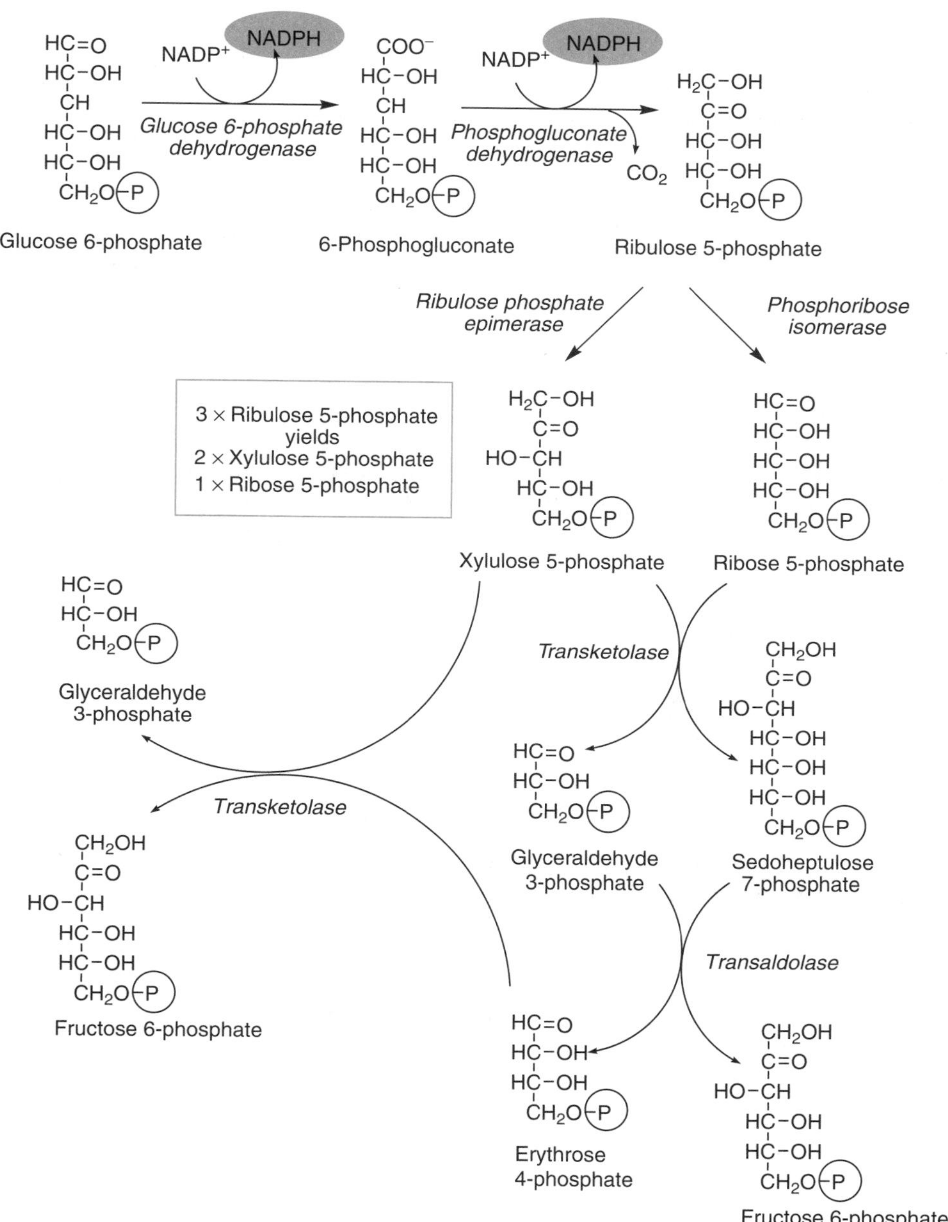

Figure 5.14 The pentose phosphate pathway (also known as the hexose monophosphate shunt).

5.4.2 The pentose phosphate pathway—an alternative to glycolysis

There is an alternative pathway for the conversion of glucose 6-phosphate into fructose 6-phosphate, the pentose phosphate pathway (sometimes known as the hexose monophosphate shunt; Figure 5.14).

Overall, the pentose phosphate pathway produces 2 mol of fructose 6-phosphate, 1 mol of glyceraldehyde 3-phosphate, and 3 mol of carbon dioxide from 3 mol of glucose 6-phosphate linked to the reduction of 6 mol of $NADP^+$ to NADPH. The sequence of reactions is as follows:

- 3 mol of glucose are oxidized to yield 3 mol of the five-carbon sugar ribulose 5-phosphate plus 3 mol of carbon dioxide.
- 2 mol of ribulose 5-phosphate are isomerized to yield 2 mol of xylulose 5-phosphate.
- 1 mol of ribulose 5-phosphate is isomerized to ribose 5-phosphate.
- 1 mol of xylulose 5-phosphate reacts with the ribose 5-phosphate, yielding (ultimately) fructose 6-phosphate and erythrose 4-phosphate.
- The other mol of xylulose-5-phosphate reacts with the erythrose 4-phosphate, yielding fructose 6-phosphate and glyceraldehyde 3-phosphate.

This is the pathway for the synthesis of ribose for nucleotide synthesis; more importantly, it is the source of about half the NADPH required for fatty acid synthesis (Section 5.6.1). Tissues that synthesize large amounts of fatty acids have a high activity of the pentose phosphate pathway. It is also important in the respiratory burst of macrophages that are activated in response to infection (Section 6.5.2.2).

5.4.2.1 The pentose phosphate pathway in red blood cells—favism

The pentose phosphate pathway is also important in the red blood cell, where NADPH is required to maintain an adequate pool of reduced glutathione, which is used to remove hydrogen peroxide.

The tripeptide glutathione (γ-glutamyl-cysteinyl-glycine; Figure 5.15) is the reducing agent for glutathione peroxidase, which reduces H_2O_2 to H_2O and O_2 (glutathione peroxidase is a selenium-dependent enzyme, Section 11.15.2.5; this explains the antioxidant role of selenium, Section 6.5.3.2).

Oxidized glutathione (GSSG) is reduced back to active GSH by glutathione reductase, which uses NADPH as the reducing agent. Glutathione reductase is a flavin-dependent enzyme, and its activity, or its activation after incubation with FAD, can be used as an index of vitamin B_2 status (Sections 2.4 and 11.7.4).

Partial or total lack of glucose 6-phosphate dehydrogenase (and hence impaired activity of the pentose phosphate pathway) is the cause of favism, an acute hemolytic anemia with fever and hemoglobinuria, precipitated in genetically susceptible people by the consumption of broad beans (fava beans) and a variety of drugs, all of which, like the toxins in fava beans, undergo redox cycling and produce hydrogen peroxide. Infection can also precipitate an attack, because of the increased production of oxygen radicals as part of the macrophage respiratory burst (Section 6.5.2.2).

Because of the low activity of the pentose phosphate pathway in affected people, there is a lack of NADPH in red blood cells, and hence an impaired ability to remove hydrogen peroxide, which causes oxidative damage to the cell-membrane lipids, leading to hemolysis. Other tissues are unaffected because there are mitochondrial enzymes that can provide a supply of NADPH; red blood cells have no mitochondria.

Favism is one of the commonest genetic defects affecting some 200 million people. It is an X-linked condition, and female carriers are resistant to malaria, an advantage that explains why defects in the gene are so widespread. A large number of variant forms of

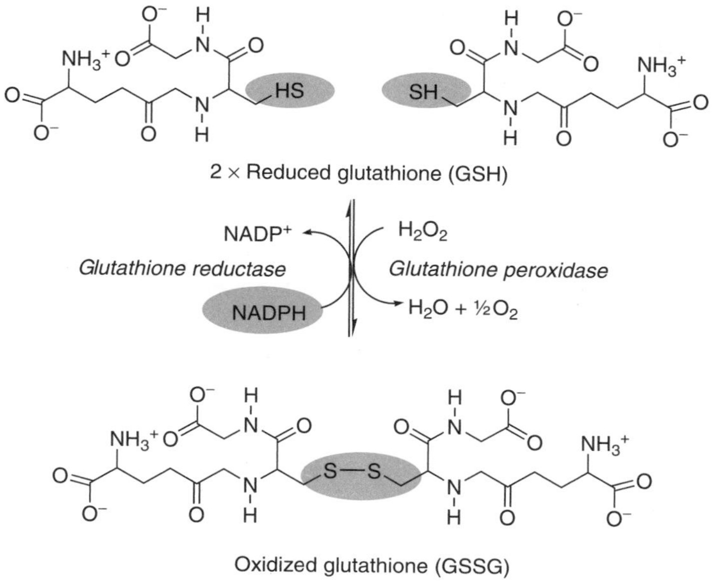

Figure 5.15 The reaction of glutathione peroxidase.

the glucose 6-phosphate dehydrogenase gene are known, some of which do not affect the activity of the enzyme significantly. There are two main types of favism:

- A moderately severe form, in which there is between 10% and 50% of the normal activity of glucose 6-phosphate dehydrogenase in red blood cells. The abnormal enzyme is unstable, so that older red blood cells have low activity, but younger cells have nearly normal activity. This means that the hemolytic crisis is self-limiting as only older red blood cells are lysed. This is the form of favism found among people of Afro-Caribbean descent. Crises are rarely precipitated by consumption of fava beans.
- A severe form, in which there is less than 10% of normal activity of glucose 6-phosphate dehydrogenase in red blood cells. Here, the problem is that the enzyme has low catalytic activity or an abnormally high K_m for $NADP^+$. In extremely severe cases, hemolytic crises can occur without the stress of toxin or infection. This is the form of favism found among people of Mediterranean descent.

5.4.3 The metabolism of pyruvate

Pyruvate arising from glycolysis (or from amino acids; Section 9.3.2) can be metabolized in three different ways, depending on the metabolic state of the body:

- Reduction to lactate (Section 5.4.1.2)
- As a substrate for gluconeogenesis (Section 5.7)
- Complete oxidation to carbon dioxide and water (Sections 5.4.3.1 and 5.4.4).

5.4.3.1 The oxidation of pyruvate to acetyl CoA

The first step in the complete oxidation of pyruvate is a multistep reaction in which carbon dioxide is lost, and the resulting two-carbon compound is oxidized to acetate. The oxidation involves the reduction of NAD^+ to NADH. Since 2 mol of pyruvate are formed from

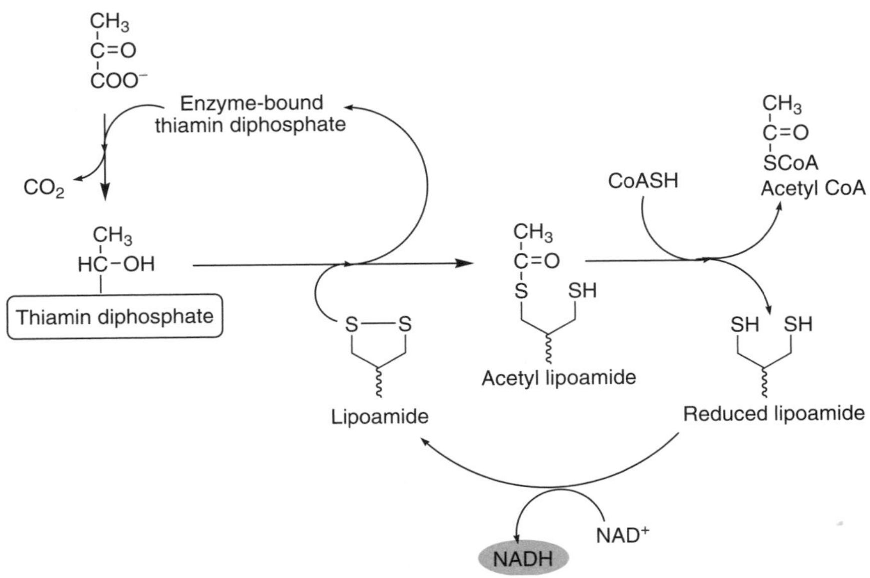

Figure 5.16 The reaction of pyruvate dehydrogenase.

each mole of glucose, this step represents the formation of 2 mol of NADH, equivalent to 5 × ATP for each mole of glucose metabolized. The acetate is released from the enzyme esterified to coenzyme A, as acetyl CoA (Figure 5.16; coenzyme A is derived from the vitamin pantothenic acid; Section 11.13.1.1).

The decarboxylation and oxidation of pyruvate to form acetyl CoA requires the coenzyme thiamin diphosphate, which is formed from vitamin B_1 (Section 11.6.2). In thiamin deficiency this reaction is impaired, and deficient subjects are unable to metabolize glucose normally. Especially after a test dose of glucose or moderate exercise they develop high blood concentrations of pyruvate and lactate. In some cases, this may be severe enough to result in life-threatening acidosis.

5.4.4 Oxidation of acetyl CoA—the citric acid cycle

The acetate of acetyl CoA undergoes a stepwise oxidation to carbon dioxide and water in a cyclic pathway, the citric acid cycle (Figures 5.17 and 5.18). This pathway is sometimes known as the Krebs cycle, after its discoverer, Sir Hans Krebs. For each mole of acetyl CoA oxidized in this pathway, there is a yield of:

- 3 × NAD^+ reduced to NADH, equivalent to 7.5 × ATP
- 1 × Flavoprotein reduced, leading to reduction of ubiquinone (Section 3.3.1.2), equivalent to 1.5 × ADP
- 1 × ADP phosphorylated to ATP, or, in liver and some other tissues, 1 × GDP phosphorylated to GTP

This is a total of 10 × ATP for each mole of acetyl CoA oxidized; since 2 mol of acetyl CoA are formed from each mole of glucose, this cycle yields 20 × ATP for each mole of glucose oxidized.

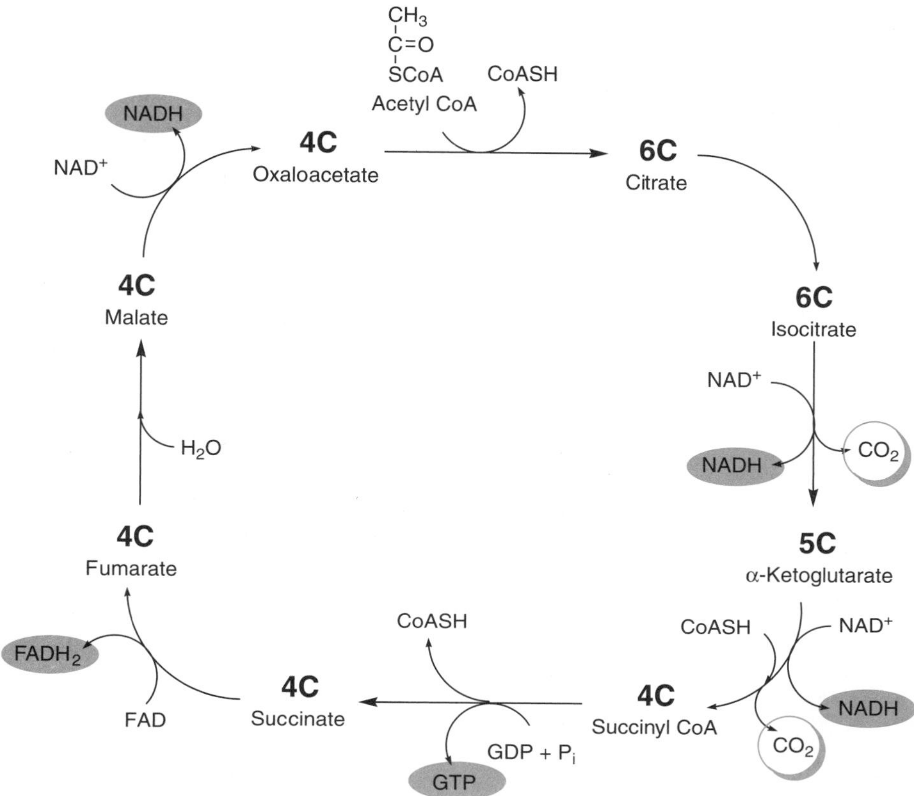

Figure 5.17 An overview of the citric acid cycle (also known as the Krebs cycle or tricarboxylic acid cycle). The reaction of succinyl CoA synthetase is linked to phosphorylation of either ADP→ATP or GDP→GTP depending on the tissue involved.

Although it appears complex at first sight, the citric acid cycle is a simple pathway. A four-carbon compound, oxaloacetate, reacts with acetyl CoA to form a six-carbon compound, citric acid. The cycle is then a series of reactions in which two carbon atoms are lost as carbon dioxide, followed by a series of oxidation and other reactions, eventually reforming oxaloacetate. The CoA of acetyl CoA is released, and is available for further formation of acetyl CoA from pyruvate.

The citric acid cycle also catalyzes the oxidation of acetyl CoA arising from other sources:

- β-Oxidation of fatty acids (Section 5.5.2)
- Ketone bodies (Section 5.5.3)
- Alcohol (Section 2.6)
- Amino acids that give rise to acetyl CoA or acetoacetate (Section 9.3.2)

Although oxaloacetate is the precursor for gluconeogenesis (Section 5.7), fatty acids and other compounds that give rise to acetyl CoA or acetoacetate cannot be used for net synthesis of glucose. As can be seen from Figure 5.18, although two carbons are added to the cycle by acetyl CoA, two carbons are lost as carbon dioxide in each turn of the cycle.

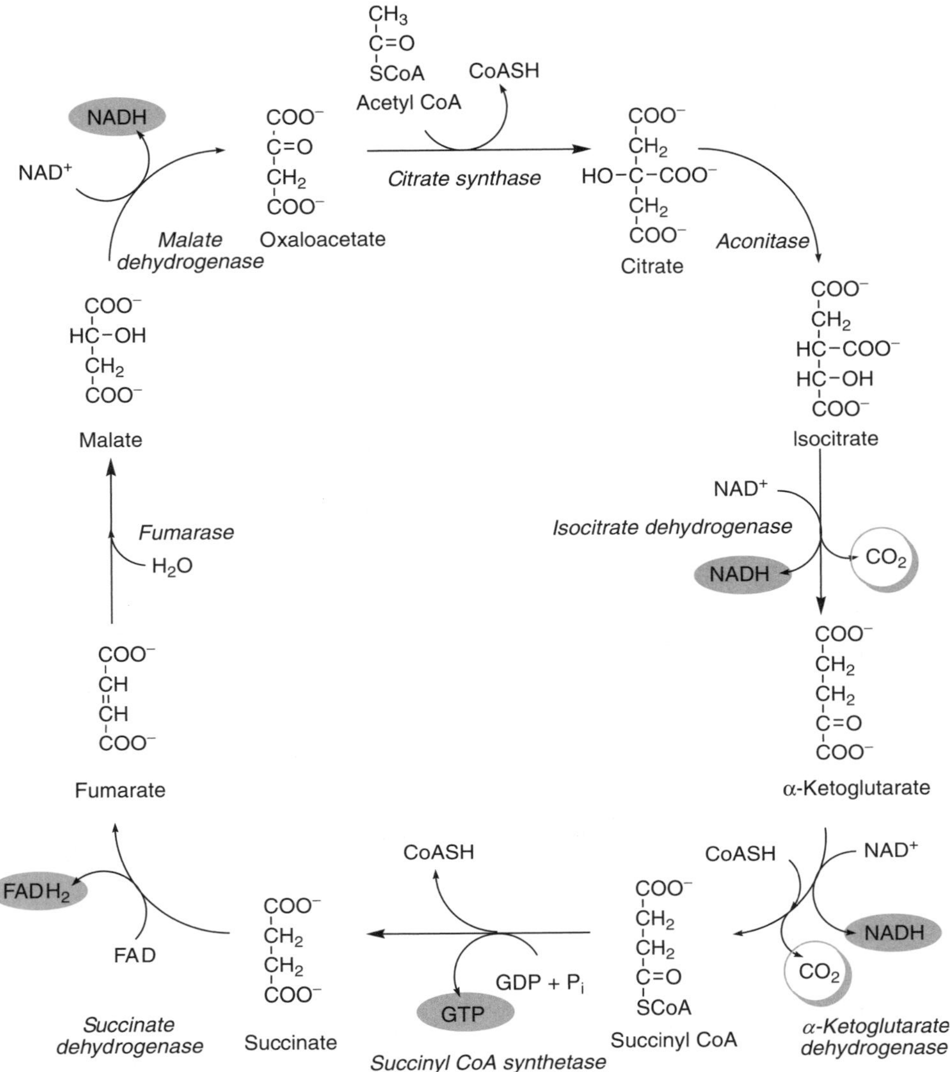

Figure 5.18 The citric acid cycle (also known as the Krebs cycle or tricarboxylic acid cycle).The reaction of succinyl CoA synthetase is linked to phosphorylation of either ADP→ATP or GDP→GTP, depending on the tissue involved.

Therefore, when acetyl CoA is the substrate there is no increase in the pool of citric acid cycle intermediates, and therefore oxaloacetate cannot be withdrawn for gluconeogenesis.

α-Ketoglutarate dehydrogenase catalyzes a reaction similar to that of pyruvate dehydrogenase—oxidative decarboxylation and formation of an acyl CoA derivative. Like pyruvate dehydrogenase, it is a thiamin diphosphate-dependent enzyme, and the reaction sequence is the same as that shown in Figure 5.16. However, thiamin deficiency does not have a significant effect on the citric acid cycle, because α-ketoglutarate can undergo transamination to yield glutamate, which is decarboxylated to γ-aminobutyric acid (GABA, Figure 5.19). In turn, GABA can undergo onward metabolism to yield succinate.

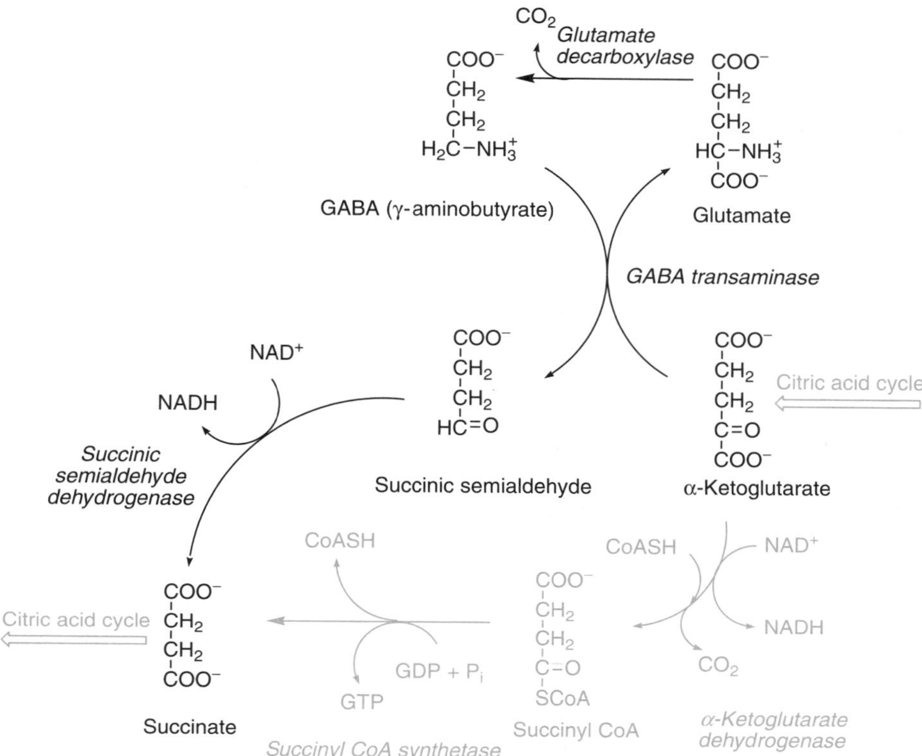

Figure 5.19 The GABA shunt—an alternative to α-ketoglutarate dehydrogenase in the citric acid cycle.

This GABA shunt thus provides an alternative to α-ketoglutarate dehydrogenase, and in thiamin deficiency there is increased turnover of GABA, permitting normal acetyl CoA oxidation and ATP formation.

The sequence of reactions between succinate and oxaloacetate is chemically the same as that involved in the β-oxidation of fatty acids (Section 5.5.2):

- Oxidation to yield a carbon–carbon double bond. Although this reaction is shown in Figure 5.18 as being linked to reduction of FAD, the coenzyme is tightly enzyme bound, and succinate dehydrogenase reacts directly with ubiquinone in the electron transport chain (Section 3.3.1.2).
- Addition of water across the carbon–carbon double bond, to yield a hydroxyl group.
- Oxidation of the hydroxyl group, linked to reduction of NAD^+, to yield an oxo-group.

5.4.4.1 *The citric acid cycle as a pathway for metabolic interconversion*

In addition to its role in oxidation of acetyl CoA, the citric acid cycle provides the link between carbohydrate, fat, and amino acid metabolism. Many of the intermediates can be used for the synthesis of other compounds:

- α-Ketoglutarate and oxaloacetate can give rise to the amino acids glutamate and aspartate, respectively (Section 9.3.1.2).

- Oxaloacetate is the precursor for glucose synthesis in the fasting state (Section 5.7).
- Citrate is the source of acetyl CoA for fatty acid synthesis in the cytosol in the fed state (Section 5.6.1).

The toxicity of ammonia (Section 9.3.1.3) is due to the activity of glutamate dehydrogenase, which forms glutamate by reaction of α-ketoglutarate with ammonium; this depletes the citric acid cycle pool of intermediates, leading to impaired activity of the cycle and reduced formation of ATP.

If oxaloacetate is removed from the cycle for glucose synthesis (Section 5.7), it must be replaced, since if there is not enough oxaloacetate available to form citrate, the rate of acetyl CoA metabolism, and hence the rate of formation of ATP, will slow down. A variety of amino acids give rise to citric cycle intermediates, thereby permitting the removal of oxaloacetate for gluconeogenesis (Section 9.3.2). In addition, the reaction of pyruvate carboxylase (Figure 5.20) is a source of oxaloacetate to maintain citric acid cycle activity.

There is a further control over the removal of oxaloacetate for gluconeogenesis. The decarboxylation and phosphorylation of oxaloacetate to form phosphoenolpyruvate uses GTP as the phosphate donor (Figure 5.20). In gluconeogenic tissues such as liver and kidney, the major mitochondrial source of GTP is the reaction of succinyl CoA synthetase. If so much oxaloacetate is withdrawn that the rate of cycle activity falls, there is not enough GTP to permit further removal. In tissues such as brain and heart, which do not carry out gluconeogenesis, there is a different isoenzyme of succinyl CoA synthetase linked to phosphorylation of ADP rather than GDP.

5.4.4.2 Complete oxidation of four- and five-carbon compounds

Although the citric acid cycle is generally regarded as a pathway for the oxidation of four- and five-carbon compounds such as fumarate, oxaloacetate, α-ketoglutarate, and succinate, arising from amino acids (Figure 5.20), it does not, alone, permit complete oxidation of these compounds. Four-carbon intermediates are not overall consumed in the cycle, since oxaloacetate is reformed. Addition of four- and five-carbon intermediates will increase the rate of cycle activity (subject to control by the requirement for ATP) only until the pool of intermediates is saturated.

Complete oxidation of four- and five-carbon intermediates requires removal of oxaloacetate from the cycle and conversion to pyruvate (Figure 5.20). This pyruvate may either undergo decarboxylation to acetyl CoA (Figure 5.16), which can be oxidized in the cycle, or may be used as a substrate for gluconeogenesis.

Oxidation of four- and five-carbon citric acid cycle intermediates thus involves a greater metabolic activity than oxidation of acetyl CoA. This has been exploited as a means of overcoming the hypothermia that occurs in patients recovering from anesthesia, by giving an intravenous infusion of the amino acid glutamate. This provides α-ketoglutarate, which will largely be used for gluconeogenesis, and hence cause an increase in metabolic activity and increased heat production.

5.5 The metabolism of fats

There are two sources of fatty acids available to tissues (Figure 5.21). In the fed state, chylomicrons assembled in the small intestine (Section 4.3.2.2) and very low density lipoproteins exported from the liver (Section 5.6.2.2) bind to lipoprotein lipase at the luminal surface of capillary epithelium. This enzyme catalyzes hydrolysis of triacylglycerols to glycerol and free fatty acids. Most of the fatty acid released enters cells and is metabolized

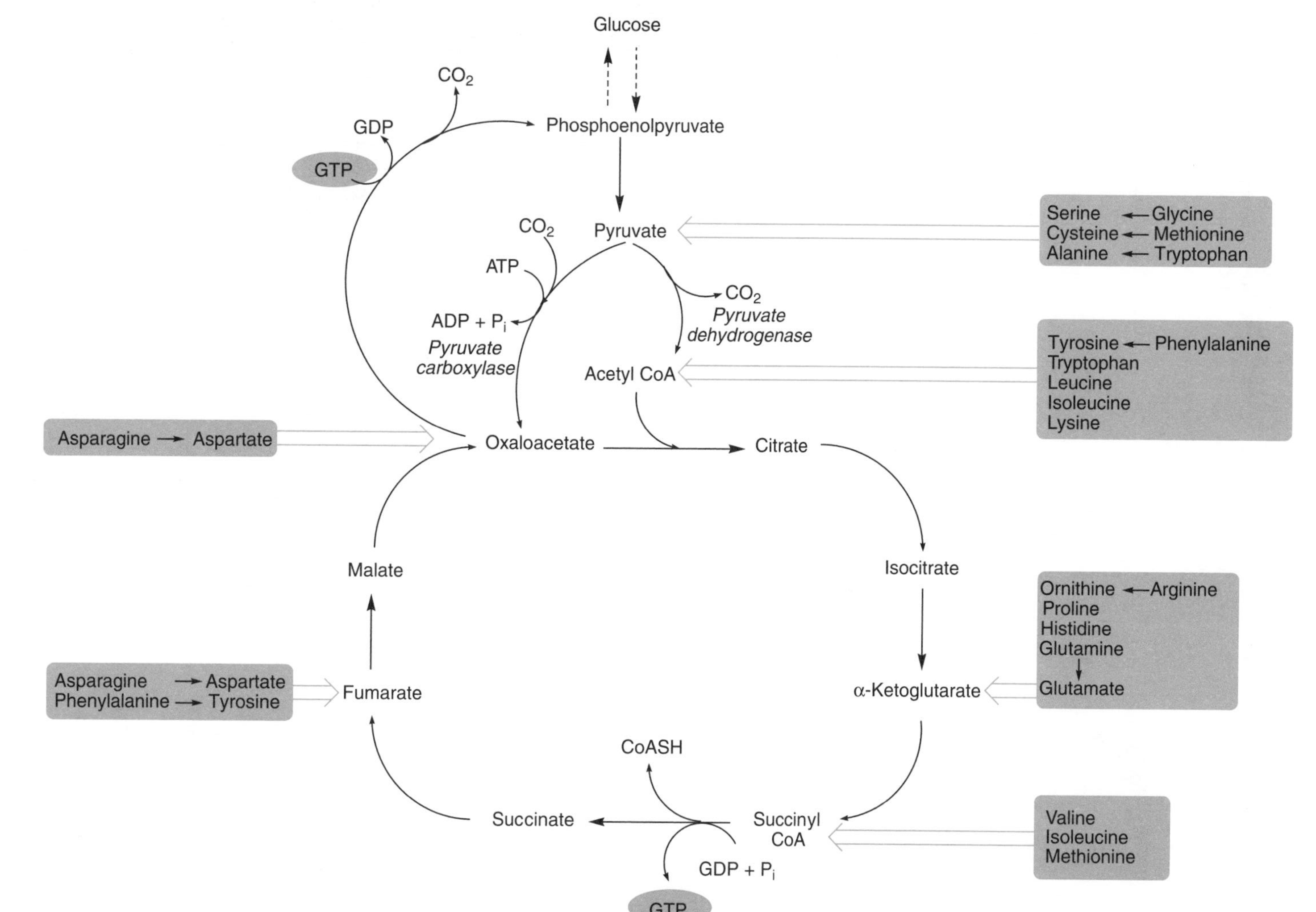

Figure 5.20 The entry of amino acid carbon skeletons into the citric acid cycle for gluconeogenesis.

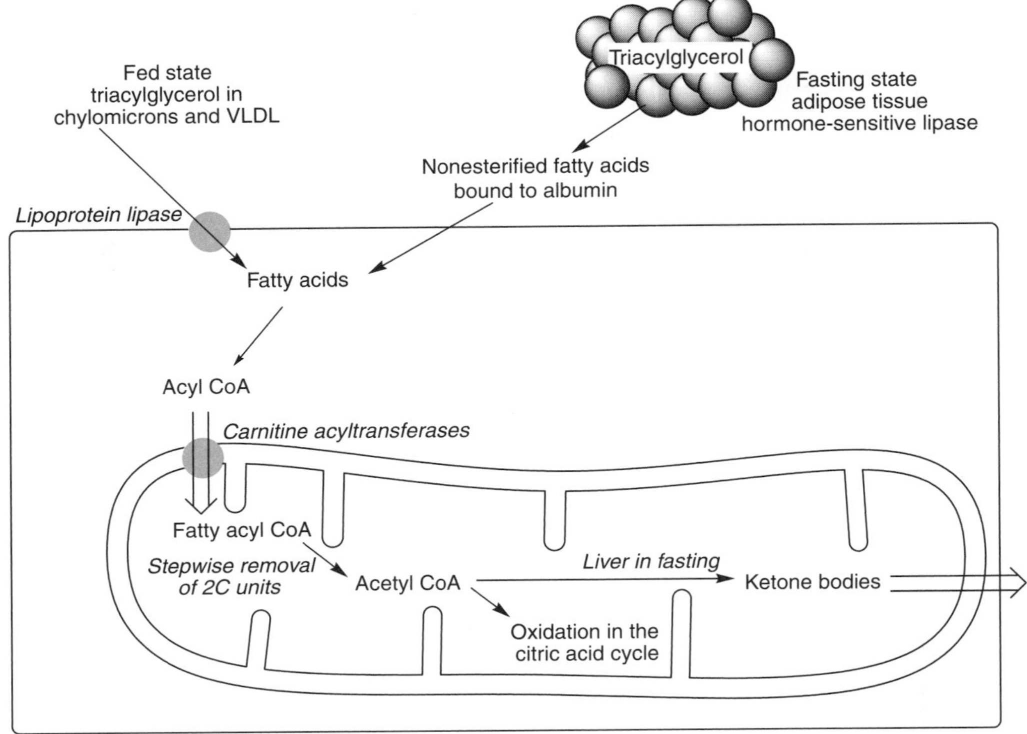

Figure 5.21 An overview of fatty acid metabolism.

(or, in adipose tissue, re-esterified to form triacylglycerol), but some remains in the bloodstream and is taken up by the liver, reesterified and exported in very low density lipoprotein; as discussed in Section 8.4.1, this is an ATP-expensive process.

In the fasting state, hormone-sensitive lipase in adipose tissue is activated in response to falling insulin secretion or the secretion of adrenaline (Section 10.5.1) and catalyzes the hydrolysis of triacylglycerol, releasing free fatty acids into the bloodstream, where they bind to albumin and are transported to tissues. Increased activity of hormone-sensitive lipase in response to compounds secreted by some tumors leads to cycling of fatty acids between adipose tissue and liver, and is a factor in the hypermetabolism seen in patients with cancer cachexia (Section 8.4.1).

The glycerol released by hormone-sensitive lipase or lipoprotein lipase is mainly transported to the liver, where it may be used either as a metabolic fuel or for gluconeogenesis. The fatty acids are oxidized in the mitochondria by the β-oxidation pathway, in which two carbon atoms at a time are removed from the fatty acid chain as acetyl CoA. This acetyl CoA then enters the citric acid cycle, together with that arising from the metabolism of pyruvate.

5.5.1 Carnitine and the transport of fatty acids into the mitochondrion

As fatty acids enter the cell, they are esterified with coenzyme A to form acyl CoA. This protects cell membranes against the lytic action of free fatty acids. However, acyl CoA cannot cross the mitochondrial membranes to enter the matrix, where the enzymes for β-oxidation are located.

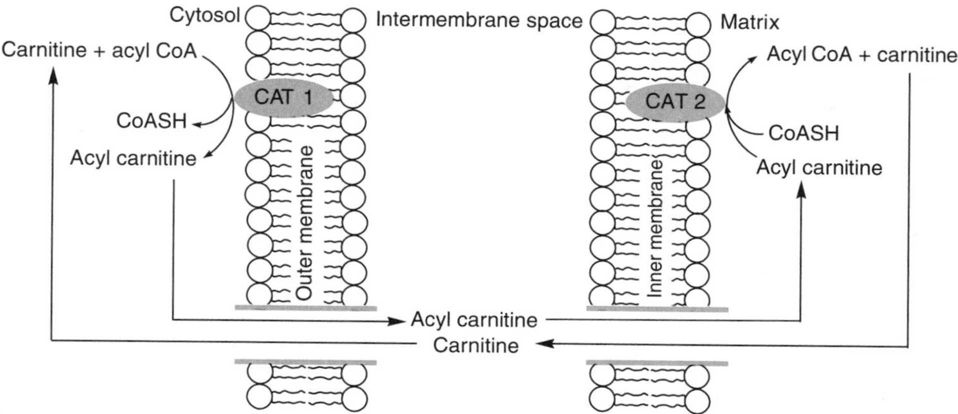

Figure 5.22 The role of carnitine in transport of fatty acids into the mitochondrion (CAT = carnitine acyltransferase).

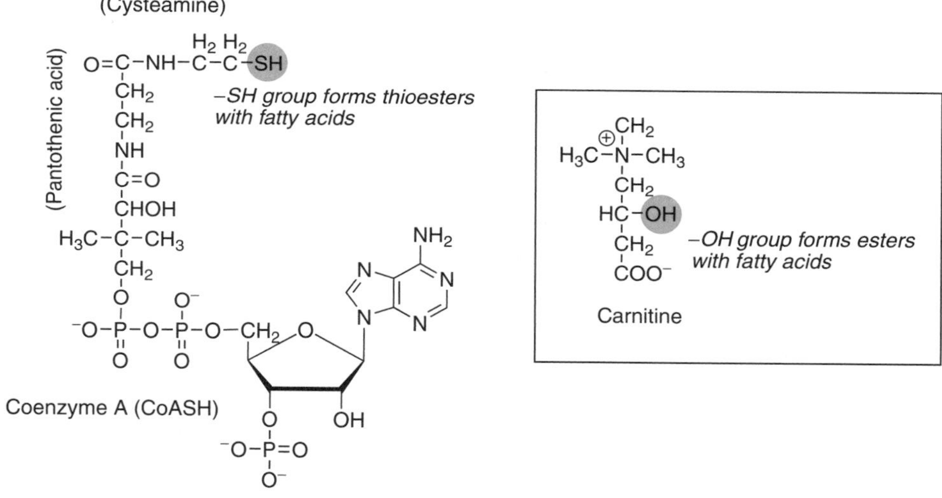

Figure 5.23 The structures of coenzyme A (CoA) and carnitine. Free coenzyme A is usually shown as CoASH to show that it has a free sulfydryl group.

On the outer face of the outer mitochondrial membrane, the fatty acid is transferred from CoA onto carnitine, forming acylcarnitine, which enters the intermembrane space through an acylcarnitine transporter (Figures 5.22 and 5.23).

Acylcarnitine can only cross the mitochondrial membranes using a countertransport system that transports acylcarnitine inward in exchange for free carnitine being transported out. Once inside the mitochondrial inner membrane, the acyl group is transferred onto CoA ready to undergo β-oxidation. This countertransport system provides regulation of the uptake of fatty acids into the mitochondrion for oxidation. As long as there is free CoA available in the mitochondrial matrix, fatty acids can be taken up, and the carnitine returned to the outer membrane for uptake of more fatty acids. However, if most of the CoA in the mitochondrion is acylated, then there is no need for further fatty uptake, and indeed, it is not possible.

This carnitine shuttle also serves to prevent mitochondrial uptake and oxidation of fatty acids synthesized in the cytosol in the fed state. Malonyl CoA (the precursor for fatty acid synthesis; Section 5.6.1) is a potent inhibitor of carnitine acyl transferase I in the outer mitochondrial membrane.

Tissues such as muscle that oxidize fatty acids, but do not synthesize them, also have acetyl CoA carboxylase and produce malonyl CoA. This controls the activity of carnitine acyl transferase I and thus controls the mitochondrial uptake and β-oxidation of fatty acids. Tissues also have malonyl CoA decarboxylase, which acts to remove malonyl CoA and thus reduces the inhibition of carnitine acyl transferase I. The two enzymes are regulated in opposite directions in response to

- Insulin, which stimulates fatty acid synthesis and reduces β-oxidation
- Glucagon, which reduces fatty acid synthesis and increases β-oxidation

Fatty acids are the major fuel for red muscle fibers, the main type involved in moderate exercise (Section 10.6). Children who lack one of the enzymes for carnitine synthesis, and are therefore reliant on a dietary intake, have poor exercise tolerance, because they have an impaired ability to transport fatty acids into the mitochondria for β-oxidation. Provision of supplements of carnitine to the affected children overcomes the problem. Extrapolation from this rare clinical condition has led to the use of carnitine as a so-called ergogenic aid to improve athletic performance. A number of studies have shown that relatively large supplements of carnitine increase the muscle content of carnitine to only a small extent, and most studies have shown no significant effect on athletic performance or endurance. This is not surprising—carnitine is readily synthesized from lysine and methionine, and there is no evidence that any dietary intake is required.

5.5.2 The β-oxidation of fatty acids

Once it has entered the mitochondria, fatty acyl CoA undergoes a series of four reactions, resulting in the cleavage of the fatty acid molecule to yield acetyl CoA and a new fatty acyl CoA, which is two carbons shorter than the initial substrate (Figure 5.24). This shorter fatty acyl CoA is a substrate for the same sequence of reactions, which is repeated until the final result is cleavage to yield two molecules of acetyl CoA. This is the pathway of β-oxidation, so called because it is the β-carbon of the fatty acid that undergoes oxidation.

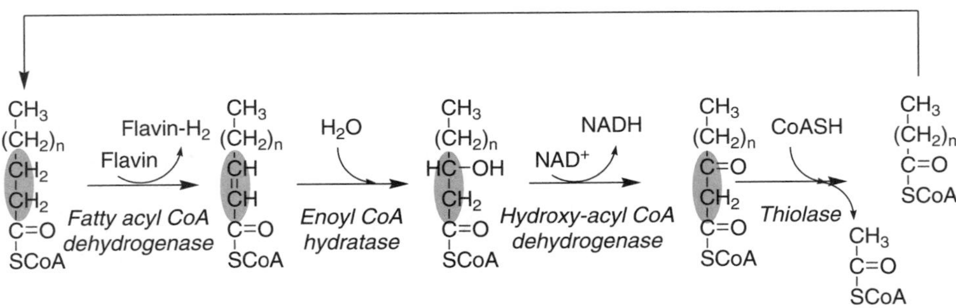

Figure 5.24 β-Oxidation of fatty acids.

The reactions of β-oxidation are chemically the same as those in the conversion of succinate to oxaloacetate in the citric acid cycle (Figure 5.18):

- Removal of two hydrogens from the fatty acid to form a carbon–carbon double bond—an oxidation reaction that is linked to the reduction of flavin—so for each double bond formed in this way there is a yield of 1.5 × ATP.
- Hydration of the newly formed double bond to form hydroxyl group.
- Oxidation of the hydroxyl group to an oxo group, linked to reduction of NAD^+, equivalent to 2.5 × ATP.
- Cleavage of the oxo-acyl CoA by coenzyme A, to form acetyl CoA and the shorter fatty acyl CoA, which undergoes the same sequence of reactions.

There are three separate sets of enzymes catalyzing these four reactions, with specificity for long-, medium-, and short-chain fatty acyl CoA derivatives. Each set of enzymes is arranged as a membrane-bound array, and the product of one is passed directly to the active site of the next. The result of this is that while short- and medium-chain fatty acyl CoA can be detected in the mitochondrial matrix, as they pass from one array of enzymes to the next, none of the intermediates of the reaction sequence can be detected—they remain enzyme bound.

The acetyl CoA formed by β-oxidation then enters the citric acid cycle (Figure 5.18). Almost all the metabolically important fatty acids have an even number of carbon atoms, so that the final cycle of β-oxidation is the conversion of a four-carbon fatty acyl CoA (butyryl CoA) to two molecules of acetyl CoA. Rare odd-carbon fatty acids yield propionyl CoA as the final product; this is carboxylated to succinyl CoA, which is an intermediate of the citric acid cycle. Because it increases the pool of four-carbon intermediates in the cycle, propionyl CoA provides a net source of carbon for gluconeogenesis.

5.5.3 Ketone bodies

Most tissues have a limited capacity for fatty acid oxidation and in the fasting state cannot meet their energy requirements from fatty acid oxidation alone. In contrast, the liver is capable of forming considerably more acetyl CoA from fatty acids than is required for its own metabolism. It takes up fatty acids from the circulation and oxidizes them to acetyl CoA, then synthesizes and exports the four-carbon ketone bodies formed from acetyl CoA to other tissues (especially heart and skeletal muscle) for use as a metabolic fuel.

Acetoacetyl CoA is formed by reaction between two molecules of acetyl CoA (Figure 5.25). This is essentially the reverse of the final reaction of fatty acid β-oxidation (Figure 5.24). Acetoacetyl CoA then reacts with a further molecule of acetyl CoA to form hydroxymethylglutaryl CoA, which is cleaved to acetyl CoA and acetoacetate.

Acetoacetate is chemically unstable and undergoes a nonenzymic reaction to yield acetone, which is only poorly metabolized. Most of it is excreted in the urine and in exhaled air—a waste of valuable metabolic fuel reserves in the fasting state. To avoid this, much of the acetoacetate is reduced to β-hydroxybutyrate before being released from the liver.

The first step in the utilization of β-hydroxybutyrate and acetoacetate in extrahepatic tissues is oxidation of β-hydroxybutyrate to acetoacetate, yielding NADH (Figure 5.26). The synthesis of β-hydroxybutyrate in the liver can thus be regarded not only as a way of preventing loss of metabolic fuel as acetone, but also effectively as a means of exporting NADH (and, therefore, effectively ATP) to extrahepatic tissues.

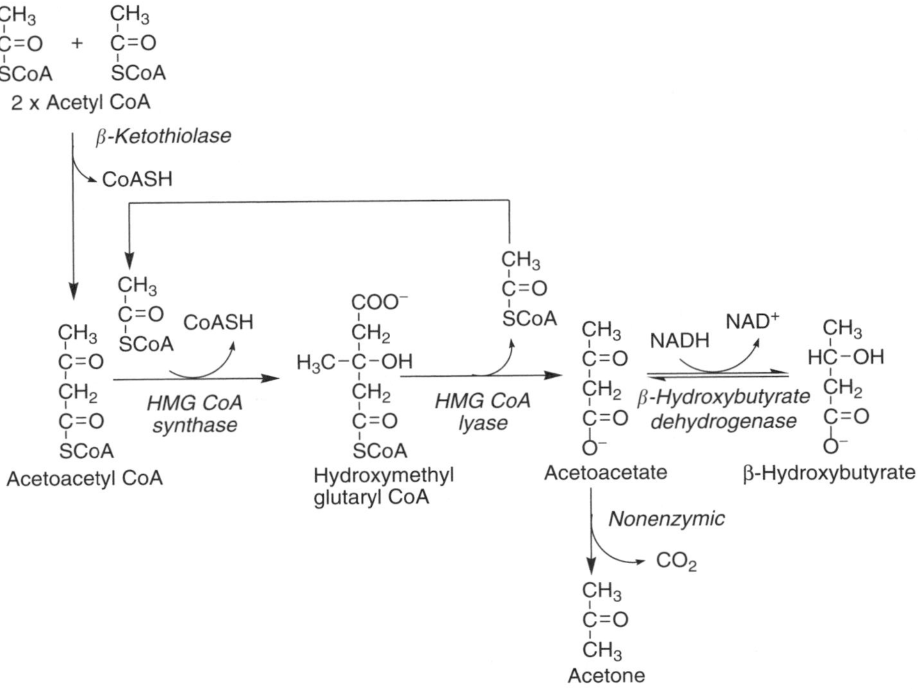

Figure 5.25 The synthesis of ketone bodies in the liver.

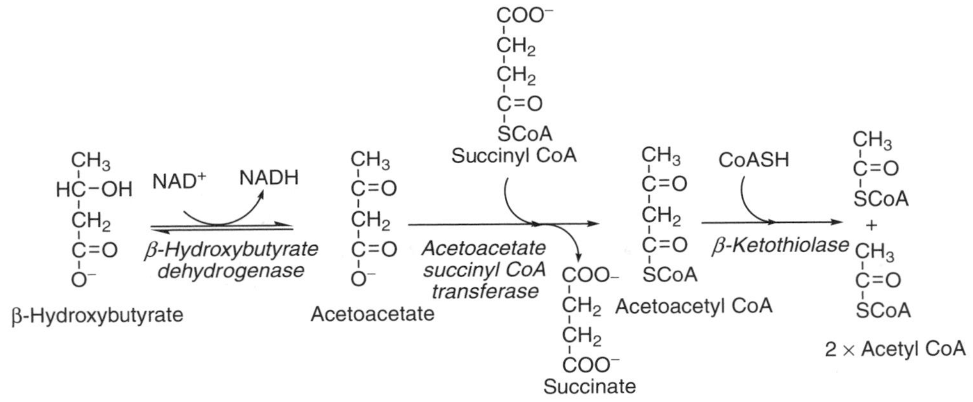

Figure 5.26 The utilization of ketone bodies in extrahepatic tissues.

The utilization of acetoacetate is controlled by the activity of the citric acid cycle. The reaction of acetoacetate succinyl CoA transferase provides an alternative to the reaction of succinyl CoA synthase (Figure 5.18), and there will only be an adequate supply of succinyl CoA to permit conversion of acetoacetate to acetoacetyl CoA as long as the rate of citric acid cycle activity is adequate. This means that even in the fasting state, there may be a need for some metabolism of glucose to provide pyruvate that can be carboxylated to oxaloacetate to maintain citric acid cycle activity.

Acetoacetate, β-hydroxybutyrate, and acetone are collectively known as the ketone bodies, and the occurrence of increased concentrations of these three compounds in the bloodstream is known as ketosis. Although acetone and acetoacetate are chemically ketones, having a –C=O grouping, β-hydroxybutyrate is not chemically a ketone. It is classified with the other two because of its metabolic relationship. Acetoacetate and β-hydroxybutyrate are also acids, and will lower blood pH, potentially leading to metabolic acidosis. See Section 10.7 for a discussion of the problems of ketoacidosis in diabetes mellitus.

5.6 *Tissue reserves of metabolic fuels*

In the fed state, as well as providing for immediate energy needs, substrates are converted into storage compounds for use in the fasting state. There are two main stores of metabolic fuels:

- Triacylglycerols in adipose tissue
- Glycogen in liver and muscle

In addition, there is an increase in the synthesis of proteins after a meal, as a result of the increased availability of metabolic fuel to provide ATP for protein synthesis (Section 9.2.3.3) and stimulation of protein synthesis by insulin.

In the fasting state, which is the normal state between meals, these reserves are mobilized and used. Glycogen is a source of glucose, while adipose tissue provides both fatty acids and glycerol from triacylglycerol. The rate of protein synthesis is slower than that of protein catabolism (Section 9.1.1), so that there is an increased supply of amino acids for gluconeogenesis.

5.6.1 *Synthesis of fatty acids and triacylglycerols*

Fatty acids are synthesized by the successive addition of two-carbon units from acetyl CoA followed by reduction. Like β-oxidation, fatty acid synthesis is a spiral sequence of reactions, with different enzymes catalyzing the reaction sequence for synthesis of short-, medium-, and long-chain fatty acids.

Unlike β-oxidation, which occurs in the mitochondrial matrix, fatty acid synthesis occurs in the cytosol. The enzymes required for fatty acid synthesis form a large multienzyme complex, arranged in a series of concentric rings around a central acyl carrier protein (ACP), which carries the growing fatty acid chain from one enzyme to the next. The functional group of the ACP is the same as that of CoA derived from the vitamin pantothenic acid and cysteamine (Figure 5.23). As the chain grows in length, so the middle, then outermost, ring of enzymes are used. Only the final 16-carbon fatty acid, and none of the intermediates, is released.

The only source of acetyl CoA is in the mitochondrial matrix, and acetyl CoA cannot cross the inner mitochondrial membrane. For fatty acid synthesis, citrate is formed inside the mitochondria by reaction between acetyl CoA and oxaloacetate (Figure 5.27), and is then transported into the cytosol, where it is cleaved to acetyl CoA and oxaloacetate. The acetyl CoA is used for fatty acid synthesis, while the oxaloacetate (indirectly) returns to the mitochondria to maintain citric acid cycle activity.

Fatty acid synthesis can only occur when there is citrate available in excess of the requirement for citric acid cycle activity for energy-yielding metabolism. Citrate is passed directly from the active site of citrate synthase to that of aconitase. It is only when isocitrate

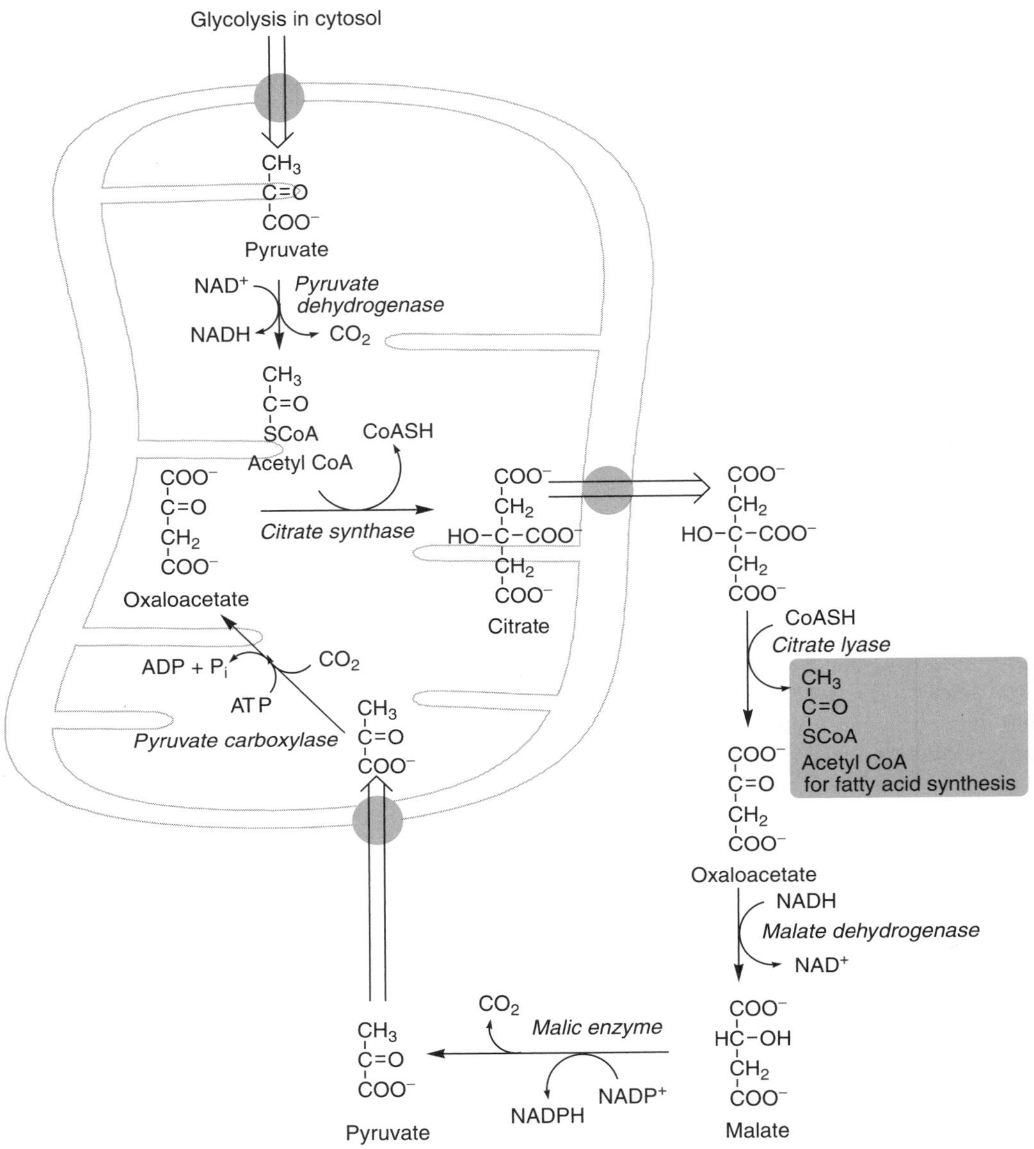

Figure 5.27 The source of acetyl CoA in the cytosol for fatty acid synthesis.

dehydrogenase is saturated, and hence aconitase is inhibited by its product, that citrate is released from the active site of citrate synthase into free solution, to be available for transport out of the mitochondria (see Problem 5.3).

Oxaloacetate cannot reenter the mitochondrion directly; it is reduced to malate, which then undergoes oxidative decarboxylation to pyruvate, linked to the reduction of $NADP^+$ to NADPH. Pyruvate enters the mitochondrion and is carboxylated to oxaloacetate in a reaction catalyzed by pyruvate carboxylase.

The first reaction in the synthesis of fatty acids is carboxylation of acetyl CoA to malonyl CoA (Figure 5.28). This is a biotin-dependent reaction (Section 11.12.2). The activity of

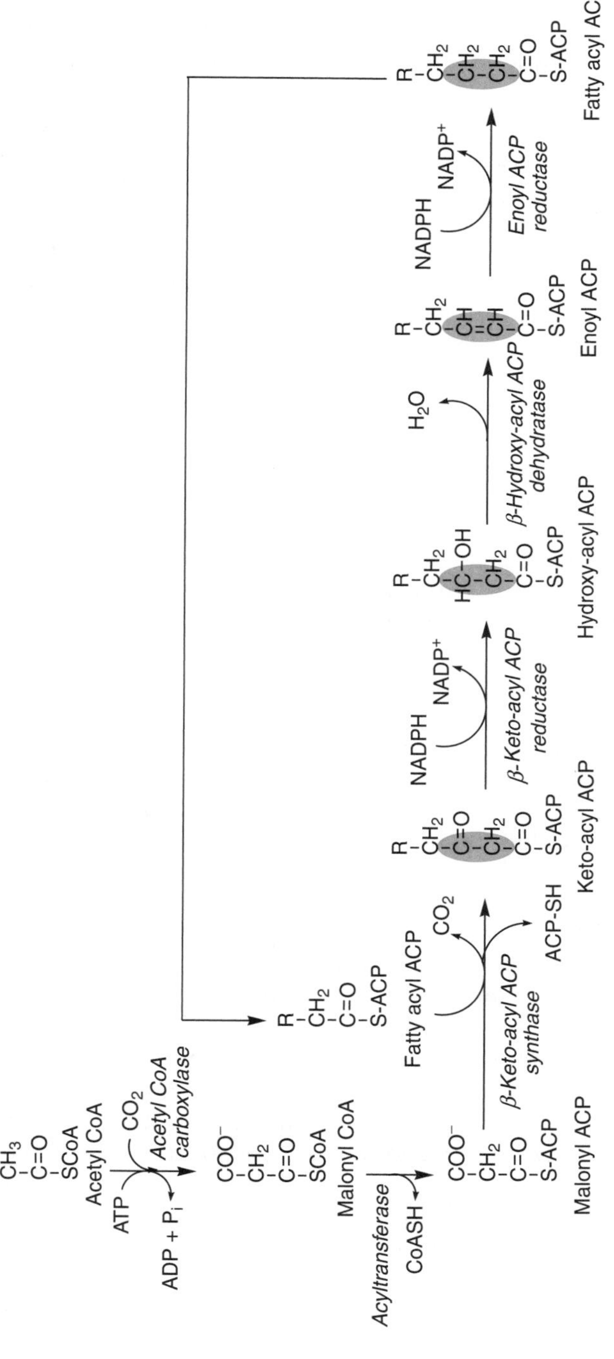

Figure 5.28 The synthesis of fatty acids.

acetyl CoA carboxylase is regulated in response to insulin and glucagon. Malonyl CoA is not only the substrate for fatty acid synthesis, but also a potent inhibitor of carnitine acyl transferase, thus inhibiting the uptake of fatty acids into the mitochondrion for β-oxidation (Section 5.5.1).

The malonyl group is transferred onto an ACP and then reacts with the growing fatty acid chain, bound to the central ACP of the fatty acid synthase complex. The carbon dioxide that was added to form malonyl CoA is lost in this reaction.

For the first cycle of reactions, the central ACP carries an acetyl group, and the product of reaction with malonyl CoA is acetoacetyl-ACP; in subsequent reaction cycles, it is the growing fatty acid chain that occupies the central ACP, and the product of reaction with malonyl CoA is a keto-acyl-ACP.

The keto-acyl-ACP is then reduced to yield a hydroxyl group. In turn, this is dehydrated to yield a carbon–carbon double bond, which is reduced to yield a saturated fatty acid chain. Thus, the sequence of reactions is the reverse of that in β-oxidation (Section 5.5.2). For both reduction reactions in fatty acid synthesis, NADPH is the hydrogen donor. One source of this NADPH is the pentose phosphate pathway (Section 5.4.2), and the other is the oxidation of malate (arising from oxaloacetate) to pyruvate, catalyzed by the malic enzyme (Figure 5.27).

The end product of cytosolic fatty acid synthesis in liver and adipose tissue is palmitate (C16:0); longer-chain fatty acids (up to C24) and unsaturated fatty acids are synthesized from palmitate in the endoplasmic reticulum and mitochondria. In lactating mammary gland fatty acid synthesis stops at myristate (C14:0), and the mammary gland does not synthesize longer-chain or unsaturated fatty acids. The polyunsaturated fatty acids in milk are derived from synthesis in the liver, and, more importantly, the maternal diet.

5.6.1.1 Unsaturated fatty acids

Although fatty acid synthesis involves the formation of an unsaturated intermediate, the next step, reduction to the saturated fatty acid derivative, is an obligatory part of the reaction sequence and cannot be omitted. The product of the fatty acid synthase multienzyme complex is always saturated. Some unsaturated fatty acids can be synthesized from saturated fatty acids by dehydrogenation to yield a carbon–carbon double bond.

Mammalian tissues have a Δ^9-desaturase, which can introduce a carbon–carbon double bond between carbons 9 and 10 of the fatty acid (counting from the carboxyl group). This will yield oleic acid (C18:1 ω9) from stearic acid (C18:0). Other mammalian desaturases permit insertion of double bonds between Δ^{9-10} and the carboxyl group, but not between Δ^{9-10} and the methyl group (see Table 4.1).

This means that fatty acids with double bonds between Δ^{9-10} and the methyl group must be provided in the diet. Linoleic acid (C18:2 ω6) is $\Delta^{9-10,\ 12-13}$, and α-linolenic acid (C18:3 ω3) is $\Delta^{9-10,\ 12-13,\ 15-16}$. Both of these are dietary essentials, and undergo chain elongation and further desaturation (between Δ^{9-10} and the carboxyl group) to yield the precursors of the eicosanoids.

The same series of enzymes catalyzes elongation and desaturation of the ω3 and ω6 families of fatty acids, and they compete with each other. Although it is considered desirable to increase intakes of polyunsaturated fatty acids (Section 6.3.2.1), there is some concern that an imbalance between intakes of ω6 polyunsaturated fatty acids (which come mainly from vegetable oils) and the ω3 series (which come mainly from fish oils) may lead to an imbalance in the synthesis of the two groups of eicosanoids synthesized from the polyunsaturated fatty acids.

5.6.1.2 Synthesis of triacylglycerol

The storage lipids in adipose tissue are triacylglycerols: glycerol esterified with three molecules of fatty acids; the three fatty acids in a triacylglycerol molecule are not always the same, and the fatty acid at carbon-2 is usually unsaturated. Triacylglycerol is synthesized in the small intestinal mucosa, liver, adipose tissue, lactating mammary gland, and skeletal muscle.

In adipose tissue, triacylglycerol is synthesized from the dietary fatty acids absorbed in lipid micelles and packaged into chylomicrons (Section 4.3.2.2). In both liver and adipose tissue, the fatty acids may be synthesized *de novo* from glucose. Adipose tissue also takes up fatty acids from chylomicrons and very low density lipoprotein; in the liver, the fatty acids may come from chylomicron remnants or free fatty acids released by the action of lipoprotein lipase that are not taken up into adipose tissue and muscle cells. In lactating mammary gland, most of the fatty acids are formed by *de novo* synthesis from glucose. Skeletal muscle also synthesizes triacylglycerol for storage between muscle fibers. In this case, all the fatty acid comes from chylomicrons and very low density lipoprotein; muscle is not capable of *de novo* fatty acid synthesis.

The substrates for triacylglycerol synthesis are fatty acyl CoA esters (formed by reaction between fatty acids and coenzyme A, linked to the conversion of ATP $\rightarrow$ AMP + pyrophosphate), and glycerol phosphate (Figure 5.29). The main source of glycerol phosphate is by reduction of dihydroxy-acetone phosphate (an intermediate in glycolysis; Figure 5.10); the liver, but not adipose tissue, can also utilize glycerol directly.

Two fatty acids are esterified to the free hydroxyl groups of glycerol phosphate, by transfer from fatty acyl CoA, forming monoacylglycerol phosphate and then diacylglycerol phosphate (or phosphatidate). Diacylglycerol phosphate is then hydrolyzed to diacylglycerol and phosphate before reaction with the third molecule of fatty acyl CoA to yield triacylglycerol. (The diacylglycerol phosphate can also be used for the synthesis of phospholipids [Section 4.3.1.2].)

Triacylglycerol synthesis incurs a considerable ATP cost; if the fatty acids are being synthesized from glucose then overall some 20% of the energy yield of the carbohydrate is expended in synthesizing triacylglycerol reserves. The energy cost is lower if dietary fatty acids are being esterified to form triacylglycerols.

The enzymes for phosphatidate synthesis, acyl CoA synthetase, glycerol 3-phosphate acyltransferase, and monoacylglycerol acyltransferase, are on both the outer mitochondrial membrane and the endoplasmic reticulum membrane. Diacylglycerol acyltransferase is only on the endoplasmic reticulum; it may use either diacylglycerol phosphate synthesized in the endoplasmic reticulum or that synthesized in mitochondria. Triacylglycerol synthesized on the endoplasmic reticulum membrane may then either enter lipid droplets in the cytosol or, in the liver and intestinal mucosa, the lumen of the endoplasmic reticulum for assembly into lipoproteins—chylomicrons in the intestinal mucosa (Section 4.3.2.2) and very low density lipoprotein in the liver (Section 5.6.2.2).

5.6.2 Plasma lipoproteins

Triacylglycerol, cholesterol, and cholesterol esters, as well as lipid-soluble vitamins, are transported in plasma complexed with proteins; there are five classes of lipoproteins, classified by their density, which in turn reflects their relative content of lipid and protein (Figure 5.30):

- Chylomicrons, the least dense of the plasma lipoproteins, are formed in the intestinal mucosa and circulate as a source of triacylglycerol in the fed state (Section 4.3.2.2).

- Very low density lipoproteins (VLDL) are assembled in the liver and circulate as a source of cholesterol and triacylglycerol for extrahepatic tissues in the fed state.
- Intermediate density lipoproteins (IDL) are formed in the circulation by removal of triacylglycerol from VLDL.

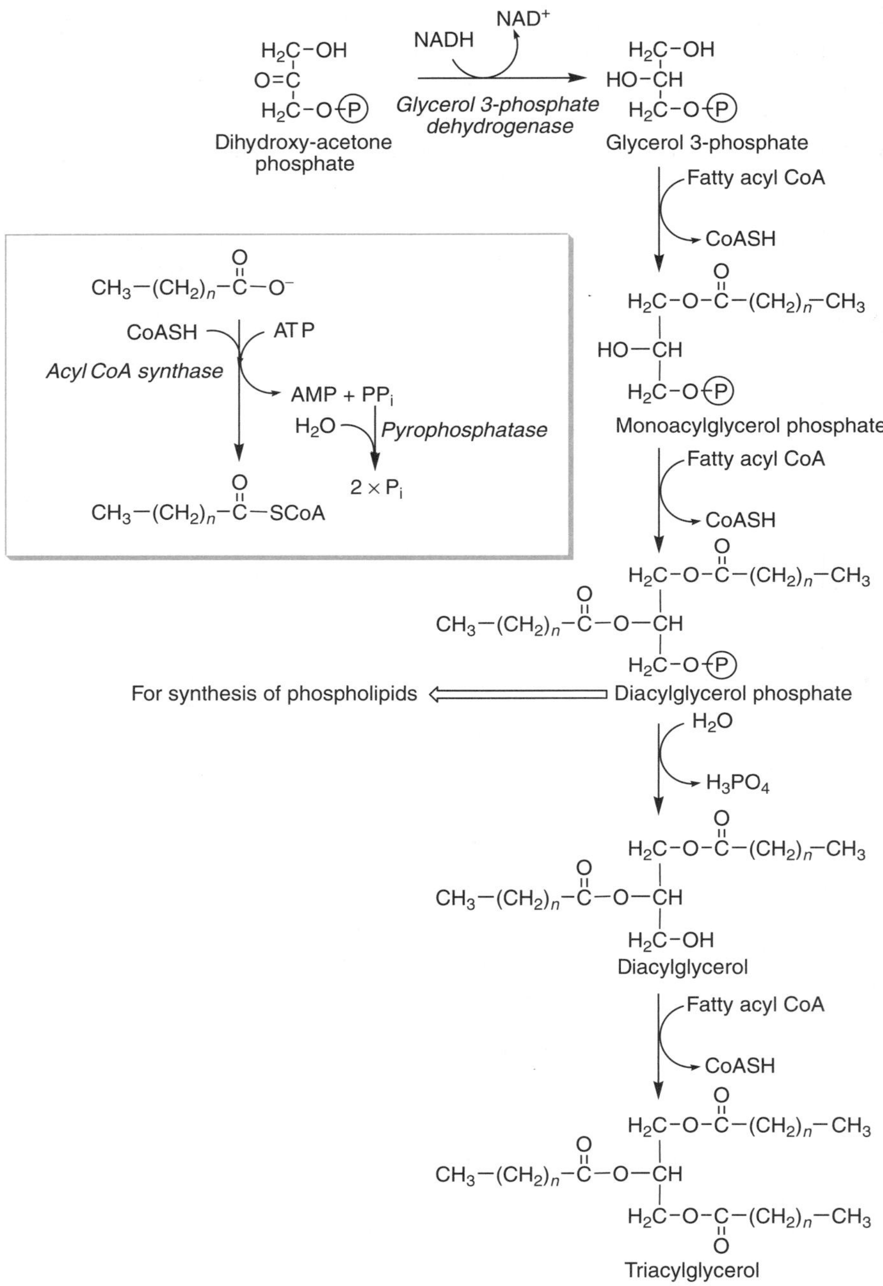

Figure 5.29 The esterification of fatty acids to form triacylglycerol.

- Low density lipoproteins (LDL) are formed in the circulation by transfer of cholesterol from HDL.
- High density lipoproteins (HDL) are synthesized in the liver and small intestine as apoproteins, and acquire lipids (and especially cholesterol) from tissues for transport back to the liver, either directly or by transfer to IDL, forming LDL.

5.6.2.1 Chylomicrons

Newly absorbed fatty acids are re-esterified to form triacylglycerol in the intestinal mucosal cells, then assembled into chylomicrons (Section 4.3.2.2), which enter the lacteal of the villus (Figure 4.2), then the lymphatic system; they enter the bloodstream (the subclavian vein) at the thoracic duct. Chylomicrons begin to appear in the bloodstream about 60 min after a fatty meal and have normally been cleared within 6–8 h by the action of lipoprotein lipase at the luminal surface of capillary blood vessels. The lipid-depleted chylomicron remnants are cleared by the liver by receptor-mediated endocytosis, followed by hydrolysis of the proteins and the residual lipids.

In the bloodstream, chylomicrons acquire three additional proteins from HDL:

- Apoprotein C-II activates lipoprotein lipase at the cell surface, permitting hydrolysis of chylomicron triacylglycerol to liberate fatty acids that are mainly taken up into adipose tissue and muscle cells.

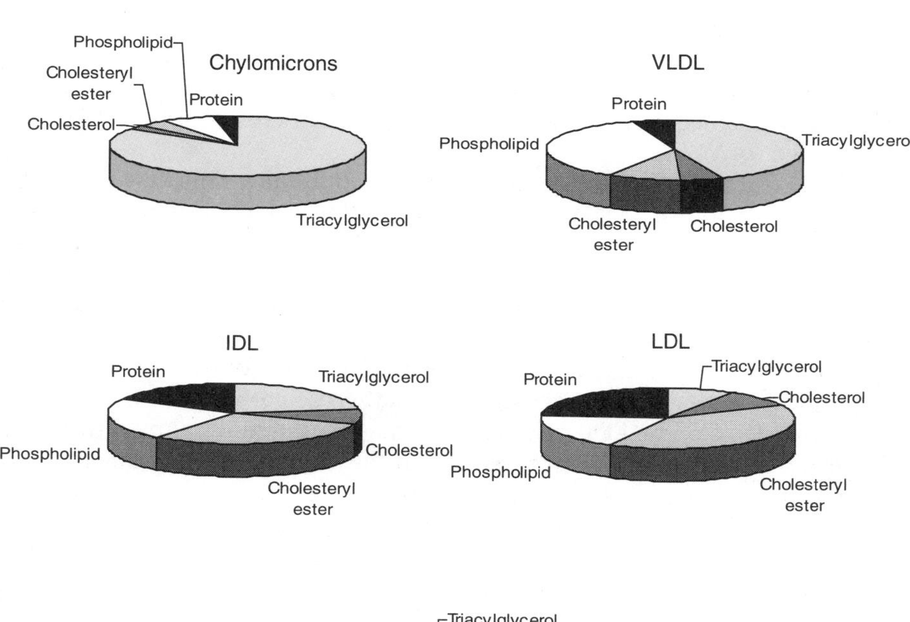

Figure 5.30 Composition of the plasma lipoproteins.

- Apoprotein C-III activates cholesterol esterase, permitting cells to take up cholesterol from chylomicron cholesteryl esters.
- Apoprotein E binds to hepatic receptors for receptor-mediated uptake of lipid-depleted chylomicron remnants.

5.6.2.2 Very low density lipoproteins, intermediate density lipoprotein, and low density lipoproteins

VLDL is assembled in the liver and contains both newly synthesized triacylglycerol, cholesterol and cholesteryl esters, and phospholipids, and also lipids from chylomicron remnants. These lipids are taken up by peripheral tissues that have cell-surface lipoprotein lipase, phospholipase, and cholesterol esterase.

As the VLDL particles are progressively depleted of lipids, they transfer apoproteins C-I and C-II to HDL, becoming IDL. IDL takes up cholesteryl esters from HDL, becoming LDL.

LDL is cleared from the circulation by receptor-mediated uptake in the liver. Both the receptor and the LDL are internalized; the LDL is hydrolyzed in lysosomes by proteases and lipases, and the receptor is recycled back to the cell surface.

Cholesterol represses synthesis of the LDL receptor, so that when there is an adequate amount of cholesterol in the liver, less LDL will be cleared. The hypocholesterolemic statin drugs both inhibit cholesterol synthesis and also increase clearance of LDL, because there is now less repression of receptor synthesis.

Elevated LDL cholesterol is one of the major factors in the development of atherosclerosis and ischemic heart disease. Two factors are involved in elevated LDL cholesterol:

- Increased synthesis and secretion of VLDL—this in turn will be a consequence of a high fat intake, since there is more lipid from chylomicron remnants to be exported from the liver in VLDL.
- Decreased clearance of LDL by receptor-mediated uptake. This may be due to:
  - Down-regulation of LDL receptor synthesis by free cholesterol in cells. Mono- and polyunsaturated fatty acids are good substrates for cholesterol esterification in cells, while saturated fatty acids are not. When saturated fatty acid levels are relatively high, less cholesterol is esterified, so that the intracellular concentration rises, repressing the synthesis of LDL receptor (see also Section 6.3.2.1).
  - Poor affinity of some genetic variants of apoprotein E for the LDL receptor. This is the basis of some genetic susceptibility to atherosclerosis.
  - Genetic defects of the LDL receptor, in some cases of familial hyperlipidemia.
  - Chemical modification of apoprotein E in the circulation, so reducing its affinity for the hepatic receptors. Commonly, this is secondary to oxidative damage to unsaturated fatty acids in LDL, hence the role of antioxidants in reducing the risk of atherosclerosis (Section 6.5.3). High levels of homocysteine (Section 11.11.3.3) can also lead to modification of apoprotein E.

LDL that is not cleared by the liver is taken up by the macrophage scavenger receptor; unlike hepatic uptake, this is an unregulated process, and macrophages can take up an almost unlimited amount of lipid from LDL. Lipid-engorged macrophages (foam cells) infiltrate blood vessel endothelium, especially when there is already some degree of endothelial damage, then undergo necrosis to form fatty streaks, which eventually develop into atherosclerotic plaque. Unesterified cholesterol and plant sterols are especially cytotoxic to macrophages.

5.6.2.3 High density lipoproteins

Peripheral tissues take up more cholesterol from VLDL than they require, and export the surplus onto HDL for return to the liver for excretion or catabolism. HDL is secreted from the liver as a lipid-poor protein and takes up cholesterol from tissues by the action of lecithin cholesterol acyltransferase at the lipoprotein surface.

Much of the cholesterol in HDL is transferred to chylomicron remnants and LDL for receptor-mediated uptake into the liver. However, cholesterol-rich HDL can also bind to a liver receptor, which has esterase activity, permitting uptake of cholesterol into the liver. The apoprotein is not internalized, as occurs with chylomicron remnants and LDL, but is released back into the circulation when most of the lipid has been removed.

5.6.3 Glycogen

In the fed state, glycogen is synthesized from glucose in both liver and muscle. The reaction is a stepwise addition of glucose units onto the glycogen that is already present (Figure 5.31).

Glycogen synthesis involves the intermediate formation of uridine diphosphate (UDP) glucose by reaction between glucose 1-phosphate and UTP (uridine triphosphate). As

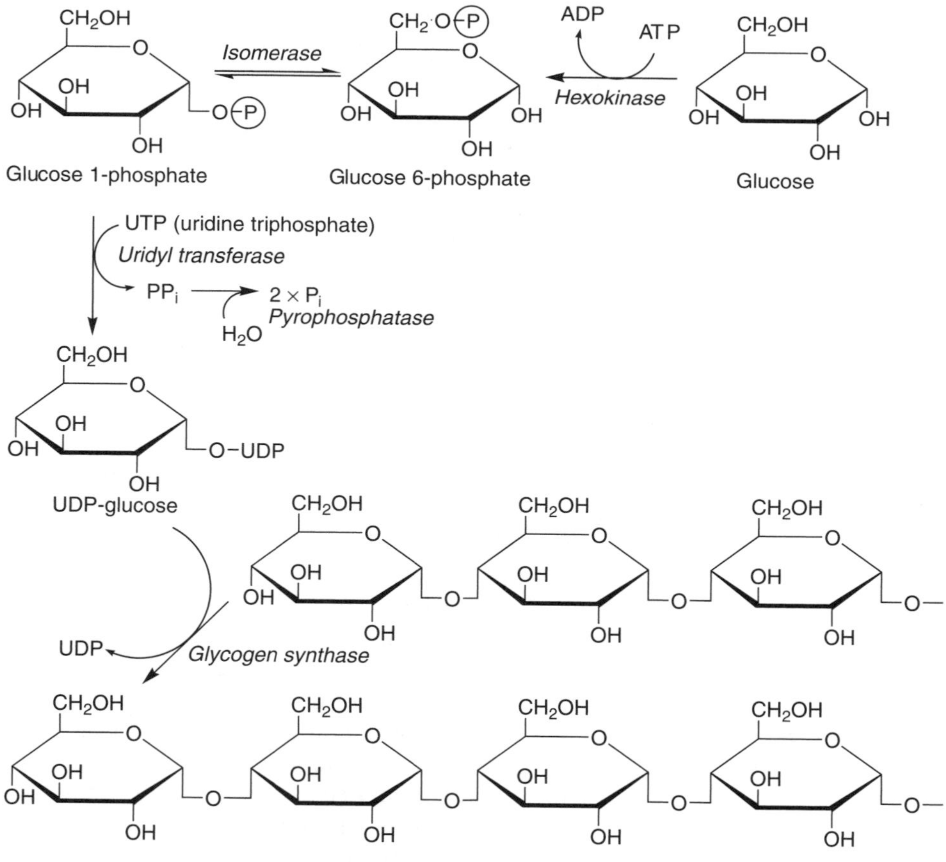

Figure 5.31 The synthesis of glycogen.

each glucose unit is added to the growing glycogen chain, UDP is released and must be rephosphorylated to UTP by reaction with ATP. There is thus a significant cost of ATP in the synthesis of glycogen: 2 mol of ATP are converted to ADP and phosphate for each glucose unit added, and overall the energy cost of glycogen synthesis may account for 5% of the energy yield of the carbohydrate stored.

Glycogen synthetase forms only the α1→4 links that form the straight chains of glycogen. The branch points are introduced by the transfer of a chain of 6–10 glucose units from carbon-4 to carbon-6 of the glucose unit at the branch point.

The branched structure of glycogen means that it traps a considerable amount of water within the molecule. In the early stages of food restriction, there is depletion of muscle and liver glycogen, with the release and excretion of this trapped water. This leads to an initial rate of weight loss that is very much greater than can be accounted for by catabolism of adipose tissue, and, of course, it cannot be sustained—once glycogen has been depleted, the rapid loss of water (and weight) will cease (Section 5.2).

5.6.3.1 Glycogen utilization

In the fasting state, glycogen is broken down by the removal of glucose units one at a time from the many ends of the molecule. The reaction is a phosphorolysis—cleavage of the glycoside link between two glucose molecules by the introduction of phosphate (Figure 5.9). The product is glucose 1-phosphate, which is then isomerized to glucose 6-phosphate. In the liver, glucose 6-phosphatase catalyzes the hydrolysis of glucose 6-phosphate to free glucose, which is exported for use especially by the brain and red blood cells.

Muscle cannot release free glucose from the breakdown of glycogen, since it lacks glucose 6-phosphatase. However, muscle glycogen can be an indirect source of blood glucose in the fasting state. Glucose 6-phosphate from muscle glycogen undergoes glycolysis to pyruvate (Figure 5.10), which is then transaminated to alanine. Alanine is exported from muscle and taken up by the liver for use as a substrate for gluconeogenesis (Section 5.7).

Glycogen phosphorylase stops cleaving α1→4 links four glucose residues from a branch point, and a debranching enzyme catalyzes the transfer of a three-glucosyl unit to the free end of another chain. The α1→6 link is then hydrolyzed by a glucosidase, releasing glucose.

The branched structure of glycogen means that there are a great many points at which glycogen phosphorylase can act; in response to stimulation by adrenaline, there is a very rapid rise in blood glucose as a result of phosphorolysis of glycogen.

Endurance athletes require a slow release of glucose 1-phosphate from glycogen over a period of hours rather than a rapid release. There is some evidence that this is achieved better from glycogen that is less branched and therefore has fewer points at which glycogen phosphorylase can act. The formation of branch points in glycogen synthesis is slower than the formation of α1→4 links, and this has been exploited in the process of "carbohydrate loading" in preparation for endurance athletic events. The athlete exercises to exhaustion, when muscle glycogen is more or less completely depleted, then consumes a high carbohydrate meal, which stimulates rapid synthesis of glycogen, with fewer branch points than normal. There is little evidence to show whether this improves endurance performance or not; such improvement as has been reported may be the result of knowing that one has made an effort to improve performance rather than any real metabolic effect.

5.7 Gluconeogenesis—the synthesis of glucose from noncarbohydrate precursors

Because the brain is largely dependent on glucose as its metabolic fuel (and red blood cells are entirely so), there is a need to maintain the blood concentration of glucose above about 3 mmol/L in the fasting state. If the plasma concentration of glucose falls below about 2 mmol/L, there is a loss of consciousness—hypoglycemic coma.

The plasma concentration of glucose is maintained in short-term fasting by the use of glycogen and by releasing free fatty acids from adipose tissues and ketone bodies from the liver, which are preferentially used by muscle, thus sparing such glucose as is available for use by the brain and red blood cells.

However, the total body content of glycogen would be exhausted within 12–18 h of fasting if there were no other source of glucose. The process of gluconeogenesis is the synthesis of glucose from noncarbohydrate precursors: amino acids from the breakdown of protein and the glycerol of triacylglycerols. It is important to note that although acetyl CoA, and hence fatty acids, can be synthesized from pyruvate (and therefore from carbohydrates), the decarboxylation of pyruvate to acetyl CoA (Figure 5.16) cannot be reversed. Pyruvate cannot be formed from acetyl CoA. Since two molecules of carbon dioxide are formed for each two-carbon acetate unit metabolized in the citric acid cycle (Figure 5.18), there can be no net formation of oxaloacetate from acetate. It is not possible to synthesize glucose from acetyl CoA; fatty acids and ketone bodies cannot serve as a precursor for glucose synthesis under any circumstances.

The main organ for gluconeogenesis is the liver; during prolonged starvation and at times of metabolic acidosis, when hepatic gluconeogenesis decreases, the kidney also makes a significant contribution. The key enzymes for gluconeogenesis are also expressed in small intestinal mucosal cells, and isotopic tracer experiments suggest that the small intestine may contribute to glucose synthesis in starvation.

The pathway of gluconeogenesis is essentially the reverse of the pathway of glycolysis, shown in Figure 5.10. However, at three steps there are separate enzymes involved in the breakdown of glucose (glycolysis) and gluconeogenesis. The reactions of pyruvate kinase, phosphofructokinase, and hexokinase cannot readily be reversed (i.e., they have equilibria that are strongly in the direction of the formation of pyruvate, fructose bisphosphate, and glucose 6-phosphate, respectively).

There are therefore separate enzymes, under distinct metabolic control, for the reverse of each of these reactions in gluconeogenesis:

- Pyruvate is converted to phosphoenolpyruvate for glucose synthesis by a two-step reaction with the intermediate formation of oxaloacetate (Figure 5.32). Pyruvate is carboxylated to oxaloacetate in an ATP-dependent reaction in which the vitamin biotin (Section 11.12.2) is the coenzyme. This reaction can also be used to replenish oxaloacetate in the citric acid cycle when intermediates have been withdrawn for use in other pathways and is involved in the return of oxaloacetate from the cytosol to the mitochondrion in fatty acid synthesis (Figure 5.26). Oxaloacetate then undergoes a phosphorylation reaction, in which it also loses carbon dioxide, to form phosphoenolpyruvate. The phosphate donor for this reaction is GTP; this provides control of the withdrawal of oxaloacetate for gluconeogenesis if citric acid cycle activity would be impaired (Section 5.4.4).
- Fructose bisphosphate is hydrolyzed to fructose 6-phosphate by a simple hydrolysis reaction catalyzed by the enzyme fructose bisphosphatase.
- Glucose 6-phosphate is hydrolyzed to free glucose and phosphate by the action of glucose 6-phosphatase.

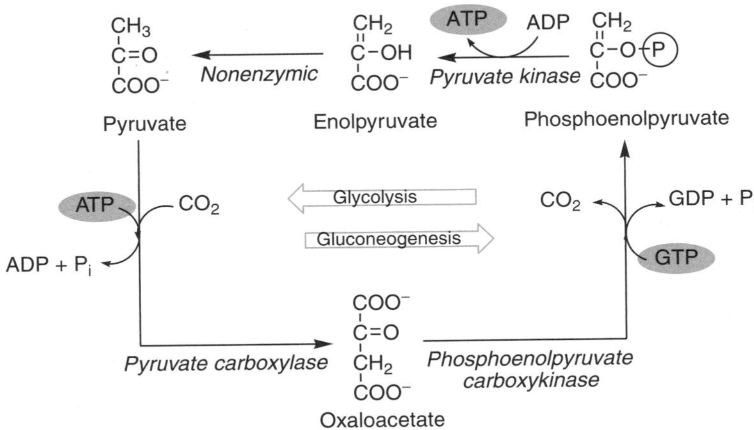

Figure 5.32 Reversal of the reaction of pyruvate kinase for gluconeogenesis: pyruvate carboxylase and phosphoenolpyruvate carboxykinase.

The other reactions of glycolysis are readily reversible and the overall direction of metabolism, either glycolysis or gluconeogenesis, depends mainly on the relative activities of phosphofructokinase and fructose bisphosphatase (Section 10.2.2).

Many of the products of amino acid metabolism can also be used for gluconeogenesis, since they are sources of pyruvate or one of the intermediates in the citric acid cycle and hence give rise to oxaloacetate (Sections 5.4.4.2 and 9.3.2). The requirement for gluconeogenesis from amino acids to maintain a supply of glucose explains why there is a considerable loss of muscle in prolonged fasting or starvation, even if there are apparently adequate reserves of adipose tissue to meet energy needs.

Key points

- Energy expenditure can be measured directly by heat output from the body or indirectly by measuring oxygen consumption or the difference in the rate of loss of ^{18}O and ^{2}H from dual isotopically labeled water.
- Measurement of carbon dioxide production as well as oxygen consumption (RQ), and urinary excretion of urea permits estimation of the relative amounts of fat, carbohydrate, and protein being metabolized.
- In fasting, when the major fuel is fatty acids, RQ is near 0.8; in the fed state, when there is ample carbohydrate available, it rises to near 1.0.
- BMR is the energy expenditure at rest under controlled conditions of thermal neutrality about 12 h after a meal; it is the energy required to maintain nerve and muscle tone, circulation and respiration, and metabolic homeostasis. It is determined by gender, age, and body weight.
- The energy cost of physical activity is expressed as the PAR—the cost of the activity as a multiple of BMR.
- A person's overall PAL is the sum of the PARs of individual activities multiplied by the time spent in each activity per 24 h.

- Diet-induced thermogenesis is the increase in metabolic activity after a meal; it is mainly the energy cost of synthesizing reserves of triacylglycerol and glycogen, as well as increased protein synthesis.
- From the composition of adipose tissue, it is possible to calculate that there will be a change of 33 g in body weight per MJ energy imbalance per day. In practice, the weight change is less than this because of adaptation to increased or decreased food intake.
- In the fed state, there is an ample supply of metabolic fuel, and reserves of fat and glycogen are formed; these are used in the fasting state to ensure a supply of fuel for tissues.
- The brain and central nervous system are largely reliant on glucose, and red blood cells and renal medulla wholly so; in the fasting state, muscle does not utilize glucose but metabolizes fatty acids released from adipose tissue reserves and ketone bodies synthesized by the liver.
- Glycolysis is the pathway by which glucose is oxidized to 2 mol of the three-carbon compound pyruvate. There is a net yield of $7 \times$ ATP per mole of glucose metabolized.
- In maximum exertion, glycolysis can proceed anaerobically with reduction of pyruvate to lactate; the net yield is then $2 \times$ ATP per mole of glucose oxidized. Resynthesis of glucose from lactate in the liver is ATP expensive; oxygen debt is the increased oxygen consumption associated with increased metabolic activity to provide the ATP needed.
- The pentose phosphate pathway provides an alternative to part of the pathway of glycolysis; it is the pathway for synthesis of ribose and also for the production of NADPH.
- Favism, due to impaired activity of glucose 6-phosphate dehydrogenase in the pentose phosphate pathway, impairs the ability of red blood cells to reduce glutathione, and hence the impaired ability to reduce H_2O_2, leading to hemolytic crisis in response to metabolic stress.
- Pyruvate is oxidized to acetyl CoA in a multistep reaction for which thiamin (vitamin B_1) provides the coenzyme. The reaction is irreversible.
- The acetate of acetyl CoA, arising from pyruvate oxidation, the oxidation of fatty acids and some amino acids, undergoes oxidation in the citric acid cycle, with a yield of $10 \times$ ATP per acetate.
- The citric acid cycle also provides the main pathway for the interconversion of four- and five-carbon compounds arising from amino acid metabolism and provision of substrates for gluconeogenesis.
- In the fed state, fatty acids are available to tissues from chylomicrons and VLDL by the action of lipoprotein lipase in capillary blood vessels. In the fasting state, fatty acids are provided by hydrolysis of adipose tissue triacylglycerol catalyzed by hormone-sensitive lipase.
- The uptake of fatty acids into the mitochondrion for oxidation requires formation of acyl carnitine, and the process is regulated by the availability of free coenzyme A inside the mitochondrion.
- The β-oxidation of fatty acids proceeds by the stepwise removal of two-carbon units as acetyl CoA with a yield of $4 \times$ ATP per acetyl CoA formed.
- Ketone bodies are synthesized in the liver in the fasting state to provide a metabolic fuel for muscle so as to spare glucose. In prolonged starvation, the brain can utilize ketone bodies to some extent.

- Fatty acids are synthesized in the fed state from acetyl CoA exported from the mitochondria as citrate. Fatty acid synthetase is a large multienzyme complex; the final product is palmitate (C16:0) and none of the intermediate compounds is released. Longer-chain fatty acids are synthesized from palmitate in the endoplasmic reticulum and mitochondria.
- Unsaturated fatty acids are synthesized by dehydrogenation of saturated fatty acids. Mammals can only insert double bonds between C-9 and the carboxyl group of a fatty acid; there is a dietary requirement for ω3 and ω6 polyunsaturated fatty acids, although precursors can undergo chain elongation and further desaturation.
- Triacylglycerol synthesis from fatty acids is relatively ATP expensive.
- Chylomicrons carry newly absorbed lipids from the small intestine to tissues; the liver clears chylomicron remnants.
- VLDL is assembled in the liver, containing triacylglycerol from chylomicron remnants and formed from newly synthesized fatty acids. In the circulation, it loses lipids and gains proteins, becoming intermediate density, then LDL.
- LDL transports cholesterol to tissues and acquires cholesterol from HDL. It is normally cleared by receptor-mediated uptake in the liver. The LDL receptor is downregulated by a high intracellular free cholesterol, and chemically modified (oxidized) LDL is not recognized by the liver receptor. It is taken up by macrophage scavenger receptors; lipid-engorged macrophages infiltrate blood vessel endothelium, forming fatty streaks that develop into atherosclerotic plaque.
- HDL collects surplus cholesterol from peripheral tissues, returning it to the liver (either directly or by transfer to LDL) for catabolism and excretion.

Problem 5.1: Winston B

Winston is a 75 kg man who takes part in a 100-m sprint. His plasma lactate was 0.5 mmol/L before the race and 11.5 mmol/L immediately after the race. When his breathing had returned to normal, after 30 min, it was 1.0 mmol/L.

Assuming that extracellular fluid is 20% of body weight, what is the total amount of lactate that he metabolizes during this 30 min?

Most of this lactate will be metabolized in the liver, undergoing gluconeogenesis, followed by release of glucose into the bloodstream, and uptake into muscle for synthesis of glycogen to replace that used during the race.

What is the total cost in moles of ATP or GTP per 2 mol of lactate converted to glycogen?

How much ATP would be required to convert all the lactate that is metabolized into muscle glycogen?

How much lactate must undergo total oxidation to CO_2 and water (via lactate dehydrogenase, pyruvate dehydrogenase, and the citric acid cycle) to provide this ATP?

The oxidation of lactate, like that of glucose, consumes 0.746 L oxygen per gram. The molecular mass of lactate is 90.1. What is his additional oxygen requirement (in liters) over the 30 min after the end of the race?

Assuming that his total energy expenditure is 14 MJ/day and that regardless of the fuel being oxidized the energy yield is 20 kJ/L oxygen consumed, what is the percentage increase in his oxygen consumption during this 30 min?

Problem 5.2: Peter C*

Peter is a 50 year old man, 174 cm tall, and weighs 105 kg. He is an engineer and works on secondment in one of the strict Islamic states in the Gulf where alcohol is prohibited. At the beginning of August, he returned to England for his annual leave. According to his family, he behaved as he usually did when on home leave, consuming a great deal of alcohol and refusing meals. He was known to be drinking 2 L of whiskey, two or three bottles of wine, and a dozen or more cans of lager each day; his only solid food consisted of sweets and biscuits.

On September 1, he was admitted to Accident and Emergency at UCL Hospital, semiconscious, and with a rapid respiration rate (40/min). His blood pressure was 90/60 and his pulse rate was 136/min. His temperature was normal (37.1°C). Emergency blood gas analysis revealed severe acidosis: pH 7.02 and base excess –23; pO_2 91 mmHg and pCO_2 10 mmHg. He was transferred to intensive care and given intravenous bicarbonate.

His pulse rate remained high and his blood pressure low, so emergency cardiac catheterization was performed; this revealed a cardiac output of 23 L/min (normal: 4–6). A chest X-ray showed significant cardiac enlargement.

Table 5.6 shows the clinical chemistry results from a plasma sample taken shortly after he was admitted.

What is the likely biochemical basis of Peter's problem, which led to his emergency hospitalization?

What additional test(s) might you request to confirm your assumption?

What emergency treatment would you suggest?

Table 5.6 Clinical Chemistry Results for a Plasma Sample from Peter C Taken in the Fasting State

mmol/L	Peter C	Reference Range
Glucose	10.6	3.5–5.0
Sodium	142	131–151
Potassium	3.9	3.4–5.2
Chloride	91	100–110
Bicarbonate	5	21–29
Lactate	18.9	0.9–2.7
Pyruvate	2.5	0.1–0.2

* This information is from the case notes of a patient in ITU at UCLH (The Middlesex Hospital); I am grateful to Dr. Hugh Montgomery for drawing my attention to this case and for permission to repeat data from the patient's notes.

Table 5.7 Oxygen Consumption by Pigeon Breast Muscle with and without Added Citrate

	Oxygen Consumed (μL)		
Incubated (min)	No Citrate	+ Citrate	Difference
30	645	682	+ 37
60	1055	1520	+ 465
90	1132	1938	+ 806

Source: Data reported by Krebs, H.A. and Johnson, W.A., *Enzymologia*, 4, 148–156, 1937.

Problem 5.3: The citric acid cycle

The key experiments that led to elucidation of the citric acid cycle (tricarboxylic acid cycle) were described by Krebs and Johnson in 1937. They measured the consumption of oxygen by a preparation of minced pigeon breast muscle incubated with various additions. The results in Table 5.7 show the volume of oxygen consumed during the incubation by 460 mg wet weight of tissue (the complete oxidation of 1 mmol of citrate to CO_2 and H_2O consumes 100 μL of O_2).

Previous studies had shown a similar effect of adding fumarate, oxaloacetate, or succinate. What conclusions can you draw from these results?

Isolated hepatocytes were incubated for 40 min in a phosphate/bicarbonate/CO_2 buffer system, with [U-^{14}C]palmitate (i.e., palmitate labeled with ^{14}C in all 16 carbon atoms), at a specific radioactivity of 10^3 dpm (radioactive disintegrations)/μmol, with and without the addition of 60 mmol/L malonate or oxaloacetate. One set of incubations was set up to act as a control, in which perchloric acid was added at the beginning of the experiment.

After collection of the CO_2 for measurement of the radioactivity incorporated, the denatured incubation mixture was extracted with a chloroform:methanol mixture to separate unmetabolized palmitate (in the organic phase) from water-soluble metabolites (which remained in the aqueous layer). The radioactivity in both phases was determined and the results are shown in Table 5.8.

Can you account for these observations? What is the water-soluble compound that accumulates in the presence of malonate?

Isolated hepatocytes were incubated with lactate, glutamate, or palmitate as substrates. At the end of the experiment, lactate, palmitate, glutamate, glucose (after acid hydrolysis of glycogen), and total ketone bodies (acetoacetate + β-hydroxybutyrate) were determined. The results have been expressed as change during the incubation, compared with similar incubations that were stopped with perchloric acid at the beginning of the experiment, and are shown in Table 5.9.

What conclusions can you draw from these results?

Isolated hepatocytes were incubated with lactate labeled with ^{14}C in carbon-2 ([^{14}C-2]lactate) or palmitate labeled with ^{14}C in all carbon

Table 5.8 Recovery of Radioactivity from [U-^{14}C]Palmitate in Isolated Hepatocytes

	Radioactivity (10^3 dpm/min/g cells)		
	CO_2	Organic Phase	Aqueous Phase
Control (unincubated)	0	10.0	0
No addition	2.3	7.5	0.2
+ Malonate	0	9.8	0.2
+ Oxaloacetate	4.8	5.0	0.2
+ Malonate + oxaloacetate	0	5.0	5.0

Table 5.9 Metabolism of Palmitate, Lactate, and Glutamate in Isolated Hepatocytes

	Change (μmol/min/g cells)			
Substrate	Lactate	Palmitate	Glutamate	Glucose
Lactate	–4.11	+0.21	0	+0.60
Palmitate	0	–0.35	0	0
Palmitate + lactate	–2.4	–0.59	0	+1.20
Glutamate	0	0	–3.42	+0.81

Table 5.10 Recovery of Radioactivity from [^{14}C-2]Lactate and [U-^{14}C] Palmitate in Isolated Hepatocytes

	Radioactivity (10^3 dpm/min/g cells)	
Substrate	CO_2	Glucose
[^{14}C-2]Lactate	3.71	1.20
[U-^{14}C]Palmitate	3.71	0
[U-^{14}C]Palmitate + glutamate	7.75	0.51

atoms ([U-^{14}C]palmitate); in each case, the specific radioactivity of the labeled substrate in the incubation medium was 10^3 dpm/μmol. In a further series of incubations with [U-^{14}C]palmitate, nonradioactive glutamate was also added. The results are shown in Table 5.10.

What conclusions can you draw from these results?

Problem 5.4: GABA metabolism in thiamin-deficient rats

GABA is a neurotransmitter; it is synthesized by decarboxylation of glutamate and inactivated by transamination to succinic semialdehyde, which is then oxidized to succinate. GABA transaminase uses ketoglutarate as the amino-acceptor, forming glutamate, which can then be decarboxylated to yield GABA. Succinate is an intermediate of the citric acid cycle. Formation of GABA can thus be considered an alternative to ketoglutarate dehydrogenase in the citric acid

Table 5.11 GABA Metabolism in Thiamin-Deficient Rats

	Control	Thiamin Deficient
Brain concentrations		
ATP µmol/g	2.8 ± 0.085	2.9 ± 0.09
Glutamate µmol/g	13.8 ± 0.29	11.3 ± 0.21[a]
Ketoglutarate µmol/g	0.14 ± 0.006	0.09 ± 0.007
GABA	1.67 ± 0.046	1.58 ± 0.031[a]
Total GABA in brain (µmol/g) after intracerebroventricular injection of [^{14}C]glutamate		
2 min after injection	1.57 ± 0.087	1.34 ± 0.063[a]
5 min after injection	2.18 ± 0.015	1.59 ± 0.038[a]
10 min after injection	2.32 ± 0.120	2.05 ± 0.057[a]
Specific radioactivity of GABA in brain (Ci/mol) after intracerebroventricular injection of [^{14}C]glutamate		
2 min after injection	105 ± 8.9	152 ± 10.1[a]
5 min after injection	127 ± 10.9	192 ± 10.0[a]
10 min after injection	61 ± 5.1	89 ± 9.5[a]

[a] Indicates results significantly different from controls by t-test.
Source: Data reported by Page, M.G. et al., *Br. J. Nutr.*, 62, 245–253, 1989.

cycle, and the pathway is sometimes known as the GABA shunt (Figure 5.19).

Page et al. (1989) reported on studies of glutamate and GABA metabolism in the brains of thiamin-deficient rats. The results are shown in Table 5.11.

What conclusions can you draw from these results?

Problem 5.5: Glucose utilization in exercising muscle

Table 5.12 shows glucose and oxygen uptake and lactate output across the gastrocnemius-plantaris muscle group of the (anesthetized) fasting dog, at rest and stimulated to twitch one or five times per second for 30 min, measured by cannulation of the femoral artery and popliteal vein.

Muscle biopsy samples showed that the glycogen concentration in the stimulated muscle was 98% of that in the unstimulated muscle at 1 twitch/s and 68% of that in the unstimulated muscle at 5 twitches/s.

What conclusions can you draw from these results?

Problem 5.6: Use of glucose and fatty acids in exercise

Figure 5.33 shows the disappearance of plasma glucose (left-hand side) and nonesterified fatty acids (right-hand side) in two separate experiments involving a student walking at moderate speed on a treadmill.

Table 5.12 Carbohydrate Metabolism in Contracting Dog Muscle

	nmol/g muscle/min		
	At Rest	1 Twitch/s	5 Twitches/s
Glucose uptake	64	215	483
Oxygen uptake	576	2592	6912
Lactate output	297	188	1112
Ratio lactate:glucose	4.6	0.87	2.3

Source: Data reported by Chaplet, C.K. and Stainsby, W.N., *Am. J. Physiol.*, 215, 995–1004, 1968.

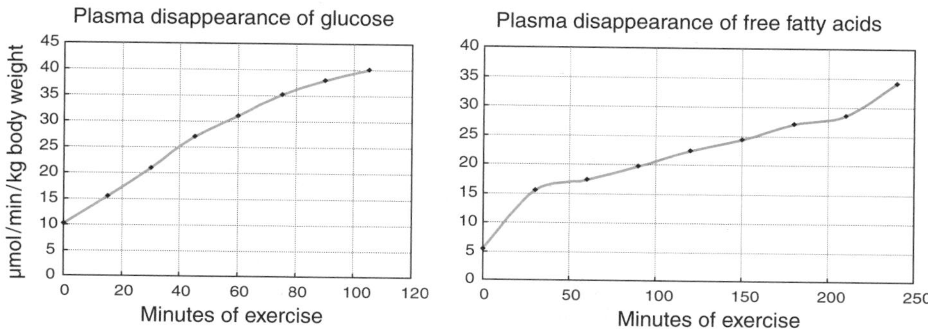

Figure 5.33 Disappearance of plasma glucose and fatty acids in exercise. (Data reported by Martin, W.H. and Klein, S., *Proc. Nutr. Soc.*, 57, 49–54, 1998.)

In the experiment in which glucose disappearance was measured, muscle glycogen was also measured by taking a muscle biopsy before and after the exercise; it fell from 111 to 39 mmol/kg during the 105 min of exercise.

What conclusions can you draw from these results?

Problem 5.7: David B

David is a 70 kg student; as part of a research project he performed exercise on a treadmill. Table 5.13 shows his oxygen consumption and carbon dioxide production at different speeds.
From these results and using information in Table 5.1, calculate:

- Energy expenditure at each speed of walking (in kJ/30 min)
- PAR at each speed
- RQ (the ratio of CO_2 produced/O_2 consumed) at each speed
- The percentage of fat and carbohydrate he is metabolizing at each speed (assuming that these are the only fuels he is utilizing)

Table 5.14 shows his oxygen consumption and carbon dioxide production walking on the treadmill at 3.5 kph for 30 min early in the morning (after an overnight fast) and again 2 h after eating breakfast.

What conclusions can you draw from these results?

Table 5.13 Oxygen Consumption and Carbon Dioxide Production during 30 min Exercise on a Treadmill at Different Speeds

						Energy (%)		
Speed (kph)	O_2 (L)	kJ/ 30 min	PAR	CO_2 (L)	RQ	Carbo-hydrate	Fat	Fat metabolized (g)
At rest	9.1		1.0	6.6				
1	14.4			10.4				
3.5	26.6			19.5				
5	33.0			26.0				
6.5	47.2			38.7				

Table 5.14 Oxygen Consumption and Carbon Dioxide Production during 30 min Exercise on a Treadmill at 3.5 kph, before and after Breakfast

				% Energy	
	O_2 (L)	CO_2 (L)	RQ	Carbohydrate	Fat
Fasting	26.6	18.9			
Fed	26.6	26.0			

Problem 5.8: Samuel W

Samuel W is an African-American recruit to the army. He was given the antimalarial drug primaquine, and suffered a delayed reaction with kidney pain, dark urine, and low red blood cell counts that led to anemia and weakness. Centrifugation of a blood sample showed a low hematocrit, and the plasma was red colored.

Similar acute hemolytic attacks have been observed, predominantly in men of Afro-Caribbean origin, in response to primaquine and a variety of other drugs, including dapsone, the antipyretic acetylphenylhydrazine, the antibacterial bactrim/septrim, sulfonamides, and sulfones, whose only common feature is that they all undergo cyclic nonenzymic reactions in the presence of oxygen to produce hydrogen peroxide and a variety of oxygen radicals that can cause oxidative damage to membrane lipids, leading to hemolysis. Moderately severe infection can also precipitate a hemolytic crisis in susceptible people.

One way of screening for sensitivity to primaquine is based on the observation that the glutathione concentration of erythrocytes from sensitive subjects is somewhat lower than that of control subjects and falls considerably on incubation with acetylphenylhydrazine.

Glutathione (GSH) is a tripeptide, γ-glutamyl-cysteinyl-glycine, which readily undergoes oxidation to form a disulfide-linked hexapeptide, oxidized glutathione (generally abbreviated to GSSG;

Table 5.15 The Effect of Incubation with 330 μmol/L Acetylphenylhydrazine on Erythrocyte Glutathione

	Controls		Samuel W	
	GSH (mmol/L)	GSSG (mmol/L)	GSH (mmol/L)	GSSG (μmol/L)
Initial	2.01± 0.29	4.2 ± 0.61	1.61	400
+ Acetylphenyl hydrazine	1.82 ± 0.24	190 ± 28	0.28	1540

Table 5.16 Glutathione Reductase (μmol product formed/min)

	Controls	Samuel W
NADPH	0.63 ± 0.06	0.64
NADH	0.01 ± 0.001	0.01

Figure 5.15). Table 5.15 shows the concentrations of GSH and GSSG in red cells from 10 control subjects and Samuel W, before and after incubation with acetylphenylhydrazine.

What conclusions can you draw from these results?

These results suggest that acetylphenylhydrazine causes the oxidation of glutathione to GSSG. This is not a simple stoichiometric oxidation of glutathione by acetylphenylhydrazine; the ratio of glutathione oxidized to acetylphenylhydrazine present is 4.7. This suggests that it is likely that acetylphenylhydrazine undergoes a cyclic redox reaction that results in the production of hydrogen peroxide, which in turn oxidizes glutathione.

In control subjects, incubation with acetylphenylhydrazine leads to a modest decrease in GSH and accumulation of GSSG; Samuel's red cells show a very considerable depletion of GSH and a very large accumulation of GSSG on incubation with acetylphenylhydrazine, suggesting that he cannot reduce GSSG back to GSH as effectively as normal. This could be due to lack of either glutathione reductase or NADPH.

The reported K_m of glutathione reductase for GSSG is 65 μmol/L and for NADPH, 8.5 μmol/L. Erythrocyte lysates were incubated with a saturating concentration of GSSG (1 mmol/L) and either NADPH or NADH (100 μmol/L). Each incubation contained the hemolysate from 0.5 mL packed cells (Table 5.16).

What conclusions can you draw from these results?

Since none of the lysates showed any significant activity with NADH, it is unlikely that there is any transhydrogenase activity in erythrocytes to reduce $NADP^+$ to NADPH at the expense of NADH. This raises the problem of the source of NADPH in erythrocytes.

The dye methylene blue will oxidize NADPH; the reduced dye then undergoes nonenzymic oxidation in air, so the addition of a relatively small amount of methylene blue will effectively deplete

Table 5.17 Production of [^{14}C]Lactate, Pyruvate, and CO_2 by 1 mL Erythrocytes Incubated for 1 h with 10 mmol/L [^{14}C]Glucose at 10 μmCi/mmol

	Control		+ Methylene Blue	
	Lactate + Pyruvate	CO_2	Lactate + Pyruvate	CO_2
[^{14}C-1]Glucose	12680 ± 110	1410 ± 15	1830 ± 20	12260 ± 130
[^{14}C-2]Glucose	14080 ± 120	ND	14120 ± 120	ND
[^{14}C-3]Glucose	14100 ± 120	ND	14090 ± 120	ND
[^{14}C-4]Glucose	14060 ± 120	ND	14080 ± 120	ND
[^{14}C-5]Glucose	14120 ± 120	ND	14060 ± 120	ND
[^{14}C-6]Glucose	14090 ± 110	ND	14100 ± 120	ND

Note: Figures show dpm, mean ± sd for five replicate incubations. ND indicates not detectable, i.e., below the limits of detection.

Table 5.18 Production of $^{14}CO_2$ by 1 mL Erythrocytes Incubated for 1 h with 10 mmol/L [^{14}C-1]Glucose at 10 μmCi/mmol

Additions	Control	+ *N*-Ethylmaleimide
None	1410 ± 70	670 ± 30
Ascorbate	8665 ± 300	2133 ± 200
Acetylphenylhydrazine	7740 ± 320	4955 ± 325
Methylene blue	12230 ± 500	11265 ± 450

Note: Figures show dpm, mean ± sd for five replicate incubations.

NADPH and would be expected to stimulate any pathway that reduces $NADP^+$ to NADPH.

Erythrocytes from control subjects were incubated with 10 mmol/L [^{14}C]glucose with or without the addition of methylene blue; all six possible positional isomers of [^{14}C]glucose were used, and the radioactivity (in lactate plus pyruvate) determined after thin layer chromatography of the incubation mixture. Each incubation contained 1 mL erythrocytes in a total incubation volume of 2 mL (Table 5.17).

What conclusions can you draw from these results?

In further studies, only the formation of $^{14}CO_2$ from [^{14}C-1]glucose was measured, with the addition of the following:

- Sodium ascorbate (which undergoes a nonenzymic reaction in air to produce H_2O_2)
- Acetylphenylhydrazine (which is known to precipitate hemolysis in sensitive subjects and depletes glutathione)
- Methylene blue (which oxidizes NADPH)

All incubations were repeated in the presence and absence of *N*-ethylmaleimide, which undergoes a nonenzymic reaction with the –SH group of reduced glutathione, and thus depletes the cell of glutathione (Table 5.18).

What conclusions can you draw from these results?

Further studies showed that Samuel's red blood cells contained only about 10% of the normal activity of glucose 6-phosphate dehydrogenase. To investigate why his enzyme activity was so low, a sample of his red blood cells was incubated at 45°C for 60 min, then cooled to 30°C, and the activity of glucose 6-phosphate dehydrogenase was determined. After the preincubation at 45°C, Samuel's red cells showed only 60% of their initial activity. In contrast, red cells from control subjects retained 90% of their initial activity after preincubation at 45°C for 60 min.

What conclusions can you draw from these results?

Problem 5.9: Alessandro DiFava

Alessandro DiFava is a Maltese boy. One day his aunt gave him a pie made from fava beans (a local delicacy), and that evening he suffered kidney pain and passed dark urine. A blood film showed a low RBC count and the plasma was red colored. This problem is not uncommon in Malta, and indeed several of Alessandro's classmates (all boys) have died when an acute crisis has been precipitated by eating fava beans, or after a moderate fever associated with an infection.

Further studies showed that Alessandro's erythrocyte glucose 6-phosphate dehydrogenase was only 10% of normal and had a very high K_m for NADP. Unlike Samuel W (Problem 5.8), his red blood cell enzyme was as stable to incubation at 45°C as that from control subjects.

What conclusions can you draw from these observations?

chapter six

Diet and health—nutrition and chronic diseases

Patterns of disease and mortality differ around the world. One of the factors that can be correlated with many of the differences is diet, although there are obviously other environmental (and genetic) factors involved. This chapter is concerned with the ways in which we can gather evidence that diet is, or may be, a factor in the development of chronic diseases (especially atherosclerosis and coronary heart disease, and cancer), and how we can extrapolate from these findings to produce guidelines for a prudent or healthful diet.

At one time, chronic diseases were known as diseases of affluence because they were seen mainly in affluent Western countries and among the wealthier sections of society. Nowadays, they are becoming major causes of morbidity and premature death in developing countries, and are more common among the poorer rather than wealthier sections of society in developed countries. They are diseases associated with a nutrition transition, from a traditional diet in which the total food was often only marginally adequate to one in which a superabundant amount of food is available, with increased intake of fat (especially saturated fat) and sugars, and decreased consumption of unrefined cereals, fruits and vegetables.

Obviously, neither undernutrition, leading to the problems discussed in Chapter 8, nor overnutrition, leading to the problems of obesity (Chapter 7), is desirable. The relative amounts of fat, carbohydrate, and protein in the diet are important, as is the mixture of different types of carbohydrate (Section 6.3.3) and fat (Section 6.3.2.1). Consumption of alcohol may have both beneficial and adverse effects on health (Section 6.3.5), and intakes of some vitamins and minerals above the levels that are adequate to prevent deficiency (Chapter 11) may be beneficial. A wide variety of compounds in foods that are not considered to be nutrients may also have beneficial effects (Section 6.6).

Objectives

After reading this chapter, you should be able to

- Explain the types of evidence that link diet with the diseases of affluence
- Describe and explain the guidelines for a prudent diet and explain the recommendations concerning dietary fat and carbohydrate
- Explain what is meant by a free radical, how oxygen radicals cause tissue damage, and the main sources of oxygen radicals
- Describe the main antioxidant nutrients and explain how they are believed to protect against cancer and heart disease
- Describe and explain the interactions between nutrition and genetics, and the ways in which early nutrition may affect patterns of gene expression and disease risk in later life
- Describe the various protective non-nutrient compounds that are found in plant foods and explain their protective actions

6.1 Chronic diseases (the "diseases of affluence")

The major causes of death in developed countries today are heart disease, high blood pressure, stroke, and cancer. These are not just diseases of old age, although it is true to say that the longer people live, the more likely they are to develop them. Heart disease is a major cause of premature death, striking a significant number of people aged under 40.

As societies develop, and socioeconomic changes and improvements in general health (especially reduction in infectious diseases) result in an increased average life expectancy of 50–60 years or more, coronary heart disease becomes more prevalent, accounting for 15%–25% of deaths. In developing countries, cardiovascular disease began to emerge as a significant cause of premature death in the 1970s and 1980s; the corresponding stage in socioeconomic development in the United States was the 1920s, and somewhat later in western Europe, where cardiovascular disease mortality mirrored that in the United States, but with a 10–20 year time lag. Since the 1980s, there has been a progressive fall in cardiovascular disease mortality in most developed countries, possibly reflecting changes in diet (Section 6.3).

Diet is, of course, only one of the differences between life in the developed countries of western Europe, North America, and Australasia and that in developing countries; there are a great many other differences in environment and living conditions. In addition, genetic variation affects susceptibility to nutritional and environmental factors (Section 6.4), and there is evidence that nutritional status *in utero* and in infancy affects responses to diet in adult life (Section 6.4.1).

It can be assumed that humans and their diet have evolved together. Certainly, we have changed our crops and farm animals by selective breeding over the last 10,000 years (more recently, by genetic modification of crop plants), and it is reasonable to assume that we have evolved by natural selection to be suited to our diet. The problem is that evolution is a slow process, and there have been major changes in food availability in most countries over only a single generation. As recently as the 1930s (very recent in evolutionary terms), it was estimated that up to one-third of households in Britain could not afford an adequate diet. Malnutrition was a serious problem, and the daily provision of 200 mL of milk to schoolchildren had a significant effect on their health and growth.

Foods that historically were scarce luxuries are now commonplace and available in surplus. Sugar was an expensive luxury until the middle of the nineteenth century; traditionally fat was also scarce, and every effort was made to save and use all the fat (dripping) from a roast joint of meat.

There are thus two separate, but related, questions to be considered:

- Is diet a factor in the etiology of diseases of affluence that are major causes of premature death in developed countries?
- Might changes in average western diets reduce the risk of developing cancer and cardiovascular disease?

6.2 Types of evidence linking diet and chronic diseases

The main evidence linking diet with chronic diseases is epidemiological; animal studies are used to test hypotheses derived from epidemiology and the effects of specific nutritional changes, and investigate biological mechanisms to explain the epidemiological findings. When there is a substantial body of evidence, then there can be intervention studies in which the diets of large numbers of people are changed (e.g., by providing supplements

Table 6.1 Secular Changes in Diet with Changes in Disease Incidence in Rural Wales

	1870	1970	
Protein	11	11	% of energy
Fat	25	42	% of energy
Sugar	4	17	% of energy
Starch	60	30	% of energy
Unsaturated fat	19	9	% of total fat
Cholesterol	130	517	mg/day
Dietary fiber	65	21	g/day

of nutrients for which there is epidemiological evidence of a protective effect) and they are followed for 5–10 or more years to see whether the intervention has any effect on disease incidence or mortality.

6.2.1 Secular changes in diet and disease incidence

The first type of evidence comes from studying changes in disease incidence and diet (as well as other factors) over time. Table 6.1 shows the changes in diet in rural southwest Wales between 1870 and 1970. This was a century during which there was a marked decrease in hunger-related diseases, and a marked increase in premature death from coronary heart disease—to the extent that in 1970 this region had one of the highest rates of coronary heart disease in Europe.

The major changes over this period were an increase in the proportion of energy derived from fat and dietary fat that was saturated (Section 4.3.1.1). At the same time, there was a considerable increase in cholesterol consumption (as a result of increased consumption of animal fats) and a significant decrease in the proportion of energy derived from starch, although sugar consumption increased considerably. Intake of cereal fiber also decreased. This suggests that increased intakes of fat (especially saturated fat), cholesterol, and sugar, along with reduced intakes of starch and cereal fiber may be factors in the development of coronary heart disease.

A similar nutrition transition is occurring now in developing countries. There is increased overall availability of food, with increased consumption of fat (especially saturated fat) and sugars and decreased consumption of complex carbohydrates, whole grain cereals, fruit and vegetables. At the same time, physical activity (and hence energy requirement) is falling as a result of increased mechanization in the workplace, increased mechanized transport, and low-activity recreation. These changes occurred over a century or more in western Europe and North America; they are now occurring over a decade or so in developing countries.

6.2.2 International correlations between diet and disease incidence

Worldwide, there are considerable differences in mortality from cancer and heart disease. Incidence of breast cancer ranges from 34 per million in the Gambia to 1002 per million in Hawaii, and prostate cancer from 12 per million in the Gambia to 912 per million among black Americans. There is also a considerable variation in the percentage of energy derived from fat—about 10% in Bangladesh and 40% in France.

Coronary heart disease accounts for 4.8% of deaths in Japan, but 31.7% of deaths in Northern Ireland. In the Seven Countries Study, the incidence of coronary heart disease over a

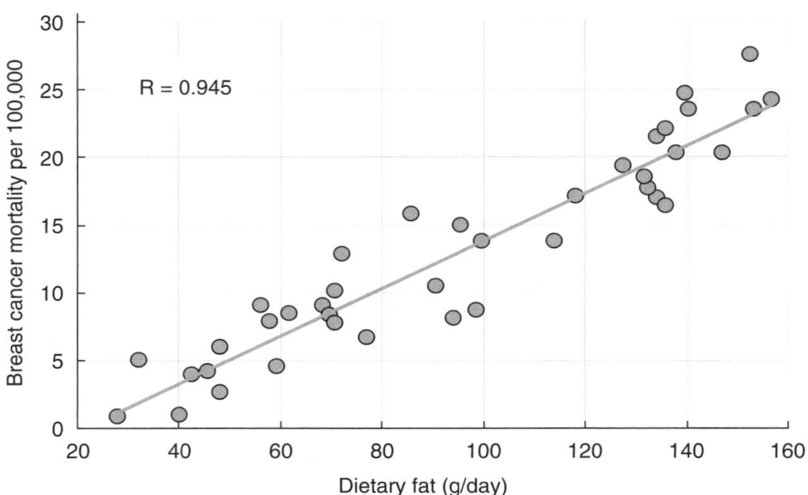

Figure 6.1 International correlation between fat intake and breast cancer in women. (From Caroll, K.K., *Cancer Res.*, 35: 3374–3383, 1975.)

15 year period was 14.4 per 1000 in Japan, compared with 120.2 per 1000 in eastern Finland; saturated fat accounted for 3% of energy intake in Japan and 22% in eastern Finland (and mean serum cholesterol was 4.3 mmol/L in Japan and 7 mmol/L in Finland).

Assuming that there are adequate and comparable data available for food consumption and disease incidence in different countries, it is possible to plot graphs such as that in Figure 6.1, which shows a highly significant positive association between fat consumption and breast cancer. It is important to note that statistical correlation does not imply cause and effect; indeed, further analysis of the factors involved in breast cancer suggests that it is not dietary fat intake but rather adiposity, or total body fat content, that is the important factor. Obviously, dietary fat intake is a significant factor in the development of obesity and high body-fat reserves (Chapter 7).

One problem in interpreting correlations between diet and disease is that national data for food availability disguise possibly large differences between cities and rural areas. In India in the 1980s some 17% of the rural poor had little or no visible oil or fat in their diet, while the urban elite received more than 30% of energy from fat; 5% of the population consumed 40% of the available fat. The food available per person in sub-Saharan Africa (excluding South Africa) fell over the period 1980–2005, but cardiovascular disease is an increasing cause of mortality in African cities.

Rather than looking at national data for food availability, some studies have measured plasma concentrations of nutrients or other more specific markers of food intake. Figure 6.2 shows a highly significant negative correlation between mortality from coronary heart disease and the serum concentration of vitamin E, suggesting that vitamin E may be protective against the development of atherosclerosis and coronary heart disease.

6.2.3 Studies of migrants

People who migrate from one country to another provide an excellent opportunity to study the effects of dietary and environmental factors on disease; their first-degree relatives who have not migrated provide a genetically matched control group for comparison.

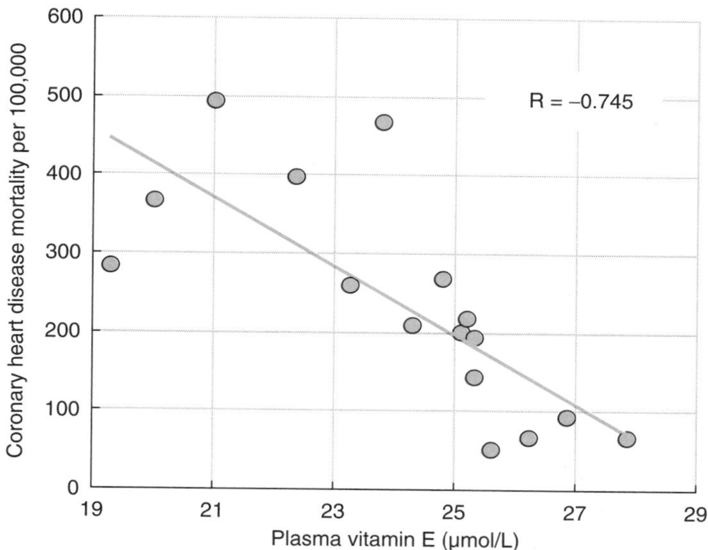

Figure 6.2 The relationship between plasma vitamin E levels and coronary heart disease. (From Gey, K.F. et al., *Am. J. Clin. Nutr.*, 53: suppl. 1, 326s–334s, 1991.)

Both breast and prostate cancers are rare in China and Japan compared with the incidence of these in the United States. Studies of people who migrated from China and Japan to Hawaii or San Francisco in the twentieth century showed that they had a considerably higher incidence of both cancers than their relatives at home who retained their traditional diet and lifestyle. There were similar differences in mortality from coronary heart disease.

Studies of immigrants in the mid-twentieth century from Poland (where gastric cancer was common and colorectal cancer rare) to Australia (where gastric cancer is rare and colorectal cancer more common) show a significant increase in colorectal cancer, while they retained the relatively high Polish incidence of gastric cancer, although second-generation Polish-Australians have the low Australian incidence of gastric cancer. This suggests that dietary or environmental factors involved in the development of colorectal cancer may act relatively late in life, while factors that predispose to gastric cancer act earlier in life. Infection with *Helicobacter pylori*, which was more common in Poland than in Australia, is a factor in gastric cancer. Diets high in salted and preserved meats are associated with higher incidence of gastric cancer, and diets high in fat and low in nonstarch polysaccharides are associated with higher incidence of colorectal cancer. As the incidence of gastric cancer in a population decreases, the incidence of colorectal cancer increases.

6.2.4 Case–control studies

An alternative way of studying relationships between diet and disease is to compare people suffering from the disease with disease-free subjects who are matched for gender, ethnicity, age, lifestyle, and as many other factors as possible. Figure 6.3 shows the results of a series of such case–control studies, which show that the serum concentration of β-carotene (Section 6.5.3.4) is significantly lower in people with a variety of cancers than in disease-free control subjects. Such data have been widely interpreted as suggesting that

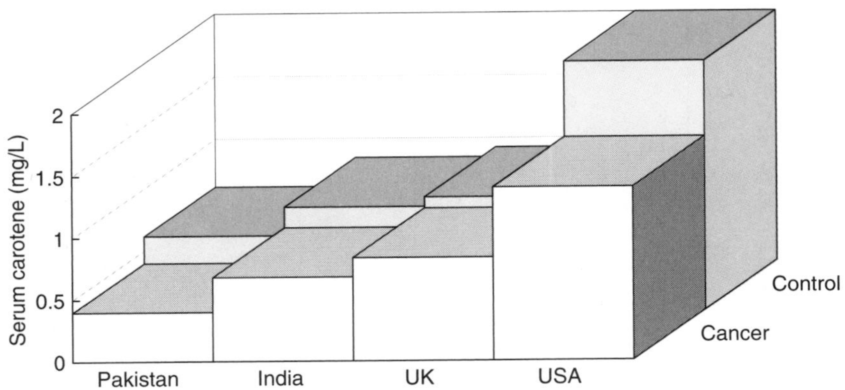

Figure 6.3 The relationship between plasma carotene and various cancers—case–control studies. (From Peto, R. et al., *Nature*, 290: 201–208, 1981.)

β-carotene has a protective effect against a variety of cancers; equally, it could be interpreted as suggesting that cancer affects carotene metabolism.

An obvious problem here is that studies of nutritional status when people present with a disease do not give us any information about their diet at the time the disease was developing. Their diet may have changed over the years and, of course, illness may affect what they eat now.

6.2.5 Prospective studies

The most useful epidemiological studies involve following a group of people over a long period of time, with assessment of their nutritional, health, and other status at the beginning of the study, and at intervals thereafter. Probably the oldest such study is the U.K. National survey of Health and Development, which has followed all 16,500 children born during one week in March 1946; further cohorts were enrolled in 1970 and 2000. The Framingham study has followed every resident of the town of Framingham, Massachusetts, from 1948; the nurses' health study in the United States is following some 85,000 nurses. In some such studies, blood and urine samples are stored, and diet and other records are available over a long period of time, so that it is possible to measure markers of nutritional status that were not considered important or relevant at the beginning of the study.

Figure 6.4 shows the results of such a prospective study in which people were grouped according to their plasma concentration of β-carotene at the beginning of the study; those with the lowest initial concentration of plasma carotene were 6.2 times more likely to die from lung cancer during the study period than those with the highest concentration. As with the case–control studies (Figure 6.3), this suggests a protective effect of β-carotene. But in this case, the subjects were presumably free from cancer at the beginning of the study, so the confounding problem—the disease may have affected carotene metabolism rather than carotene affecting the chance of developing cancer—is not there.

The European Prospective Investigation into Cancer and Nutrition (EPIC) is a multicenter prospective study of more than half a million subjects, with blood samples available for 75%, and by 2006 24,000 cases of cancer were recorded. Early results suggest a protective effect of both fish and nonstarch polysaccharide against colorectal cancer, an increased risk associated with consumption of red and processed meat, as well as an association

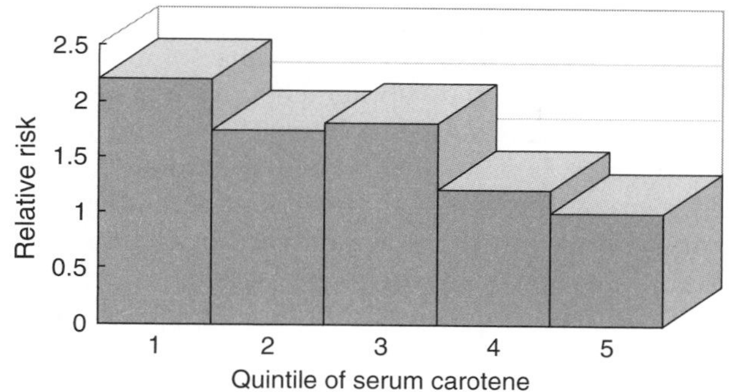

Figure 6.4 The relationship between plasma carotene and lung cancer—a prospective study. (From Peto, R. et al., *Nature*, 290: 201–208, 1981.)

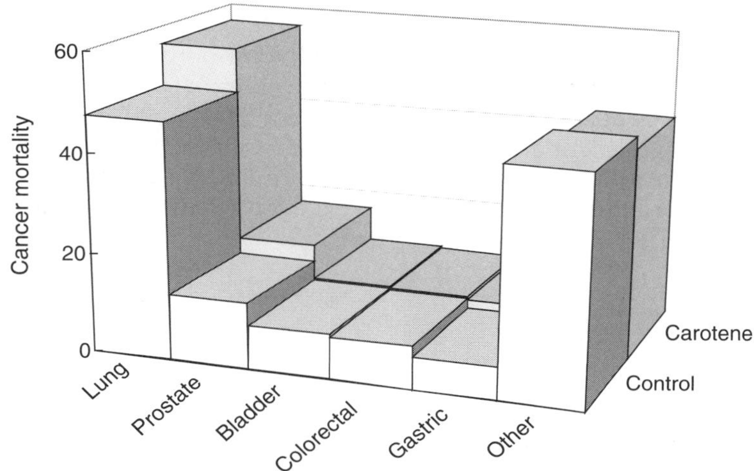

Figure 6.5 The effects of β-carotene supplementation on death from lung and other cancers. (From Alpha-Tocopherol Beta-Carotene Cancer Prevention Study Group, *New Engl. J. Med.*, 330: 1029–1035, 1994.)

between saturated fat intake and breast cancer, and an apparent protective effect of fruit consumption with respect to lung cancer.

6.2.6 Intervention studies

The next step is to test the hypothesis that has been derived from epidemiological studies, backed by plausible biological or chemical mechanisms, that a nutritional supplement or a change in diet will reduce the risk of developing a disease. Figure 6.5 shows the results of such an intervention trial in Finland in the 1980s to test the protective effect of β-carotene against lung cancer. Altogether, some 10,000 smokers were involved—half received supplements of β-carotene and half did not, and they were followed for 5–10 years. The results were disappointing—not only did the supplements not reduce the incidence of lung cancer in the test group, but there was an increased incidence of lung, prostate, and bladder cancer among those receiving β-carotene. A similar intervention trial of β-carotene in the United States involving 18,000 people, who either were smokers or had been exposed to asbestos, was terminated early because of a 46% excess death rate from lung cancer among those receiving the supplements. As a result of these two trials, the advice from the U.K. Food Standards Agency Expert Group on Vitamins and Minerals is that smokers should avoid supplements that contain β-carotene.

Figure 6.2 is typical of a large number of epidemiological studies that have suggested that supplements of vitamin E may be protective against cardiovascular disease. There have been a number of intervention trials with vitamin E supplements. Figure 6.6 shows the results of a meta-analysis of all such trials; in most of the trials of relatively high doses of vitamin E supplements, there is increased all-cause mortality among the intervention group.

6.3 Guidelines for a prudent diet

Diet is not the only factor in the development of chronic disease; many other factors, including heredity, multiple environmental factors, smoking, and exercise (or the lack of it), are also involved. While people can take decisions about diet, smoking, and exercise, they can do little about the stresses of city life, environmental pollution, or the other problems of industrial society and nothing, of course, to change their genetic makeup, which determines the extent to which they are at risk from environmental and nutritional factors (Section 6.4).

There is general agreement among nutritionists and medical scientists about changes in the average Western diet that would be expected to reduce the prevalence of chronic disease (see Table 6.2) and the public health message can be summarized in either the diet pyramid or the balanced plate shown in Figure 6.7.

6.3.1 Energy intake

Obesity involves both an increased risk of premature death from a variety of causes and increased morbidity from conditions such as diabetes, varicose veins, and arthritis (Section 7.2.2). However, people who are significantly underweight are also at increased

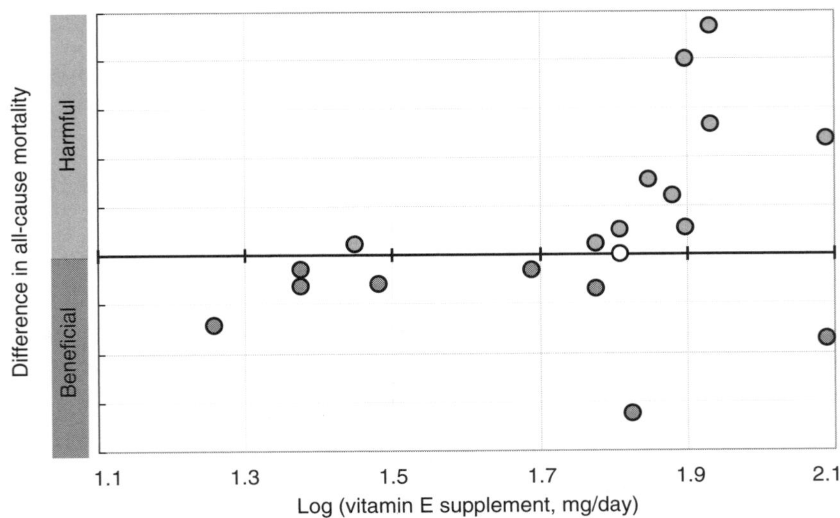

Figure 6.6 The effects of vitamin E supplementation on all-cause mortality in various intervention trials. (From Miller E.R. et al., *Ann. Intern. Med.*, 142: 37–46, 2005.)

Table 6.2 Guidelines for a Prudent Diet

	% of Energy
Total fat	15–30
Saturated fatty acids	<10
Polyunsaturated fatty acids	6–10
ω6 polyunsaturated fatty acids	5–8
ω3 polyunsaturated fatty acids	1–2
Trans-fatty acids	<1
Monounsaturated fatty acids	By difference
Total carbohydrate	55–75
Free sugars	<10
Protein	10–15
	Amount per Day
Cholesterol	<300 mg
Sodium chloride	<5 g
Sodium	<2 g
Fruit and vegetables (excluding tubers such as potatoes, yams, and cassava)	>400 g
Dietary fiber[a]	>25 g
Nonstarch polysaccharide[a]	>20 g

[a] This is the amount of fiber or nonstarch polysaccharide that would be provided by consuming the desirable amount of fruits and vegetables, and whole grain cereals.
Source: Diet, Nutrition, and the Prevention of Chronic Diseases, WHO Technical Report series 916, WHO, Geneva, 2003.

risk of illness as a result of undernutrition (see Chapter 8). For people whose body weight is within the desirable range, energy intake should be adequate to maintain a reasonably constant body weight, with an adequate amount of exercise. The benefits of exercise extend beyond weight control and energy balance, and include improved cardiovascular and respiratory function, muscle tone, and bone and joint health. The recommendation is to aim for 30 min of moderately vigorous exercise each day. Energy expenditure in physical activity and appropriate levels of energy intake are discussed in Section 5.1.

Figure 6.8 shows the average percentage of energy intake from fat, carbohydrate, protein, and alcohol in the diets of adults in Britain in the 1990s compared with the guidelines for a prudent diet.

6.3.2 Fat intake

Dietary fat includes not only the obvious fat in the diet (the visible fat on meat, cooking oil, butter or margarine spread on bread), but also the hidden fat in foods. This latter may be either the fat naturally present in foods (e.g., the fat between the muscle fibers in meat, the oils in nuts, cereals, and vegetables) or fat used in cooking and manufacture of foods. There are two problems associated with a high intake of fat:

- The energy yield of fat (37 kJ/g) is more than twice that of protein (16 kJ/g) or carbohydrate (17 kJ/g). This means that foods that are high in fat are also concentrated energy sources. Excessive energy intake is easier on a high-fat diet, and hence a high-fat diet can be a factor in the development of obesity (see Chapter 7).

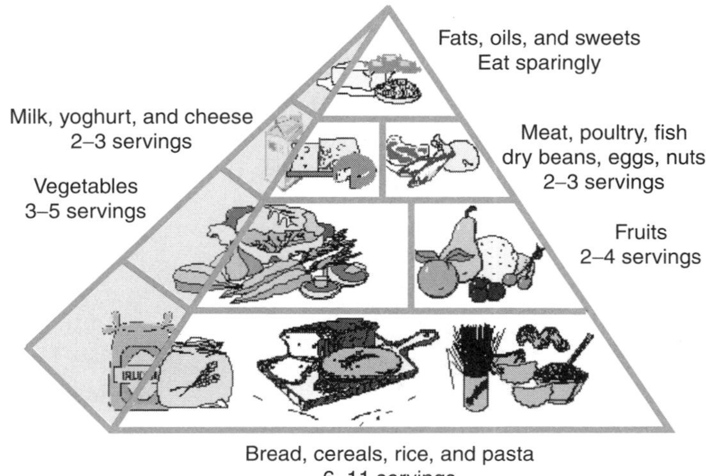

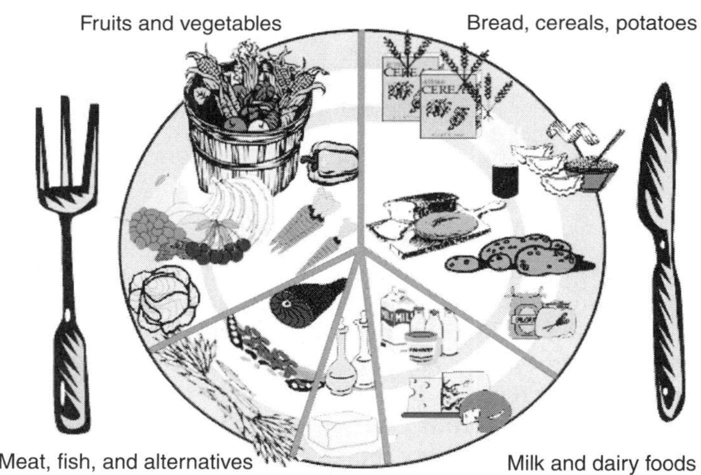

Figure 6.7 The food pyramid and balanced plate.

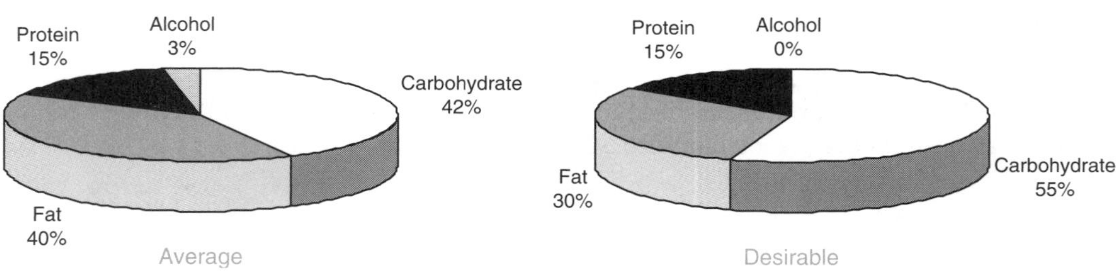

Figure 6.8 Average and desirable percentage of energy intake from different metabolic fuels.

- There is epidemiological evidence that fat intake is correlated with premature death from a variety of conditions, including especially atherosclerosis and ischemic heart disease, and cancer of the colon, prostate, breast, and uterus.

Diets that provide about 30% of energy from fat are associated with the lowest risk of ischemic heart disease. There is no evidence that a fat intake below 30% of energy intake confers any additional benefit, although a very low-fat diet is specifically recommended as part of treatment for some pathological hyperlipidemias. The wide range of desirable fat intake in Table 6.2 reflects the fact that for people whose habitual fat intake is 15%–20% of energy (as in many developing countries), there is no evidence that increasing fat intake will confer any benefits, and it may well be detrimental.

6.3.2.1 Type of fat in the diet

Figure 6.9 shows the relationship between the plasma concentration of cholesterol, specifically cholesterol in plasma low density lipoproteins (LDL; Section 5.6.2.2), and premature death from ischemic heart disease. The main dietary factor affecting the plasma concentration of cholesterol is the intake of fat.

Both the total intake of fat and, more importantly, the relative amounts of saturated and unsaturated fatty acids affect the concentration of LDL cholesterol. Figure 6.10 shows the results of a number of studies of the effects of different types of dietary fat on serum LDL cholesterol. In these studies, the effects of fats rich in saturated and polyunsaturated fatty acids were compared with a control diet containing an equivalent amount of monounsaturated fatty acids, so that monounsaturated fatty acids appear to be neutral, but are clearly beneficial when they replace saturated fatty acids. LDL cholesterol:

- Increases by a factor related to 2 times the intake of saturated fatty acids
- Decreases by a factor related to 1 time the intake of polyunsaturated fatty acids
- Increases by a factor related to the square root of cholesterol intake

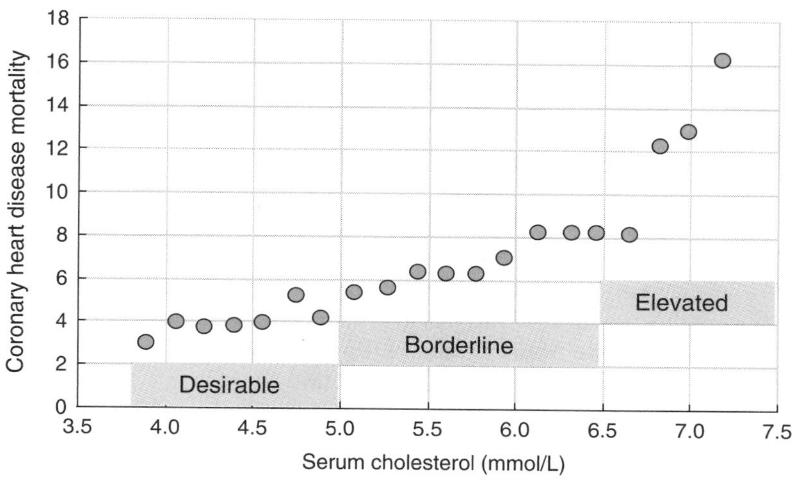

Figure 6.9 The relationship between serum cholesterol and coronary heart disease mortality. (From the Multiple Risk Factor Intervention Trial Research Group, *J. Am. Med. Assoc.*, 248: 1465–1475, 1982.)

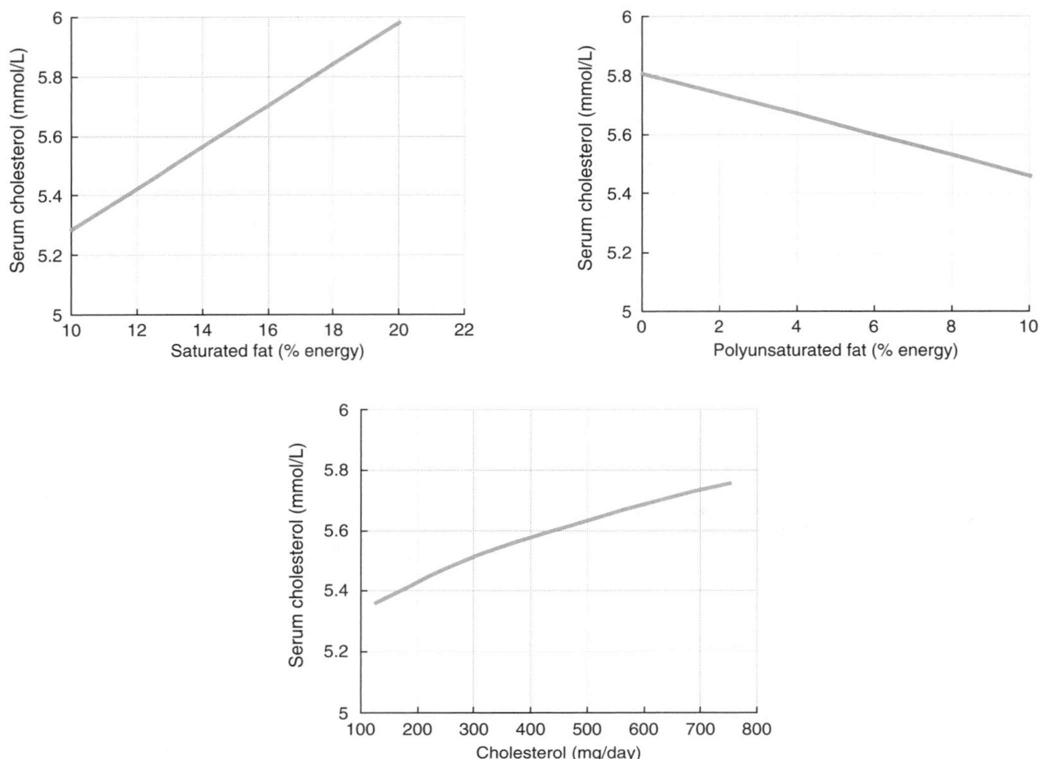

Figure 6.10 The effects of dietary saturated and polyunsaturated fatty acids (compared with monounsaturated fatty acids) and cholesterol on serum cholesterol. (From Keys, A. et al., *Metabolism*, 14: 747–787, 1965.)

As discussed in Section 5.6.2.2, mono- and polyunsaturated fatty acids are good substrates for cholesterol esterification in cells, while saturated fatty acids are not. When saturated fatty acid levels are relatively high, less cholesterol is esterified, so that the intracellular concentration rises, repressing the synthesis of LDL receptor. Not all saturated fatty acids have the same effect on LDL cholesterol. Myristic and palmitic acids have the greatest effect, since they down-regulate expression of the LDL receptor in the same way as does cholesterol (Section 5.6.2.2), while stearic (C18:0) has little effect, because it is rapidly desaturated to oleic acid.

Diets that are relatively rich in polyunsaturated fatty acids result in decreased synthesis of fatty acids in the liver (Section 5.6.1); this means that there is less export of lipids from the liver in very low density lipoproteins (Section 5.6.2.2), which are the precursors of LDL in the circulation. Polyunsaturated fatty acids (or their derivatives) act via nuclear receptors (Section 10.4) to reduce the transcription of the genes coding for acetyl CoA carboxylase and other key enzymes of fatty acid synthesis (Section 5.6.1).

In addition, the polyunsaturated fatty acids in fish oil (the ω3 series long-chain polyunsaturated fatty acids; Section 4.3.1.1) have further protective effects. The Italian GISSI trial was a secondary prevention trial of fish oil supplements in people who had survived a myocardial infarction. After 3.5 years of follow-up, there was a 20% reduction in total deaths and a 30% reduction in cardiovascular mortality. The main action of ω3 polyunsaturated fatty acids is to reduce the expression of adhesion molecules on blood platelets

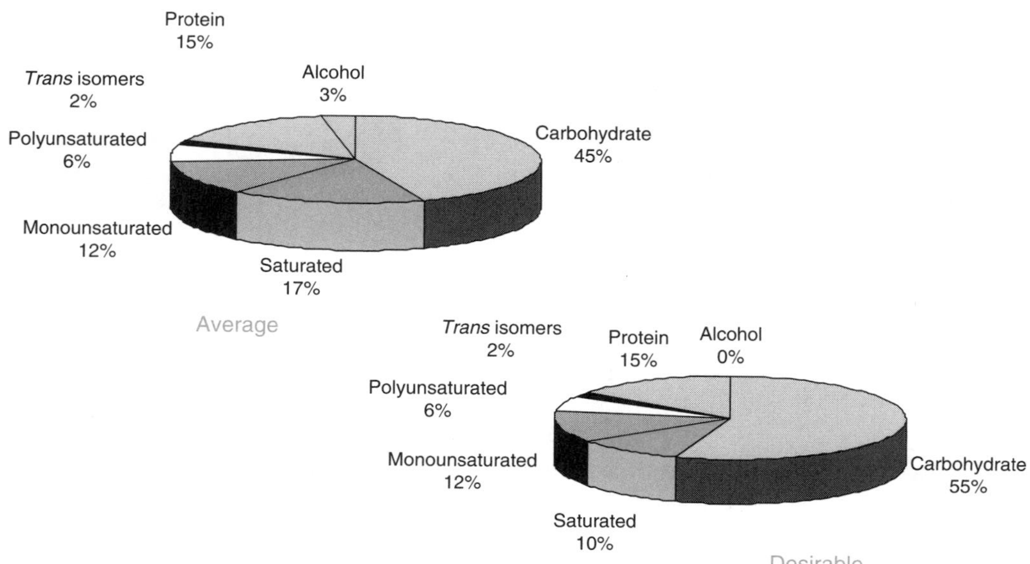

Figure 6.11 Average and desirable percentage of energy intake from different types of fat.

(thus reducing the risk of blood clot formation) and on blood vessel endothelium (thus reducing the adhesion of macrophages—a key step in the development of atherosclerosis). By contrast, ω6 polyunsaturated fatty acids (especially linoleic acid) may increase the expression of adhesion molecules. The balance between ω3 and ω6 polyunsaturated fatty acids is important, and there is concern that the increasing use of vegetable oils rich in ω6 polyunsaturated fatty acids leads to an excessively high ratio of ω6 to ω3 (see Table 6.2).

Epidemiological evidence suggests that a high intake of saturated fatty acids is associated with impaired glucose tolerance, and the development of type II diabetes mellitus and metabolic syndrome (Section 7.2.3). Intervention studies have shown an improvement in glucose tolerance and insulin sensitivity when saturated fatty acids are replaced by polyunsaturated fatty acids, although when total fat intake is more than about 37% of energy intake there is little effect.

Figure 6.11 shows the average proportions of energy from saturated, monounsaturated, and polyunsaturated fatty acids in the dietary fat in the United Kingdom in the 1990s, and the desirable proportions. As a general rule, animal foods (meat, eggs, and milk products) are rich sources of saturated fats, while oily fish and vegetables are rich sources of unsaturated fats.

The recommendation is to reduce intake of saturated fats considerably more than just in proportion with the reduction in total fat intake. Total fat intake should be 30% of energy intake, with no more than 10% from saturated fats (compared with the average of 17% of energy from saturated fat). Average intakes of 6% of energy from polyunsaturated and 12% from monounsaturated fats match what is considered desirable on the basis of epidemiological studies. About 1%–2% of average energy intake is accounted for by the *trans* isomers of unsaturated fatty acids (Section 4.3.1.1); ideally they should not exceed 1%. However, there are two sources of *trans* isomers of fatty acids in the diet:

- Those formed during the hydrogenation of oils in the manufacture of solid fats have a more adverse effect on plasma lipoproteins than saturated fatty acids.

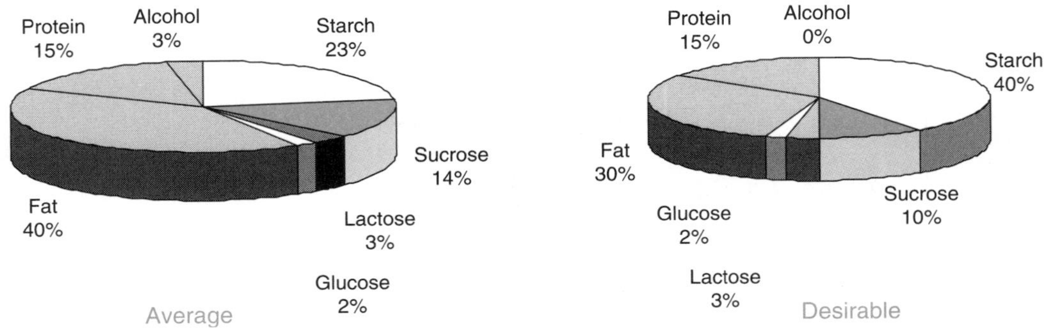

Figure 6.12 Average and desirable percentage of energy intake from different types of carbohydrate.

- Those found in fat from ruminants as a result of rumen bacterial metabolism appear to have little adverse effect on plasma lipoproteins.

6.3.3 Carbohydrate intake

If the total energy intake is to remain constant, as it should for people who are not overweight, and the proportion derived from fat is to be reduced from 40% of energy intake to 30%, then the proportion derived from another metabolic fuel must be increased. It is not considered desirable to increase the proportion derived from protein above 15% of energy intake, so the proportion derived from carbohydrates should increase from 45% to 55%. This should be achieved by increasing the intake of starches, not sugars (Figure 6.12).

6.3.3.1 Sugars in the diet

Average intakes of sugars (especially sucrose) are generally considered to be higher than is desirable. The adverse effects of an excessive intake of sugars include the following:

- *Dental decay*: Although many sugars in free solution (extrinsic sugars; Section 4.2.1) will promote the growth of oral bacteria that produce acids and cause dental decay, sucrose specifically promotes the growth of plaque-forming oral bacteria.
- *Obesity*: Sugars added to foods increase the energy yield of the food and the pleasure of eating (Section 1.3.3.1), so it is relatively easy to consume an excessive amount. In addition, as discussed in Sections 5.4.1 and 10.2.2, the fructose derived from sucrose enters glycolysis after the main regulatory point and results in excessive synthesis of fatty acids.
- *Diabetes mellitus*: Sugars and other carbohydrates with a high glycemic index (Section 4.2.2) lead to a higher postprandial insulin response, which results in increased lipogenesis and secretion of very low density lipoprotein from the liver (Section 5.6.2.2). This has been associated with the development of insulin resistance and noninsulin-dependent (type II) diabetes (Section 10.7). There is a genetic predisposition to type II diabetes, and it is difficult to determine the relative importance of heredity and sucrose consumption, or the effects of sucrose *per se* and obesity.
- *Atherosclerosis and coronary heart disease*: There is some evidence that a high consumption of sucrose is a factor in the development of atherosclerosis and coronary heart disease, although the evidence is less convincing than that for the effects of a high (saturated) fat intake.

It is considered desirable that sucrose should provide no more than 10% of energy (compared with the current average >14%). Intakes of other sugars (mainly glucose and fructose in fruits and lactose from milk) are considered to be appropriate.

6.3.3.2 *Undigested carbohydrates (dietary fiber and nonstarch polysaccharides)*

The residue of plant cell walls is not digested by human enzymes, but provides bulk in the diet (and hence in the intestines). It is measured by weighing the fraction of foods that remains after treatment with a variety of digestive enzymes. This is what is known as dietary fiber. It is a misleading term, since not all the components of dietary fiber are fibrous; some are soluble and form viscous gels. A more precise analytical method permits measurement of the specific polysaccharides other than starch (Section 4.2.1.6) that are the main constituents of dietary fiber; the results of such analysis are quoted as nonstarch polysaccharides.

The two methods of analysis give different results. Measurement of nonstarch polysaccharides in the diet gives average intakes in Britain of between 11 and 13 g/day, compared with an intake of dietary fiber of about 20 g/day as measured by the less specific method. Nonstarch polysaccharides are found only in foods of vegetable origin, and vegetarians have a higher intake than omnivores.

Nonstarch polysaccharides have little nutritional value in their own right since they are compounds that are not digested or absorbed to any significant extent. Nevertheless, they are a valuable component of the diet, and some of the products of fermentation by colonic bacteria can be absorbed and utilized as metabolic fuel. Starch that is (relatively) resistant to digestion in the small intestine (Section 4.2.2.1) is also a substrate for bacterial fermentation.

The main products of bacterial fermentation of nonstarch polysaccharides and resistant starch are short-chain fatty acids such as propionate and butyrate. These provide a major metabolic fuel for colon enterocytes and have an antiproliferative effect on tumor cells in culture. There is epidemiological evidence that they provide protection against the development of colorectal cancer.

Diets low in nonstarch polysaccharides are associated with the excretion of a small bulk of feces, constipation, and straining while defecating. This has been linked with the development of hemorrhoids, varicose veins, and diverticular disease of the colon. These diseases are more common in Western countries where people generally have a relatively low intake of nonstarch polysaccharide than in parts of the world where the intake is higher.

A number of compounds that are believed to be involved in causing or promoting cancer of the colon occur in the contents of the intestinal tract, either because they are present in foods or as a result of bacterial metabolism. They are adsorbed by cellulose and other nonstarch polysaccharides, and so cannot interact with the cells of the gut wall but are eliminated in the feces, thus providing protection against potential carcinogens.

Although epidemiological studies show that diets high in nonstarch polysaccharides are associated with a low risk of colon cancer, such diets also provide relatively large amounts of fruit and vegetables, and are therefore rich in vitamins C and E and carotene, which may have protective effects against the development of cancers (Section 6.5.3). Furthermore, because they provide more fruits and vegetables and less meat, such diets are also relatively low in saturated fats, and there is evidence that a high intake of saturated fats is a separate risk factor for colon cancer.

The bile salts required for the absorption of dietary fat are synthesized in the liver from cholesterol (Section 4.3.2.1). Normally, about 90%–95% of the 30 g of bile salts secreted daily is reabsorbed and reutilized. Nonstarch polysaccharides adsorb bile salts, so that they are excreted in the feces. This means that there has to be increased synthesis *de novo* from cholesterol to replace the lost bile salts, thus reducing the total body content of cholesterol.

A total intake of about 20 g/day of nonstarch polysaccharides is recommended (equivalent to about 25 g/day of dietary fiber). In general, this should come from fiber-rich foods—whole grain cereals and wholemeal cereal products, fruits, and vegetables—rather than supplements. This is because besides the nonstarch polysaccharides, these foods are valuable sources of a variety of nutrients. There is no evidence that intakes of nonstarch polysaccharides over 20 g/day confer any benefit other than in the treatment of established bowel disease. Above this level of intake, it is likely that people would reach satiety (or at least feel full, or even bloated) without eating enough food to satisfy their energy needs. This may be a problem for children fed on a diet that is very high in fiber—they may be physically full but still physiologically hungry.

6.3.4 Salt

There is a physiological requirement for the mineral sodium, and salt (sodium chloride) is the main dietary source of sodium. One of the basic senses of taste is for saltiness—a pleasant sensation (Section 1.3.3.1). However, average intakes of salt are considerably higher than the physiological requirement for sodium. Most people are able to cope with this excessive intake adequately by excreting the excess, but people with a genetic predisposition to develop high blood pressure are sensitive to the amount of sodium in their diet. About 10% of the population is salt sensitive, and there is a relationship between sodium intake and the increase in blood pressure that occurs with increasing age. As shown in Table 6.2, salt intake should not exceed 5 g/day (or 2 g of sodium). Obesity (Chapter 7) and alcohol (Section 6.3.5) have a greater effect on blood pressure than salt intake.

6.3.5 Alcohol

A high intake of alcoholic drinks can be a factor in causing obesity, both as a result of the energy yield of the alcohol itself and also because of the relatively high carbohydrate content of many alcoholic beverages (but see Problem 7.3). People who satisfy much of their energy requirement from alcohol frequently show vitamin deficiencies, because they are meeting their energy needs from drink, and therefore not eating enough foods to provide adequate amounts of vitamins and minerals. Deficiency of vitamin B_1 is especially a problem among heavy drinkers (Section 11.6.3 and Problem 5.2).

In moderate amounts, alcohol has an appetite-stimulating effect and may also help the social aspect of meals. Furthermore, there is good epidemiological evidence that modest consumption of alcohol is protective against atherosclerosis and coronary heart disease. However, alcohol in excess has harmful effects, not only in the short term, when drunkenness may have undesirable consequences, but also in the longer term.

Figure 6.13 shows the relationship between alcohol consumption and mortality from various causes—it is a classical "J-shaped" curve, with a protective effect for modest consumption compared with abstinence, but a sharp increase in mortality with excessive consumption.

Opinions differ as to whether the protective effect of modest alcohol consumption is due to the alcohol itself or some other constituent of alcoholic beverages. Figure 6.14 shows that there are differences between the effects of wine, beer, and spirits regardless of the amount of alcohol consumed. Some studies have shown the same protective effects for

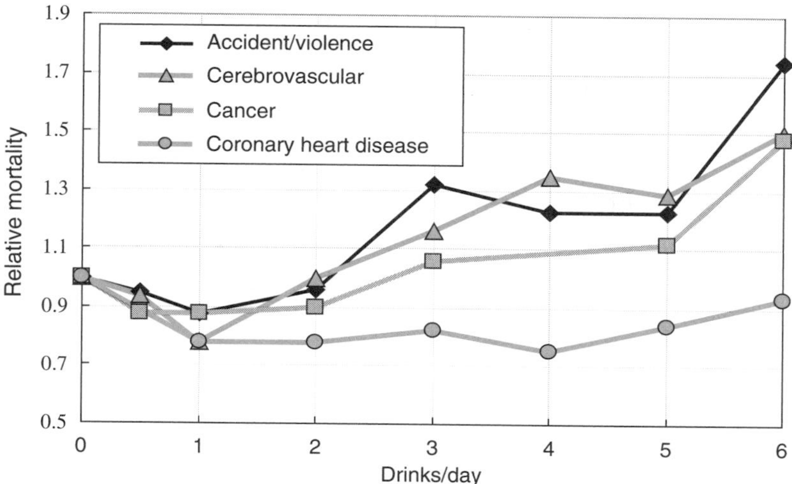

Figure 6.13 The effects of habitual alcohol consumption on mortality from various causes. (From Boffetta, P. and Garfinkel, L., *Epidemiology*, 1: 342–348, 1990.)

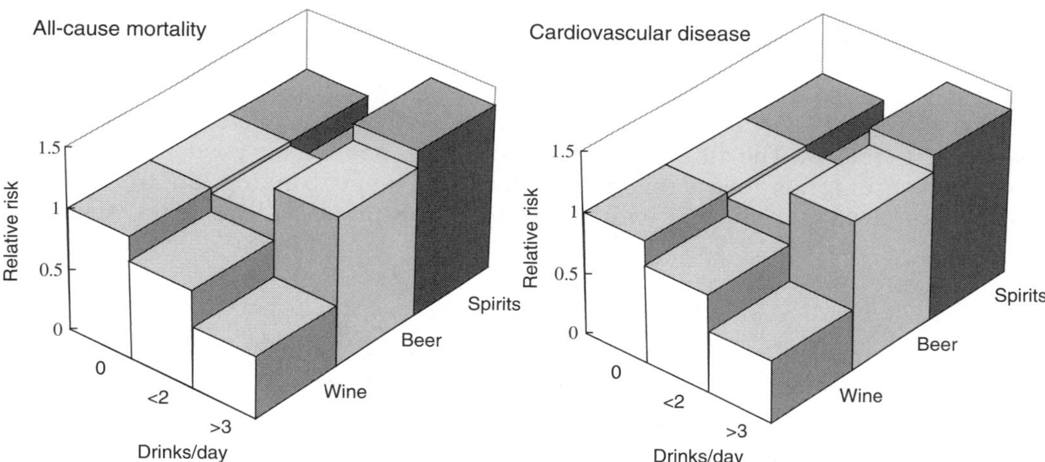

Figure 6.14 The effects of different alcoholic beverages on mortality. (From Grøbbæk, M. et al., *Br. Med. J.*, 310: 1165–1169, 1995.)

red wine and dealcoholized wine, suggesting that alcohol is not the protective factor; the various polyphenols in red wine may well have an antioxidant action (Section 6.5.3.6).

One problem in interpreting the data on alcohol consumption is that those who do not consume alcohol will include not only those who for religious or other reasons choose to abstain from alcohol, but also those whose health has already been damaged by excessive consumption. Habitual excess consumption of alcohol is associated with long-term health problems, including loss of mental capacity, liver damage, cancer of the esophagus, and hypertension. Continued abuse can lead to physical and psychological addiction.

Table 6.3 Prudent Upper Limits of Alcohol Consumption

Royal College of Physicians	
Men	21 units (168 g alcohol)/week
Women	14 units (112 g alcohol)/week
Department of Health (1995)	
Men	4 units (32 g alcohol)/day
Women	3 units (24 g alcohol)/day

Table 6.4 Amounts of Beverages Providing 1 Unit of Alcohol

8 g absolute alcohol
½ pint of beer (300 mL)
1 glass of wine (100 mL)
single measure of spirits (25 mL)

The infants of mothers who drink more than a very small amount of alcohol during pregnancy are at risk of congenital abnormalities, and heavy alcohol consumption during pregnancy can result in the fetal alcohol syndrome—low birth weight and lasting impairment of intelligence, as well as congenital deformities.

The guidelines on alcohol intake are summarized in Table 6.3, and the alcohol content of beverages in Table 6.4. The difference between the daily and weekly prudent upper limits of alcohol consumption reflects the greater danger of binge drinking (the whole week's intake in one evening) compared with more modest consumption through the week.

6.4 Nutritional genomics: interactions between diet and genes

Although diet and other environmental factors are important in the etiology of chronic diseases, one of the main factors in both cancer and cardiovascular disease is genetic. In many cases, the genetic factor influences the extent to which an individual is sensitive to the long-term health effects of the diet, so that there is a considerable interaction between genes and diet. The long-term aim of nutritional genomic research is to identify which people are likely to be susceptible to the adverse effects of, for example, saturated fat intake, and who are not, and so to be able to develop individualized nutritional advice.

When a variant of a gene is found relatively widespread in the population, it is known as a genetic polymorphism (as opposed to rare variants or mutations that are the cause of classical inborn errors of metabolism affecting only a very small number of people). A number of genetic polymorphisms affect the extent to which different metabolic and nutritional insults affect health:

- About 10% of the population is sensitive to the hypertensive effect of excessive salt intake (Section 6.3.4).
- About 10% of the population is genetically at risk of iron overload (Section 4.5.3.1) as a result of polymorphisms in the HFE gene (responsible for detecting iron status), hepcidin, or the transferrin receptor.

- Polymorphisms of various apoproteins of the plasma lipoproteins and of LDL receptor and cholesterol ester transfer protein account for much of the variance in atherosclerosis (Section 5.6.2.2).
- Polymorphisms of the insulin receptor substrate (Section 10.3.4) explain much of the inherited susceptibility to type II diabetes mellitus (Section 10.7).
- Polymorphisms of the vitamin D receptor explain much of the susceptibility to osteoporosis (Section 11.3.3).
- Polymorphisms of methylene tetrahydrofolate reductase are associated with elevated blood homocysteine and a higher-than-normal requirement for folic acid, a factor in neural tube defects and cardiovascular disease (Section 11.11.3.3).
- A number of polymorphisms occur in the untranscribed regions of genes, affecting the extent of gene expression rather than the activity of the protein product.

6.4.1 Epigenetic modifications

Unlike polymorphisms, which are inherited, epigenetic modifications are changes to the genome that do not involve changes to the base sequence of DNA (Section 9.2.1), but methylation of cytosine residues that results in changes in the extent to which a gene is expressed. This is part of the normal process of cell and tissue differentiation in development, the silencing of some genes, and switching on of others. Folate (Section 11.11.3) is required for these methylation reactions, and there is evidence that impaired methylation as a result of low folate status is a factor in the development of some cancers, and possibly some neurodegenerative diseases.

Nutrition *in utero* and in early life may also affect the extent to which different genes are silenced or expressed, so affecting health in later life. There is good evidence that moderately low birth weight (at the lower end of the normal range) is associated with a greater risk of obesity, diabetes mellitus, and the metabolic syndrome (Section 7.2.3), as a result of early adaptation leading to greater metabolic efficiency and persistent metabolic programming.

6.5 Free radicals, oxidative damage, and antioxidant nutrients

One of the theories to explain the etiology of cardiovascular disease, cancer, autoimmune diseases, and some of the neurodegenerative diseases is that the initiating factor is tissue damage (to lipids, proteins, or DNA) caused by free radicals, and that compounds that can quench free radicals may be protective. The main tissue-damaging radicals are oxygen radicals (sometimes known as reactive oxygen species), and it is usual to talk of oxidative damage as a result of radical action and consider protective compounds to be antioxidants.

Free radicals are highly reactive, unstable, molecular species that have an unpaired electron in the outermost shell. They exist for an extremely short time, of the order of nanoseconds (10^{-9} s) or less, before they react with another molecule, either gaining or losing a single electron, to achieve a stable configuration. However, this in turn generates another radical, so radical reactions are self-perpetuating. To show that a compound is a free radical, its chemical formula is shown with a dot (·) to represent the unpaired electron—for example, the hydroxyl radical is $\cdot OH$.

If two radicals react together, each contributes its unpaired electron to the formation of a new, stable bond. This means that the chain reaction, in which reaction of radicals with other molecules generates new radicals, is quenched. Since radicals are short-lived and are present in low concentrations in cells, it is rare for two radicals to react together in this way.

Some radicals are relatively stable. This applies especially to those that have aromatic rings or conjugated double-bond systems. An unpaired electron can be delocalized through such a system of double bonds, and the resultant radical is less reactive and longer lived than most radicals. Compounds that are capable of forming stable radicals are important in quenching radical chain reactions. Vitamins C (Section 11.14) and E (Sections 6.5.3.3 and 11.4) and carotene (Section 6.5.3.4) form stable radicals and are generally regarded as having a protective antioxidant action.

6.5.1 Tissue damage by oxygen radicals

Radicals may interact with any compounds present in the cell, and the result may be initiation of cancer, heritable mutations, atherosclerosis and coronary heart disease, or autoimmune disease. The most important and potentially damaging of such interactions are the following:

1. Interactions with DNA in the nucleus (Section 9.2.1), causing chemical changes to the nucleic acid bases or breaks in the DNA strand. This damage may result in heritable mutations if the damage is to ovaries or testes, or the induction of cancer in other tissues. While much damage to DNA is detected and repaired by the DNA repair system in cells, some will escape detection.
2. Interactions with individual amino acids in proteins. This results in a chemical modification of the protein, which may therefore be recognized as foreign by the immune system, leading to the production of antibodies against the modified protein that will also react with the normal, unmodified body protein. This can be a cause of autoimmune disease. Some modified amino acids (e.g., dihydroxyphenylalanine) are capable of undergoing nonenzymic redox cycling, resulting in the production of more oxygen radicals.
3. Interactions with unsaturated fatty acids in cell membranes, this leads to the formation of dialdehydes, which react with DNA, causing chemical modification, and hence may result in either heritable mutations or initiation of cancer. Dialdehydes can also react with amino acids in proteins, leading to modified proteins that stimulate the production of autoantibodies.
4. Interactions with unsaturated fatty acids or amino acids in plasma lipoproteins (Section 5.6.2.2). Oxidized LDL is not recognized by the LDL receptors in the liver but is taken up by scavenger receptors in macrophages. Macrophage uptake of LDL is unregulated, and the cells become engorged with lipid. These lipid-rich macrophages (called foam cells, because of their microscopic appearance) then infiltrate the epithelium of blood vessel walls, leading to the development of fatty streaks and, eventually, atherosclerosis.

6.5.2 Sources of oxygen radicals

Ionizing radiation such as X-rays, radiation from radioactive isotopes, and ultraviolet rays from sunlight cause lysis of water to yield hydroxyl radicals. In addition, oxygen radicals arise in the body in four main ways as described below.

6.5.2.1 Reoxidation of reduced flavins

The reoxidation of reduced flavin coenzymes (Sections 3.3.1.2 and 11.7.2) involves formation of a number of radicals as transient intermediates. Since radicals are unpredictable, some always escape from the normal reaction sequence. Overall, some 3%–5% of the 30 mol of oxygen consumed by an adult each day is converted to oxygen radicals rather than undergoing complete reduction to water in the mitochondrial electron transport chain (Section 3.3.1.2). There is thus a total daily formation of some 1.5 mol of reactive oxygen species that are potentially able to cause damage to tissues.

6.5.2.2 The macrophage respiratory burst

The cytotoxic action of macrophages is due to production of halogen and oxygen radicals. This means that infection can lead to a considerable increase in the total radical burden in the body. This may be an important factor in the etiology of the protein-energy deficiency disease, kwashiorkor (Section 8.5.1); infection is a common precipitating factor in undernourished children.

Stimulation of macrophages leads to a considerable increase in the consumption of glucose (the respiratory burst), which is metabolized by the pentose phosphate pathway (Section 5.4.2), leading to increased production of NADPH. The respiratory burst oxidase (NADPH oxidase) is a flavoprotein that transfers electrons from NADPH onto cytochrome b_{558}, which then reduces oxygen to superoxide. The reaction is

$$\text{NADPH} + 2\text{O}_2 \rightarrow \text{NADP}^+ + 2{\cdot}\text{O}_2^- + 2\text{H}^+$$

The respiratory burst oxidase is a transmembrane multienzyme complex that is activated in response to

- Complement fragment C_{5a}, which arises from the antibody–antigen reaction
- Peptides containing *N*-formyl-Met-Leu-Phe, which may be bacterial or arise from the mitochondria of damaged tissue
- Cytokines and other signaling molecules released in response to infection, including platelet-activating factor, leukotrienes, and interleukins

6.5.2.3 Formation of nitric oxide

Production of nitric oxide (NO•), by hydroxylation of arginine, is a part of normal cell signaling. In addition to being a radical, and hence potentially damaging in its own right, nitric oxide can react with superoxide to form peroxynitrite, which in turn decays to yield the more damaging hydroxyl radical. Nitric oxide was first discovered as the endothelium-derived relaxation factor, and this loss of nitric oxide by reaction with superoxide may be an important factor in the development of hypertension.

6.5.2.4 Nonenzymic formation of radicals

A variety of transition metal ions react with oxygen or hydrogen peroxide in solution, generating hydroxyl radicals:

$$\text{M}^{n+} + \text{H}_2\text{O}_2 \rightarrow \text{M}^{(n+1)+} + {\cdot}\text{OH} + \text{OH}^-$$

Physiologically important ions include iron, copper, cobalt, and nickel.

Metal ions are not normally present in free solution to any significant extent, but are bound to transport proteins (in plasma) or storage proteins and enzymes (in cells). Thus, iron is bound to transferrin (in plasma), and hemosiderin and ferritin (in tissues); copper is bound to ceruloplasmin (in plasma); metallothionein (in plasma) binds a wide variety of metal ions. The adverse effects of iron overload (Section 4.5.3.1) are the result of free iron, not bound to storage proteins, undergoing nonenzymic reactions to produce oxygen radicals.

6.5.3 Antioxidant nutrients and non-nutrients—protection against radical damage

Apart from avoiding exposure to ionizing radiation, there is little that can be done to prevent the formation of radicals since they are the result of normal metabolic processes and responses to infection. There are, however, a number of mechanisms to minimize the damage done by radical action. Since the important radicals are oxygen radicals, and the damage done is oxidative damage, the protective compounds are known collectively as antioxidants.

Compounds such as vitamin E (Sections 6.5.3.3 and 11.4), carotene (Section 6.5.3.4), and ubiquinone (Section 3.3.1.2) owe their antioxidant action to the fact that they can form stable radicals, in which an unpaired electron can be delocalized. Such stable radicals persist long enough to undergo reaction to yield nonradical products. However, because they are stable, they are also capable of penetrating further into cells or lipoproteins, hence causing damage to DNA in the nucleus or lipids in the core of the lipoprotein. Therefore, as well as being protective antioxidants, these compounds are also capable of acting as potentially damaging pro-oxidants, especially at high concentrations. This may explain the disappointing results of trials of β-carotene against lung cancer, and the increased mortality seen in most intervention trials with high-dose vitamin E (Section 6.2.6).

6.5.3.1 Superoxide dismutase, peroxidases, and catalase

Superoxide is a substrate for the enzyme superoxide dismutase, which catalyzes the reaction

$$\cdot O_2^- + H_2O \rightarrow O_2 + H_2O_2$$

In turn, hydrogen peroxide is removed by catalase and a variety of peroxidases:

$$2H_2O_2 \rightarrow 2H_2O + O_2$$

As a further protection, many of the reactions in the cell that generate superoxide or hydrogen peroxide occur in the peroxisomes—intracellular organelles that also contain superoxide dismutase, catalase, and peroxidases.

6.5.3.2 Glutathione peroxidase

Lipid peroxides formed by radical action on unsaturated fatty acids in membranes and LDL can be reduced to unreactive alcohols by the enzyme glutathione peroxidase, with the oxidation of the tripeptide glutathione (γ-glutamyl-cysteinyl-glycine; GSH) to the disulfide-linked GSSG. In turn, oxidized glutathione is reduced back to the active peptide by glutathione reductase (Figure 5.15).

Glutathione reductase has selenium at the catalytic site as a selenocysteine residue (Section 11.15.2.5); this explains the role of selenium as an antioxidant nutrient. Glutathione reductase is a flavoprotein and is especially sensitive to riboflavin (vitamin B_2)

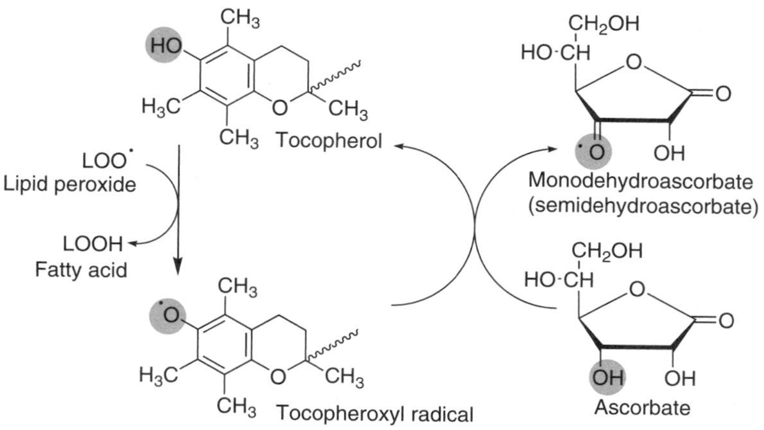

Figure 6.15 The antioxidant role of vitamin E.

depletion; measurement of glutathione reductase activation by its coenzyme added *in vitro* is a method of assessing riboflavin status (Section 2.7.3).

6.5.3.3 Vitamin E

Vitamin E (Section 11.4) forms a stable radical that can persist long enough to undergo reaction to yield nonradical products. Tocopherol reacts with lipid peroxides to form stable fatty acids and the tocopheroxyl radical, which then reacts with ascorbate (vitamin C) at the surface of the cell or lipoprotein, regenerating tocopherol, and forming the stable monodehydroascorbate radical (Figure 6.15).

There is epidemiological evidence that intakes of vitamin E higher than those required to prevent deficiency, and probably higher than can be achieved from normal diets, may have significant protective action against the development of atherosclerosis and cardiovascular disease (Figure 6.2). However, intervention trials with vitamin E supplements have been disappointing, and most high-dose trials have shown an increased overall mortality (Figure 6.6). This reflects the fact that the stable tocopheroxyl radical can penetrate deeper into plasma lipoproteins and tissues and so cause more damage. There is experimental evidence that vitamin E-depleted LDL is less susceptible to lipid peroxidation than native LDL.

6.5.3.4 Carotenes

A variety of carotenes, including both those that are precursors of vitamin A and those that are not (Section 11.2.2), can act as radical-trapping antioxidants under conditions of low oxygen tension. There is epidemiological evidence from a variety of studies that high blood levels of carotene are associated with low incidence of a variety of cancers (Sections 6.2.4 and 6.2.5). However, the results of intervention studies have been disappointing; in two major trials there was increased lung cancer mortality among people taking supplements of β-carotene (Section 6.2.6). Here, the problem may be not only that carotene can form a stable radical that penetrates deeper into tissues, but also that while it is an antioxidant at low partial pressures of oxygen (as occur in most tissues), it is an autocatalytic pro-oxidant at higher partial pressures of oxygen (as in the lungs).

6.5.3.5 Vitamin C

Vitamin C can act at the surface of cells or lipoproteins to reduce the tocopheroxyl radical back to tocopherol, forming the stable monodehydroascorbate radical (Figure 6.15). It can also react with superoxide and hydroxyl radicals:

$$\text{ascorbate} + {}^{\bullet}O_2^- + H^+ \rightarrow H_2O_2 + \text{monodehydroascorbate}$$

$$\text{ascorbate} + {}^{\bullet}OH + H^+ \rightarrow H_2O + \text{monodehydroascorbate}$$

The resultant monodehydroascorbate can then undergo enzymic reduction back to ascorbate, or a nonenzymic reaction between 2 mol of monodehydroascorbate to yield ascorbate and dehydroascorbate (Figure 6.16). Dehydroascorbate may then either be reduced to ascorbate, or be oxidized to diketogulonate.

Although ascorbate has a protective role in the reactions shown above, it can also be a source of oxygen radicals, and hence potentially damaging:

$$\text{ascorbate} + O_2 \rightarrow {}^{\bullet}O_2^- + \text{monodehydroascorbate}$$

$$\text{ascorbate} + Cu^{2+} \rightarrow Cu^+ + \text{monodehydroascorbate}$$

$$Cu^+ + H_2O_2 \rightarrow Cu^{2+} + {}^{\bullet}OH + OH^-$$

It is unlikely that high intakes of vitamin C will result in significant radical formation, since once intake rises above 100–120 mg/day, the vitamin is excreted quantitatively in urine. However, there is some evidence that vitamin C supplements increase coronary heart disease mortality in diabetics; like excessively high concentrations of glucose, vitamin C can glycate proteins, including LDL (Section 10.7.1).

6.5.3.6 Non-nutrient antioxidants

A number of other compounds that are not nutrients, but are formed in the body as normal metabolites also provide protection against radical damage. Such compounds include uric acid (the end product of the metabolism of purines) and the coenzyme ubiquinone (Section 3.3.1.2). The latter is sometimes marketed as "vitamin Q," but it can be synthesized in the body, and there is no evidence that it is a dietary essential or that an increase above the amount that is normally present in tissues confers any benefit.

In addition to the protective nutrients and normal metabolites, a wide variety of compounds that are naturally present in plant foods also have antioxidant action. These are mainly polyphenols, which are capable of forming stable radicals that persist long enough to undergo reaction to nonradical products. However, they are also potentially capable of undergoing nonenzymic redox cycling, leading to increased formation of oxygen radicals. It is possible that the epidemiological evidence suggesting a protective effect of vitamin E and β-carotene is misleading, since the plasma concentrations of these two nutrients may be simply a marker for the consumption of fruits and vegetables that are sources of polyphenols and other protective compounds.

6.6 Other protective compounds in foods

Some compounds present in plant foods that are not normally considered nutrients, in that they are not dietary essentials, may have other protective effects, including:

- Inhibition of cholesterol synthesis or absorption, which is potentially beneficial with respect to atherosclerosis

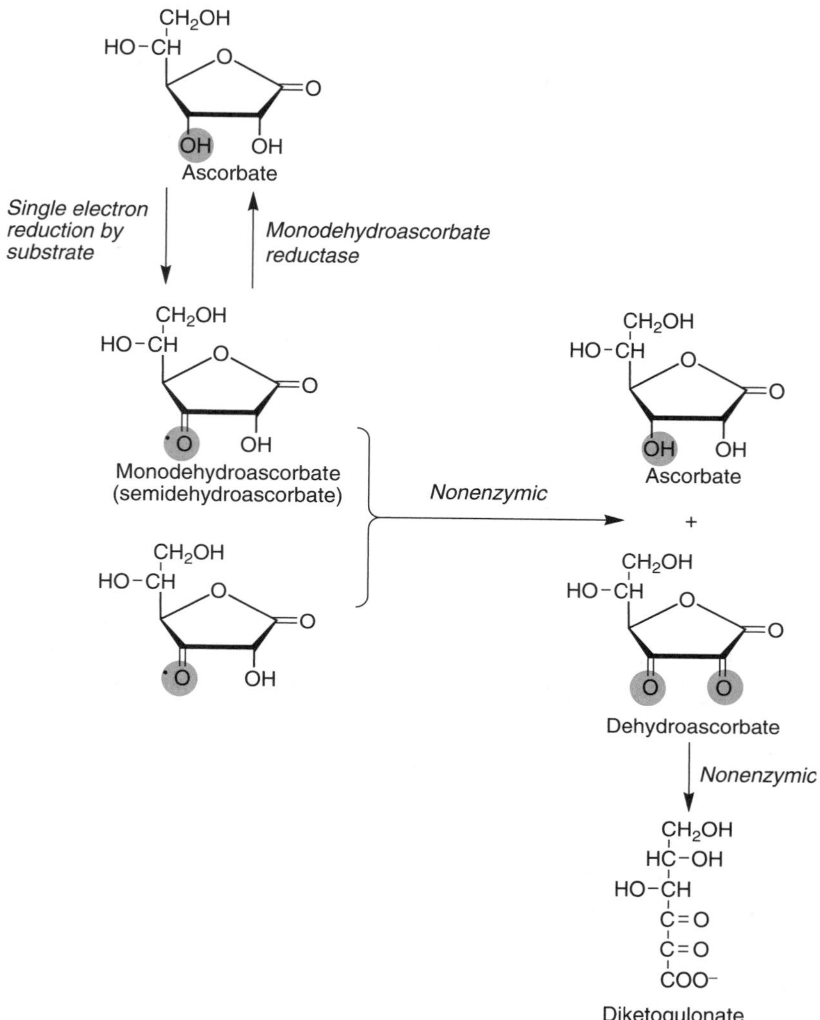

Figure 6.16 Metabolism of the monodehydroascorbate radical to nonradical products.

- Decreased metabolic activation or increased conjugation and excretion of potentially carcinogenic compounds
- Antiestrogenic actions that may be beneficial with respect to hormone-dependent cancer of the breast and uterus

Collectively, these compounds are known as phytochemicals or phytoceuticals. They are not classified as nutrients because they do not have a clear function in the body, and deficiency does not lead to specific lesions. Nevertheless, they are important in the diet and provide a sound basis for increasing intake of fruits and vegetables, quite apart from the beneficial effects of increased intake of nonstarch polysaccharides, vitamins and minerals, and reduced intake of fat (especially saturated fat).

6.6.1 Inhibition of cholesterol absorption or synthesis

Plant sterols and stanols (Figure 4.13) inhibit the absorption of cholesterol from the small intestine. In addition to 3–500 mg of dietary cholesterol, about 2 g of cholesterol is secreted each day in the bile (Section 4.3.2.1), almost all of which is normally reabsorbed. Inhibition of cholesterol absorption is therefore likely to have a more marked hypocholesterolemic effect than might be expected simply by considering the dietary intake. A number of products such as margarine, yogurts, and cream have been marketed that contain plant sterols or stanol esters; there is good evidence that they reduce LDL cholesterol and could therefore be expected to reduce atherosclerosis and coronary heart disease.

The rate-limiting step of cholesterol synthesis is the reduction of hydroxymethylglutaryl (HMG) CoA to mevalonic acid, catalyzed by HMG CoA reductase. Cholesterol acts to repress synthesis of HMG CoA reductase and so do a number of other compounds derived from mevalonic acid (Figure 6.17). Such compounds include the following:

- The tocotrienol vitamers of vitamin E, which have an unsaturated side chain. This means that the tocotrienols, although they have low vitamin activity (Sections 11.4.1 and 11.4.3.1), may have a quite different protective effect with respect to atherosclerosis.
- Ubiquinone (Figure 3.19).
- Squalene, the last noncyclic intermediate in cholesterol synthesis. Olive oil is an especially rich source. However, although it inhibits HMG CoA reductase, squalene is also a precursor of cholesterol and it is not clear what effect it has on LDL cholesterol.

6.6.2 Inhibition of carcinogen activation and increased conjugation of activated metabolites

Foreign compounds (and a number of endogenous metabolites, including steroid hormones) undergo two stages of metabolism before excretion:

- Phase I metabolism is metabolic activation leading to the introduction of reactive groups. Many such reactions involve hydroxylation catalyzed by cytochromes of the P_{450} family.
- Phase II metabolism is conjugation of these reactive groups, with glucuronic acid, amino acids, or sulfate, to increase water solubility and permit urinary excretion.

Although phase I metabolism is considered to be catabolic and part of the inactivation of steroid hormones, it also results in the production of active carcinogens from a number of otherwise inactive compounds. A number of compounds present in fruits and vegetables either inhibit phase I metabolism or activate phase II metabolism or both.

6.6.2.1 Allyl sulfur compounds

Onions, leeks, garlic, and other *Allium* spp. synthesize cysteine sulfoxide derivatives (allyl sulfur compounds) as a mechanism of protection against attack by pests. When the plant cells are damaged, the enzyme alliinase is released. It catalyzes a series of reactions to form thiosulfinates and a variety of organic mono-, di-, and trisulfates, and thiols. In onions, the major product is thiopropanal-*S*-oxide, a potent lachrymator.

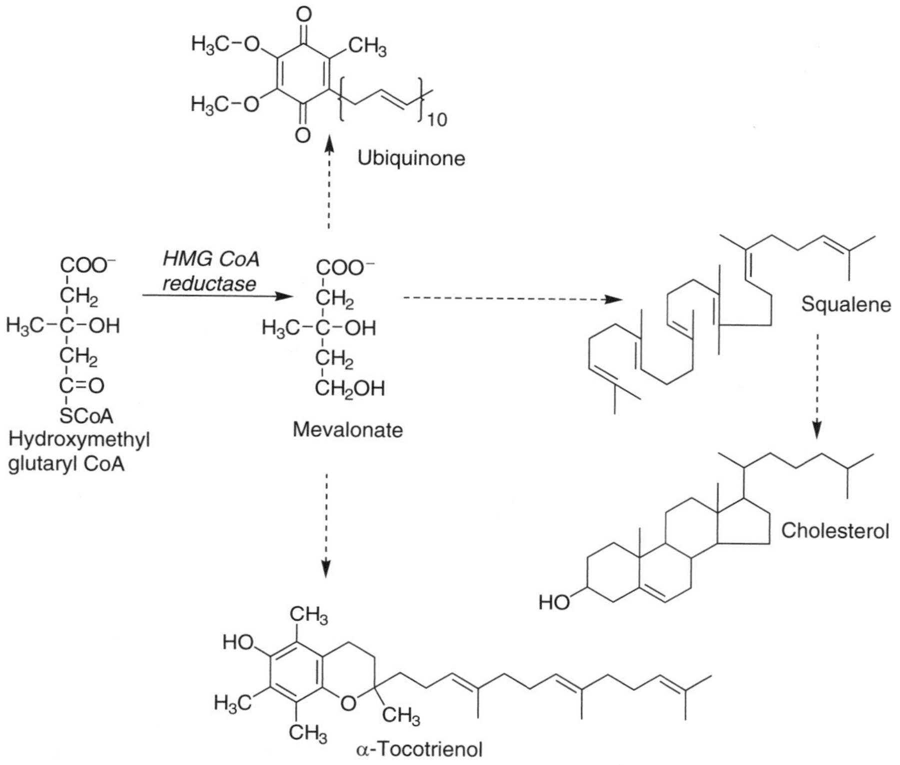

Figure 6.17 Compounds synthesized from mevalonate that reduce cholesterol synthesis by inhibiting HMG CoA reductase.

These allyl sulfur compounds lower the activity of microsomal cytochrome P_{450} by four different mechanisms:

- Acting as substrates and inhibiting the enzyme by mechanism-dependent (suicide) inhibition (Section 2.3.4.1)
- Antagonizing the induction of cytochrome P_{450} by ethanol (see Problem 5.4)
- Slowing the translation of cytochrome P_{450} mRNA with no effect on transcription (Section 9.2.3)
- Increasing the clearance of potential carcinogens and metabolites, by induction of glutathione *S*-transferases

6.6.2.2 Glucosinolates

Glucosinolates (Figure 6.18) occur in brassicas (e.g., cabbage, cauliflower, broccoli, and brussels sprouts) and some other plants. The enzyme myrosinase in vacuoles in the plant cell is released when cells are damaged; it catalyzes cleavage of glucosinolates to yield a variety of isothiocyanates, thiocyanates, and nitriles plus the aglycones.

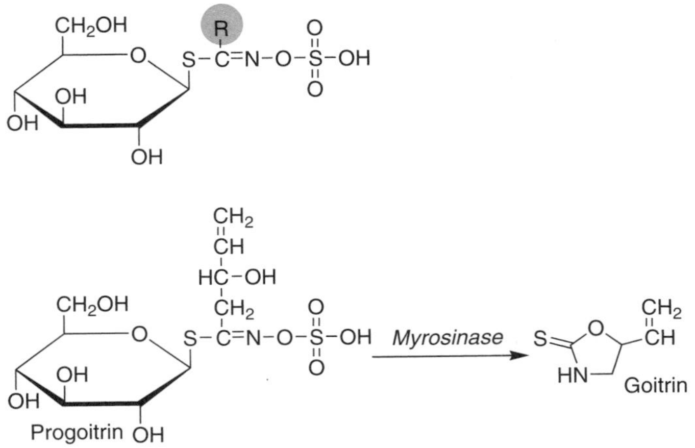

Progoitrin
Myrosinase
Goitrin

Figure 6.18 The glucosinolates.

Intestinal bacteria have a similar enzyme, so glucosinolates from cooked vegetables yield similar products.

Like the allyl sulfur compounds in *Allium* spp., the aglycones of glucosinolates lower the activity of microsomal cytochrome P_{450} by:

- Direct enzyme inhibition
- Down-regulation of enzyme synthesis—it is not known whether this is at the level of transcription or translation

They also increase the clearance of potential carcinogens and metabolites by induction of glutathione *S*-transferases and quinone reductase.

There is a potential hazard associated with excessive consumption of brassicas—a number of the glucosinolates have a goitrogenic action, reducing synthesis of the thyroid hormones (Section 11.15.3.3). Two mechanisms are involved:

- Thiocyanate (SCN^-) competes with iodide for tissue uptake and is goitrogenic when iodine intakes are marginal.
- Oxazolidine-2-thiones (e.g., goitrin; Figure 6.18) inhibit thyroxine synthesis by inhibition of iodination of mono-iodotyrosine to di-iodotyrosine. They are goitrogenic regardless of iodine nutritional status.

Goiter is a well-known problem in cattle fed on brassicas, but there is no evidence of reduced thyroid hormone status in people consuming, e.g., 150 g of sprouts per day for several weeks. However, iodine deficiency goitre was a problem in the Netherlands (a country that cannot be considered to be upland, over limestone soil or inland, the usual criterion on for iodine deficiency; Section 11.15.3.3) until the introduction of iodide enrichment of flour at the beginning of the twentieth century. The traditional Dutch diet included a considerable amount of sauerkraut (fermented cabbage)—to such an extent that during the sixteenth and seventeenth centuries, when seafarers from most countries suffered from scurvy (vitamin C deficiency; Section 11.14.3) during long voyages of exploration, the Dutch mariners did not.

6.6.2.3 Flavonoids

There are six main groups of flavonoids (Figure 6.19) in plants; most occur as glycosides (with a variety of sugars) and are hydrolyzed to aglycones by digestive enzymes. They serve both to protect plants against attack and also as the pigments of many plants (especially the anthocyanin pigments of berry fruits). They were at one time considered to be vitamins (vitamin P), although there is no evidence that they are dietary essentials; then during the 1970s were considered to be mutagens and carcinogens because they are polyphenols and can undergo redox cycling with the production of oxygen radicals. Since the 1990s, they have been considered potentially protective antioxidants, because they can form relatively stable radicals that persist long enough to undergo reaction to nonradical products.

The flavonoids are also inhibitors of phase I reactions and activators of phase II reactions. In addition, they can form inactive complexes with a number of carcinogens. Epidemiological evidence suggests a beneficial effect of a high intake of flavonoids with respect to cardiovascular disease (accounting for perhaps 8% of the international variation in coronary heart disease), although there is no epidemiological evidence of a negative association with cancer. Intakes of flavonoids are estimated to be around 23 mg/day, of which almost half comes from tea; onions, apples, and red wine are also good sources.

6.6.3 Phytoestrogens

A number of compounds that are widely distributed in plants as glycosides and other conjugates have weak estrogenic action, although they are not chemically steroids. They all have two hydroxyl groups that are in the same position relative to each other as the hydroxyl groups in estradiol (Figure 6.20), so that they bind to estradiol receptors. The amounts present in plants increase in response to microbial and insect attack, suggesting that they function as antimicrobial or antifungal agents in plants. Legumes, especially soybeans, are rich sources.

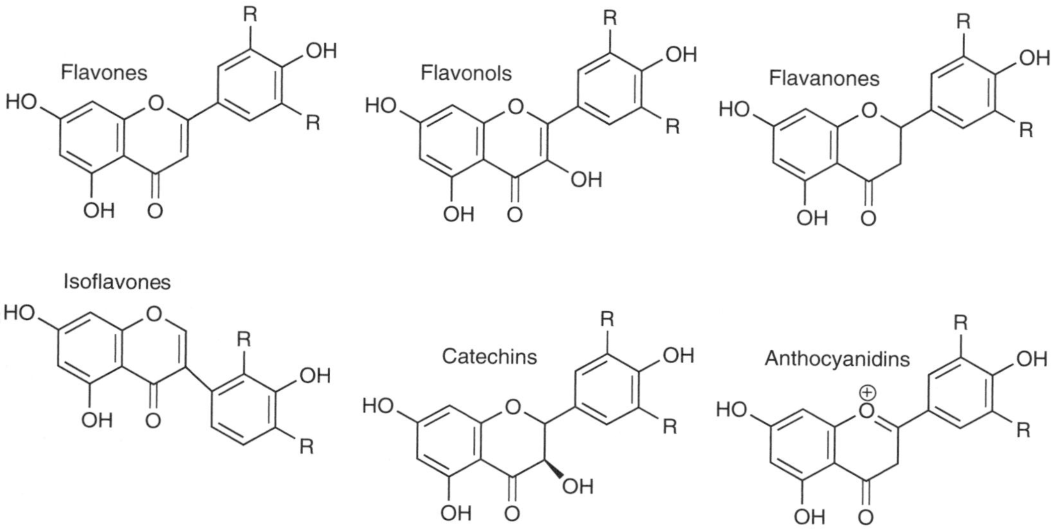

Figure 6.19 The flavonoids.

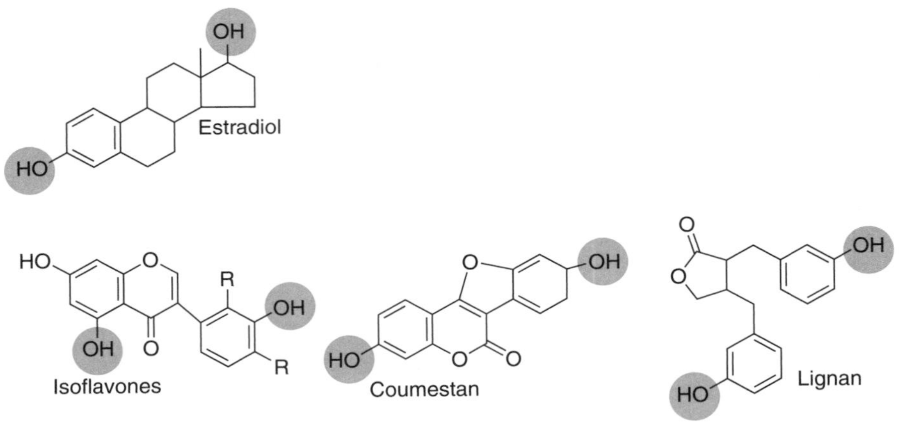

Figure 6.20 Phytoestrogens—nonsteroidal compounds that have two hydroxyl groups in the correct orientation to bind to the estradiol receptor.

The phytoestrogens produce typical and reproducible estrogen responses with an activity 1/500–1/1000 of that of estradiol. They may be agonistic or antagonistic to estradiol when both are present at the target tissue (isoflavones are mainly antagonistic, lignans are mainly agonistic). They compete with estradiol for receptor binding, but the phytoestrogen-receptor complex does not undergo normal activation, so it has only a weak effect on the hormone response element of DNA (Section 10.4).

Phytoestrogens also reduce circulating free estradiol because they increase the synthesis of sex hormone binding globulin in liver—more hormone is bound to globulin and therefore less is available for uptake into target tissues. Vegetarians have higher levels of circulating sex hormone binding globulin than omnivores. The correlation between adiposity and breast cancer is almost certainly due to synthesis of estradiol in adipose tissue; enterolactone and some of the other flavonoid phytoestrogens inhibit aromatase and will therefore reduce synthesis of estradiol in adipose tissue.

In Japan, where the traditional diet contains relatively large amounts of phytoestrogens from soybean products, there is a low incidence of cancer of the breast and prostate, as well as an unexpectedly low incidence of osteoporosis (Section 11.15.1.1), despite lower peak bone density of Japanese women compared with European or American women. While some prospective and case–control studies show a protective effect of soybean consumption with respect to breast cancer, others do not.

6.6.4 Miscellaneous actions of phytochemicals

Salicylates are irreversible inhibitors of cyclooxygenase, and hence inhibit the synthesis of thromboxane A_2 and have an anticoagulant action. They occur in many fruits (and red wine) in amounts similar to the dose of aspirin recommended to prevent excessive blood clotting in patients at risk of thrombosis.

The allyl sulfur compounds (Section 6.6.2.1) in garlic inhibit platelet coagulation and have a potentially beneficial effect with respect to thrombosis. Terpenes such as limonene (in peel oil of citrus fruits, and aromatic oils of caraway, dill, etc.), myrecene (in nutmeg), and zingiberine (in ginger) are polyisoprene derivatives that inhibit isoprenylation of the

P21-*ras* oncogene product; isoprenylation is essential for action of the ras protein, which is known to be associated with pancreatic cancer. Genistein (but not other phytoestrogens) inhibits cell proliferation by inhibiting the tyrosine kinase activity of the epithelial growth factor receptor.

Key points

- Evidence that diet is a factor in the etiology of chronic diseases comes from various types of epidemiological studies, supported by plausible biological mechanisms, but controlled intervention trials are needed to test any hypotheses developed from epidemiological data and mechanistic studies.
- For people whose weight is within the desirable range, energy intake should be adequate to maintain a reasonably constant body weight, with a desirable level of physical activity.
- Fat should provide no more than 30% of energy.
- Saturated fatty acids raise serum cholesterol and polyunsaturated fatty acids lower it compared with monounsaturated fatty acids.
- The balance between ω3 and ω6 polyunsaturated fatty acids is important.
- Saturated fatty acids should provide no more than 10% of energy intake. *Trans* isomers of unsaturated fatty acids should provide no more than 1% of energy.
- The reduction in fat intake should be balanced by increased carbohydrate intake, up to 55% of energy, mainly as starches. Free sugars should provide no more than about 10% of energy intake.
- Undigested carbohydrates (resistant starch and nonstarch polysaccharides or dietary fiber) have a number of potential health benefits, and higher intakes are associated with lower risk of colorectal cancer.
- About 10% of the population is sensitive to the hypertensive effects of salt, and salt intakes should not exceed 5 g/day.
- Moderate alcohol consumption may provide health benefits, but habitual intake should not exceed 4 units/day for men or 3 units/day for women.
- Genetic polymorphisms may explain the differences in sensitivity to various dietary and metabolic factors implicated in the etiology of chronic diseases.
- Free radicals are highly reactive molecular species with an unpaired electron. Oxygen radicals can cause damage to nucleic acids, lipids, and proteins, leading to mutation, initiation of cancer, development of autoimmune disease, and atherosclerosis and coronary heart disease.
- Oxygen radicals are formed in the normal reoxidation of reduced flavins, the macrophage respiratory burst, as a result of nitric oxide synthesis, in a variety of nonenzymic reactions of metal ions, and as a result of lysis of water by ionizing radiation.
- Protection against radical damage is provided by enzymes that reduce superoxide, hydrogen peroxide, and lipid peroxides, as well as vitamins C and E and β-carotene, which form relatively stable radicals that persist long enough to undergo reaction to nonradical products.
- Epidemiological studies suggest that β-carotene is protective against various cancers, but intervention trials have shown increased death from lung cancer among people taking β-carotene supplements. This is mainly because β-carotene is an antioxidant

at low partial pressure of oxygen, but an oxidant at high partial pressures of oxygen, as occur in the lungs.
- Epidemiological studies suggest that vitamin E is protective against atherosclerosis and coronary heart disease, but many intervention studies have shown increased death among people taking vitamin E supplements. This is mainly because the stable vitamin E radical can penetrate deeper into tissues and plasma lipoproteins, and cause more damage.
- A variety of other compounds found in plant foods, not normally considered to be nutrients, may provide protection in various ways against the development of chronic disease.

Problem 6.1: Healthy elderly people eating the wrong foods

The guidelines for a prudent diet (Section 6.3) can be summarized as:

- Fat to provide 30% of energy
- Saturated fat to provide 10% of energy (1/3 of total fat)
- Sucrose to provide 10% of energy

A study of healthy elderly people (aged between 70 and 75) in Roskilde in Denmark found that:

- 5% of them received more than 50% of energy from fat
- 22% had an intake of more than 50% of their fat as saturated fat
- 90% received more than 10% of energy from sugar
- 46% of the men were smokers

What explanation can you suggest for these results?

Problem 6.2: Adverse effects of lowering serum cholesterol

Figure 6.11 shows that there is a clear relationship between elevated serum cholesterol and risk of premature death from coronary heart disease. Table 6.5 shows the results of a meta-analysis of trials of various interventions to lower serum cholesterol.

Can you account for the disappointing results of the intervention trials?

Table 6.5 Relative Mortality in Cholesterol-Lowering Intervention Trials

	Relative Mortality
Cardiovascular disease	0.85
All-causes	1.07
Cancer (only in drug trials[a])	1.43
Not illness related	1.76

[a]These were trials with the earlier cholesterol lowering drugs, not the more modern statins.
Source: Muldoon, M.F. et al., *Br. Med. J.*, 301: 309–314, 1990.

Problem 6.3: A change in cooking oil

In 1987 the government of Mauritius, concerned about the high incidence of coronary heart disease, changed the formulation of the main cooking oil, from one based on palm oil (46% saturated, 41% monounsaturated, and 13% polyunsaturated fatty acids) to one based on soybean oil (31% saturated, 33% monounsaturated, and 36% polyunsaturated). Total fat intake was unchanged at 23.6% of energy, as was cholesterol intake at 85.5 mg/1000 kcal.

In 1996, Uusitalo et al. (*Br. Med. J.*, 313, 1044–1046) reported that there had been a significant fall in average serum cholesterol among adults in the country. However, to date there has been no report of any change in death from coronary heart disease.

Can you account for this?

chapter seven

Overweight and obesity

If the intake of metabolic fuels (i.e., the total intake of food) is greater than is required to meet energy expenditure, the result is storage of the excess, largely as triacylglycerol in adipose tissue (Section 5.2). This chapter is concerned with the problems associated with excessive accumulation of body fat: overweight and obesity—a serious public health problem worldwide. There has been a considerable increase in the prevalence of obesity in all countries over the past two decades, to the extent that WHO talks of a global epidemic of obesity. In 2005, it was estimated that for the first time in human history, there were more overweight and obese people in the world than those who were hungry and underfed; many developing countries have the problems of undernutrition (Chapter 8) and overnutrition at the same time. Perhaps more seriously, metabolic programming (Section 6.4.1) as a result of (marginal) undernutrition *in utero* and in early life is a major factor in the development of obesity and the metabolic syndrome in later life (Section 7.2.3).

Objectives

After reading this chapter, you should be able to

- Explain what is meant by desirable body weight, calculate body mass index, and determine whether it is within the desirable range or not
- Describe the methods that are available to determine body fat content and distribution
- Describe the health hazards associated with overweight and obesity, and explain the association between obesity and insulin resistance in the metabolic syndrome
- Explain the causes and treatment of obesity

7.1 Desirable body weight

Figure 7.1 shows the results of one of the early prospective studies to determine desirable ranges of weight. 750,000 people were classified by weight, then followed up for 15 years. Those who were most overweight were twice as likely to die as those whose weight was around the average.

People who were significantly below average weight at the beginning of the study were also more at risk of premature death. However, this may be because those people who were significantly underweight were already seriously ill (Section 8.4), rather than implying that a moderate degree of underweight is undesirable or poses any health hazards.

7.1.1 Body mass index

Many of the early studies of overweight and premature mortality used relatively complex tables of weight for height, sometimes also corrected for skeletal frame size. A simpler solution is to calculate the body mass index (BMI), sometimes also called Quetelet's index, after the nineteenth century mathematician who first demonstrated its usefulness. BMI

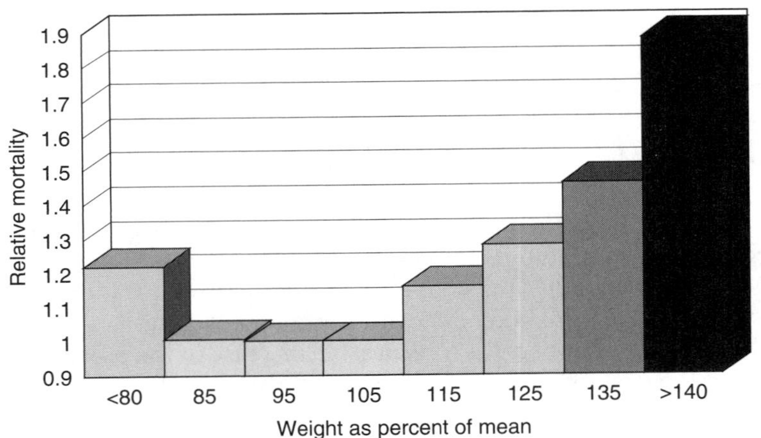

Figure 7.1 Excess mortality with obesity. (From data reported by Garfinkel, L., *Cancer*, 58, 1826–1829, 1986.)

Table 7.1 Classification of Overweight and Obesity by Body Mass Index

	BMI	Excess Weight (kg)	Percentage of Desirable Weight
Desirable	20–25	–	100
Acceptable, but not desirable	25–27	<5	100–110
Overweight	25–30	5–15	110–120
Obese	30–40	15–25	120–160
Severely obese	>40	>25	>160

Note: BMI = weight (kg)/height^2 (m).

is calculated from the weight (in kg) divided by the square of the height (in meters), that is, BMI = weight (kg)/height^2 (m). The desirable range, associated with optimum life expectancy, is between 20 and 25. Values of BMI below 18.5 are associated with undernutrition (Section 8.2). Table 7.1 and Figure 7.2 show the classification of overweight and obesity by BMI.

Most people gain weight as they grow older. There is some evidence that a modest increase in BMI (by 1 unit/decade) may be associated with better health. Tables 7.2 and 7.3 show the acceptable ranges of BMI at different ages.

Although BMI provides a useful way of assessing weight relative to height, and for most people a high BMI reflects excessive adipose tissue, it does not provide useful information for people like bodybuilders, whose high BMI is due to increased muscle mass, not adipose tissue.

7.1.2 Measurement of body fat

The important factor for health is the proportion of body weight that is fat. This is termed adiposity. A number of techniques are available for assessing adiposity, although most of them are research techniques and are not appropriate for routine screening of the general public.

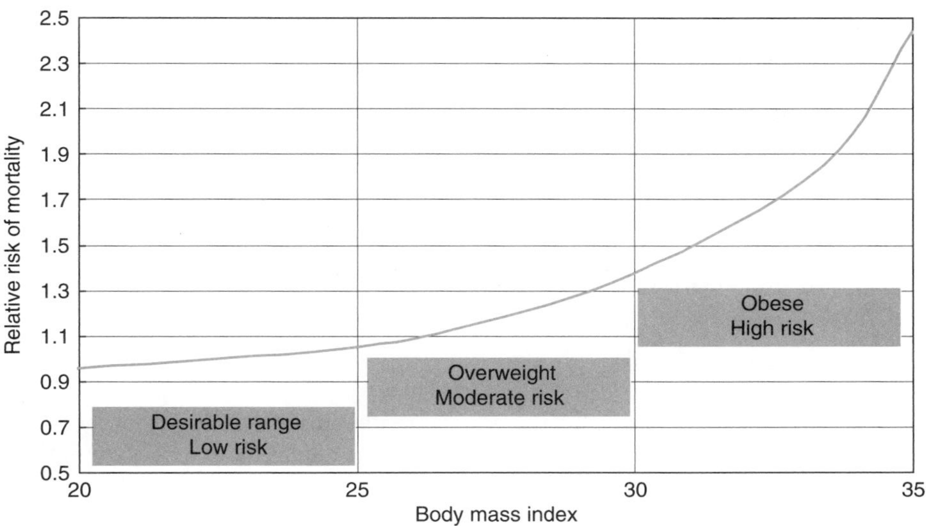

Figure 7.2 Excess mortality with obesity as defined by body mass index.

Table 7.2 Desirable Range of Body Mass Index for Children and Adolescents

	Boys		Girls	
Age	5th Centile	85th Centile	5th Centile	85th Centile
5	1.8	16.8	13.5	1.8
6	13.8	17	13.4	17.1
7	13.8	17.4	13.4	17.6
8	1.8	17.9	13.5	18.3
9	14	18.6	13.7	191
10	14.2	19.4	14	19.9
11	14.5	20.2	14.4	20.8
12	15	21	14.8	21.7
13	15.4	21.8	15.3	22.6
14	16	22.6	15.8	2.3
15	16.5	2.4	16.3	24
16	17.1	24.2	1.8	24.7
17	17.7	24.9	17.2	25.2
18	18.2	25.6	17.5	25.7
19	18.8	26.4	17.8	26.1

Note: Body mass index = weight (kg)/height^2 (m).
Source: US National Center for Health Statistics body mass index for age percentiles (http://www.cdc.gov/growth charts).

7.1.2.1 Determination of body density

The density of body fat is 0.9 g/mL, while that of the fat-free body mass is 1.10 g/mL. This means that if the density of the body can be measured, then the proportion of fat and lean tissue can be calculated.

Density is determined either by weighing in air, and again totally submerged in water, or by measuring the volume of the body by its displacement of water when submerged. Neither

Table 7.3 Acceptable Ranges of Body Mass Index with Age

Age (years)	Acceptable BMI
19–24	19–24
25–34	20–25
35–44	21–26
45–54	22–27
55–64	23–28
>65	24–29

Note: BMI = weight (kg)/height^2 (m).

procedure is particularly pleasant for the experimental subject, and considerable precision is necessary in the measurements; if 10% of body weight is fat, which is extremely low, the density is 1.08 g/mL, while at 50% fat, which is very high, the density is 1.00 g/mL.

While direct determination of body density is the standard, against which all the other techniques discussed below must be calibrated, it is clearly a research technique and not appropriate for general use.

7.1.2.2 Determination of total body water or potassium

The fat content of the body can be determined by estimating the fat-free mass of the body. This can be done by measuring total body water (fat-free tissue is 73% water) by giving a dose of water labeled with ^2H or ^{18}O, and then measuring the dilution of the label in urine or saliva.

Alternatively, the total body content of potassium can be measured. Potassium occurs only in the fat-free mass of the body, and the radioactive isotope ^{40}K occurs naturally. It is a weak γ-emitter, and total body potassium can be determined by measuring the γ-radiation of the appropriate wavelength emitted by the body. This requires total enclosure in a shielded whole-body counter for about 15 min to achieve adequate precision, and because of this, and the cost of the equipment required, again, this is purely a research technique.

7.1.2.3 Imaging techniques

Fat, bone, and lean tissues absorb X-rays and ultrasound to different extent, and therefore either an X-ray or an ultrasound image will permit determination of the amounts of different tissues in the body, by measuring the areas (or volumes if scanning techniques are used) occupied by each type of tissue. Such imaging techniques permit determination not only of the total amount of fat in the body, but also its distribution; it is adipose tissue within the abdominal cavity, rather than subcutaneous adipose tissue, that is the main health hazard (Section 7.2.2.1).

7.1.2.4 Measurement of whole-body electrical conductivity and impedance

Fat is an electrical insulator, while lean tissue, being a solution of electrolytes, will conduct an electric current. If electrodes are attached to the hand and the foot, and an extremely small alternating electric current (typically 80 μA at 50 MHz) is passed between them, measurement of the fall in voltage permits calculation of the conductivity or impedance of the body. The percentage of fat and lean tissue can be calculated from equations based on a series of studies in which this technique has been calibrated against direct determination of density (Section 7.1.2.1).

Measurement of either total body electrical conductivity (TOBEC) or bioelectrical impedance (BIE) has been used mainly in research, but many gyms and fitness centers now have the equipment to measure body fat in this way.

7.1.2.5 Measurement of skinfold thickness

Where equipment is not available to determine body fat by electrical conductivity or impedance, the thickness of subcutaneous adipose tissue is measured as an index of total body fat content, using standardized calipers that exert a moderate pressure (10 g/mm^2 over an area of 20–40 mm^2). For greatest precision, the mean of the skinfold thickness at four sites is calculated:

- Over the triceps, at the mid-point of the upper arm
- Over the biceps, at the front of the upper arm, directly above the cubital fossa, at the same level as the triceps site
- Subscapular, just below and laterally to the angle of the shoulder blade, with the shoulder and arm relaxed
- Suprailiac, on the midaxillary line immediately superior to the iliac crest

The desirable ranges of mean skinfold thickness are 3–10 mm for men and 10–22 mm for men and women. However, the important factor for health is intraabdominal fat, which cannot be estimated from skinfold thickness. A combination of skinfold measurements with measurement of the waist:hip circumference ratio gives an indication of the relative amounts of subcutaneous and intra-abdominal fat.

7.2 The problems of overweight and obesity

Overweight and obesity are a major problem in most developed countries (Figure 7.3); and in developing countries, there are problems of both obesity and undernutrition at the same time (Figures 7.4 and 7.5).

There is a worrying increase in the prevalence of overweight and obesity. In 2003 (the most recent year for which data are available), almost two-thirds of adults in Britain were classified as overweight (BMI > 25); 24% of men and 26% of women were classified as obese (BMI > 30). The proportion of men who were classified as obese had increased fourfold and the proportion of women who were obese threefold over a 20 year period (Figure 7.6). This increase in the prevalence of overweight and obesity is occurring worldwide, and there is no evidence that the rate of increase is slowing.

7.2.1 Social problems of obesity

Historically, a moderate degree of overweight was considered desirable; when food was scarce, fatness was a visible sign of wealth. There was also a survival advantage in having reserves of fat in order to survive periods of food shortage or famine. As food supplies have become more assured, perceptions have changed. Fatness is no longer regarded as a sign of wealth; indeed, obesity is more common among lower socioeconomic groups in developed countries, although in developing countries it is still mainly confined to the

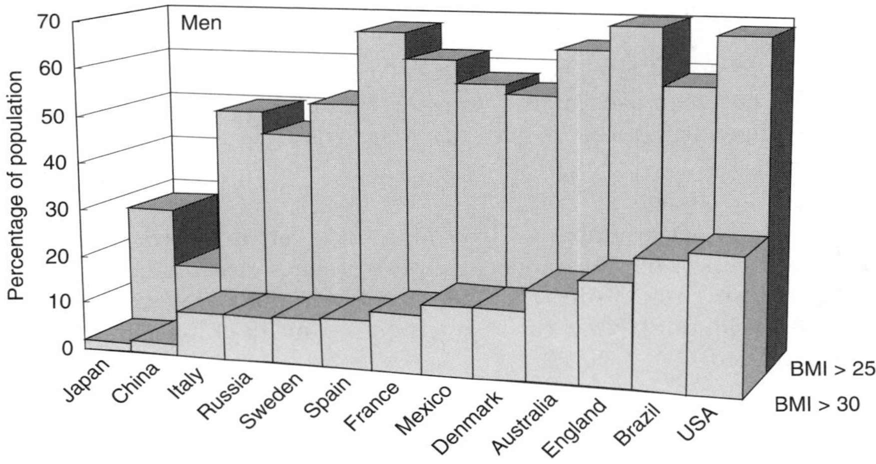

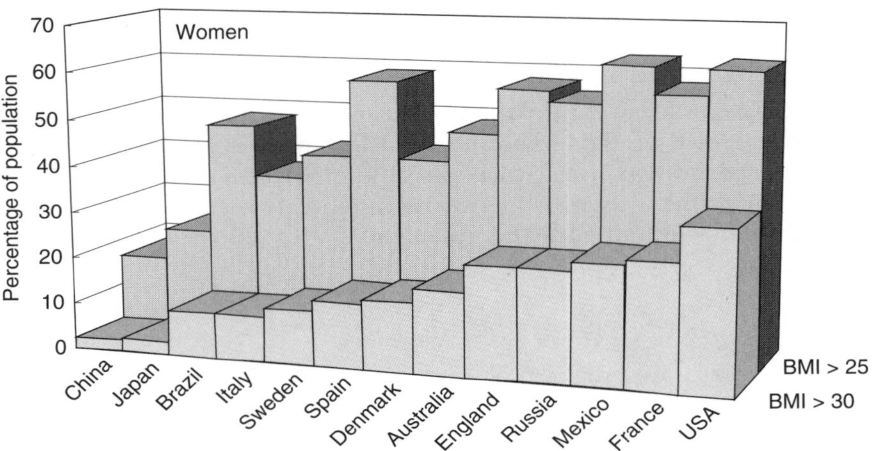

Figure 7.3 Overweight and obesity in selected countries in 2003. (From World Health Organization data.)

wealthier sections of the population. No longer are the overweight envied; rather, they are likely to be mocked, reviled, and made deeply unhappy by the unthinking comments and prejudices of their lean companions.

Because society at large considers obesity undesirable, and fashion emphasizes slimness, many overweight and obese people have problems of a poor self-image and low self-esteem. Obese people are certainly not helped by the all-too-common prejudice against them, the difficulty of buying clothes that will fit, and the fact that they are often regarded as a legitimate butt of crude and cruel humor. This may lead to a sense of isolation and withdrawal from society, and may frequently result in increased food consumption, for comfort, thus resulting in yet more weight gain, a further loss of self-esteem, further withdrawal, and more eating for compensation.

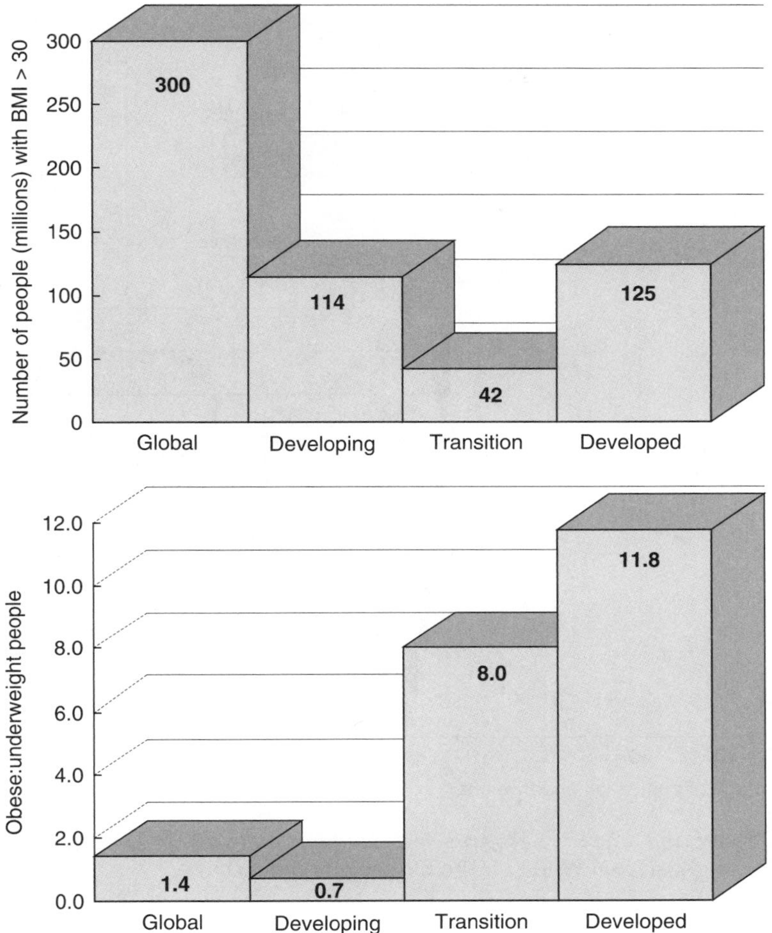

Figure 7.4 Obesity in developed and developing countries in 2003. (From World Health Organization data.)

The psychological and social problems of the obese spill over to people of normal weight as well. There is continual advertising pressure for "slimness," and newspapers and magazines are full of propaganda for slimness, and "diets" for weight reduction. This may be one of the factors in the development of major eating disorders such as anorexia nervosa and bulimia (Section 8.3.1.1).

7.2.2 The health risks of obesity

The major causes of death associated with obesity are:

- Cancer, especially breast, prostate, and colorectal cancers
- Atherosclerosis, coronary heart disease, high blood pressure, and stroke
- Type II diabetes mellitus
- Respiratory diseases

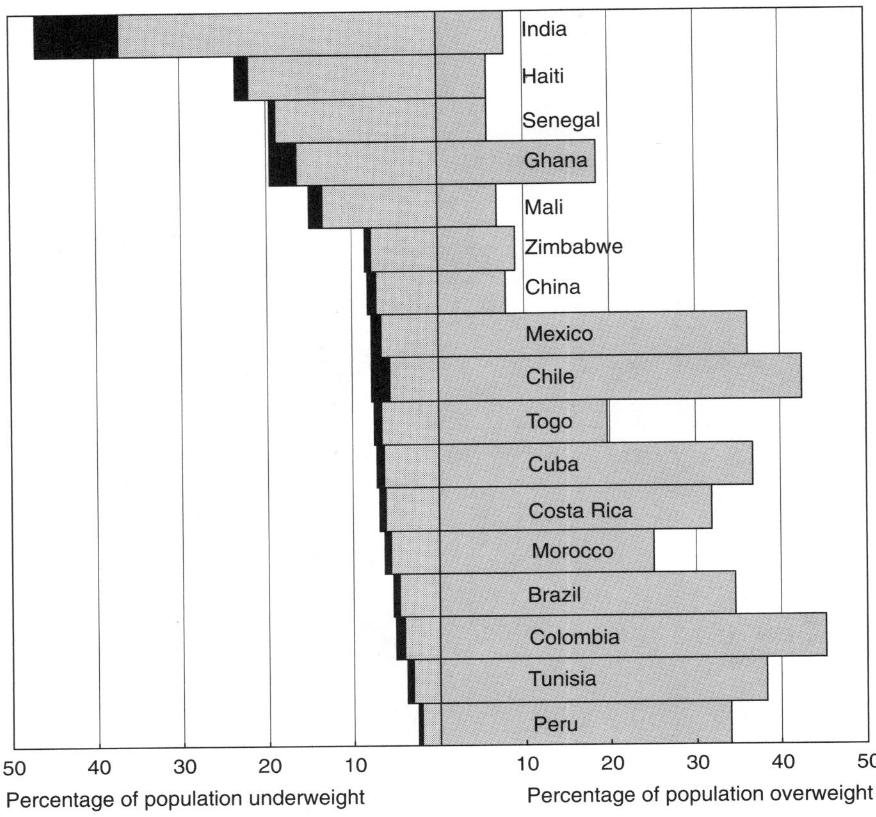

Figure 7.5 Obesity and underweight in selected countries in 2003 (dark shading shows those seriously underweight). (From World Health Organization data.)

In addition to the diseases caused by, or associated with, obesity, obese people are considerably more at risk of death during surgery and postoperative complications. There are three main reasons for this:

- Surgery is longer and more difficult when the surgeon has to cut through large amounts of subcutaneous and intra-abdominal adipose tissue.
- Induction of anesthesia is more difficult when veins are not readily visible through subcutaneous adipose tissue, and maintenance of anesthesia is complicated by the solubility of anesthetic agents in fat, so that there is a large buffer pool in the body, and adjustment of the dose is difficult.
- Most importantly, anesthesia depresses lung function (as does being in a supine position) in all subjects. Obese people suffer from impaired lung function under normal conditions, largely as a result of adipose tissue in the upper body segment; total lung capacity may be only 60% of that in lean people and the mechanical workload on the respiratory muscles may be twice that of lean people. Therefore, they are especially at risk during surgery.

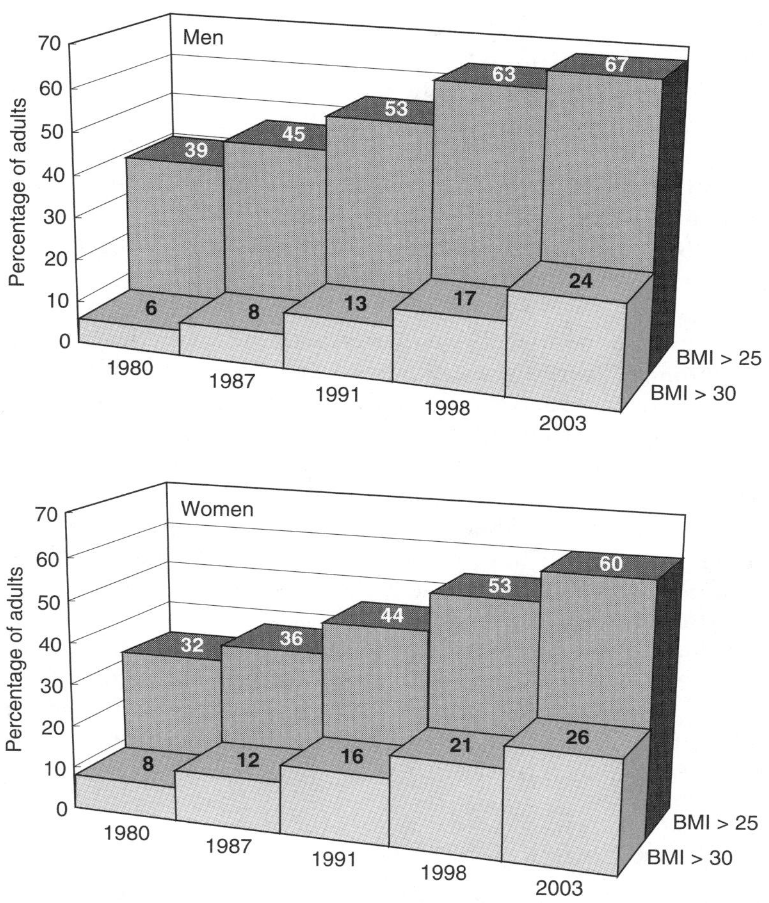

Figure 7.6 The increasing prevalence of overweight and obesity in the United Kingdom, 1980–2003. (From UK Department of Health data.)

Because of their impaired lung function, obese people are more at risk of respiratory distress, pneumonia, and bronchitis than are lean people. In addition, excess body weight is associated with increased morbidity from conditions such as the following:

- Arthritis of the hips and knees, associated with the increased stress on weight-bearing joints. In addition, there is increased synthesis of nitric oxide in response to leptin action, and this has been implicated in the destruction of cartilage. Rheumatoid arthritis may also be exacerbated in obese people as a result of the immunodulatory inflammatory actions of leptin.
- Varicose veins and hemorrhoids, associated with increased intra-abdominal pressure, and possibly because of a low intake of dietary fiber (Sections 4.2.1.6 and 6.3.3.2) and hence straining on defecation, rather than directly a result of obesity.
- Obesity in childhood and adolescence is associated with lower bone mineral density and increased risk of developing osteoporosis (Section 11.15.1.1) in later life.

7.2.2.1 The distribution of excess adipose tissue

The adverse effects of obesity are not only due to the excessive amount of body fat, but also because of its distribution in the body. Measurement of the waist:hip ratio provides a convenient way of defining two patterns of adipose tissue distribution:

- Predominantly in the upper body segment (thorax and abdomen)—the classical male pattern of obesity, sometimes called apple-shaped obesity
- Predominantly in the lower body segment (hips)—the classical female pattern of obesity, sometimes called pear-shaped obesity

It is the male pattern of abdominal obesity that is associated with the major health risks. In most studies of coronary heart disease, there is a threefold excess of men compared with women, a difference that persists even when the data are corrected for risk factors such as blood pressure, cholesterol in low density lipoproteins, BMI, smoking, and physical activity. However, if the data are corrected for the waist:hip ratio, there is only a 1.4-fold excess of men over women.

Figure 7.7 shows the effects of body weight and waist:hip ratio on the prevalence of diabetes in women, and Figure 7.8 shows that increased intra-abdominal fat is associated with insulin resistance (and hence ultimately the development of diabetes) even in people whose BMI is within the desirable range.

Abdominal adipose tissue produces less leptin than does subcutaneous adipose tissue, so that abdominal fat will have less effect on the long-term regulation of food intake and energy expenditure (Section 1.3.2). In addition, it has a higher lipolytic activity, so that more nonesterified fatty acid is secreted by abdominal adipose tissue, which is a factor in insulin resistance (Section 7.2.3.1).

7.2.3 Obesity and the metabolic syndrome

It has become apparent in recent years that not only is obesity a cause of considerable morbidity and mortality, but it can be considered to be a disease in its own right also, since

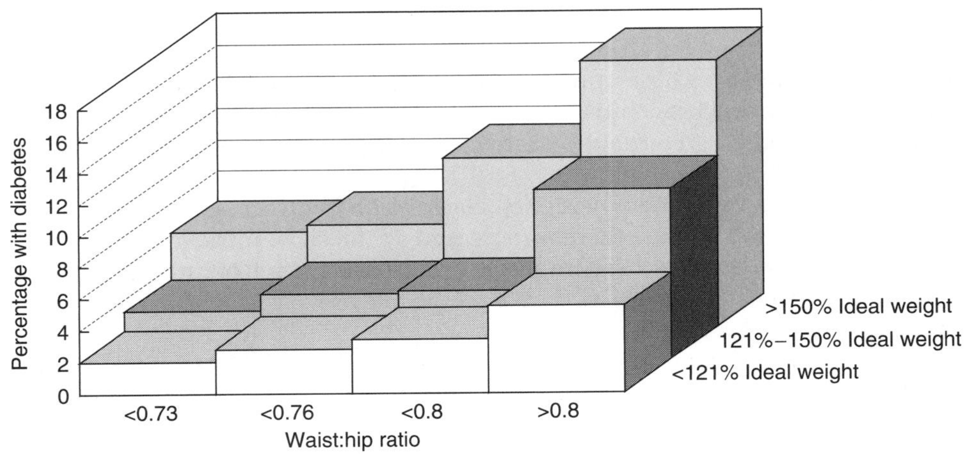

Figure 7.7 The effects of obesity and abdominal adiposity on the prevalence of diabetes. (From data reported by Hartz, A.J. et al., *Am. J. Epidemiol.*, 119, 71–80, 1984.)

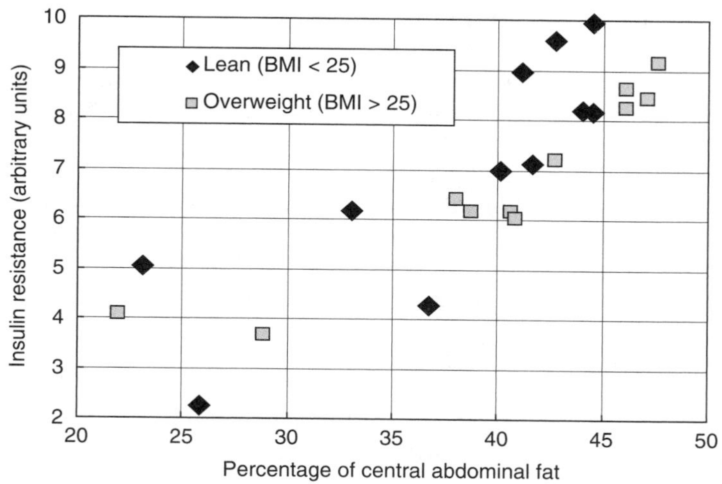

Figure 7.8 The effect of abdominal adiposity in lean and obese subjects on insulin resistance. (From data reported by Wilkin, T.J., in *Adult Obesity: A Paediatric Challenge*, Voss, L.D. and Willkin, T.J., Eds., Taylor & Francis, London, 2003, chap.4.)

obesity (and especially intra-abdominal obesity) is associated with chronic low-grade inflammation. Adipose tissue not only stores triacylglycerol and secretes leptin but also secretes a number of inflammatory cytokines (sometimes known as adipocytokines or adipokines) as well as adiponectin (Section 7.2.3.2), angiotensinogen (which is converted to angiotensin in the circulation and raises blood pressure), and macrophage attractants (Section 7.2.3.3).

The metabolic syndrome is characterized by obesity (and especially abdominal obesity) associated with the following:

- High blood pressure
- Insulin resistance—hyperglycemia with inappropriately high levels of insulin
- Low levels of high-density lipoproteins (HDL), but high plasma triacylglycerol and high levels of small, dense low-density lipoproteins (LDL) (Section 5.6.2)
- Elevated plasma concentrations of nonesterified fatty acids
- Low-grade systemic inflammation with high levels of circulating inflammatory cytokines
- Increased oxidative stress
- Increased risk of atherosclerosis and cardiovascular disease

7.2.3.1 Insulin resistance and hyperinsulinism

Abdominal obesity is associated with resistance of tissues to the rapid metabolic actions of insulin (Section 10.3.4), and in response to hyperglycemia there is increased synthesis and secretion of insulin—hyperinsulinemia. However, there is no impairment of the slower mitogenic actions of insulin, so that these responses are exaggerated by the hyperinsulinemia. Among other effects, this leads to increased proliferation of vascular smooth muscle, leading to atherosclerosis and hypertension.

A number of factors account for this insulin resistance:

- Visceral adipose tissue has high lipolytic activity and releases nonesterified fatty acids, which inhibit glucose metabolism and may also inhibit the insulin receptor signaling pathway (Section 10.3.4).
- Leptin antagonizes some actions of insulin.
- Various cytokines secreted by adipose tissue may cause insulin resistance, including tumor necrosis factor (TNF-α), interleukins IL-1 and IL-6, monocyte chemotactic protein, and resistin.
- Cortisol is synthesized in adipose tissue in an unregulated manner, and acts to increase hepatic gluconeogenesis and glucose release (Section 5.7), and lipolysis and release of nonesterified fatty acids in adipose tissue.

As insulin resistance continues, the ability of the pancreatic β-islet cells to synthesize and secrete insulin is exceeded, and the result is frank diabetes mellitus (Section 10.7).

7.2.3.2 Adiponectin

Adiponectin is a collagen-like protein that is synthesized in, and secreted by, adipose tissue. It is induced during the differentiation of adipocytes, but its secretion is inversely proportional to adipose tissue mass, so that plasma levels are low in obesity. The main actions of adiponectin are the following:

- To decrease the expression of vascular adhesion molecules and so reduce infiltration of macrophages into blood vessel endothelium
- To inhibit the proliferation of vascular smooth muscle cells and hence again reduce infiltration of macrophages into the endothelium
- To enhance insulin action by increasing the insulin-induced phosphorylation of the insulin receptor substrate (Section 10.3.4)
- To increase oxidation of glucose and fatty acids by activating 5′AMP kinases (Section 10.2.2.1) and increasing the expression of enzymes involved in fatty acid transport and oxidation (Section 5.5.2)
- To increase energy expenditure in nonshivering thermogenesis by increasing the expression of uncoupling proteins (Section 3.3.1.5)

7.2.3.3 Macrophage infiltration of adipose tissue

Both adipocytes and adipocyte precursor cells secrete chemotactic agents that attract macrophages to infiltrate the tissue. Macrocytes secrete a variety of cytokines, including interleukins and tumor necrosis factor α, which stimulate preadipocytes and endothelial cells to secrete further macrophage attractants. They also cause phosphorylation of serine residues in the insulin receptor and its substrate, and impair insulin signaling.

As a result of increased macrophage activation in adipose tissue, there is a considerable degree of oxidative stress associated with increased synthesis of the respiratory burst oxidase (Section 6.5.2.2) and reduced activity of antioxidant enzymes (Section 6.5.3.1).

7.2.3.4 Excessive synthesis of cortisol

Glucocorticoid hormones are synthesized in adipose tissue. The enzyme 11β-hydroxysteroid dehydrogenase converts inactive cortisone into active cortisol. This leads to both elevated blood pressure, and hyperglycemia and insulin resistance. Cortisol produced in adipose tissue acts in that tissue, increasing lipolysis and the release of nonesterified fatty acids.

Transgenic mice that overexpress 11β-hydroxysteroid dehydrogenase in adipose tissue gain weight, mainly as abdominal adipose tissue. They are hyperglycemic and hyperinsulinemic with insulin resistance; plasma nonesterified fatty acids and triacylglycerol are increased; plasma leptin is increased, but there is leptin resistance, and the expression of uncoupling proteins in brown adipose tissue (Section 3.3.1.5) is decreased.

7.3 The causes and treatment of obesity

The cause of obesity is an intake of metabolic fuels greater than is required for energy expenditure, so that excess is stored, largely as fat in adipose tissue reserves. The simple answer to the problem of obesity is therefore to reverse the balance: reduce food intake and increase physical activity, and hence energy expenditure. Three factors explain the rapid increase in the prevalence of obesity over the past 2 to 3 decades: lower levels of physical activity, increased availability of food, and failure of appetite control.

7.3.1 Energy expenditure

In developing countries, energy expenditure has fallen as increased mechanization has replaced physical labor; in almost all countries there has been an increase in sedentary leisure activities, at the expense of active recreation.

A desirable physical activity level (PAL) for fitness is 1.7 times the basal metabolic rate (BMR) (Section 5.1.3.2), but in Britain the average PAL is only 1.4—physical activity accounts for only 40% more energy expenditure than BMR. Sometimes, the problem can be attributed to a low rate of energy expenditure despite a reasonable level of physical activity. There is a range of individual variations as much as 30% above and below the average BMR (Section 5.1.3.1). This means that some people will have a very low BMR and hence a very low requirement for food. Despite eating very little compared with those around them, they may gain weight. Equally, there are people who have a relatively high BMR and are able to eat a relatively large amount of food without gaining weight.

Lean people can increase their energy expenditure to match their food intake; leptin (Section 1.3.2) increases the activity of mitochondrial uncoupling proteins (Section 3.3.1.5). The result of this is an increased rate of metabolism of metabolic fuels, and increased heat output from the body, especially after meals and while asleep.

Other people seem to be much more energy efficient, and their body temperature may drop slightly while they are asleep. This means that they are using less metabolic fuel to maintain body temperature, and so are able to store more as adipose tissue. Such people tend to be overweight. (This response, lowering body temperature and metabolic rate to conserve food, is seen in a more extreme form in animals that hibernate. During their long winter sleep, these animals have a very low rate of metabolism, and hence a low rate of utilization of the fuel they have stored in adipose tissue reserves.)

7.3.2 Availability of food

In most countries, there has been an increase in the total amount of food available, even in developed countries that had superabundant food 30 years ago (see PowerPoint presentation 7 on the CD). There has been a very considerable increase in the availability of fat and sugars, especially in ready prepared meals and food from fast-food restaurants. Between 1977 and 1996, the amount spent on meals outside the home in the United States increased from 30% to 40% of total food expenditure, but this represented almost a doubling

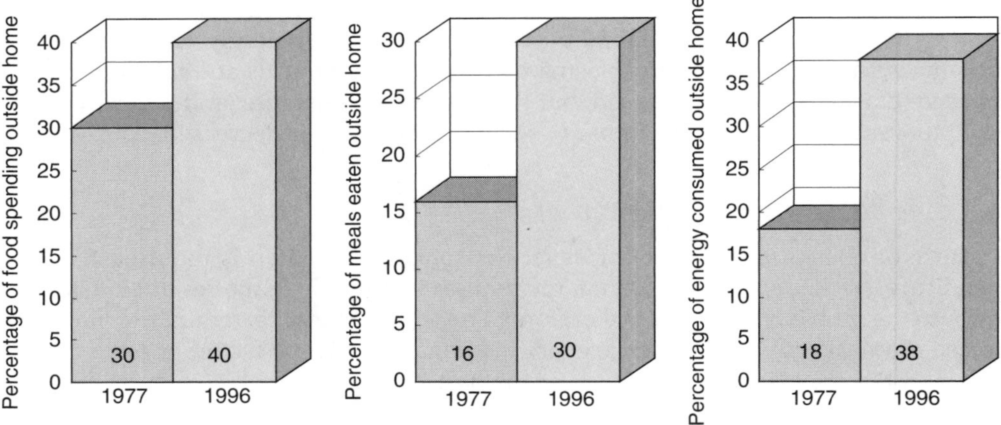

Figure 7.9 US food consumption away from home. (From data reported by Critser, G., *Fatland—How Americans Became the Fattest People in the World*, Penguin Books, London, 2003.)

of the number of meals, and more than a doubling of the percentage of energy intake from meals outside the home (Figure 7.9). Part of this is explained by the high energy density of such meals, and part by the increase in portion sizes coupled with constant or reduced prices; many standard servings are now considerably larger than the standard serving sizes defined by the USDA for food labeling.

Increased use of high fructose syrups to replace sucrose in manufactured foods may also be important, since fructose enters glycolysis after the main regulatory step, and results in increased synthesis of fatty acids and triacylglycerol in liver and adipose tissue (Section 5.4.1).

7.3.3 Control of appetite

Most people manage to balance their food intake with energy expenditure remarkably precisely. Indeed, even people who are overweight or obese are in energy balance when their weight is more or less constant. As discussed in Section 1.3.2, leptin is central to the control of both food intake and energy expenditure, and there are a number of mechanisms involved in short-term control of food intake, with regulation of both hunger and satiety.

Very rarely, people are overweight or obese as a result of a physical defect of the appetite control centers in the brain, for example, some tumors can cause damage to the satiety center, so that the patient feels hunger, but not the sensation of satiety, and has no physiological cue to stop eating. A very small number of children who are pathologically obese have defects in their leptin receptors or downstream signaling from the leptin receptor, so that they have little or no control over their appetite and energy expenditure.

More commonly, obesity can be attributed to a psychological failure of appetite control. At its simplest, this can be blamed on the variety of attractive foods available. People can easily be tempted to eat more than they need, and it may take quite an effort of willpower to refuse a choice morsel. Even when hunger has been satisfied, the appearance of a different dish can stimulate appetite. Experimental animals that normally do not become obese can be persuaded to overeat and become obese by providing them with a "cafeteria" array of attractive foods.

A number of studies comparing severely obese people with lean people have shown that they do not respond to the normal cues for hunger and satiety. Rather, in many cases, it is the sight of food that prompts them to eat, regardless of whether they are "hungry" or not. If no food is visible, they will not feel hungry; conversely, if food is still visible they will not feel satiety. There have been no similar studies involving more moderately overweight people, so it is not known whether this failure of appetite regulation is a general problem or whether it only affects severely obese people with BMI > 40.

7.3.4 How obese people can be helped to lose weight

In considering the treatment of obesity, two different aspects of the problem must be considered:

- The initial problem, which is to help the overweight or obese person to reduce his or her weight to within the desirable range, where life expectancy is maximum.
- The long-term problem of helping the now lean person to maintain desirable body weight. This is largely a matter of education, increasing physical activity, and changing eating habits. The same guidelines for a prudent diet (Section 6.3) apply to the slimmed-down, formerly obese, person as to anyone else.

The aim of any weight-reduction regime is to reduce the intake of food to below the level needed for energy expenditure, so that body reserves of fat will have to be used. The theoretical maximum possible rate of weight loss is 230 g/MJ energy imbalance per week; for a person with an energy expenditure of 10 MJ/day, total starvation would result in a loss of 2.3 kg/week. In practice, the rate of weight loss is lower than this theoretical figure, because of the changes in metabolic rate and energy expenditure that occur with changes in both body weight and food intake (Section 5.2).

Very often, the first 1 or 2 weeks of a weight-reducing regime are associated with a very much greater loss of weight than this. Obviously, this cannot be due to loss of fat. It is because of loss of the water associated with glycogen (Section 4.2.1.5). Although it is not sustained, the initial rapid rate of weight loss can be extremely encouraging for the obese person. The problem is to ensure that he or she realizes that it will not, and indeed cannot, be sustained. It also provides excellent advertising copy for less than totally scrupulous vendors of slimming regimes, who make truthful claims about the weight loss in the first week or two, and omit any information about the later weeks and months needed to achieve goal weight.

7.3.4.1 Starvation

More or less total starvation has been used in a hospital setting to treat seriously obese patients, especially those who are to undergo elective surgery. Vitamins and minerals have to be supplied (Chapter 11), as well as fluid, but an obese person can lose weight at about the predicted rate of 2–2.5 kg/week, if starved completely. There are two major problems with total starvation as a means of rapid weight loss:

- The problem of enforcement. It is very difficult to deprive someone of food and prevent them finding more or less devious means of acquiring it—by begging or stealing from other patients, visitors, and hospital volunteers, or even by walking down to the hospital shop or outpatients' cafeteria.
- As much as half the weight lost in total starvation may be protein from muscle and other tissues to provide a source of amino acids for gluconeogenesis to maintain

blood glucose (Section 5.7). This is not desirable; the stress of surgery causes a considerable loss of protein (Section 9.1.2.2), and it would be highly undesirable to start this loss before surgery.

7.3.4.2 Very low-energy diets

Many of the problems associated with total starvation can be avoided by feeding a very low energy intake, commonly 1–1.5 MJ/day, in specially formulated meal replacements that provide adequate intakes of vitamins and minerals. Such regimes have shown excellent results in the treatment of severe obesity. There is very much less loss of tissue protein than in total starvation, and people feel less hungry than if they are starved completely.

If very low-energy diets are used together with a program of exercise, the rate of weight loss can be close to the theoretical maximum of 2–2.5 kg/week. Such diets should probably be regarded as a treatment of last resort, for people with a serious problem of obesity that does not respond to more conventional diet therapy. These diets do not provide appropriate education in changes to diet for long-term maintenance of reduced weight.

7.3.4.3 Conventional diets

For most people, the problem is not one of severe morbid obesity, but a more modest excess body weight. Even for people who have a serious problem of obesity, it is likely that less drastic measures than those discussed above will be beneficial. The aim is to reduce energy intake to below expenditure, and so ensure the utilization of adipose tissue reserves. To anyone who has not tried to lose weight, the answer would appear to be simply to eat less. Obviously it is not so simple; a vast array of diets, slimming regimes, and special foods are available.

The ideal approach to the problem of obesity and weight reduction would be to provide people with the information that they need to choose an appropriate diet for themselves. This is not easy. It is not simply a matter of reducing energy intake, but of ensuring at the same time that intakes of protein, vitamins, and minerals are adequate. The preparation of balanced diets, especially when the total energy intake is to be reduced, is a skilled task, and a major function of the professional dietitian. Furthermore, there is the problem of long-term compliance with dietary restrictions—the diet must not only be low in energy and high in nutrients, it must also be attractive and pleasant to eat in appropriate amounts.

A simple way of helping people to select an appropriate diet for weight reduction is to offer three lists of foods:

- Energy-rich foods, which should be avoided. These are generally foods rich in fat and sugar, but providing little in the way of vitamins and minerals. Such foods include oils and fats; fried foods; fatty cuts of meat, cakes, biscuits; alcoholic beverages, etc. They should be eaten sparingly, if at all.
- Foods that are relatively high in energy yield, but also good sources of protein, vitamins, and minerals. They should be eaten in moderate amounts.
- Foods that are generally rich sources of vitamins and minerals, high in starch and nonstarch polysaccharide, and low in fat and sugars (i.e., nutrient dense). These can be eaten (within reason) as much as is wanted.

An alternative method is to provide people with a series of meal plans and menus, designed to be nutrient dense and energy low, and providing sufficient variety from day to day to ensure compliance. To make this less rigid and prescriptive, it is easy to provide a list of foods with "exchange points," permitting one food to be substituted for another. At its simplest, such a list would give portions of foods with approximately the same energy yield. A more elaborate exchange list calculates "points" for foods based on their energy yield, nutrient density, and total or saturated fat content. The consumer is given a target number of "points" to be consumed each day, depending on gender, physical activity, and the amount of weight to be lost, and can make up a diet to meet this target. An advantage of this is that foods that might be considered forbidden in a simple energy-counting diet can be permitted—but a single portion may constitute a whole day's points.

An interesting variant of the exchange points system also allocates (negative) points to physical activity, so promoting physical activity as well as sound eating habits.

7.3.4.4 Very low carbohydrate (ketogenic) diets

From time to time there is a fashion for very low carbohydrate diets for weight reduction, typically allowing less than 20 g of carbohydrate per day in the initial stages, but with unlimited fat and protein. Such diets are effective, but the subjects become ketotic and feel unwell. Three factors explain the efficacy of such diets:

- In response to a high protein diet, there is a considerable increase in the rate of whole body protein turnover, which is ATP expensive (Section 9.2.3.3), resulting in increased energy expenditure.
- A high protein intake increases the expression of neuropeptide Y in the hypothalamic appetite control centers (Section 1.3.1), thus increasing satiety.
- To maintain an adequate supply of glucose for the central nervous system and red blood cells, there has to be considerable gluconeogenesis from amino acids; again this is ATP expensive (Section 5.7), resulting in increased energy expenditure.

Although very low carbohydrate diets are effective for weight loss, they are unlikely to be useful for long-term maintenance of desirable body weight, and they run counter to all advice on what constitutes a prudent diet for health (Section 6.3). Not only are they undesirably high in fat, but there is also some evidence that excessively high intakes of protein may pose long-term health hazards.

7.3.4.5 Low glycemic index diets

Carbohydrates with a low glycemic index (Section 4.2.1) lead to a slower rise in blood glucose after a meal, and hence to less insulin secretion. As a result, there is less synthesis of fatty acids and triacylglycerol.

Although sucrose has a low glycemic index, because it yields 1 mol of glucose and 1 mol of fructose, and so has less effect on blood glucose than an equivalent amount of glucose, it is misleading to consider it to be beneficial in the same way as low glycemic starches are beneficial, because of the effect of fructose in increasing fatty acid synthesis (Section 5.4.1).

7.3.4.6 High fiber diets

One of the problems raised by many people who are restricting their food intake is that they continually feel hungry. Quite apart from true physiological hunger, the lack of bulk in the gastrointestinal tract may be a factor here. This problem can be alleviated by increasing the intake of dietary fiber or nonstarch polysaccharide (Section 4.2.1.6)—increased amounts of whole grain cereal products, fruits, and vegetables. Such regimes are certainly successful and again represent essentially a more extreme version of the general advice for a prudent diet. Soluble nonstarch polysaccharides (plant mucilages and gums) increase the viscosity of the intestinal contents, and slow the absorption of the products of digestion, thus effectively decreasing the glycemic index of a meal.

It is generally desirable that the dietary sources of nonstarch polysaccharides should be ordinary foods, rather than "supplements." However, as an aid to weight reduction, a number of preparations of dietary fiber are available. Some of these are more or less ordinary foods, but contain added fiber, which gives texture to the food, and increases the feeling of fullness and satiety. Some of the special slimmers' soups, biscuits, etc. are of this type. They are formulated to provide about one-third of a day's requirement of protein, vitamins, and minerals, but with a low energy yield. They are supposed to be taken in place of one meal each day, and to aid satiety they contain carboxymethylcellulose or another nondigested polysaccharide.

7.3.4.7 "Diets" that probably will not work

Weight reduction depends on reducing the intake of metabolic fuels, but ensuring that the intake of nutrients is adequate to meet requirements. Equally important is the problem of ensuring that the weight that has been lost is not replaced—in other words, eating patterns must be changed after weight has been lost to allow for maintenance of a body weight with a well-balanced diet.

There is a bewildering array of different diet regimes on offer to help the overweight and obese to lose weight. Some of these are based on sound nutritional principles and provide about half the person's energy requirement, with adequate amounts of protein, vitamins, and minerals. They permit a sustained weight loss of about 1–1.5 kg/week.

Other "diets" are neither scientifically formulated nor based on sound nutritional principles, and indeed frequently depend on pseudoscience in an attempt to give them some validity. They frequently make exaggerated claims for the amount of weight that can be lost and rarely provide a balanced diet. Publication of testimonials from "satisfied clients" cannot be considered to be evidence of efficacy, and publication in a book that is a best seller or in a magazine with wide circulation, cannot correct the underlying flaws of many of these "diets."

Some of the more outlandish diet regimes depend on such unscientific principles as eating protein and carbohydrates at different meals (so-called food combining)—ignoring the fact that "carbohydrate" foods such as bread and potatoes provide a significant amount of protein as well (see Figure 9.3). Others depend on a very limited range of foods. The most extreme allow the client to eat bananas, grapefruit, or peanuts (or some other food) in unlimited amounts, but little else. Other diet regimes ascribe almost magical properties to certain fruits (e.g., mangoes and pineapples), again with a very limited range of other foods allowed.

The idea is that if someone is permitted to eat as much they wish of only a very limited range of foods, even desirable and much-liked foods, they will end up eating very little, because even a favorite food soon palls if this is all that is permitted. In practice, these "diets" do neither good nor harm. People get so bored that they give up before there can be any significant effect on body weight, or any adverse effects of a very unbalanced diet. This is all to the good—if people did stick to such diets for any length of time, they might well encounter problems of protein, vitamin, and mineral deficiency.

One persistent myth is that obesity (and its adverse health consequences) is the result of accumulation in the body (and especially the gastrointestinal tract) of toxins derived from foods. There are a number of so-called "detox" diets that depend on a period of more or less total fasting, sometimes combined with herbal extracts or eating only one type of fruit, together with drinking large volumes of water.

7.3.4.8 Slimming patches

BMR is controlled to a considerable extent by the thyroid hormone tri-iodothyronine, and iodine deficiency (Section 11.15.3.3) results in impaired synthesis of thyroid hormone, a low metabolic rate, and ready weight gain. Pathological overactivity of the thyroid gland results in increased synthesis and secretion of thyroid hormone, and an increased BMR, with weight loss.

The synthesis of thyroid hormone is regulated, and in the absence of thyroid disease, provision of additional iodine does not increase hormone secretion except in people who were iodine deficient. Nevertheless, there are people who market various iodine-rich preparations to aid weight loss. Foremost among these are the so-called slimming patches, which contain seaweed extract as a source of iodine that is supposed to be absorbed from a small patch applied to the skin. There is no evidence that such patches have any beneficial effect at all.

7.3.4.9 Sugar substitutes

The average consumption of sugar is higher than is considered desirable (Section 6.3.3.1), and omitting sugar from tea and coffee would make a significant contribution to reduction of energy intake—a teaspoon of sugar is 5 g of carbohydrate, and thus provides 80 kJ—in each of six cups of tea or coffee a day, two spoons of sugar would thus account for some 960 kJ, almost 10% of the average person's energy expenditure. Quite apart from this obvious sugar, there is a great deal of sugar in beverages, for example, a standard 330 mL can of lemonade provides 20 g of sugar (= 320 kJ).

Because many people like their tea and coffee sweetened, and to replace the sugar in lemonades, etc., a number of intense sweeteners are used as sugar substitutes. These are synthetic chemicals that are very much sweeter than sugar, but are not metabolic fuels. Even those that can be metabolized (e.g., aspartame, which is an amino acid derivative) are taken in such small amounts that they make no significant contribution to intake. All these compounds have been extensively tested for safety, but as a result of concerns about possible hazards, some are not permitted in some countries, although they are widely used elsewhere.

Sugar alcohols such as sorbitol are poorly absorbed from the small intestine and therefore have only about half the energy yield of other carbohydrates (Sections 4.2.2.1 and 4.2.2.3). Unlike intense sweeteners, they can be used in manufacture of jam, sweets, and other foods, where they provide the same bulk and have the same osmotic preservative effect as sugars, but at half the energy yield.

7.3.4.10 Fat substitutes

In addition to low-fat versions of conventional foods (e.g., leaner cuts of meat used in manufactured foods and minced meat, skimmed and semiskimmed milk, and cheese and yogurt made from skimmed or semiskimmed milk), there are a number of fat substitutes available for food manufacture. Some of these are based on modified starch or protein, and are useful in the manufacture of very low-fat spreads (to replace butter or margarine), and salad dressings and dips. Fatty acid esters of sucrose (Olestra™ or Olean™) can be used for frying foods in the same way as oils and fats that are fatty acid esters of glycerol (Section 4.3.1), but they are not hydrolyzed by digestive enzymes and so have no nutritional value.

7.3.4.11 Pharmacological treatment of obesity

A number of compounds act either to suppress the activity of the hunger center in the hypothalamus or stimulate the satiety center. Sometimes this is an undesirable side effect of drugs used to treat disease and can contribute to the undernutrition seen in chronically ill people (Section 8.4). As an aid to weight reduction, especially in people who find it difficult to control their food intake, drugs that suppress appetite may be useful. Four compounds have been used as appetite suppressants: fenfluramine (and the D-isomer, dexfenfluramine), phentermine, diethylpropion, and mazindol. The combination of phentermine and fenfluramine was withdrawn in the 1990s, after a number of reports associating it with cardiac damage, and there is evidence of psychiatric disturbance and possible problems of addiction with other drugs. None of these appetite suppressants is now legally available in most countries.

The South African succulent plant, *Hoodia gordonii*, has been traditionally used by the San people of the Kalahari to stave off hunger, and a steroid glycoside has been isolated from the plant that has an anorectic action in experimental animals. However, there is no evidence from clinical trials that it is effective, or safe, for weight reduction in human beings.

A number of compounds have been marketed as "carbohydrate blockers," which are supposed to act by inhibiting amylase (Section 4.2.2.1), and so reducing the digestion of starch. There is no evidence that they are effective, and none has been licensed for pharmaceutical use. Similarly, there is no evidence of efficacy of compounds that are marketed as "fat burners," which are supposed to increase the rate at which fat is metabolized; if they were effective they would increase metabolic rate to such an extent that the consumer would have a persistent fever.

Inhibitors of pancreatic lipase (Section 4.3.2) reduce lipid digestion and absorption, and some (e.g., Xenical) have been licensed for use in morbidly obese patients who have made a serious effort to lose weight by more conventional means. The problem with their use is that undigested fat in the gastrointestinal tract can cause discomfort, and if enough is present, foul-smelling fatty diarrhea (steatorrhea).

7.3.4.12 Surgical treatment of obesity

Severe obesity may be treated by surgical removal of much of the excess adipose tissue—a procedure known as liposuction. Two further surgical treatments have also been used, but there is a considerable risk in undertaking any surgery in obese people (Section 7.2.2):

- Intestinal bypass surgery, in which the jejunum is connected to the distal end of the ileum, so bypassing most of the small intestine where the digestion and absorption of food occurs (Section 4.1). The resultant malabsorption means that the subject can, and indeed must, eat a relatively large amount of food, but will only absorb a small proportion. There are severe side effects of intestinal bypass surgery, including persistent foul-smelling diarrhea and flatulence, and failure to absorb medication, as well as problems of mineral and vitamin deficiency. This procedure has been more or less abandoned in most centers.
- Gastroplasty, in which the physical capacity of the stomach is reduced to half or less. This limits the amount of food that can be consumed at any one meal. While the results of such surgery appear promising, long-term follow-up suggests that a significant number of patients experience serious side effects, including micronutrient deficiencies.

7.3.4.13 Help and support

Especially for the severely obese person, weight loss is a lengthy and difficult experience. Friends and family can be supportive, but frequently specialist help and advice are needed.

To a great extent, this is the role of the dietitian and other health care professionals. In addition, there are a number of organizations, normally of formerly obese people, who can offer a mixture of professional, nutritional, and dietetic advice together with practical help and counseling. The main advantage of such groups is that they provide a social setting, rather than the formal setting of the dietitian's office in an outpatient clinic, and fellow members have experienced similar problems. Many people find the sharing of the problems and experiences of weight reduction extremely helpful.

Key points

- Obesity is a major problem of public health in developed countries, and increasingly so in developing countries; worldwide there are now more overweight and obese people than undernourished.
- BMI provides a convenient way of classifying ranges of body weight. There is a considerable increase in premature mortality among people who are obese (BMI > 30).
- Various ways can be used to assess the total body fat content, but only imaging techniques permit differentiation between subcutaneous fat and abdominal (interorgan) fat. Excess abdominal fat poses a more serious threat to health than does subcutaneous fat.
- Obese people are more likely to suffer from a range of physical illnesses and experience social problems; they are more at risk of death during surgery.
- Abdominal obesity leads to the development of insulin resistance, which develops into frank diabetes mellitus.
- Obesity is associated with chronic low-grade inflammation and increased oxidative stress.
- The underlying cause of obesity is low levels of physical activity coupled with plentiful availability of food, especially food that is high in fat and sugars. High fructose consumption may be a contributor to excessive synthesis of fatty acids.
- Effective treatment of obesity requires not only energy restriction to lose weight, but changes to diet habits and physical activity to maintain reduced weight. The most successful slimming regimes are those that are somewhat more restricted versions of the general advice for a prudent diet.

Problem 7.1: Janice W

Janice is a 40-year-old woman who is 162 cm tall and weighs 85 kg.

What is her BMI? Is this within the desirable range?
How much weight could she lose per MJ energy deficit?

For the purpose of these calculations, you may assume that all the weight loss will be adipose tissue: 15% water, 5% protein (with an energy yield of 17 kJ/g), and 80% triacylglycerol (with an energy yield of 37 kJ/g). You should ignore the (probably considerable) loss of muscle tissue to provide amino acids for gluconeogenesis.

Her total energy expenditure is 10 MJ/day. Assuming that she maintains her habitual level of physical activity, how much weight could she expect to lose per week:

(1) If she reduced her food intake by 10%
(2) If she halved her food intake
(3) If she replaced all meals with a specially formulated, very low-energy diet providing 2 MJ/day
(4) If she starved completely

For a woman aged 40 and weighing 85 kg, BMR will be about 7.6 MJ/day. What is her PAL?

Rather than reducing her food intake, she decides that she would prefer to increase her physical activity. What would be the effect on her body weight per week of walking moderately briskly for 1 h/day (PAR = 3.0)?

After her exercise, she is thirsty and drinks a pint of lager. The energy yield of lager is 130 kJ/100 mL. What is the effect of this drink on her overall energy balance and weight loss?

Problem 7.2: Do people lose weight as they grow older?

Figure 7.10 shows the mean BMI of people of different ages in the United Kingdom in 1993 and 2003. It suggests that people over the age of 55 lose weight as they age. Is this so?

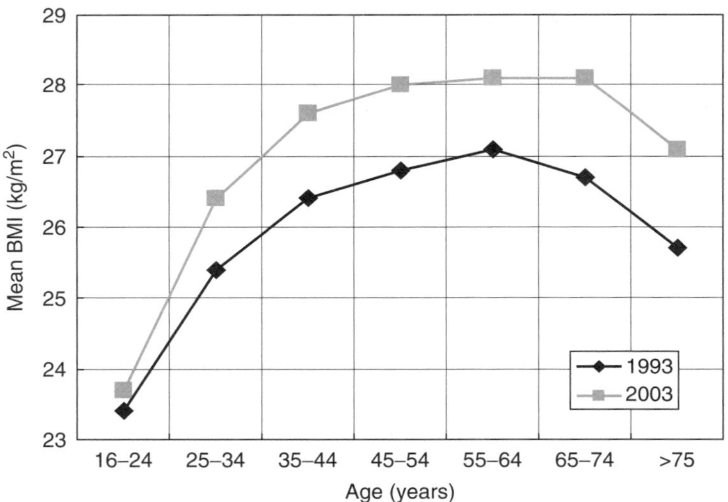

Figure 7.10 Mean body mass index at different ages. (From UK Department of Health data.)

Table 7.4 Alcohol Consumption and Body Mass Index

Alcohol Consumption (g/day)	Body Mass Index (kg/m²)	Total Energy Intake (kJ/day)	Nonalcohol Energy Intake (kJ/day)
0	26.8	6276	6276
0–5	25.1	–	–
5–15	23.4	–	–
15–25	23.0	–	–
25–50	22.8	7036	5938

Source: Data reported by Colditz, G.A. et al., *Am. J. Clin. Nutr.*, 54, 49–55, 1991.

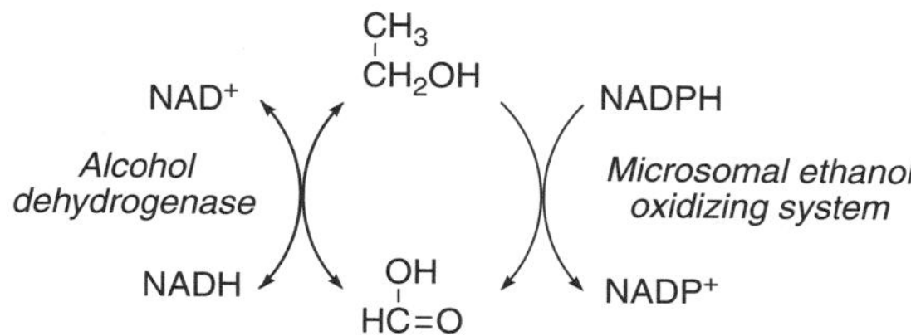

Figure 7.11 The oxidation of ethanol (see also Figure 2.21).

Problem 7.3: The case of the "missing calories"

Table 7.4 shows the results of a study of food and alcohol intake and BMI in 89,538 women—a part of the Nurses' Health Study.

The energy yield of alcohol is 29 kJ/g. What appears to be the relationship between BMI, energy intake, and alcohol consumption? What explanations can you offer for these observations?

Figures 7.11 and 2.21 show the two possible pathways of alcohol metabolism.

chapter eight

Protein-energy malnutrition—problems of undernutrition

If the intake of metabolic fuels is lower than is required to meet energy expenditure, the body's reserves of fat, carbohydrate (glycogen), and protein are used. Undernutrition may develop because of either inadequate food intake (due to lack of food or pathological disorders of appetite) or increased metabolic rate as a result of cancer and other chronic diseases. Especially in lean people, who have small reserves of body fat, there can be a large loss of tissue protein (to provide substrates for gluconeogenesis) when food intake is inadequate. As the deficiency continues, there is increasing loss of tissue, until eventually essential tissue proteins are catabolized as metabolic fuels—a process that obviously cannot continue for long.

Objectives

After reading this chapter, you should be able to

- Explain what is meant by protein-energy malnutrition and differentiate between marasmus and kwashiorkor
- Explain why marasmus can be considered to be the predictable outcome of prolonged negative energy balance
- Describe the groups of people in developed countries who are at risk of protein-energy malnutrition
- Describe the features of cachexia and explain how it differs from marasmus
- Describe the features of kwashiorkor and explain how it differs from marasmus

8.1 Problems of deficiency

Humans have evolved in a hostile environment in which food has always been scarce. Only in the past half century has there been a surplus of food, and in much of sub-Saharan Africa, food is still in short supply. Indeed, although food available per head of population has increased in most countries, in many sub-Saharan African countries it has decreased over the past decade (see PowerPoint presentation 8 on the CD). Figure 8.1 shows the numbers of people who are so undernourished that they have a body mass index (BMI) < 17; while most of these people are in developing countries, a significant number of people in developed countries are also undernourished.

Despite the advances in food production during the latter part of the twentieth century, up to 210 million people are at risk from protein-energy malnutrition. More importantly, as shown in Figures 8.2 and 8.3, the world population will increase from the present 6.5 billion to 8 billion by 2021, and most of this increase will be in less developed countries. It is unlikely that food production can be increased to the same extent.

Deficiency of individual nutrients is also a major problem—the total amount of food may be adequate to satisfy hunger, but the quality of the diet is inadequate. Deficiencies of

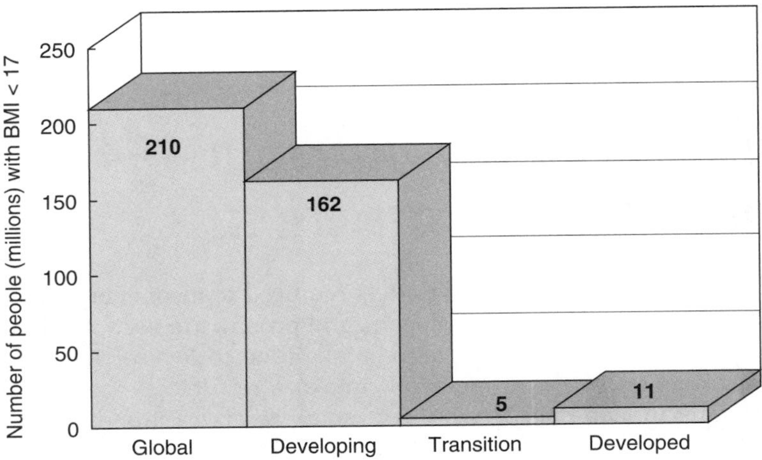

Figure 8.1 Number of people with BMI less than 17. (From United Nations Food and Agriculture Organization data.)

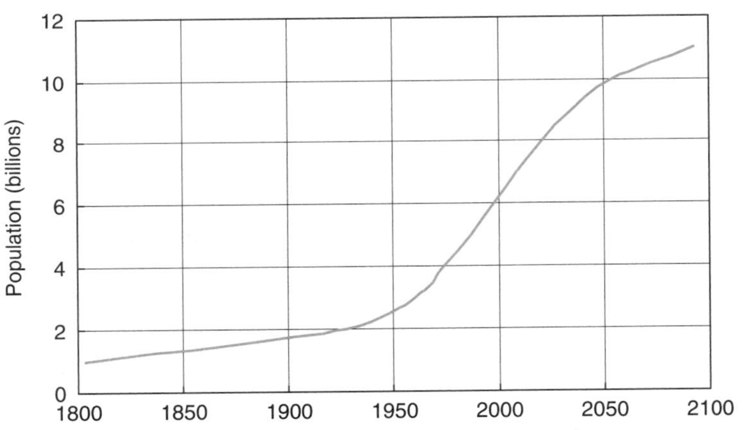

Figure 8.2 World population growth. (From World Health Organization data.)

vitamin A (Section 11.2.4), iron (Section 11.15.2.3), and iodine (Section 11.15.3.3) are major public health problems worldwide and are priority targets for the World Health Organization. Deficiency of vitamins B_1 (Section 11.6.3) and B_2 (Section 11.7.3) continues to be a problem in parts of Asia and Africa, and selenium deficiency (Section 11.15.2.5) is a significant problem in large regions of China, and elsewhere.

8.2 Protein-energy malnutrition

The terms *protein-energy malnutrition* and *protein-energy deficiency* are widely used to mean a general lack of food as opposed to specific deficiencies of vitamins or minerals (discussed in Chapter 11). The problem is not one of protein deficiency, but rather a deficiency of

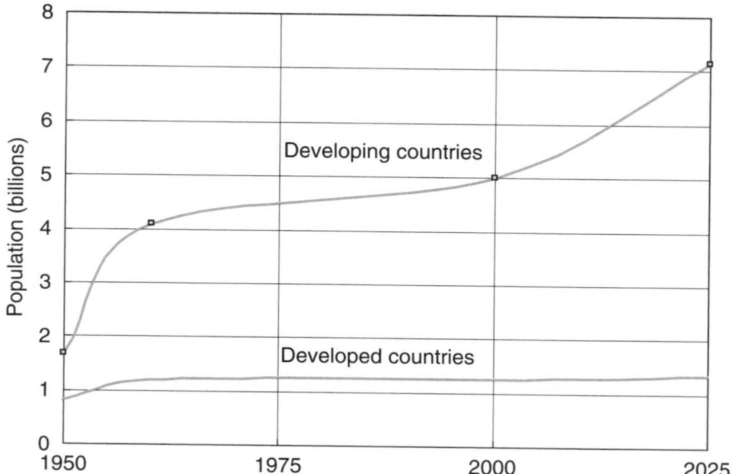

Figure 8.3 Population growth in developed and developing countries. (From World Health Organization data.)

Table 8.1 Classification of Protein-Energy Malnutrition by Body Mass Index

BMI	
20–25	Desirable range
18.5–20	Underweight but acceptable
17–18.4	Moderate protein-energy malnutrition
16–17	Moderately severe protein-energy malnutrition
<16	Severe protein-energy malnutrition

Note: BMI = weight (kg)/height^2 (m).

metabolic fuels. Indeed, there may be a relative excess of protein, in that protein that might be used for tissue protein replacement, or for growth in children, is being used as a fuel because of the deficiency of energy intake.

This was demonstrated in a series of studies in India in the early 1980s. Children whose intake of protein was marginally adequate were given additional carbohydrate (as sugary drinks). They showed an increase in growth and the deposition of new body protein. This was because their previous energy intake was inadequate; increasing their energy intake both spared dietary protein for the synthesis of tissue proteins and provided an adequate energy source to meet the high energy cost of protein synthesis (Section 9.2.3.3). The body's first requirement, at all times, is for an adequate source of metabolic fuels. Only when energy requirements have been met can dietary protein be used for tissue protein synthesis.

The severity of protein-energy malnutrition in adults can be assessed from the BMI (the ratio of weight [kg]/height^2 [m]; Section 7.1.1) as shown in Table 8.1.

There are two extreme forms of protein-energy malnutrition:

- *Marasmus* can occur in both adults and children, and occurs in vulnerable groups of the population in developed countries as well as in developing countries.

Table 8.2 Classification of Protein-Energy Malnutrition in Children

	No Edema	Edema
60%–80% of expected weight for age	Underweight	Kwashiorkor
<60% of expected weight for age	Marasmus	Marasmic kwashiorkor

- *Kwashiorkor* only affects children and has only been reported in developing countries. The distinguishing feature of kwashiorkor is that there is fluid retention, leading to edema.

Protein-energy malnutrition in children can be classified by the deficit in weight compared with what would be expected for age and also the presence or absence of edema, as shown in Table 8.2. The most severely affected group, and therefore the priority group for intervention, are those suffering from marasmic kwashiorkor—they are both severely undernourished and edematous.

8.3 Marasmus

Marasmus is a state of extreme emaciation; the name is derived from the Greek for wasting. It is the predictable outcome of prolonged negative energy balance with severe depletion of all body energy reserves.

Not only have fat reserves been exhausted, but there is wastage of muscle also, and as the condition progresses there is loss of protein from the heart, liver, and kidneys, although as far as possible essential tissue proteins are protected. Protein synthesis is energy expensive (Section 9.2.3.3), and in marasmus there is a considerable reduction in the rate of protein synthesis, although catabolism continues at the normal rate (Section 9.1.1). The amino acids released by the catabolism of tissue proteins are substrates for gluconeogenesis to maintain a supply of glucose for the brain and red blood cells (Section 5.7).

As a result of the reduced protein synthesis, there is a considerable impairment of immune responses, so that undernourished people are more at risk from infections than those who are adequately fed. Diseases that are minor childhood illnesses in developed countries can often prove fatal to undernourished children in developing countries. Measles is commonly cited as the cause of death, although it would be more correct to give the true cause of death as malnutrition.

One of the proteins secreted by the liver, which is most severely affected by protein-energy malnutrition, is the plasma-retinol-binding protein, which transports vitamin A from liver stores to its sites of action (Section 11.2.2.2). As a result, there are clinical signs of vitamin A deficiency; although there may be adequate reserves in the liver, they cannot be mobilized because of lack of the binding protein.

A more serious effect of protein-energy malnutrition is impairment of cell proliferation in the intestinal mucosa (Section 4.1). The villi are shorter than usual, and in severe cases the intestinal mucosa is almost flat. This results in a considerable reduction in the surface area of the intestinal mucosa, and hence a reduction in the absorption of such nutrients as are available from the diet. As a result, diarrhea is a common feature of protein-energy malnutrition. Thus, not only does the undernourished person have an inadequate intake of food, but the absorption of what is available is impaired, so compounding the problem.

Undernutrition also results in reduced muscle strength and increased fatigability, leading to inactivity and inability work, and may also predispose to falls. Reduced strength of the respiratory muscles predisposes to chest infections and impairs recovery from chest infections, as well as leading to a poor prognosis under general anesthesia. At the same time, inactivity predisposes to sores and thromboembolism, impaired thermogenesis leads to hypothermia, and reduced protein synthesis impairs wound healing. Even when not accompanied by physical illness, undernutrition causes apathy, depression, self-neglect, hypochondriasis, loss of libido, and deterioration in social interactions.

8.3.1 Causes of marasmus and vulnerable groups of the population

In developing countries, the cause of marasmus is either a chronic shortage of food or the more acute problem of famine, where there will be very little food available at all. All too frequently, famine comes after a long-term shortage of food, so its effects are all the more rapid and serious.

A lack of food is unlikely to be a problem in developed countries, although the most socially and economically disadvantaged in the community are at risk. In Britain, 2% of adults have a BMI < 18.5, and one survey showed that 40% of consecutive hospital admissions were at least mildly undernourished.

Two further factors may cause undernutrition: disorders of appetite and impairment of the absorption of nutrients.

8.3.1.1 Disorders of appetite: anorexia nervosa and bulimia

While obesity is a major public health problem (Section 7.2.2), one effect of the publicity about obesity is to put pressure on people to reduce their body weight, even if they are within the acceptable and healthy weight range. In some cases, the pressure for slimness may be a factor in the development of anorexia nervosa, bulimia, and other eating disorders, although the evidence suggests that media and peer pressure activates the desire for thinness in people who are vulnerable because of low self-esteem and dissatisfaction with their body image, but does not cultivate it otherwise. The group most at risk is adolescent girls; at any time some 25% are dieting to lose weight, whether they need to or not, and 50% think they are too fat. Similar disturbances of eating behavior can occur in older women, and (more rarely) in adolescent boys and men. One cause of the problem in adolescent girls is a reaction to the physical changes of puberty. By refusing food, the girl believes that she can delay or prevent these changes. To a considerable extent this is so. Breast development slows down or ceases as the energy balance becomes more negative. When body weight falls below about 45 kg, menstruation ceases, because of the lower secretion of leptin from the reduced amount of adipose tissue (Section 1.3.2).

The main feature of anorexia nervosa is a refusal to eat—with the obvious result of very considerable weight loss. Despite all evidence and arguments to the contrary, the anorectic subject is convinced that she is overweight and restricts her eating very severely. Dieting becomes the primary focus of her life. She has a preoccupation with, and often a considerable knowledge of, food, and frequently has a variety of stylized compulsive behavior patterns associated with food. As a part of her pathological obsession with thinness, the anorectic subject frequently takes a great deal of strenuous exercise, often exercising to exhaustion in solitude. She will go to extreme lengths to avoid eating, and frequently when forced to eat will induce vomiting soon afterward. Many anorectics also make excessive use of laxatives.

Surprisingly, many anorectic people are adept at hiding their condition, and it is not unknown for the problem to remain unnoticed even in a family setting. Food is played with, but little or none is actually eaten; excuses are frequently made to leave the table in the middle of the meal, perhaps on the pretext of going into the kitchen to prepare the next course.

Some anorectic subjects also exhibit a further disturbance of eating behavior—bulimia or binge eating. After a period of eating very little, they suddenly eat an extremely large amount of food (40 MJ or more in a single meal, compared with an average daily requirement of 8–12 MJ), frequently followed by deliberate induction of vomiting and heavy doses of laxatives. This is followed by a further prolonged period of anorexia.

Bulimia also occurs in the absence of anorexia nervosa—a person of normal weight will consume a very large amount of food (commonly 40–80 MJ over a period of a few hours), again followed by induction of vomiting and excessive use of laxatives. In severe cases, such binges may occur five or six times a week.

It is estimated that about 2% of adolescent girls go through at least a short phase of anorexia, and another 3% have a borderline eating disorder. In most cases, anorexia is self-limiting, and normal eating patterns are reestablished as the emotional crises of adolescence resolve. Other people may require specialist counseling and treatment, and in an unfortunate few problems of eating behavior persist into adult life.

8.3.1.2 *Malabsorption*

Any clinical condition that impairs the absorption of nutrients from the intestinal tract will lead to undernutrition, despite an apparently adequate intake. Obviously, major intestinal surgery will result in a reduction in the amount of intestine available for the digestion and absorption of nutrients. Here the problem is known in advance, and precautionary measures can be taken: a period of intravenous feeding, to supplement normal food intake, and careful counseling by a dietitian, so as to ensure adequate nutrient intake despite the problems.

A variety of infectious diseases can cause malabsorption and diarrhea. In many cases, this lasts only a few days and so has no long-term consequences. However, some intestinal parasites can cause long-lasting diarrhea and damage to the intestinal mucosa, leading to malnutrition if the infection remains untreated for too long.

8.3.1.3 *Food intolerance and allergy*

The problem of disaccharide intolerance was discussed in Section 4.2.2.2. Food allergies, involving an immune response and the production of antibodies—as opposed to intolerance, which does not—result from the absorption of relatively large intact peptides derived from dietary proteins (Section 4.4.3.2). Allergic reactions to foods may include dermatitis, eczema and urticaria, asthma, allergic rhinitis, muscle pain, rheumatoid arthritis, and migraine, as well as effects on the gastrointestinal tract. In severe cases, exposure to a food can cause potentially fatal anaphylactic shock. These reactions are likely to impair the sufferer's appetite and may contribute to undernutrition. There can be serious damage to the intestinal mucosa, leading to severe malabsorption, and hence malnutrition despite an apparently adequate intake of food. Allergy to nut proteins (and especially peanuts) has become a common problem, and other common allergens include cow's milk, eggs, shellfish, strawberries, and kiwifruit; laws in many countries now require that potential allergens from a standard list that may be present in the food must be declared on the label.

In general, once the offending food has been identified, the patient's condition has stabilized and body weight has been restored, continuing treatment is relatively easy, although avoidance of some common foods may provide significant problems. It is the identification of the offending food that provides the greatest problem, and frequently calls for lengthy investigations, maintaining the patient on a very limited range of foods, then gradually introducing additional foods, until the offending item is identified.

Patients with food intolerances or allergies are generally extremely ill after they have eaten the offending food, and this may persist for several days. Even after the offending foods have been identified, and the patient's condition has been stabilized, there may be continuing problems of appetite and eating behavior.

Celiac disease is an allergy to one specific protein in wheat—the gliadin fraction of gluten. There is a gradient in the prevalence of celiac disease across Europe, with the lowest rates in the Middle East, where wheat was first introduced as a dietary staple, and the highest in Ireland, where wheat only became a major food in the late nineteenth century.

There is a considerable loss of intestinal mucosa and flattening of the intestinal villi, so that the appearance of the intestine is similar to that seen in marasmus. This reduction in the absorptive surface of the intestine leads to persistent fatty diarrhea (steatorrhea) and a failure to absorb nutrients. The result is undernutrition, and severe emaciation can occur in patients with untreated celiac disease. Once the diagnosis is established, and the immediate problems of undernutrition have been dealt with, treatment is by avoidance of all wheat- and rye-based products; oats are also sometimes a problem. In practice, this is less easy than it sounds—apart from the obvious foods, like bread and pasta, wheat flour is used in a great many food products. There is therefore a need for counseling from a dietitian, and careful reading of labels for lists of ingredients. A number of products have the symbol of the Celiac Society on the label, to show that they are known to be free from gluten, and therefore safe for patients to eat.

8.4 Cachexia

Patients with advanced cancer, HIV infection and AIDS, and a number of other chronic diseases, are frequently undernourished. Physically they show all the signs of marasmus, but there is considerably more loss of body protein than occurs in starvation. The condition is called cachexia from the Greek for "in a poor condition." A number of factors contribute to the problem:

- The patients are extremely sick and because of this appetite may be impaired.
- Many of the drugs used in chemotherapy can cause nausea, loss of appetite, and alteration of the senses of taste and smell (Section 1.3.3.1), so that foods that were appetizing are now unappetizing or even aversive.
- Chemotherapy and radiotherapy inhibit cell division, leading to reduced cell proliferation in the intestinal mucosa, villous atrophy, and malabsorption (Section 8.3.1.2).
- There is a considerable increase in basal metabolic rate, to the extent that patients are described as being hypermetabolic.
- A number of cytokines increase the rate of breakdown of tissue protein. This is a major difference from marasmus, in which protein synthesis is reduced, but catabolism is unaffected.

8.4.1 Hypermetabolism in cachexia

Many tumors metabolize glucose anaerobically to release lactate. This is then used for gluconeogenesis in the liver; there is a cost of 4 mol of ATP and 2 mol of GTP for each mole of glucose reformed from lactate (Figure 5.13), and hence there has to be an increased rate

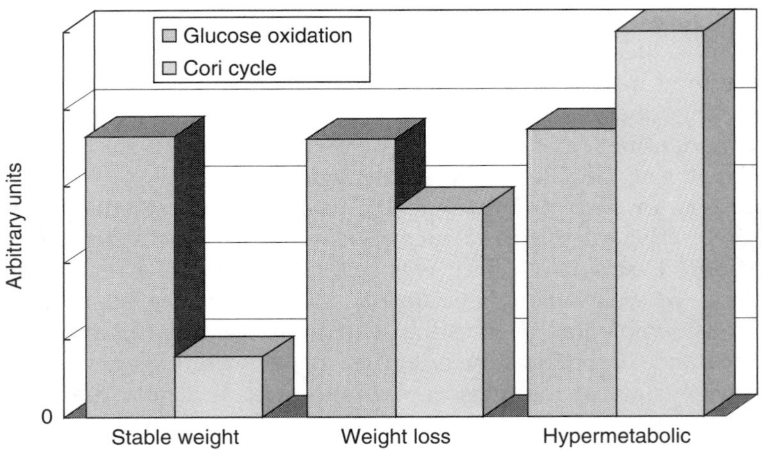

Figure 8.4 Glucose cycling in patients with cancer cachexia.

of metabolism in the liver to provide this ATP and GTP (see Problems 5.1 and 8.1). Figure 8.4 shows the increase in glucose cycling in patients with advanced cancer.

The cytokines secreted in response to many tumors and in inflammatory diseases stimulate mitochondrial uncoupling proteins (Section 3.3.1.4), leading to thermogenesis and hence increased oxidation of metabolic fuels. An increase in body temperature of 1°C is equivalent to a 13% increase in metabolic rate.

Hormone-sensitive lipase in adipose tissue (Section 10.5.1) is activated by a small proteoglycan produced by tumors that cause cachexia. This results in increased liberation of fatty acids from adipose tissue, with reesterification to triacylglycerols (which are exported in VLDL; Section 5.6.2.2) in the liver—futile cycling of lipids. The esterification of fatty acids requires 6 mol ofATP per mole of triacylglycerol formed (Section 5.6.1.2).

8.4.2 Increased protein catabolism in cachexia

As in marasmus, protein synthesis is impaired as a result of low availability of ATP. In addition, there is a considerable depletion of individual amino acids, resulting in an incomplete mixture of amino acids available for protein synthesis (Section 9.1.2.2), for three main reasons:

- Many tumors have a high requirement for glutamine and leucine.
- There is increased utilization of alanine and other amino acids as a result of the stimulation of gluconeogenesis by tumor necrosis factor.
- Interferon-γ induces indoleamine dioxygenase and depletes tissue pools of tryptophan.

Unlike marasmus, cachexia is characterized by an increase in the rate of protein catabolism as well as reduced synthesis. Tumor necrosis factor causes increased protein catabolism by increasing both the expression of ubiquitin and the activity of the ubiquitin-dependent protease (section 9.1.1.1). The proteoglycan produced by tumors that cause cachexia also stimulates protein catabolism; in this case the mechanism is unknown.

8.5 Kwashiorkor

Kwashiorkor was first described in Ghana, West Africa, in 1932—the word is the Ga name for the condition. In addition to the wasting of muscle tissue, loss of intestinal mucosa (leading to diarrhea), and impaired immune responses seen in marasmus, children with kwashiorkor show a number of characteristic features that distinguish this disease:

- Fluid retention and hence severe edema, associated with a decreased concentration of plasma proteins. The puffiness of the limbs, due to the edema, masks the severe wasting of muscles.
- Enlargement of the liver due to the accumulation of abnormally large amounts of fat in the liver, to the extent that instead of its normal reddish-brown color, the liver is pale yellow when examined postmortem or during surgery. The metabolic basis for this fatty infiltration of the liver is not known. It is the enlargement of the liver which causes the paradoxical "pot-bellied" appearance of children with kwashiorkor; together with the edema, they appear, from a distance, to be plump, yet they are starving.
- Characteristic changes in the texture and color of the hair. This is most noticeable in African children—instead of tightly curled black hair, children with kwashiorkor have sparse, wispy hair, which is less curled than normal, and poorly pigmented—it is often reddish or even grey.
- A sooty, sunburn-like skin rash.
- A characteristic expression of deep misery.

8.5.1 Factors in the etiology of kwashiorkor

The underlying cause of kwashiorkor is an inadequate intake of food, as is the case for marasmus. Kwashiorkor traditionally affects children aged between 3 and 5. In many societies a child continues to suckle until about this age, when the next child is born. As a result, the toddler is abruptly weaned, frequently onto very unsuitable food. In some societies, children are weaned onto a dilute gruel made from whatever is the local cereal; in others the child may be fed on the water in which rice has been boiled—it may look like milk, but has little nutritional value. Sometimes the child is given little or no special treatment, but has to compete with the rest of the family for its share from the stewpot. A small child has little chance of getting an adequate meal under such conditions, especially if there is anyway not much food for the whole family.

There is no satisfactory explanation for the development of kwashiorkor rather than marasmus. At one time it was believed that it was due to a lack of protein, with a more or less adequate intake of energy. However, analysis of the diets of children suffering from kwashiorkor shows that this is not so. Furthermore, children who are protein deficient have a slower rate of growth and are therefore stunted (Section 9.1.2.1); as shown in Figure 8.5, children with kwashiorkor are less stunted than those with marasmus. Finally, many of the signs of kwashiorkor, and especially the edema, begin to improve early in treatment, when the child is still receiving a low-protein diet (Section 8.5.2).

Very commonly, an infection precipitates kwashiorkor in children whose nutritional status is inadequate, even if they are not yet showing signs of malnutrition. Indeed, pediatricians in developing countries expect an outbreak of kwashiorkor a few months after an outbreak of measles.

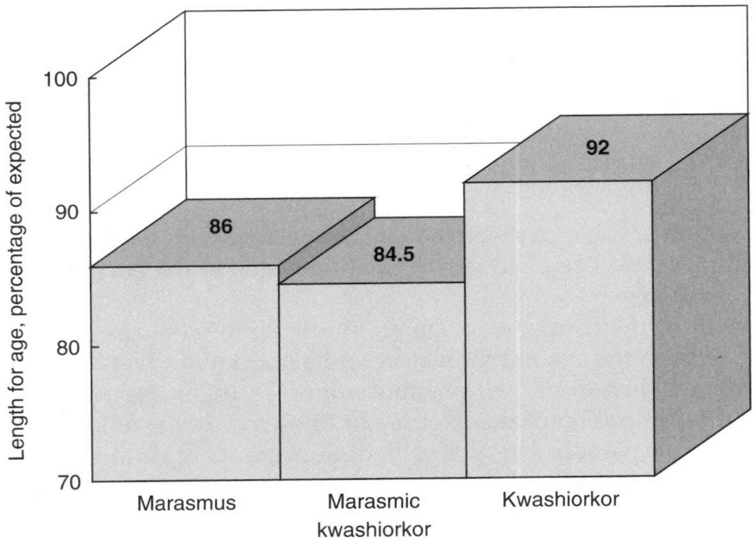

Figure 8.5 Stunting of growth in kwashiorkor, marasmus, and marasmic kwashiorkor.

The most likely precipitating factor is that superimposed on general food deficiency, there is a deficiency of the antioxidant nutrients such as zinc, copper, carotene, and vitamins C and E (Section 6.5.3). The respiratory burst in response to infection leads to the production of oxygen and halogen radicals as part of the cytotoxic action of stimulated macrophages (Section 6.5.2.2). The added oxidant stress of an infection may well trigger the sequence of events that leads to the development of kwashiorkor.

8.5.2 Rehabilitation of malnourished children

The intestinal tract of the malnourished child is in a very poor state. This means that the child is not able to deal at all adequately with a rich diet or a large amount of food. Rather, treatment begins with small frequent feeding of liquids—a dilute sugar solution for the first few days, followed by diluted milk, and then full strength milk. This may be achieved by use of a nasogastric tube, so that the dilute solution can be provided at a slow and constant rate throughout the day and night. Where such luxuries are not available, the malnourished infant is fed from a teaspoon, a few drops at a time, more or less continually.

Once the patient has begun to develop a more normal intestinal mucosa (when the diarrhea ceases), ordinary foods can gradually be introduced. Recovery is normally rapid in children, and they soon begin to grow at a normal rate.

Key points

- Although food available per head of population has increased in most countries (apart from sub-Saharan Africa), undernutrition remains a problem, and predicted population growth is unlikely to be matched by further increases in food production.
- Protein-energy malnutrition is a lack of total food, and not specifically of protein.
- Marasmus is the predictable outcome of prolonged energy depletion: loss of adipose tissue reserves and wasting of muscle as a result of decreased protein synthesis.

- Cachexia in chronic diseases resembles marasmus, but in addition there is hypermetabolism and increased protein catabolism.
- Kwashiorkor involves edema as well as wasting; the trigger to develop kwashiorkor in an undernourished child is probably radical damage, superimposed on general undernutrition.

Problem 8.1: Arthur N

Arthur is a 75-year-old man, 170 cm tall, and weighs 50 kg. He has advanced cancer and has lost 2 kg of body weight over the past 4 weeks.

What is his BMI? Is it within the desirable range?

His mean skinfold thickness is 1.9 mm, suggesting that he has negligible reserves of adipose tissue, and he shows considerable wasting of muscle, so we can assume that most of his weight loss is muscle. The composition of muscle is 79% water, 17% protein (at 17 kJ/gm), and 3% fat (at 37 kJ/gm).

What was his overall energy deficit over the past 4 weeks (total energy deficit and average per day)?

For his age and body weight, BMR would be expected to be between 4.7 and 4.9 MJ/day. His BMR was determined by measuring oxygen consumption with a respirometer; regardless of the fuel being oxidized, 1 L of oxygen is equivalent to 20 kJ. His oxygen consumption was 11.2 L/h. What is his BMR (in MJ/day)?

Assuming the mean BMR for his age and weight is 4.8 MJ/day, what is his daily energy deficit now?

How much intravenous glucose would be required daily to restore energy balance and prevent further weight loss (energy yield of glucose × 16 kJ/g)?

What volume of 5% glucose would be required?

Problem 8.2: David Blaine

In autumn 2003, David Blaine survived for 44 days without food, suspended in a Perspex box above Tower Bridge in London. If we had been able to perform some experiments, we could have observed his metabolic adaptation to starvation.

His oxygen consumption was measured at the beginning and end of the 44 days. From the following data, calculate his energy expenditure (effectively his resting metabolic rate, since he was not particularly active):

Day 1	18.0 L oxygen/h
Day 44	14.5 L oxygen/h

Why did his metabolic rate change over 44 days?

He ate no food at all; what was his total energy deficit over 44 days?

Adipose tissue is 80% triacylglycerol, 5% protein, 15% water. What is the energy yield of 1 kg of adipose tissue?

Assuming that he lost *only* adipose tissue, what was his expected weight loss over 44 days?

Why is it not correct to assume that he lost only adipose tissue?

What metabolic fuels were available for tissue metabolism, and what were their sources during the first 1–2 days of the fast?

What metabolic fuels were available for tissue metabolism, and what were their sources after 5–6 days of the fast?

His urinary excretion of urea was measured during the fast:

Day 1	112 mmol/24 h
Day 10	142 mmol/24 h
Day 43	117 mmol/24 h

Why did his excretion of urea increase, then fall again?

chapter nine

Protein nutrition and metabolism

The need for protein in the diet was demonstrated early in the nineteenth century when it was shown that animals fed only on fats, carbohydrates, and mineral salts were unable to maintain their body weight and showed severe wasting of muscle and other tissues. It was known that proteins contain nitrogen (mainly in the amino groups of their constituent amino acids; Section 4.4.1), and methods for measuring the total amount of nitrogenous compounds in foods and excreta were soon developed.

Objectives

After reading this chapter, you should be able to

- Explain what is meant by the terms nitrogen balance and dynamic equilibrium
- Describe the processes involved in tissue protein catabolism
- Explain the basis for current recommendations for protein intake and for essential and nonessential amino acids
- Explain what is meant by protein nutritional value or quality and why it is of little importance in most diets
- Describe the processes involved in protein synthesis, outline the flow of information from DNA → RNA → protein, and explain the energy cost of protein synthesis
- Describe and explain the pathways by which the amino nitrogen of amino acids is metabolized and explain the importance of transamination
- Describe and explain the metabolism of ammonia and the synthesis of urea
- Describe the metabolic fates of the carbon skeletons of amino acids

9.1 Nitrogen balance and protein requirements

Figure 9.1 shows an overview of protein metabolism; in addition to the dietary intake of about 80 g of protein, almost the same amount of endogenous protein is secreted into the intestinal lumen. There is a small fecal loss equivalent to about 10 g of protein per day; the remainder is hydrolyzed to free amino acids and small peptides that are absorbed (Section 4.4.3). The fecal loss of nitrogen is partly composed of undigested dietary protein but the main contributors are intestinal bacteria and shed mucosal cells, which are only partially broken down, and the protective mucus secreted by intestinal mucosal goblet cells (Figure 4.2). Mucus is especially resistant to enzymic hydrolysis and contributes a considerable proportion of inevitable losses of nitrogen, even on a protein-free diet.

There is a small pool of free amino acids in the body in equilibrium with proteins that are being catabolized and synthesized. A small proportion of this amino acid pool is used for synthesis of a variety of specialized metabolites (including hormones and neurotransmitters, purines, and pyrimidines). An amount of amino acids equivalent to that absorbed is oxidized, with the carbon skeletons being used for gluconeogenesis

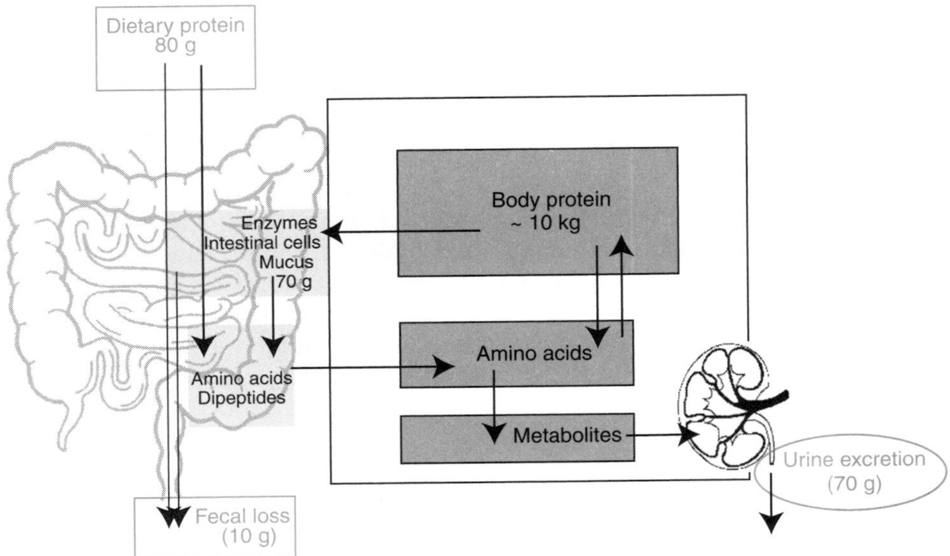

Figure 9.1 An overview of protein metabolism.

(Sections 9.3.2 and 5.7) or as metabolic fuels, and the nitrogen being excreted mainly as urea (Section 9.3.1.4).

The state of protein nutrition, and the overall state of body protein metabolism, can be determined by measuring the dietary intake of nitrogenous compounds and the output of nitrogenous compounds from the body. Although nucleic acids contain nitrogen (Section 9.2.1), protein is the major dietary source of nitrogenous compounds and measurement of total nitrogen intake gives a good estimate of protein intake. Nitrogen constitutes 16% of most proteins and therefore the protein content of foods is calculated on the basis of milligrams of nitrogen times 6.25, although for some foods with an unusual amino acid composition other factors are used.

The output of nitrogen from the body is largely in the urine and feces, but significant amounts may also be lost in sweat and shed skin cells and in longer-term studies the growth of hair and nails must be taken into account. Obviously, any loss of blood or tissue will involve a loss of protein. While the intake of nitrogenous compounds is mainly as protein, the output is mainly as urea (Section 9.3.1.4), with a number of other products of amino acid metabolism as shown in Table 9.1.

The difference between intake and output of nitrogenous compounds is known as nitrogen balance. Three states can be defined:

- An adult in good health and with an adequate intake of protein excretes the same amount of nitrogen each day as is taken in from the diet (with minor fluctuations from day to day). This is nitrogen balance or nitrogen equilibrium: intake = output, and there is no change in the total body content of protein.
- In a growing child, a pregnant woman, or someone recovering from protein loss, the excretion of nitrogenous compounds is less than the dietary intake—there is a net retention of nitrogen in the body. This is positive nitrogen balance: intake > output, and there is a gain in total body protein.

Table 9.1 Average Daily Excretion of Nitrogenous Compounds in Urine

Urea	10–35 g	150–600 mol	Depends on the intake of protein
Ammonium	340–1200 mg	20–70 mmol	Depends on the state of acid–base balance
Amino acids, peptides, and conjugates	1.3–3.2 g	–	
Protein	<60 mg	–	Significant proteinuria indicates kidney damage
Uric acid	250–750 mg	1.5–4.5 mmol	Major product of purine metabolism
Creatinine	1.8 g (Male) 1.2 g (Female)	16 mmol (Male) 10 mmol (Female)	Depends on muscle mass
Creatine	<50 mg	<400 mmol	Higher levels indicate muscle catabolism

- In response to trauma or infection (Section 9.1.2.2), or if the intake of protein is inadequate to meet requirements, the excretion of nitrogenous compounds is greater than the intake—there is a net loss of nitrogen from the body. This is negative nitrogen balance: intake < output, and there is a loss of body protein.

9.1.1 Dynamic equilibrium

The proteins in the body are continually being broken down and replaced; this is dynamic equilibrium. As shown in Table 9.2, some proteins (especially enzymes that have a role in controlling metabolic pathways) turn over with a half-life of minutes or hours; others last days or weeks before they are broken down. Some proteins turn over only very slowly—for example, the connective tissue protein collagen has a half-life of almost a year.

There is normally no change in total body protein in an adult. Nevertheless, if an isotopically labeled amino acid is given, the process of turnover can be followed. As shown in Figure 9.2, the label rapidly becomes incorporated into newly synthesized proteins and is gradually lost as the proteins are broken down. The rate at which the label is lost from an individual protein depends on the rate at which that protein is broken down and replaced; the time for the labeling to fall to half its peak is the half-life of that protein.

Protein breakdown occurs at a more or less constant rate throughout the day, and an adult catabolizes and replaces some 3–6 g of protein per kilogram of body weight per day. Turnover is also important in growing children, who synthesize considerably more protein each day than their gain in total body protein. Children recovering from severe protein-energy malnutrition (Chapter 8) and increasing their body protein rapidly still synthesize 2–3 times more protein than the overall gain.

Although an adult may be in overall nitrogen balance, this is the average of periods of negative balance in the fasting state and positive balance in the fed state. Protein synthesis is energy expensive (Section 9.2.3.3), and in the fasting state the rate of synthesis is lower than that of catabolism. There is a loss of tissue protein, which provides amino acids for gluconeogenesis (Section 5.7). In the fed state, when there is an abundant supply of metabolic fuel, in response to stimulation by insulin, protein synthesis increases and exceeds breakdown, so that what is observed is an increase in tissue protein, replacing that which was lost in the fasting state.

Even in severe undernutrition the rate of protein breakdown remains more or less constant, while the rate of replacement synthesis falls, as a result of the low availability of metabolic

Table 9.2 Half-Lives of Some Proteins

Protein	Half-Life
Ornithine decarboxylase	11 min
Lipoprotein lipase	1 h
Tyrosine transaminase	1.5 h
Phosphoenolpyruvate carboxykinase	2 h
Tryptophan oxygenase	2 h
HMG CoA reductase	3 h
Glucokinase	12 h
Alanine transaminase	0.7–1 d
Serum albumin	3.5 d
Arginase	4–5 d
Lactate dehydrogenase	16 d
Adult collagen	300 d
Infant collagen	1–2 d and 150 d

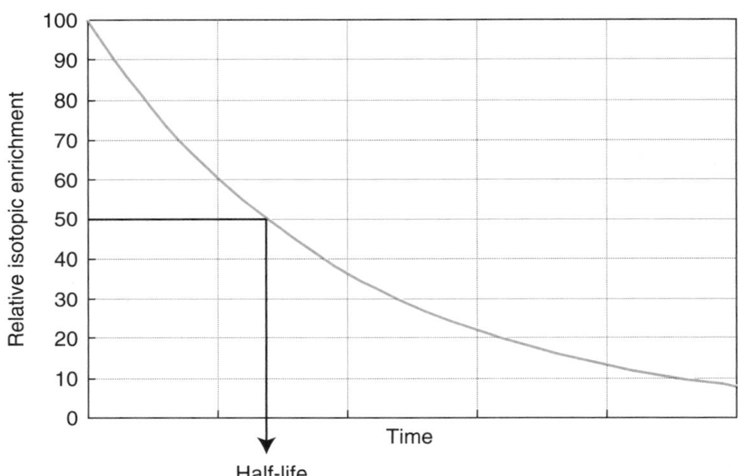

Figure 9.2 Determination of the half-life of body proteins using [^{15}N]amino acids.

fuels (Section 8.3). It is only in cachexia (Section 8.4.2) that there is increased protein catabolism as well as reduced replacement synthesis.

9.1.1.1 Mechanisms involved in tissue protein catabolism

The catabolism of tissue proteins is a highly regulated process; as shown in Table 9.1, different proteins are catabolized (and replaced) at very different rates. A number of proteins that contain the sequence Lys-Phe-Glu-Arg-Gly are targeted for lysosomal uptake and hydrolysis. Lysosomal cathepsins are proteases with a broad range of specificities, leading to complete hydrolysis of proteins to free amino acids. They also hydrolyze proteins in organisms that have entered the cell by phagocytosis and in subcellular organelles that have been engulfed by phagosomes, and are involved in the hydrolysis of cell proteins after cell death, when they are released into the cytosol.

The major system for targeted protein catabolism is the ubiquitin–proteasome system, which catalyzes ATP-dependent proteolysis. It also has roles in antigen processing and control of the cell cycle. Ubiquitin is a small peptide (M_r 8500), which is attached to target proteins by the ATP-dependent formation of a peptide bond from its carboxyl terminal to the ε-amino group of a lysine residue. Further molecules of ubiquitin are then attached by forming peptide bonds between the carboxyl terminal of one ubiquitin and the amino terminal of another, leading to polyubiquitination of the target protein. Polyubiquitinylated proteins are substrates for the proteasome (also known as the multifunctional protease). This is a multienzyme complex that accounts for about 1% of the total soluble protein of cells; different subunits have specificity for esters of different amino acids, leading to complete hydrolysis of the targeted protein.

The increased rate of protein catabolism seen in cachexia (Section 8.4.2) is the result of activation of the ubiquitin–proteasome system in response to cytokines, and studies with inhibitors of the system have shown some success in reducing protein catabolism in cachectic patients.

9.1.2 Protein requirements

It is the continual catabolism of tissue proteins that creates the requirement for dietary protein. Although some of the amino acids released by breakdown of tissue proteins can be reused, especially in the fasting state most are metabolized (Section 9.3), yielding carbon skeletons that can be used as metabolic fuels or for gluconeogenesis (Section 5.7) and urea (Section 9.3.1.4), which is excreted. This means that there is a need for dietary protein to replace metabolic losses, even in an adult who is not growing. In addition, protein is lost from the body in mucus, enzymes, and other proteins that are secreted into the gastrointestinal tract and are not completely digested and reabsorbed.

Current estimates of protein requirements are based on studies of the amount required to maintain nitrogen balance. If the intake is not adequate to replace the protein that has been broken down, then there is negative nitrogen balance—a greater output of nitrogen from the body than the dietary intake. Once the intake is adequate to meet requirements, nitrogen balance is restored. The proteins that have been broken down can be replaced and any surplus intake of protein can be used as a metabolic fuel. Intakes above requirement do not result in positive nitrogen balance except after a period of protein loss; nitrogen equilibrium is maintained with a higher level of output to match the higher intake.

Such studies show that for adults, the average daily requirement is 0.66 g of protein per kilogram of body weight. Allowing for individual variation, the reference intake (Section 11.1.1) is 0.8 g/kg body weight, or 56 g/day for a 70 kg adult. Average intakes of protein by adults in developed countries are considerably greater than requirements, of the order of 80–100 g/day. The reference intake of protein is sometimes called the safe level of intake, meaning that it is safe and (more than) adequate to meet requirements, not implying that there is any hazard from higher levels of intake, although there is some evidence that excessively high intakes of protein may be associated with chronic diseases.

Protein requirements can also be expressed as a proportion of energy intake. The energy yield of protein is 17 kJ/g and the reference intake of protein represents some 8%–9% of energy intake. In Western countries, protein provides about 14%–15% of energy intake.

It is unlikely that adults in most countries will suffer from protein deficiency if they are eating enough food to meet their energy requirements. As shown in Figure 9.3, the major dietary staples, which are generally considered as sources of carbohydrate, also provide significant amounts of protein. Even among people in Western countries who eat

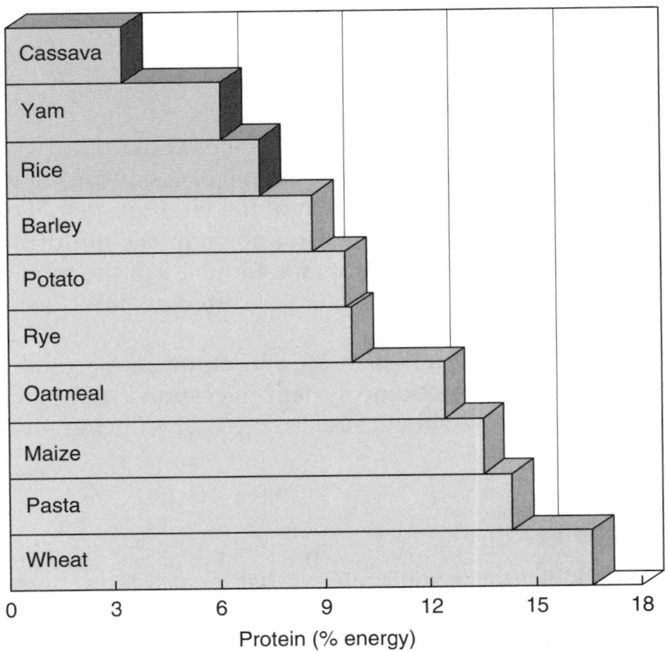

Figure 9.3 Protein as percentage of energy in dietary staples. Protein requirements of an adult are met when the diet provides 8%–9% of energy from protein. Of the major dietary staples, only cassava, yam, and (marginally) rice fail to provide this much protein.

meat, fish, and eggs (which are generally regarded as rich protein sources), about 25% of protein intake comes from cereals and cereal products, with an additional 10% from fruit and vegetables.

Only cassava, yam, and rice provide insufficient protein (as a percentage of energy) to meet adult requirements. The shortfall in protein provided by a diet based on yam or rice would be made up by small amounts of other foods that are sources of protein—this may be either small amounts of meat and fish or legumes and nuts, which are rich vegetable sources of protein. With diets based largely on cassava, there is a more serious problem in meeting protein requirements.

9.1.2.1 Protein requirements of children

Because children are growing and increasing the total amount of protein in the body, they have a proportionally greater requirement than adults. A growing child should be in positive nitrogen balance. However, the need for protein for growth is relatively small compared with the requirement for protein turnover. Table 9.3 shows protein requirements at different ages. Children in Western countries consume more protein than is needed to meet their requirements, but in developing countries protein intake may well be inadequate to meet the requirement for growth.

A protein-deficient child will grow more slowly than one receiving an adequate intake of protein—this is stunting of growth. The protein-energy deficiency diseases—marasmus and kwashiorkor (Section 8.3)—result from a general lack of food (and hence metabolic fuels) and not a specific deficiency of protein.

Table 9.3 Reference Intakes of Protein

Age (years)	Average Requirement	Reference Intake g/day
0–0.5	–	9.1
0.5–1.0	9	11
1–3	11	13
4–8	15	19
Males		
9–13	27	34
14–18	44	52
19–30	46	56
>31	46	56
Females		
9–13	28	34
14–18	38	46
19–30	38	46
>31	38	46
Pregnancy	50	71
Lactation	60	71

Source: Standing Committee on the Scientific Evaluation of Dietary Reference Intakes, Food and Nutrition Board, Institute of Medicine in *Dietary Reference Intakes for Energy, Carbohydrate, Fiber, Fat, Fatty Acids, Cholesterol, Protein and Amino Acids*, National Academy Press, Washington, DC, 2002.

9.1.2.2 Protein losses in trauma and infection—requirements for convalescence

One of the metabolic reactions to a major trauma, such as a burn, a broken limb, or surgery, is an increase in the net catabolism of tissue proteins. As shown in Table 9.4, apart from the loss of blood associated with injury, as much as 750 g of protein (about 6%–7% of the total body content) may be lost over 10 days. Even prolonged bed rest results in a considerable loss of protein, because there is atrophy of muscles that are not used. Muscle protein is catabolized as normal, but without the stimulus of exercise less is replaced.

This protein loss is mediated by the hormone cortisol, which is secreted in response to stress, and the cytokines that are secreted in response to trauma. Four mechanisms are involved:

- Induction of tryptophan dioxygenase (Section 11.8.2) and tyrosine transaminase by cortisol. This results in depletion of the tissue pools of these two amino acids, leaving an unbalanced mixture that cannot be used for protein synthesis (Section 9.2.3).
- In response to cytokine action there is an increase in metabolic rate, leading to an increased rate of oxidation of amino acids as metabolic fuel, thus reducing the amount available for protein synthesis.
- Some cytokines cause an increase in the rate of protein catabolism as occurs in cachexia (Section 8.4.2).
- A variety of plasma proteins synthesized in increased amounts in response to cytokine action (the acute phase proteins) are richer in two amino acids, cysteine and threonine, than most tissue proteins. This leads to depletion of tissue pools of these two amino acids, again leaving an unbalanced mixture that cannot be used for protein synthesis.

Table 9.4 Protein Losses over 10 Days after Trauma or Infection

	Tissue Loss	Blood Loss	Catabolism	Total
Fracture of femur	–	200	700	900
Muscle wound	500–750	150–400	750	1350–1900
35% burns	500	150–400	750	1400–1650
Gastrectomy	20–180	20–10	625–750	645–850
Typhoid fever	–	–	675	685

Source: Cuthbertson, D.P., in *Human Protein Metabolism* (Vol. II), Academic Press, New York, 1964, 373–414.

The lost protein has to be replaced during recovery, and patients who are convalescing will be in positive nitrogen balance. However, this does not mean that a convalescent patient requires a diet that is richer in protein than usual. As discussed in Section 9.1.2, average protein intakes are twice requirements; a normal diet will provide adequate protein to permit replacement of the losses due to illness and hospitalization.

9.1.3 Essential amino acids

Early studies of nitrogen balance showed that not all proteins are nutritionally equivalent. More of some than others is needed to maintain nitrogen balance. This is because different proteins contain different amounts of the various amino acids (Section 4.4.1). The body's requirement is not simply for protein but for the amino acids that make up proteins in the correct proportions to replace the body proteins.

There are nine essential or indispensable amino acids, which cannot be synthesized in the body (Table 9.5). If one of these is provided in inadequate amounts, then regardless of the total intake of protein, it will not be possible to maintain nitrogen balance since there will not be enough of this limiting amino acid for protein synthesis to replace all losses from turnover.

For infants, a tenth amino acid, arginine, is essential. Although adults can synthesize adequate amounts of arginine to meet their requirements, the capacity for arginine synthesis is low in infants and may not be adequate to meet the requirements for growth. Because the pathway of arginine synthesis is also the pathway for synthesis of urea for excretion of excess nitrogen (Section 9.3.1.4), infants are susceptible to hyperammonemia if fed an excessively high protein intake.

Two amino acids, cysteine and tyrosine, can only be synthesized in the body from essential precursors—cysteine from methionine and tyrosine from phenylalanine. The dietary intakes of cysteine and tyrosine thus affect the requirements for methionine and phenylalanine; if more of either is provided in the diet, then less will have to be synthesized from the essential precursor.

The remaining amino acids are considered nonessential or dispensable; they can be synthesized from metabolic intermediates as long as there is enough total protein in the diet. If one of these amino acids is omitted from the diet, nitrogen balance can still be maintained. Only three amino acids, alanine, aspartate, and glutamate, can be considered to be truly dispensable; they are synthesized from common metabolic intermediates (pyruvate, oxaloacetate, and α-ketoglutarate, respectively; Section 9.3.1.2). The remaining amino acids are generally considered to be nonessential, but under some circumstances the requirement may outstrip the capacity for synthesis:

- A high intake of compounds that are excreted as glycine conjugates will increase the requirement for glycine considerably.

Table 9.5 Essential and Nonessential Amino Acids

Essential	Essential Precursor	Nonessential	Semiessential
Histidine		Alanine	Arginine
Isoleucine		Aspartate	Asparagine
Leucine		Glutamate	Glutamine
Lysine			Glycine
Methionine	Cysteine		Proline
Phenylalanine	Tyrosine		Serine
Threonine			
Tryptophan			
Valine			

- In response to severe trauma, there is an increased requirement for proline for collagen synthesis for healing.
- In surgical trauma and sepsis, the requirement for glutamine increases. A number of studies have shown improved healing after major surgery if additional glutamine is provided.

Early studies of essential amino acid requirements were based on the amounts required to maintain nitrogen balance in young adults. Interestingly, for reasons that are not clear, these relatively short-term studies did not show a requirement for histidine. More recent studies have measured the rate of whole-body protein turnover using isotopically labeled amino acids. These show that the maximum rate of protein turnover is achieved with intakes of the essential amino acids some threefold higher than required to maintain nitrogen balance. What is not clear is whether the maximum rate of protein turnover is essential or even desirable.

Other studies have estimated essential amino acid requirements by measuring the oxidation (and hence irreversible loss) of isotopically labeled amino acids. These again suggest higher requirements than those derived from studies of nitrogen balance. However, because stable isotopes are used, the experiments involve administration of a relatively large amount of a single amino acid, which may well distort normal metabolic pools, so that there is an excess of the test amino acid to be catabolized.

9.1.3.1 Protein quality and complementation

A protein that contains at least as much of each of the essential amino acids as is required will be completely useable for tissue protein synthesis, while one that is relatively deficient in one or more of the essential amino acids will not. More of the latter will be required to maintain nitrogen balance or growth.

The limiting amino acid of a protein is the essential amino acid that is present in the lowest amount relative to the requirement. In animal and most vegetable proteins, the limiting amino acid is methionine (correctly, the sum of methionine plus cysteine, because cysteine is synthesized from methionine and providing adequate cysteine reduces the requirement for methionine). In cereal proteins, the limiting amino acid is lysine.

The nutritional value or quality of individual proteins depends on whether or not they contain the essential amino acids in the amounts that are required. A number of different ways of determining protein quality have been developed:

- Biological value (BV) is the proportion of absorbed protein that is retained in the body. A protein that is completely useable (e.g., egg and human milk) has a BV of 0.9–1; meat and fish, 0.75–0.8; wheat protein, 0.5; and gelatin (which completely lacks tryptophan), 0.

- Net protein utilization (NPU) is the proportion of dietary protein that is retained in the body (i.e., it takes account of the digestibility of the protein). By convention it is measured at 10% dietary protein, at which level the experimental animal can utilize all of the protein as long as the balance of essential amino acids is correct.
- Protein efficiency ratio (PER) is the gain in weight of growing animals per gram of protein eaten.
- Relative protein value (RPV) is the ability of a test protein, fed at various levels of intake, to support nitrogen balance compared with a standard protein.
- Chemical score is based on chemical analysis of the amino acids present in the protein; it is the amount of the limiting amino acid compared with the amount of the same amino acid in egg protein (which is completely useable for tissue protein synthesis).
- Protein score (or amino acid score) is again based on chemical analysis but uses a reference pattern of amino acid requirements as the standard. This provides the basis for the legally required way of expressing protein quality in North America—the protein digestibility corrected amino acid score (PDCAAS).

While protein quality is important when considering individual foods, it is not relevant when considering total diets because different proteins are limited by different amino acids and hence have a relative excess of others. The result of mixing different proteins in a diet is an unexpected increase in the nutritional value of the mixture. Wheat protein is limited by lysine and has a protein score of 0.6, while pea protein is limited by methionine and cysteine and has a protein score of 0.4. A mixture of equal amounts of these two individually poor-quality proteins has a protein score of 0.82—as high as that of meat.

The result of this complementation between proteins that are individually of low quality is that most diets have very nearly the same protein quality, regardless of the protein quality of individual foods. The average Western diet has a protein score of 0.73, while the poorest diets in developing countries—with a restricted range of foods and very little milk, meat, or fish—have a protein score of 0.6.

9.1.3.2 Unavailable amino acids and protein digestibility

Chemical analysis of the amino acid content of proteins overestimates their nutritional value because not all the amino acids are released by digestive enzymes (Section 4.4.3) and hence available for absorption. The most important problems arise with lysine, which can form peptide bonds from its ε-amino group to side chain carboxyl groups of aspartate and glutamate (Figure 4.21). These bonds are hydrolyzed by strong acid used in chemical analysis but are not substrates for human digestive enzymes, so that the lysine is not available for absorption. At the same time, the presence of these cross-links inhibits the intestinal proteases, so that several amino acids on either side of the cross-link are also not liberated.

The ε-amino group of lysine can also react nonenzymically with glucose and other carbohydrates, again rendering the amino acid unavailable for absorption. In foods, this is the basis of the nonenzymic browning reaction (Maillard reaction) that gives many cooked foods their characteristic flavor. A similar reaction occurs *in vivo* in poorly controlled diabetes mellitus, and glycation of proteins underlies many of the problems associated with poor glycemic control (Section 10.7.1).

9.2 Protein synthesis

The information for the amino acid sequence of each of the 30,000–40,000 different proteins in the body is contained in the DNA in the nucleus of each cell. As required, a working copy

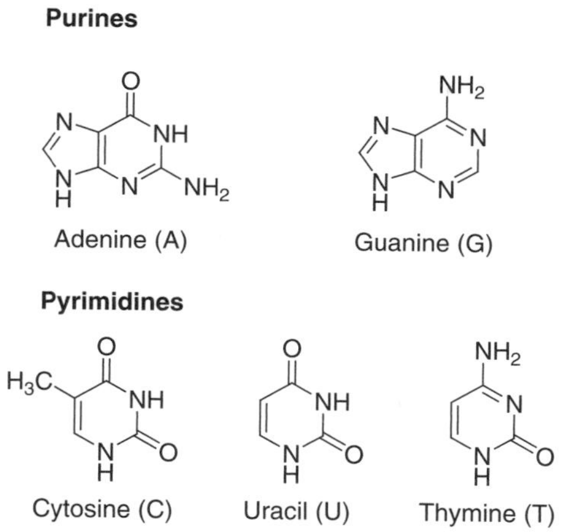

Figure 9.4 The nucleic acid bases.

Table 9.6 Nomenclature of Nucleic Acid Bases, Nucleosides, and Nucleotides

		RNA		DNA	
	Base	Nucleoside	Nucleotide	Deoxynucleoside	Deoxynucleotide
A	Adenine	Adenosine	Adenylate	Deoxyadenosine	Deoxyadenylate
G	Guanine	Guanosine	Guanylate	Deoxyguanosine	Deoxyguanylate
U	Uracil	Uridine	Uridylate	–	–
T	Thymine	–	–	Deoxythymidine	Deoxythymidylate
C	Cytosine	Cytidine	Cytidylate	Deoxycytidine	Deoxycytidylate

of the information for an individual protein (the gene for that protein) is transcribed as messenger RNA (mRNA) and this is then translated during protein synthesis on the ribosomes.

The information in DNA and RNA is provided by the sequence of purines and pyrimidines (Figure 9.4) along the chain; collectively these are known as the bases. A base esterified to a sugar is a nucleoside and the phosphorylated nucleoside is a nucleotide (Table 9.6). Both DNA and RNA are linear polymers of nucleotides. In RNA the sugar is ribose, while in DNA it is deoxyribose.

9.2.1 *The structure and information content of DNA*

As shown in Figure 9.5, DNA is a linear polymer of nucleotides. It consists of a backbone of deoxyribose linked by phosphodiester bonds between carbon-3 of one sugar and carbon-5 of the next. The bases of the nucleotides project from this sugar phosphate backbone. There are of two strands of deoxyribonucleotides, held together by hydrogen bonds between a purine (adenine or guanine) and a pyrimidine (thymine or cytosine); adenine forms two hydrogen bonds with thymine and guanine forms three hydrogen bonds with cytosine. Because of this hydrogen bonding, there is always an equal amount of adenine and thymine, and guanine and cytosine—the ratio A:G equals C:T.

The double strand coils into a helix, the so-called double helix (Figure 9.6). The two strands of a DNA molecule run in opposite directions—where one strand has a 3′ hydroxyl group at the end, on the complementary strand there is a free 5′ hydroxyl group. The information of DNA is always read from the 3′ end toward the 5′ end.

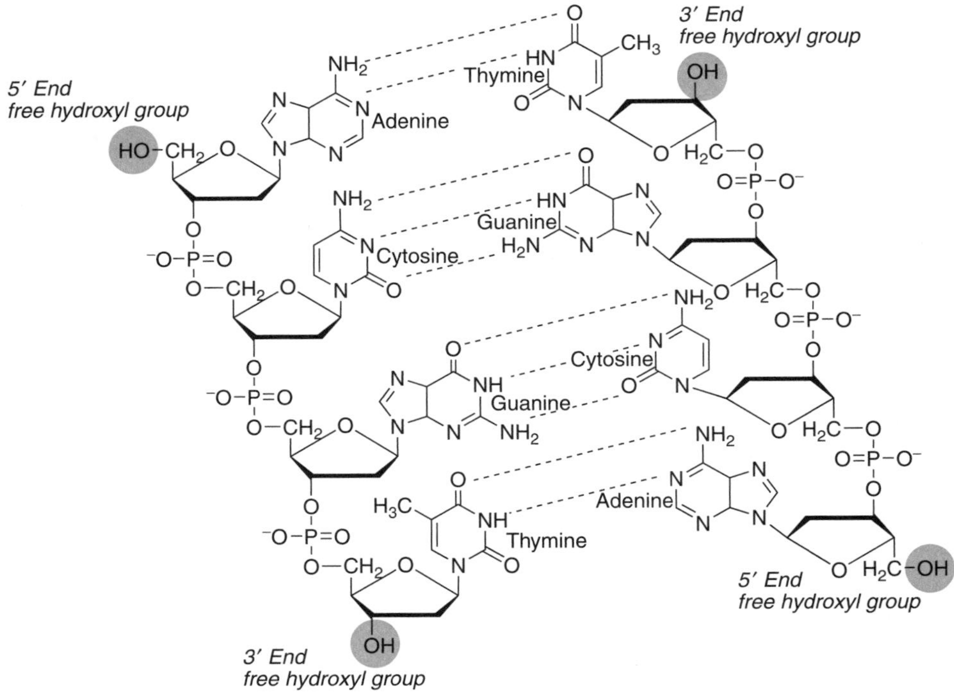

Figure 9.5 The structure of DNA.

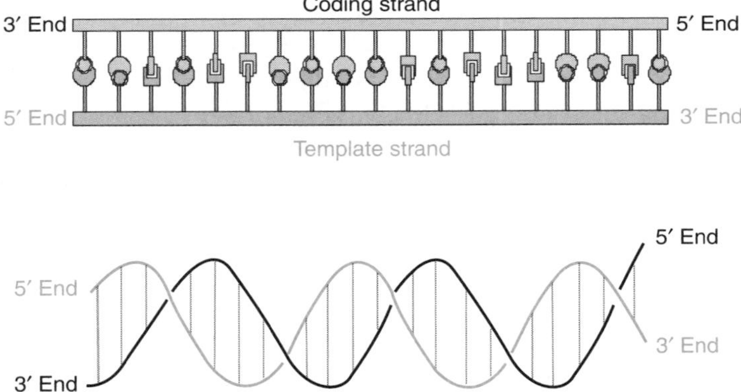

Figure 9.6 The structure of DNA—hydrogen bonding between bases and coiling of the chains to form the double helix.

If stretched out, the DNA in a single cell would be about 2 m long; to fit within the nucleus, the DNA helix is supercoiled and then wound around histones (basic proteins) to form nucleosomes. There are short linking regions between nucleosomes, which are mutation hotspots, suggesting that as well as permitting packaging of DNA, histones also protect it from damage. The chains of nucleosomes are then wound around other proteins and folded to form chromosomes.

Only about 3%–5% of the DNA in a human cell carries information for genes; the remainder consists mainly of the following:

- Control regions, which promote or enhance the expression of individual genes and include regions that respond to hormones and other factors that control gene expression (Section 10.4), as well as sites for the initiation and termination of DNA replication.
- Spacer regions, both between and within genes, which carry no translatable message but serve to link those regions that do carry a translatable message. When such regions occur within a gene sequence, they are called introns.
- Pseudogenes, which seem to be genes that have undergone mutation in our evolutionary past and are now untranslatable. Presumably, these are a reminder of evolutionary history.

9.2.1.1 DNA replication

Prior to cell division, all the DNA in the 46 chromosomes has to be replicated, so that each daughter cell will have a full complement of chromosomes and genetic information. DNA replication occurs by separating the two strands of the double helix in a relatively short region at a time, then pairing deoxynucleotides along the separated strands to synthesize two new strands complementary to each original strand of DNA. This is so-called semiconservative replication—each new DNA molecule has one old strand and one newly synthesized strand (Figure 9.7). This process occurs at a large number of replication sites in each chromosome at the same time.

Because each base to be incorporated into the newly synthesized DNA chain is fitted in by hydrogen bonding to the complementary base in an existing strand of DNA, the process has a high degree of fidelity. Nevertheless, mispairing of bases occurs in about 1 in 10^7 base pairs, and if uncorrected would lead to mutations and loss of genetic information. A separate DNA polymerase has a proofreading function; it detects a mispaired base by distortion of the smooth shape of the newly formed regions of double helix. The offending base is then excised and replaced by the correct one.

9.2.1.2 The genetic code

The information in DNA, contained in a code made up of only four letters (A, G, C, and T), carries the information for the 21 different amino acids that make up the 30,000–40,000 different proteins that are to be synthesized. The bases are read in groups of three, rather

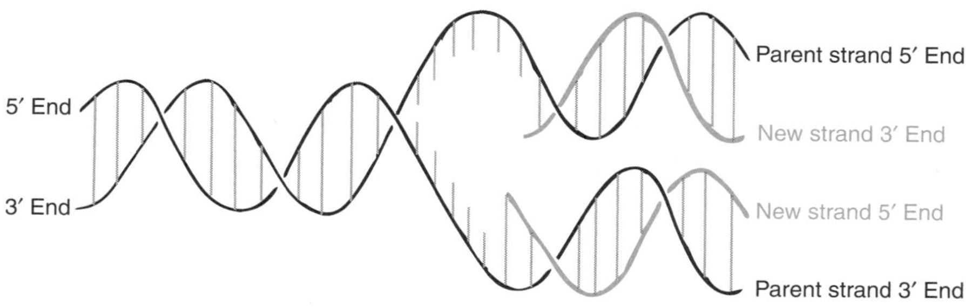

Figure 9.7 Semiconservative replication of DNA.

Table 9.7 The Genetic Code Showing the Codons in mRNA

Amino Acid		Codon(s)
Alanine	Ala	GCU GCC GCA GCG
Arginine	Arg	CGU CGC CGA CGG AGA AGG
Asparagine	Asn	AAU AAC
Aspartic acid	Asp	GAU GAC
Cysteine	Cys	UGU UGC
Glutamic acid	Glu	GAA GAG
Glutamine	Gln	CAA CAG
Glycine	Gly	GGU GGC GGA GGG
Histidine	His	CAU CAG
Isoleucine	Ile	AUU AUC AUA
Leucine	Leu	UUA UUG CUU CUC CUA CUG
Lysine	Lys	AAA AAG
Methionine	Met	AUG
Phenylalanine	Phe	UUU UUC
Proline	Pro	CCU CCC CCA CCG
Serine	Ser	UCU UCC UCA UCG AGU AGC
Threonine	Thr	ACU ACC ACA ACG
Tryptophan	Trp	UGG
Tyrosine	Tyr	UAU UAC
Valine	Val	GUU GUC GUA GUG
Stop		UAA UAG UGA[a]

[a]UGA also codes for selenocysteine in a specific context.

than singly. Each group of three nucleotides is a codon—a single unit of the genetic code. Since a codon can contain any one of the four bases in each position, there are 64 possible codons, but there is a need for only 22—one for each amino acid and one to signal the end of the message.

As can be seen from Tables 9.7 and 9.8, most amino acids are coded for by more than one codon, i.e., the code is degenerate and there are apparently redundant codons. This provides a measure of protection against mutations; in many cases, a single base change in a codon will not affect the amino acid that is incorporated into the protein, and therefore will have no functional significance.

Three codons (UAA, UAG, and UGA) do not code for amino acids but act as stop signals to show the end of the message to be translated and so terminate protein synthesis. UGA also codes for the selenium analog of cysteine, selenocysteine (Section 11.15.2.5). It is normally read as a stop codon, but in the presence of a specific sequence in the untranslated region of mRNA it is read as coding for selenocysteine.

9.2.2 Ribonucleic acid

In RNA, the sugar is ribose rather than deoxyribose as in DNA, and RNA contains the pyrimidine uracil where DNA contains thymine (Figure 9.8). There are three main types of RNA in the cell:

- Messenger RNA (mRNA) is synthesized in the nucleus as a copy of one strand of DNA (the process of transcription; Section 9.2.2.1). After some editing of the message, it is transferred into the cytosol where it binds to ribosomes. The information carried by the mRNA is then translated into the amino acid sequence of the protein.

Table 9.8 The Genetic Code Showing the Codons in mRNA

	Second Base				
First Base	U	C	A	G	**Third Base**
U	Phe	Ser	Tyr	Cys	U
U	Phe	Ser	Tyr	Cys	C
U	Leu	Ser	stop	stop[a]	A
U	Leu	Ser	stop	Trp	G
C	Leu	Pro	His	Arg	U
C	Leu	Pro	His	Arg	C
C	Leu	Pro	Gln	Arg	A
C	Leu	Pro	Gln	Arg	G
A	Ile	Thr	Asn	Ser	U
A	Ile	Thr	Asn	Ser	C
A	Ile	Thr	Lys	Arg	A
A	Met	Thr	Lys	Arg	G
G	Val	Ala	Asp	Gly	U
G	Val	Ala	Asp	Gly	C
G	Val	Ala	Glu	Gly	A
G	Val	Ala	Glu	Gly	G

[a] UGA also codes for selenocysteine in a specific context.

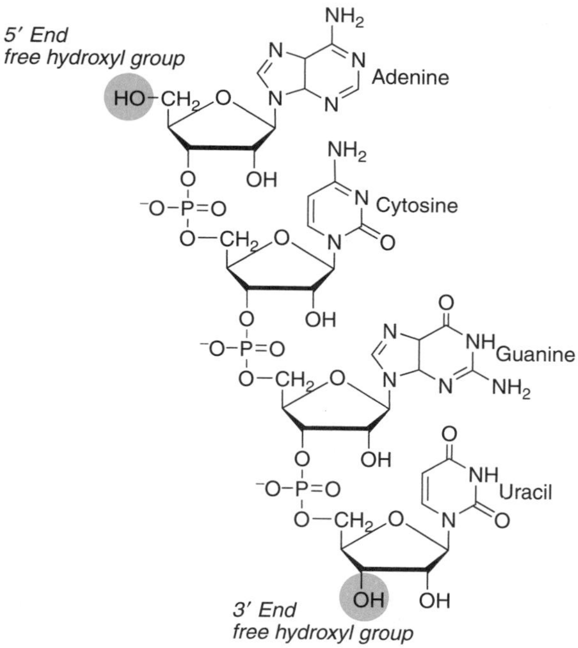

Figure 9.8 The structure of RNA.

- Ribosomal RNA (rRNA) is part of the structure of the ribosomes on which protein is synthesized (Section 9.2.3.2).
- Transfer RNA (tRNA) provides the link between mRNA and the amino acids required for protein synthesis on the ribosome (Section 9.2.3.1).

9.2.2.1 Transcription to form messenger RNA

In the transcription of DNA to form mRNA (Figure 9.9), a part of the desired region of DNA is separated from its protective proteins, uncoiled, and the two strands of the double helix are separated. A copy of one DNA strand (the template strand) is then synthesized by binding the complementary nucleotide triphosphate to each base of DNA in turn, followed by condensation to form the phospho-diester link between ribose moieties. The sequence of bases in the resultant RNA is thus identical to that in the coding strand of DNA, except that where DNA contains thymidine, RNA contains uridine.

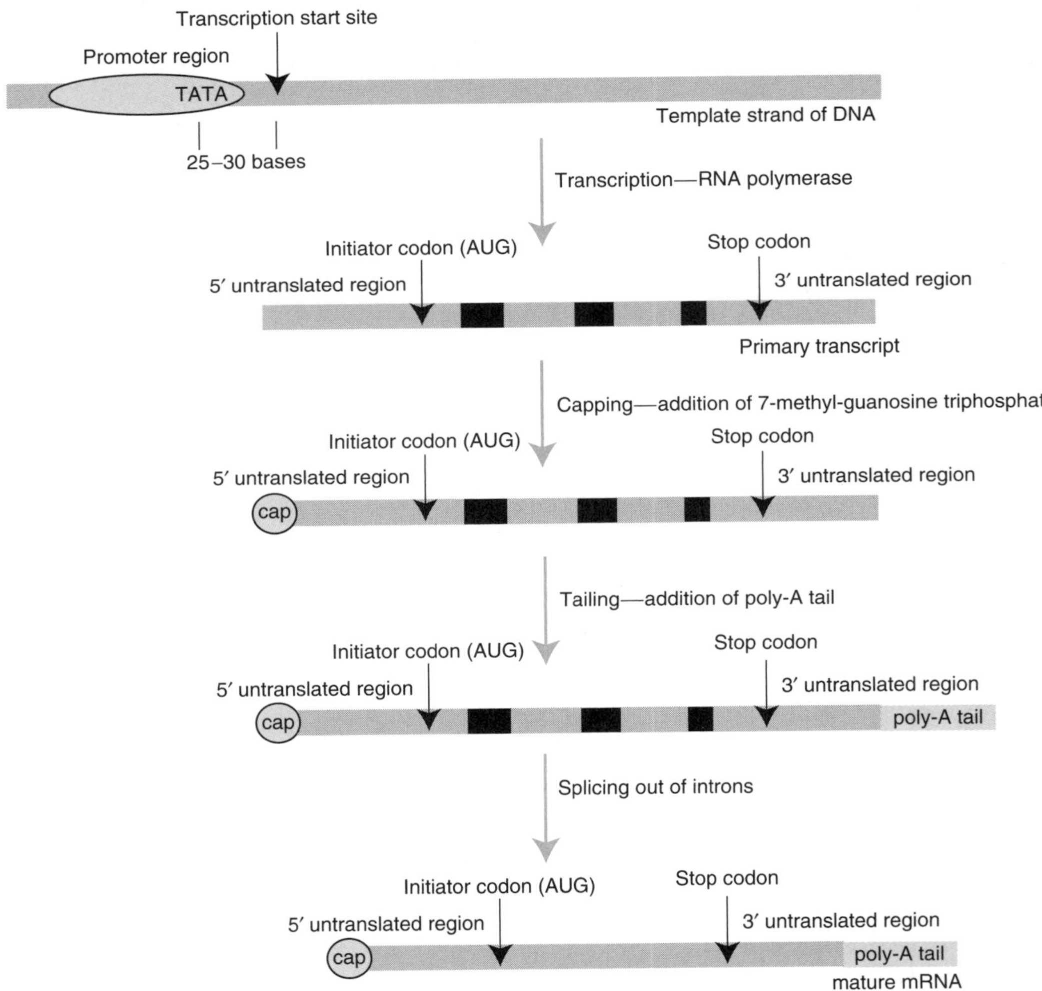

Figure 9.9 Transcription and posttranscriptional processing to yield mRNA.

Upstream of the region of DNA that contains a gene, there is a promoter region that includes the sequence TATA. Transcription factors bind to this TATA box, resulting in activation of RNA polymerase and initiation of transcription some 25–30 base pairs downstream from the TATA box. Much of the noncoding DNA that was described above as pseudogenes consists of regions that were once genes, but having lost their TATA boxes, or their promoter regions, are now untranscribable.

Further control regions (enhancer regions and hormone response elements) may be found upstream, downstream, or in the middle of a gene. These act to increase the rate at which the gene is transcribed.

The primary transcript is a complete copy of the template strand of DNA and undergoes posttranscriptional processing:

- The 5′ end of the RNA is blocked by addition of the unusual base 7-methyl-guanosine triphosphate. This is called the "cap" and has a role in the initiation of protein synthesis (Section 9.2.3.2). The 5′ end of the RNA is the first to be synthesized, and the cap is added before transcription has been completed.
- A tail of up to 250 adenosine residues is added to the 3′ end of the RNA after the termination codon. This poly-A tail stabilizes the mRNA and provides protection against hydrolysis by RNase in the cytosol. It is also useful to molecular biologists, since mRNA can readily be isolated by binding the poly-A tail to a suitable medium.
- Introns are regions of the DNA within a gene that do not carry coding information for the protein to be synthesized. The final step in RNA processing is to excise the introns and splice together the coding regions (exons) to provide a continuous sequence that will be translated. In a number of cases, there may be alternative ways of splicing the same primary transcript in different tissues—the same gene can give rise to different proteins as a result of removing different introns and sometimes also removing exons.

9.2.3 *Translation of mRNA—the process of protein synthesis*

The process of protein synthesis consists of translating the message carried by the sequence of bases on mRNA into amino acids, and then forming peptide bonds between the amino acids to form a protein. This occurs on the ribosome and requires a variety of enzymes as well as specific tRNA molecules for each amino acid.

9.2.3.1 *Transfer RNA*

The key to translating the message carried by the codons on mRNA into amino acids is tRNA. There are 56 different types (species) of tRNA in the cell. They all have the same general structure, RNA twisted into a cloverleaf shape and consisting of some 70–90 nucleotides (Figure 9.10). About half the bases in tRNA are paired by hydrogen bonding, which maintains the shape of the molecule. The 3′ and 5′ ends of the molecule are adjacent to each other as a result of this folding.

The different species of tRNA have many regions in common with each other, and all have a -CCA tail at the 3′ end, which reacts with the amino acid. Two regions are important in providing the specificity of the tRNA species:

- The anticodon, a sequence of three bases at the base of the cloverleaf. The bases in the anticodon are complementary to the bases of the codon of mRNA, and each species

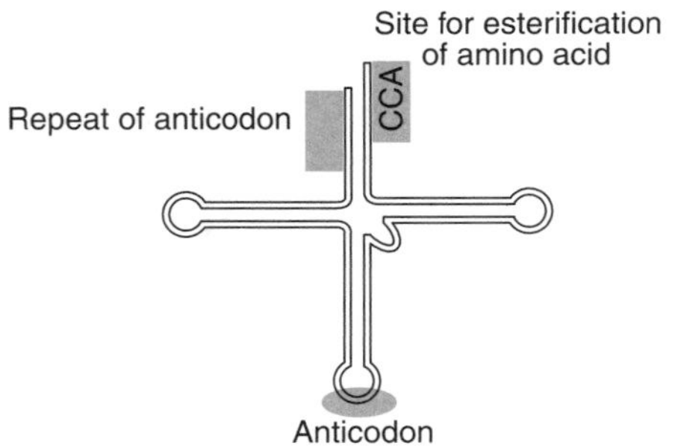

Figure 9.10 Transfer RNA.

of tRNA binds specifically to one codon or, in some cases, two closely related codons for the same amino acid.
- The region at the 5′ end of the molecule, which repeats the information contained in the anticodon.

Amino acids bind to activating enzymes (aminoacyl-tRNA synthetases), which recognize both the amino acid and the appropriate tRNA molecule. The first step is reaction between the amino acid and ATP to form aminoacyl AMP, releasing pyrophosphate. The amino acyl AMP then reacts with the -CCA tail of tRNA to form aminoacyl-tRNA, releasing AMP.

The specificity of these enzymes is critically important to the process of translation. Each enzyme recognizes only one amino acid but will react with all the various tRNA species that carry an anticodon for that amino acid. Mistakes are extremely rare. The easiest possible mistake would be the attachment of valine to the tRNA for isoleucine or vice versa, because of the close similarity between the structures of these two amino acids (Figure 4.18). However, it is only about once in every 3000 times that this mistake occurs. Aminoacyl-tRNA synthetases have a second active site that checks that the correct amino acid has been attached to the tRNA and if not, hydrolyzes the newly formed bond, releasing tRNA and the amino acid.

9.2.3.2 Protein synthesis on the ribosome

The ribosome consists of two subunits composed of RNA and a variety of proteins. It permits the binding of the anticodon region of aminoacyl-tRNA to the codon on mRNA and aligns the amino acids for formation of peptide bonds. As shown in Figure 9.11, the ribosome binds to mRNA and has two tRNA binding sites. One, the P site, contains the growing peptide chain attached to tRNA, while the other, the A site, binds the next aminoacyl-tRNA to be incorporated into the peptide chain.

The first codon of mRNA to be translated (the initiator codon) is always AUG, the codon for methionine. This means that the amino terminal of all newly synthesized proteins is methionine, although this is often removed in posttranslational modification of the protein (Section 9.2.3.4).

An initiator methionine-tRNA forms a complex with the small ribosomal subunit, then together with a variety of initiation factors (enzymes and other proteins) binds to the initiator codon of mRNA, then to a large ribosomal subunit to form the complete ribosome. AUG is the only codon for methionine, and elsewhere in mRNA it binds the normal methionine-tRNA. It is only adjacent to the 5′ cap that AUG binds the initiator methionine-tRNA.

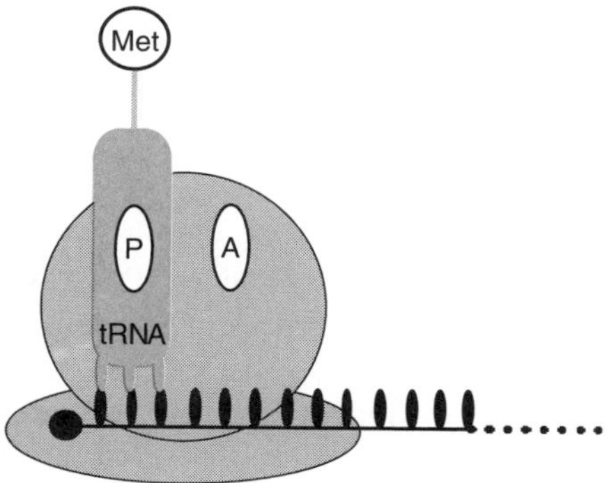

(a) Initiation: methionyl-tRNA binds to P site

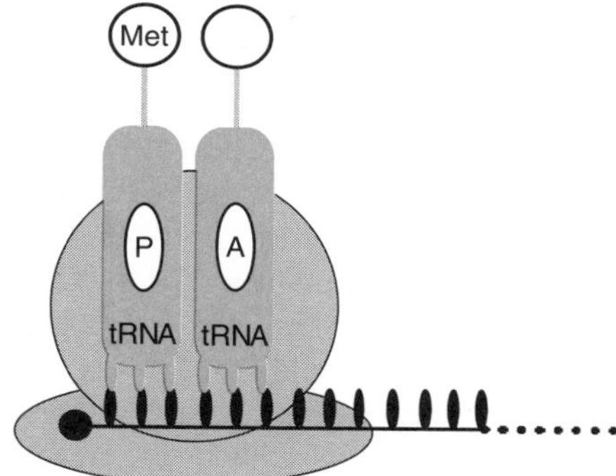

(b) Second aminoacyl-tRNA binds to A site

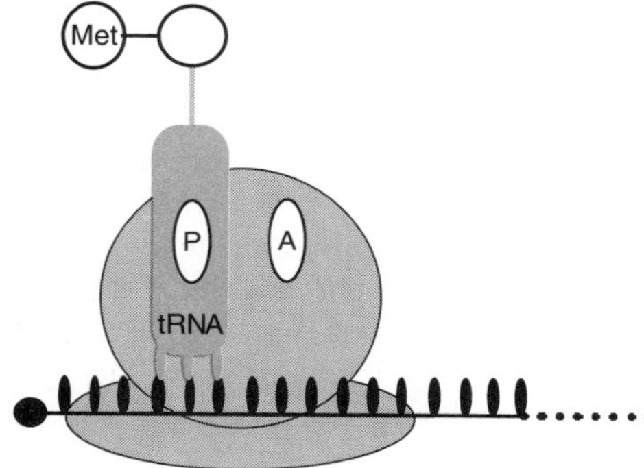

(c) Transfer of Met from tRNA to form peptide bond to second amino acid; movement of tRNA with nascent peptide to P site

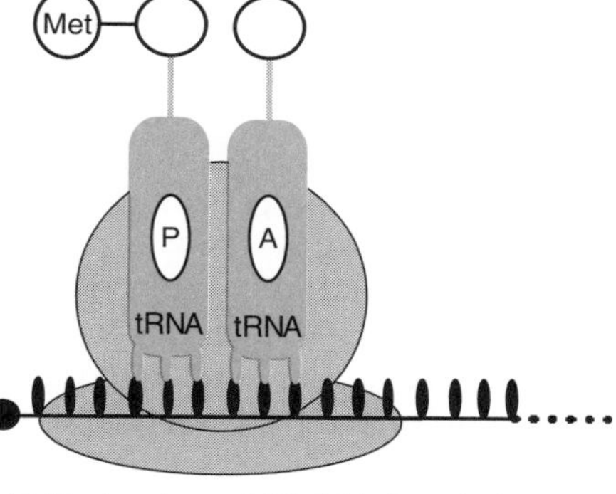

(d) Next aminoacyl-tRNA binds to A site; steps (c) and (d) repeated until a stop codon is at the A site

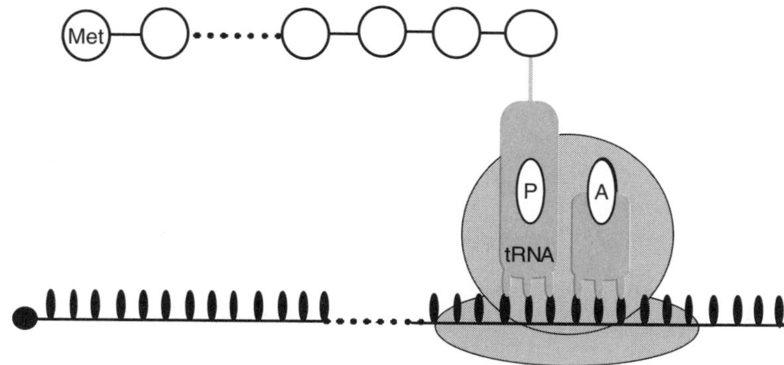

(e) Termination factor binds to stop codon at A site; nascent peptide released and ribosome disassembles, ready to translate another molecule of mRNA

Figure 9.11 Ribosomal protein synthesis.

After the ribosome has been assembled, with the initiator tRNA bound at the P site and occupying the AUG initiator codon, the next aminoacyl-tRNA binds to the A site of the ribosome, with its anticodon bound to the next codon in the sequence.

The methionine is released from the initiator tRNA at the P site, and forms a peptide bond to the amino group of the aminoacyl-tRNA at the A site of the ribosome. The initiator tRNA is then released from the P site and the growing peptide chain attached to its tRNA moves from the A site to the P site. Since the peptide chain is attached to tRNA, which occupies a codon on the mRNA, this means that as the peptide chain moves from the A site to the P site the whole assembly moves one codon along the mRNA.

As the growing peptide chain moves from the A site to the P site, and the ribosome moves along the mRNA chain, the next aminoacyl-tRNA occupies the A site, covering its codon. The growing peptide chain is transferred from the tRNA at the P site, forming a peptide bond to the amino acid at the A site. Again, the free tRNA at the P site is released and the growing peptide attached to tRNA moves from the A site to the P site, moving one codon along the mRNA as it does so.

The stop codons (UAA, UAG, and UGA) are not read by tRNA but by protein release factors. These occupy the A site of the ribosome and hydrolyze the peptide–tRNA bond. This releases the finished protein from the ribosome. As the protein leaves, the two subunits of the ribosome separate and leave the mRNA; they are now available to bind another initiator tRNA and begin the process of translation over again.

Just as several molecules of RNA polymerase can transcribe a gene at the same time, several ribosomes translate a molecule of mRNA at the same time. As the ribosomes travel along the ribosome, each has a longer growing peptide chain than the next. Such assemblies of ribosomes on a molecule of mRNA are called polysomes. Proteins that are to be exported from the cell have a sequence of hydrophobic amino acids at the amino terminal. This signal peptide draws the nascent polypeptide chain into the rough endoplasmic reticulum while it is being synthesized, so that polysomes translating mRNA for proteins to be exported are attached to the rough endoplasmic reticulum.

Termination and release of the protein from the ribosome requires the presence of a stop codon and protein release factors. However, protein synthesis will also come to a halt if there is not enough of one of the amino acids bound to tRNA. In this case, the growing peptide chain is not released from the ribosome, but remains in arrested development until the required aminoacyl-tRNA is available. This means that if the intake of one of the essential amino acids is inadequate, then protein synthesis will cease once supplies are exhausted.

9.2.3.3 The energy cost of protein synthesis

Protein synthesis is an energy-expensive process. There is a cost of 4 ATP equivalents per peptide bond synthesized (2.8 kJ per gram of protein synthesized):

- Formation of the aminoacyl-tRNA requires the formation of aminoacyl-AMP, with the release of pyrophosphate, so that for each amino acid attached to tRNA there is a cost equivalent to 2ATP → ADP + phosphate.
- The binding of each aminoacyl-tRNA to the A site of the ribosome involves the hydrolysis of GTP → GDP + phosphate, which is equivalent to ATP → ADP + phosphate.
- Movement of the growing peptide chain from the A site of the ribosome to the P site again involves the hydrolysis of ATP → ADP + phosphate.

Allowing for active transport of amino acids into cells (Section 3.2.2.6) increases this to 3.6 kJ per gram of protein synthesized, and allowing for the nucleoside triphosphates required for mRNA synthesis gives a total cost of 4.2 kJ per gram of protein synthesized.

In the fasting state, when the rate of protein synthesis is relatively low, about 9% of total energy expenditure (i.e., about 12% of the basal metabolic rate) is accounted for by protein synthesis. After a high carbohydrate meal, the rate of protein synthesis increases and accounts for 12% of energy expenditure. A high protein intake increases protein synthesis (and catabolism) further, and after a high-protein meal protein turnover accounts for almost 20% of energy expenditure.

9.2.3.4 Posttranslational modification of proteins

The signal peptide of proteins that are exported from the cell is cleaved as part of the posttranslational processing in the rough endoplasmic reticulum and Golgi apparatus. Many other proteins also lose short peptides from the amino or the carboxyl terminal, and the initial (amino terminal) methionine is removed from most newly synthesized proteins.

Many proteins contain carbohydrates and lipids covalently bound to amino acid side chains. Others contain covalently bound prosthetic groups, such as vitamins and their derivatives, metal ions, or heme. The attachment of these non-amino acid parts of the protein is part of the process of posttranslational modification to yield the active protein.

Some proteins contain unusual amino acids for which there are no codons and no tRNA. These are formed by modification of the protein after translation is complete. When the protein is catabolized, these modified amino acids cannot be reutilized but are either metabolized or excreted unchanged. Such amino acids include the following:

- Methyl-histidine in the contractile proteins of muscle.
- Hydroxyproline and hydroxylysine in the connective tissue proteins via a reaction that requires vitamin C as a cofactor. This explains why wound healing, which requires new synthesis of connective tissue, is impaired in vitamin C deficiency (Section 11.14.3; see Problem 9.3).
- Interchain links in collagen and elastin, formed by the oxidation of lysine residues. This reaction is catalyzed by a copper-dependent enzyme, and copper deficiency leads to fragility of bones and loss of the elasticity of connective tissues (Section 11.15.2.2 and see Problem 4.4). Measurement of urinary excretion of small peptides containing these cross-link compounds provides an index of bone turnover.
- γ-Carboxyglutamate in several of the blood-clotting proteins and in osteocalcin in bone. The formation of γ-carboxyglutamate requires vitamin K (Section 11.5.2; see Problem 9.2). Measurement of circulating the concentration of undercarboxylated prothrombin provides a sensitive index of vitamin K nutritional status.

9.3 The metabolism of amino acids

An adult has a requirement for a dietary intake of protein because there is continual oxidation of amino acids both as a source of metabolic fuel and, more importantly, for gluconeogenesis in the fasting state. In the fed state, amino acids in excess of immediate requirements for protein synthesis are oxidized and the carbon skeletons are used mainly for synthesis of fatty acids. Overall, for an adult in nitrogen balance, the total amount of amino acids being metabolized will be equal to the total intake of amino acids in dietary proteins.

Amino acids are also required for the synthesis of a variety of metabolic products, including:

- Purines (synthesized from glycine) and pyrimidines (synthesized from aspartate) for nucleic acid synthesis

- Heme, synthesized from glycine
- The catecholamine neurotransmitters, dopamine, noradrenaline, and adrenaline, synthesized from tyrosine
- The thyroid hormones thyroxine and triiodothyronine, synthesized from tyrosine (Section 11.15.3.3)
- Melanin, the pigment of skin and hair, synthesized from tyrosine
- The nicotinamide ring of the coenzymes, NAD and NADP, synthesized from tryptophan (Section 11.8.2)
- The neurotransmitter serotonin (5-hydroxytryptamine), synthesized from tryptophan
- The neurotransmitter histamine, synthesized from histidine
- The neurotransmitter GABA (γ-aminobutyrate), synthesized from glutamate (Figure 5.19)
- Carnitine (Section 5.5.1), synthesized from lysine and methionine
- Creatine (Section 3.2.3.1), synthesized from arginine, glycine, and methionine
- The phospholipid bases ethanolamine and choline (Section 4.3.1.2), synthesized from serine and methionine (acetyl choline is a neurotransmitter)
- Taurine, synthesized from cysteine

In general, the amounts of amino acids required for synthesis of these products are small compared with the requirement for maintenance of nitrogen balance and protein turnover.

9.3.1 Metabolism of the amino nitrogen

The initial step in the metabolism of amino acids is the removal of the amino group ($-NH_3^+$), leaving the carbon skeleton of the amino acid. Chemically, these carbon skeletons are keto-acids (more correctly, they are oxo-acids). A keto-acid has a $-C=O$ group in place of the $HC-NH_3^+$ group of an amino acid; the metabolism of keto-acids is discussed in Section 9.3.2.

9.3.1.1 Deamination

Some amino acids can be directly oxidized to their corresponding keto-acids, releasing ammonia—the process of deamination (Figure 9.12). There is a general L-amino acid oxidase that catalyzes the deamination of most amino acids, but it has a low activity and is relatively unimportant in amino acid metabolism.

Kidneys contain D-amino acid oxidase, which acts to deaminate, and hence detoxify, the small amounts of D-amino acids that arise from bacterial proteins. The keto-acids resulting from the action of D-amino acid oxidase on D-amino acids can undergo transamination (Section 9.3.1.2) to yield the L-isomers. This means that to a limited extent, D-amino acids can be isomerized and used for protein synthesis. Although there is evidence from experimental animals that D-isomers of (some of) the essential amino acids can be used to maintain nitrogen balance, there is little information on their utilization in humans.

Four amino acids are deaminated by specific enzymes:

- Glycine is deaminated to glyoxylate and ammonium ions by glycine oxidase.
- Glutamate is deaminated to ketoglutarate and ammonium ions by glutamate dehydrogenase.
- Serine is deaminated and dehydrated to pyruvate by serine deaminase (sometimes called serine dehydratase).
- Threonine is deaminated and dehydrated to oxo-butyrate by threonine deaminase.

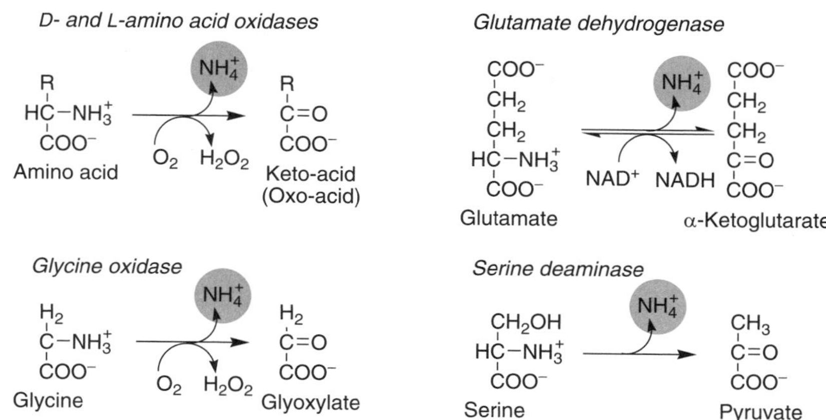

Figure 9.12 Deamination of amino acids.

9.3.1.2 Transamination

Most amino acids are not deaminated but undergo transamination, in which the amino group is transferred onto the enzyme, leaving the keto-acid. In the second half of the reaction, the enzyme transfers the amino group onto an acceptor, which is a different keto-acid, thus forming the amino acid corresponding to that keto-acid. This is a typical ping-pong reaction sequence (Section 2.3.3.2). The acceptor for the amino group at the active site of the enzyme is pyridoxal phosphate, the metabolically active coenzyme derived from vitamin B_6 (Section 11.9.2), forming pyridoxamine phosphate as an intermediate in the reaction. The reaction of transamination is shown in Figure 9.13 and the keto-acids corresponding to the amino acids in Table 9.9.

Transamination is a reversible reaction, so that if the keto-acid can be synthesized in the body, so can the amino acid. Essential amino acids (Section 9.1.3) are those for which the only source of the keto-acid is the amino acid itself. Three of the keto-acids listed in Table 9.9 are common metabolic intermediates; they are the precursors of the three amino acids that can be considered completely dispensable in that there is no requirement for them in the diet (Section 9.1.3):

- Pyruvate—the keto-acid of alanine
- α-Ketoglutarate—the keto-acid of glutamate
- Oxaloacetate—the keto-acid of aspartate

The reversibility of transamination has been exploited in the treatment of patients in renal failure. The conventional treatment is to provide them with a very low-protein diet, so as to minimize the total amount of urea that has to be excreted (Section 9.3.1.4). However, they still have to be provided with the essential amino acids. If they are provided with the essential keto-acids, they can synthesize the corresponding essential amino acids by transamination, so further reducing their nitrogen burden. The only amino acid for which this is not possible is lysine—the keto-acid corresponding to lysine undergoes rapid nonenzymic condensation to pipecolic acid, which cannot be metabolized further.

If the acceptor keto-acid in a transamination reaction is α-ketoglutarate, then glutamate is formed and can readily be oxidized back to α-ketoglutarate and ammonium, catalyzed by glutamate dehydrogenase. Similarly, if the acceptor keto-acid is glyoxylate then the

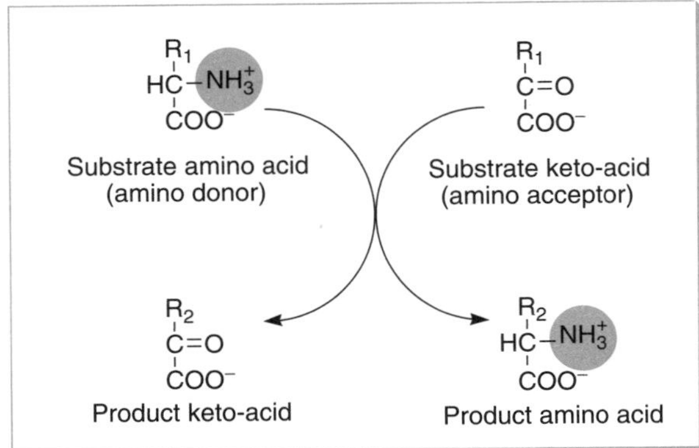

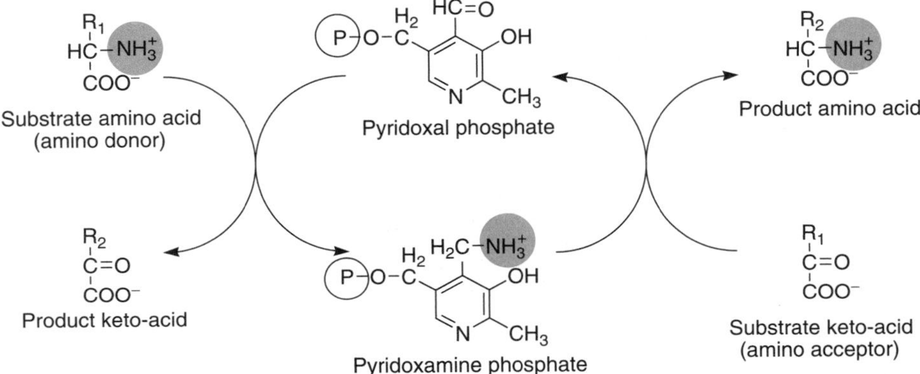

Figure 9.13 Transamination of amino acids.

product is glycine, which can be oxidized back to glyoxylate and ammonium catalyzed by glycine oxidase. Thus, by means of a variety of transaminases and using the reactions of glutamate dehydrogenase and glycine oxidase, all the amino acids can, indirectly, be converted to their keto-acids and ammonium (Figure 9.14). Aspartate can also act as an intermediate in the indirect deamination of a variety of amino acids (see Figure 9.18).

9.3.1.3 *The metabolism of ammonia*

The deamination of amino acids (and a number of other reactions in the body) results in the formation of ammonium ions. Ammonium is highly toxic. The normal plasma concentration is less than 50 μmol/L; an increase to 80–100 μmol/L (far too little to have any detectable effect on plasma pH) results in disturbance of consciousness and in patients whose blood ammonium rises above 200 μmol/L, ammonia intoxication leads to coma and convulsions and may be fatal.

At any time, the total amount of ammonium being formed in various tissues that must be transported to the liver is greatly in excess of the toxic level. As it is formed in peripheral tissues, ammonium is metabolized to yield glutamine by the reactions of glutamate dehydrogenase and glutamine synthetase (Figure 9.15). Glutamine is transported in the bloodstream to the liver and kidneys.

Table 9.9 Transamination Products of the Amino Acids

Amino Acid	Keto-Acid
Alanine	Pyruvate
Arginine	α-Keto-γ-guanidoacetate
Aspartic acid	Oxaloacetate
Cysteine	β-Mercaptopyruvate
Glutamic acid	α-Ketoglutarate
Glutamine	α-Keto-glutaramic acid
Glycine	Glyoxylate
Histidine	Imidazolepyruvate
Isoleucine	α-Keto-β-methylvalerate
Leucine	α-Keto-isocaproate
Lysine	α-Keto-ε-aminocaproate → pipecolic acid
Methionine	*S*-methyl-β-thiol α-oxopropionate
Ornithine	Glutamic-γ-semialdehyde
Phenylalanine	Phenylpyruvate
Proline	γ-Hydroxypyruvate
Serine	Hydroxypyruvate
Threonine	α-Keto-β-hydroxybutyrate
Tryptophan	Indolepyruvate
Tyrosine	*p*-Hydroxyphenylpyruvate
Valine	α-Keto-isovalerate

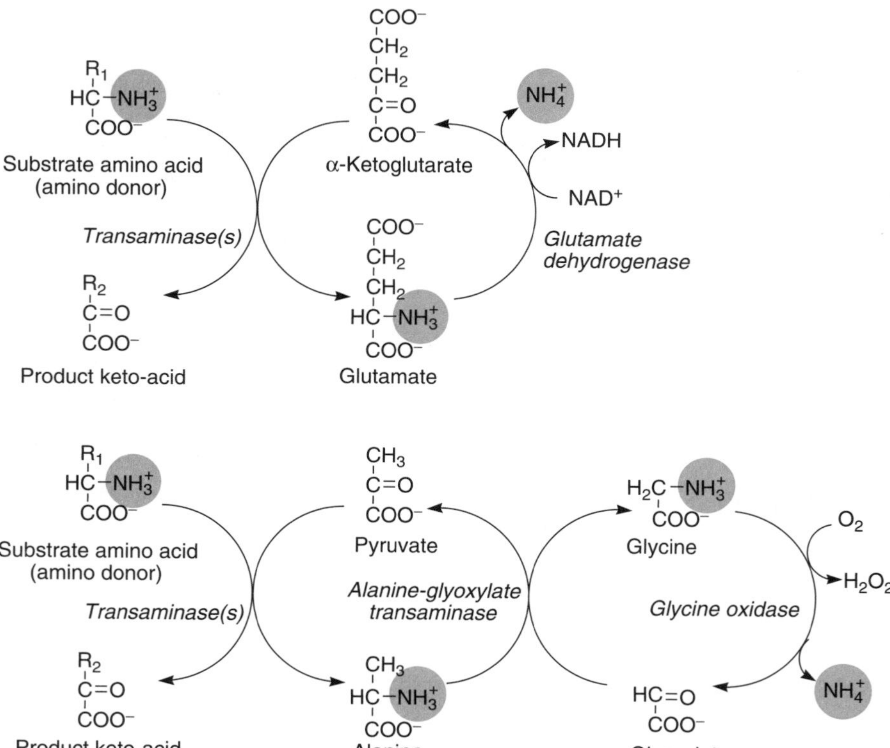

Figure 9.14 Transdeamination of amino acids—transamination linked to oxidative deamination.

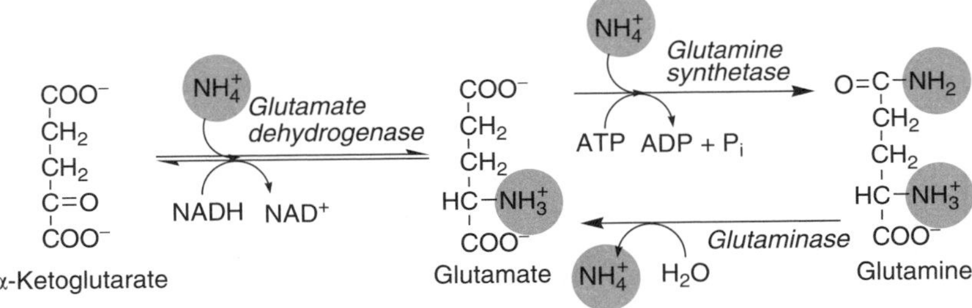

Figure 9.15 The synthesis of glutamate and glutamine from ammonium, and hydrolysis of glutamine by glutaminase.

It is the formation of glutamate from α-ketoglutarate that explains the neurotoxicity of ammonium. As ammonium concentrations in the nervous system rise, the reaction of glutamate dehydrogenase depletes the mitochondrial pool of α-ketoglutarate, resulting in impairment of the activity of the citric acid cycle (Section 5.4.4), and so impairing energy-yielding metabolism and ATP formation.

In the liver, glutamine may either be used directly as a source of nitrogen in a variety of pathways (including the synthesis of purines and pyrimidines) or may be hydrolyzed by glutaminase to yield glutamate and ammonium, which is used as the nitrogen donor in other pathways. Glutaminase is also found in the kidneys, where it acts as a source of ammonium ions to neutralize excessively acidic urine.

9.3.1.4 *The synthesis of urea*

In the liver, ammonium arising from either the hydrolysis of glutamine or the reaction of adenosine deaminase (Section 9.3.1.5) is the substrate for synthesis of urea, the main nitrogenous excretion product. The pathway for urea synthesis is shown in Figure 9.16. The key compound is ornithine, which acts as a carrier on which the molecule of urea is built up. At the end of the reaction sequence, urea is released by the hydrolysis of arginine, yielding ornithine to begin the cycle again. Although urea is an excretory end-product of nitrogen metabolism, it is reabsorbed in the distal renal tubules, where it maintains an osmotic gradient for the reabsorption of water.

The total amount of urea synthesized each day is severalfold higher than the amount that is excreted. Urea diffuses readily from the bloodstream into the large intestine, where it is hydrolyzed by bacterial urease to carbon dioxide and ammonium. Much of the ammonium is reabsorbed and used in the liver for the synthesis of glutamate and glutamine, and then a variety of other nitrogenous compounds (Figure 9.17). Studies with ^{15}N urea show that a significant amount of label is found in essential amino acids. This may reflect intestinal bacterial synthesis of amino acids or the reversibility of the transamination of essential amino acids.

The urea synthesis cycle is also the pathway for the synthesis of the amino acid arginine. Ornithine is synthesized from glutamate and then undergoes the reactions shown in Figure 9.16 to form arginine. Although the whole pathway of urea synthesis occurs only in the liver, the sequence of reactions leading to the formation of arginine also occurs in the kidneys, which are the main source of arginine in the body.

Infants have relatively low activity of the urea synthesis cycle enzymes, which explains why at times of rapid growth arginine is an essential amino acid (Section 9.1.3). Young infants cannot be fed undiluted cow's milk, because it provides more protein (as percentage

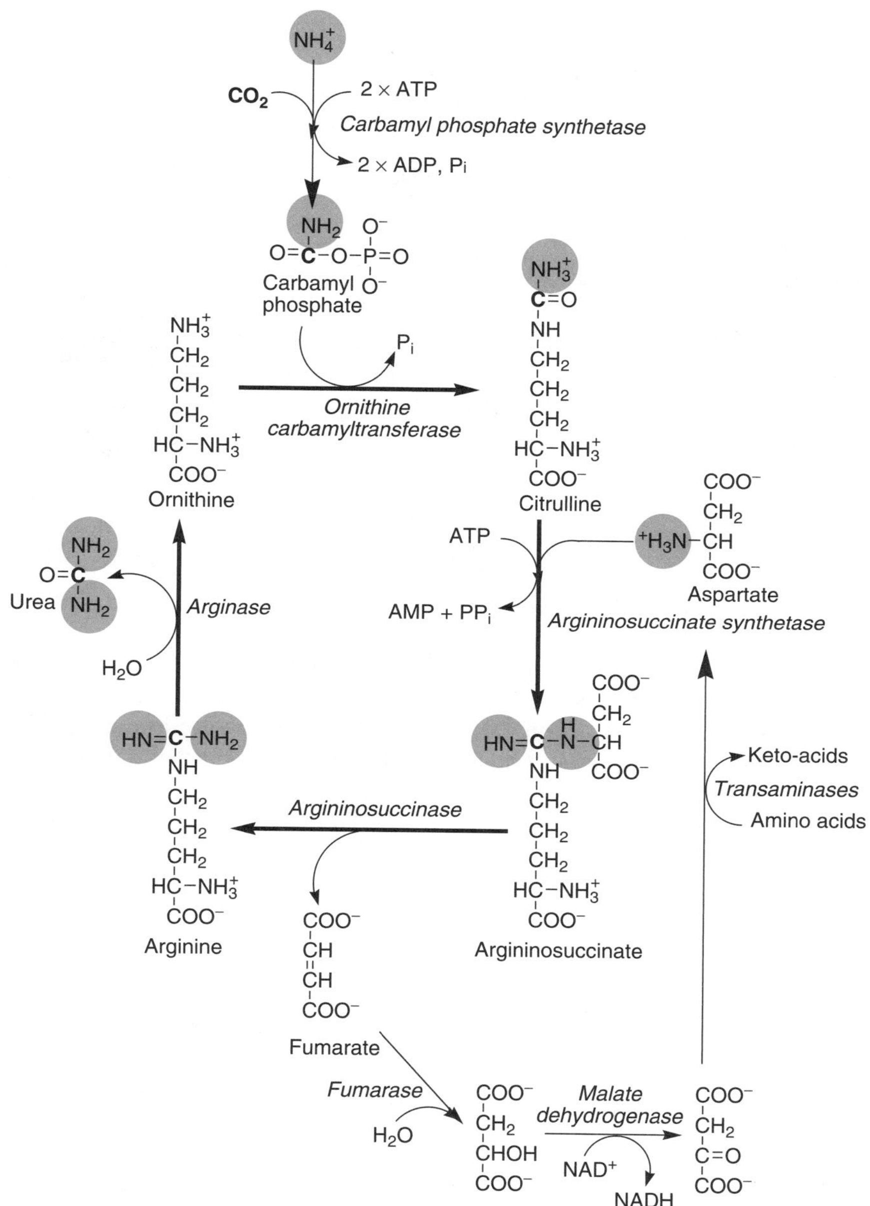

Figure 9.16 The synthesis of urea.

of energy) than human milk and more than they can use for protein synthesis. The excess protein exceeds their capacity for urea synthesis and they are at risk of hyperammonemia. Infant formula is manufactured by diluting cows milk to an appropriate protein concentration, then adding lactose to increase the energy yield to that of human milk.

The precursor for ornithine synthesis is *N*-acetyl glutamate, which is also an obligatory activator of carbamyl phosphate synthetase. This provides a regulatory mechanism—if *N*-acetyl glutamate is not available for ornithine synthesis (and hence there would be impaired activity

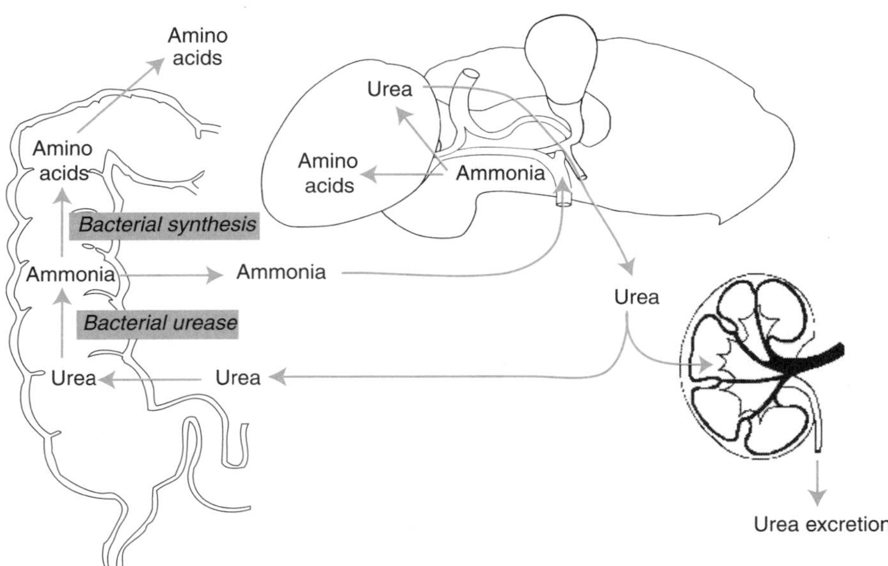

Figure 9.17 Enterohepatic cycling of urea.

of the urea synthesis cycle), then ammonium is not incorporated into carbamyl phosphate. This can be a cause of hyperammonemia in a variety of metabolic disturbances that lead to either a lack of acetyl CoA for *N*-acetyl glutamate synthesis or an accumulation of propionyl CoA, which is a poor substrate for, and hence an inhibitor of, *N*-acetyl glutamate synthetase.

9.3.1.5 Incorporation of nitrogen in biosynthesis

Amino acids are the only significant source of nitrogen for synthesis of nitrogenous compounds such as heme, purines, and pyrimidines. Three amino acids are especially important as nitrogen donors:

- Glycine is incorporated intact into purines, heme and other porphyrins, and creatine (Section 3.2.3.1).
- Glutamine—the amide nitrogen is transferred in an ATP-dependent reaction, replacing an oxo-group in the acceptor with an amino group.
- Aspartate undergoes an ATP- or GTP-dependent condensation reaction with an oxo-group, followed by cleavage to release fumarate.

Reactions in which aspartate acts as a nitrogen donor in this way result in a net gain of ATP since the fumarate is hydrated to malate, then oxidized to oxaloacetate, which is then available to undergo transamination to aspartate (Figure 9.18). Adenosine deaminase converts adenosine monophosphate back into inosine monophosphate, liberating ammonia. This sequence of reactions thus provides a pathway for the deamination of a variety of amino acids, linked to transamination, similar to those shown in Figure 9.14 for transamination linked to glutamate dehydrogenase or glycine oxidase.

9.3.2 The metabolism of amino acid carbon skeletons

Acetyl CoA and acetoacetate arising from the carbon skeletons of amino acids may either be used for fatty acid synthesis (Section 5.6.1) or oxidized as metabolic fuel, but cannot under

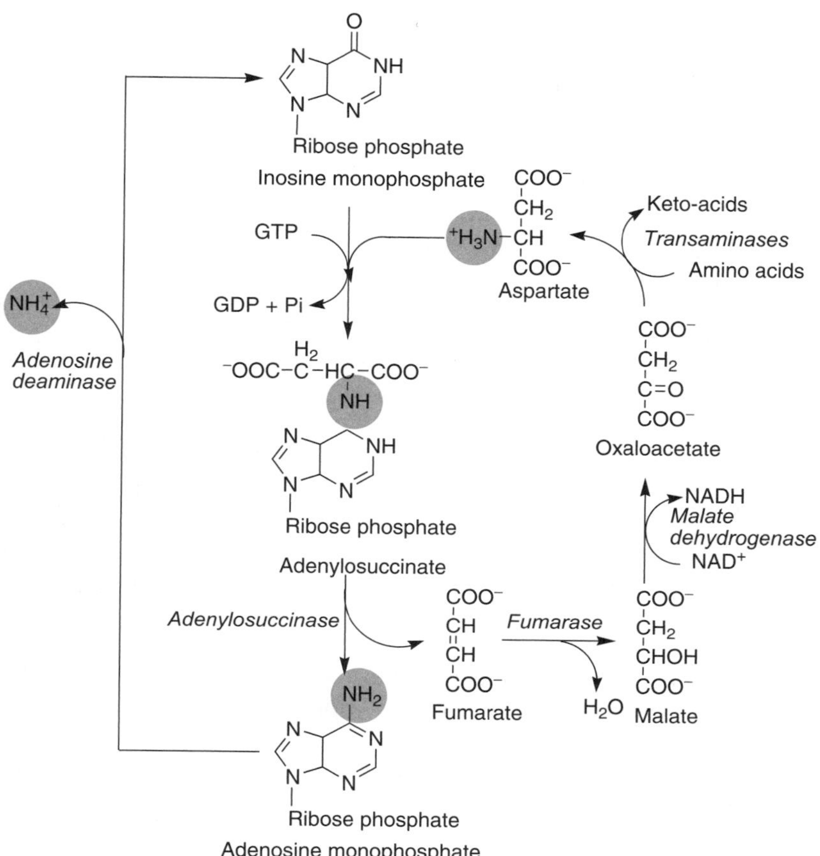

Figure 9.18 The role of aspartate as a nitrogen donor in synthetic reactions and of adenosine deaminase as a source of ammonium ions.

any circumstances be utilized for the synthesis of glucose (gluconeogenesis; Section 5.7). Amino acids that yield acetyl CoA or acetoacetate are termed ketogenic. Those amino acids that yield intermediates that can be used for gluconeogenesis are termed glucogenic. Only two amino acids (leucine and lysine) are purely ketogenic; three others (tryptophan, isoleucine, and phenylalanine) yield both glucogenic and ketogenic fragments; the other amino acids are purely glucogenic (Table 9.10).

The principal substrate for gluconeogenesis is oxaloacetate, which undergoes the reaction catalyzed by phosphoenolpyruvate carboxykinase to yield phosphoenolpyruvate (Figure 5.32). The onward metabolism of phosphoenolpyruvate to glucose is essentially the reverse of glycolysis (Figure 5.10).

The points of entry of amino acid carbon skeletons into central metabolic pathways are shown in Figure 5.20. Those that give rise to ketoglutarate, succinyl CoA, fumarate, or oxaloacetate can be regarded as directly increasing the tissue pool of citric acid cycle intermediates, and hence permitting the withdrawal of oxaloacetate for gluconeogenesis. Those amino acids that give rise to pyruvate also increase the tissue pool of oxaloacetate, because pyruvate can be carboxylated to oxaloacetate in the reaction catalyzed by pyruvate carboxylase (Section 5.7).

Table 9.10 Metabolic Fates of the Carbon Skeletons of Amino Acids

	Glucogenic Intermediates	**Ketogenic Intermediates**
Alanine	Pyruvate	–
Glycine → serine	Pyruvate	–
Cysteine	Pyruvate	–
Tryptophan	Pyruvate	Acetyl CoA
Arginine → ornithine	α-Ketoglutarate	–
Glutamine → glutamate	α-Ketoglutarate	–
Proline → glutamate	α-Ketoglutarate	–
Histidine → glutamate	α-Ketoglutarate	–
Methionine	Propionyl CoA	–
Isoleucine	Propionyl CoA	Acetyl CoA
Valine	Succinyl CoA	–
Asparagine → aspartate	Oxaloacetate or fumarate	–
Aspartate	Oxaloacetate or fumarate	–
Phenylalanine → tyrosine	Fumarate	Acetoacetate
Leucine	–	Acetoacetate and acetyl CoA
Lysine	–	Acetyl CoA

Gluconeogenesis is an important fate of amino acid carbon skeletons in the fasting state, when the metabolic imperative is to maintain a supply of glucose for the central nervous system and red blood cells. However, in the fed state, the carbon skeletons of amino acids in excess of requirements for protein synthesis will mainly be used for formation of acetyl CoA for fatty acid synthesis and storage as adipose tissue triacylglycerol.

Key points

- Nitrogen balance is the difference between the dietary intake of nitrogenous compounds (mainly protein) and excretion of nitrogenous compounds. In an adult, the normal state is nitrogen equilibrium; intake = output.
- Positive nitrogen balance is normal in growth and pregnancy, and after a period of protein loss from the body.
- Negative nitrogen balance occurs in response to trauma and when the intake of protein (or essential amino acids) is inadequate.
- There is continual catabolism of proteins and replacement synthesis. Different proteins turn over at different rates, and those that are regulatory enzymes have short half-lives.
- Protein requirements are estimated by determining the intake required to maintain nitrogen balance. For an adult, the average requirement is 0.66g/kg body weight, equivalent to 8% of energy intake. Deficiency is unlikely in adults because most starchy dietary staples provide more than 8% of energy as protein.
- Nine amino acids cannot be synthesized in the body and are dietary essentials; of the remainder, two are synthesized from essential amino acid precursors, and under some circumstances the demand for others may exceed the capacity to synthesize them. Only three amino acids—alanine, aspartate, and glutamate—can be considered completely dispensable, since they are synthesized from intermediates of carbohydrate metabolism.

- The nutritional value of a protein is determined by its content of essential amino acids compared with the amounts required for tissue protein synthesis. A deficit in one protein is complemented by a relative excess in others, so the protein quality of most diets is similar.
- DNA contains the information for synthesis of all tissue proteins; a copy of a gene is made by transcription to mRNA and this is translated into the amino acid sequence during protein synthesis on the ribosome.
- Protein synthesis is energy expensive, accounting for about 8% of energy expenditure in the fasting state and up to 20% after a meal.
- Amino acids in excess of requirements for protein synthesis and those arising from protein catabolism in the fasting state are deaminated to keto-acids either directly or by deaminases linked to transaminases. Transamination is the process of transferring the amino group from an amino acid onto the keto-acid corresponding to another amino acid. The intermediate carrier of the amino group is the coenzyme pyridoxal phosphate, derived from vitamin B_6.
- Ammonium arising from deamination of amino acids is toxic; it is transported in the bloodstream as glutamine. Urea is synthesized in the liver as the main end product of nitrogen metabolism.
- Carbon skeletons of amino acids may be glucogenic or ketogenic.

Problem 9.1: Amino acid output by muscle in the fasting state

In the fasting state, the liver releases glucose into the circulation as a metabolic fuel for the central nervous system and red blood cells. Some of this glucose arises from the breakdown of liver glycogen, but much arises by gluconeogenesis from amino acids. These amino acids are mainly derived from the breakdown of muscle protein. Although muscle contains a large amount of glycogen, this cannot be released as glucose since muscle lacks glucose 6-phosphatase.

Figure 9.19 shows the results of experiments to measure the uptake of amino acids by the liver (by cannulating the hepatic artery and veins) and the output of amino acids by skeletal muscle (by cannulating the femoral artery and vein) in a group of healthy volunteers. The results are shown as the arteriovenous difference. A positive value shows net uptake by the liver; a negative value, net output of the amino acid from muscle. Although the results are not shown, there was also a net output of glucose by the liver.

Table 9.11 shows the approximate amino acid composition of muscle protein.

Can you account for the difference between the amino acid output from muscle and the amino acid composition of muscle proteins?

Problem 9.2: A problem of bleeding cows and chickens, rat poison, and patients with thrombosis

During the 1920s, a new disease of cattle involving fatal bleeding appeared at about the same time over a wide area of prairie land in North America. It was eventually traced to feeding the animals on hay made from sweet clover (*Melilotus alba* and *M. officinalis*) that had

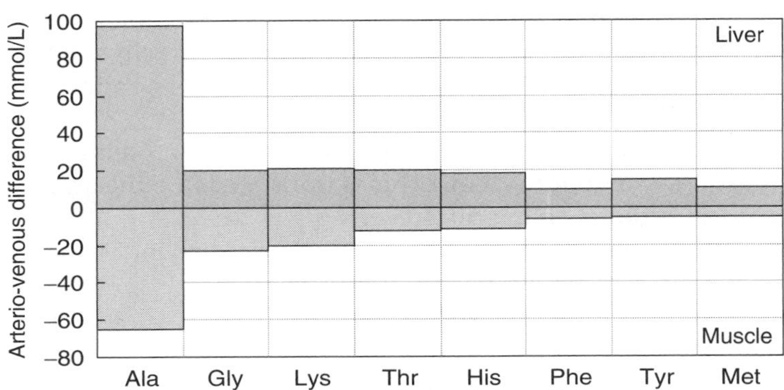

Figure 9.19 Arteriovenous differences in amino acids across the liver (arterio hepatic venous difference) and skeletal muscle (arterio femoral venous difference). A positive arteriovenous difference means uptake of amino acids by the tissue, a negative difference means output of amino acids by the tissue. (From Felig, P. and Wahren, J., *Fed. Proc.*, 33: 1092–1097, 1974.)

Table 9.11 Approximate Amino Acid Content of Muscle Protein

Amino Acid	mg/g N
Ala	370
Gly	330
Lys	590
Thr	280
His	170
Phe	250
Tyr	230
Met	170

"mysteriously gone bad." After eating the hay, the animals suffered a decline in blood clotting (over about 15 days), followed by the development of internal hemorrhage, which was generally fatal after 30–50 days. The disease was caused only by feeding the animals on spoilt sweet clover hay and was called "sweet clover disease." It could be treated by removing the spoilt hay from the animals' diet and transfusing them with blood freshly drawn from normal healthy animals.

What conclusions can you draw from these observations?

The addition of oxalate or citrate to blood will chelate calcium ions and prevent clotting. Addition of a solution of calcium chloride to oxalated normal plasma results in rapid clotting; addition of calcium chloride to oxalated plasma from calves with sweet clover disease did not result in clotting.

What conclusions can you draw from this observation?

Partially purified prothrombin was prepared from the blood of either healthy animals or those with sweet clover disease, and tested on blood from an affected animal; the results are shown in Table 9.12.

Table 9.12 Clotting Time of Blood from a Calf Affected by Sweet Clover Disease When Treated with the Prothrombin Fraction from a Normal Animal or an Affected Animal

	Prothrombin Fraction Prepared from Plasma of			
	Normal calf			Affected calf
mL added	0.5	1.0	2.5	0.5
min to clot	60	45	20	>360

Source: Roderick, L.M., *Am. J. Physiol.*, 96: 413–425, 1931.

What conclusions can you draw from these results?

The toxin present in spoiled sweet clover hay was identified as dicumarol (Figure 11.10); it is formed by the oxidation of coumarin naturally present in sweet clover. Once dicumarol was available in adequate amounts, its mode of action could be investigated; early studies showed that there was a dose-dependent impairment of blood clotting, but with a latent period of 12–24 h before any effect became apparent.

What conclusions can you draw from this observation? Why do you think dicumarol was adopted for use in low doses to reduce blood clotting in patients at risk of thrombosis and in larger amounts as a rat poison?

Further research at the University of Wisconsin resulted in the synthesis of a variety of compounds related to dicumarol that were more potent and had fewer side effects. The most successful of these compounds was called Warfarin (from the initials of the Wisconsin Alumnus Research Fund, which supported the research, see Figure 11.10); it is still the most widely used anticoagulant in clinical use and a commonly used rodenticide.

In 1929, Dam and coworkers* in Copenhagen fed chickens on a fat-free diet and reported the development of subcutaneous and intramuscular hemorrhages as well as impaired blood clotting. They went on to demonstrate that a fat-soluble compound in vegetables, grains, and animal liver would normalize blood clotting when fed to deficient chickens. They proposed the name vitamin K (Section 11.5) for this new nutrient and defined a unit of biological activity as that amount required on three successive days to normalize blood clotting in a deficient animal.

Why do you think the response to vitamin K in deficient animals takes several days to develop?

In 1952, an army recruit attempted suicide by taking rat poison containing Warfarin. On admission to a hospital, he had numerous subcutaneous hemorrhages and was suffering from nosebleeds. His prothrombin time was 54s compared with a normal value of 14s. (The prothrombin time is the time taken for the formation of a fibrin clot in citrated plasma after the addition of calcium ions and thromboplastin to activate the extrinsic clotting system.) He was given

*Dam, H. *Biochem. Z.* 215: 475, 1929.

20 mg of vitamin K intravenously daily for 10 days, after which he recovered, with a normal prothrombin time.

What does this suggest about the way in which Warfarin affects blood clotting?

In animals treated with Warfarin, it is possible to isolate a protein that reacts with the antiserum to prothrombin but has no biological activity. During Warfarin treatment, the concentration of this abnormal, inactive prothrombin in plasma increases and that of active prothrombin decreases. The abnormal prothrombin is less negatively charged than normal prothrombin and does not migrate as rapidly towards the anode on electrophoresis. The addition of calcium ions to a sample of normal prothrombin reduces its electrophoretic mobility but has no effect on the electrophoretic mobility of the abnormal prothrombin. Providing high intakes of vitamin K to Warfarin-treated animals normalizes their blood clotting and leads to disappearance of the abnormal prothrombin and reappearance of active prothrombin with normal calcium-binding capacity.

What conclusions can you draw from these results?

The results of studies of the synthesis of prothrombin in the postmitochondrial supernatant fraction from the liver of vitamin-K deficient rats, incubated with vitamin K added *in vitro*, are shown in Table 9.13.

What conclusions can you draw from these results?

A novel amino acid present in prothrombin is not present in the abnormal prothrombin (now called preprothrombin) formed in vitamin K deficiency or on treatment with Warfarin—γ-carboxyglutamate (abbreviated to Gla). There are 10 Gla residues in the amino terminal region of active prothrombin and these form a binding site for four calcium ions.

All the codons for amino acids are known. How is γ-carboxyglutamate incorporated into prothrombin? What is the likely role of vitamin K in this process?

It has been known for some years that vitamin K must be reduced to its hydroquinone for activity in prothrombin synthesis. In rats

Table 9.13 Prothrombin Synthesis by Postmitochondrial Supernatant Fraction from Liver of Vitamin-K Deficient Rats

Incubation Conditions	Relative Prothrombin Activity (%)
No vitamin K	7 ± 1
+20 μg vitamin K per mL	100
+20 μg vitamin K per mL+cycloheximide	94 ± 1
+20 μg vitamin K per mL+ 2-chlorophytyl-menaquinone	18 ± 1
+20 μg vitamin K per mL+Warfarin	87 ± 3
+20 μg vitamin K per mL, anaerobic	0

Source: From Shah, D.V. and Suttie, J.W., *Biochem. Biophys. Res. Commun.*, 60: 1397–1402, 1974.

treated with Warfarin and given [^{14}C]vitamin K, more than 50% of the radioactivity was found in a new compound—vitamin K epoxide, which has the biological activity of vitamin K in deficient animals. A very small amount is present in the liver of normal animals.

Can you propose the sequence of reactions that vitamin K undergoes in the synthesis of prothrombin? Which step is likely to be inhibited by Warfarin? Can you explain why high intakes of vitamin K will overcome the inhibition of prothrombin synthesis caused by Warfarin?

The classical way of assessing vitamin K nutritional status was by determination of prothrombin time. Can you suggest a more sensitive way of detecting marginal vitamin K deficiency?

Problem 9.3: Vitamin C and collagen synthesis

The vitamin C deficiency disease, scurvy (Section 11.14.3), is characterized by fragility of the blood vessel walls and small subcutaneous hemorrhages around hair follicles (petechial hemorrhages), as well as inflammation of the gums and loss of the dental cement (and hence loss of teeth) and poor healing of wounds. In advanced cases, there is intense deep-bone pain and there may be degenerative changes in the heart, leading to cardiac emergency. In some cases, there are also mood changes (indeed, *scurvy* is the old English word for ill-tempered). It was known from the studies of Lind in 1757 that fresh orange and lemon juice would prevent or cure scurvy; studies during the early part of the twentieth century identified the protective or curative factor as ascorbic acid or vitamin C (see Figure 11.25).

Studies in the 1940s showed that in vitamin C deficiency, there was poor healing of wounds and the scar tissue was weak with little collagen present. The results of studies of the formation of collagen in granulomatous tissue from guinea pigs at different levels of vitamin C nutrition in response to subcutaneous injection of carrageenan are shown in Table 9.14.

What conclusions can you draw from these results?

Isolated fibroblasts synthesize and secrete collagen. If they are incubated with only a low concentration of vitamin C, they secrete a very small amount of collagen and a soluble, gelatine protein accumulates in the rough endoplasmic reticulum. Similarly, incubation of fibroblasts under anaerobic conditions or in the presence of iron-chelating

Table 9.14 Percent Composition of Granulatomous Tissue in Vitamin C Deficient Guinea Pigs after Subcutaneous Injection of Carageenan

	Control Animals	Vitamin C Deficient
Collagen	11.6 ± 0.64	2.3 ± 0.14
Water	66.0	85.0

Source: Robertson, W.v.B. and Schwartz, B., *J. Biol. Chem.*, 201: 689–696, 1953.

compounds also prevents the secretion of normal collagen and leads to the accumulation of the soluble gelatine-like protein in the rough endoplasmic reticulum.

What conclusions can you draw from these observations?

One of the characteristic features of collagen is its relatively high content of hydroxy-proline (Hyp). Table 9.15 shows the incorporation of radioactivity into guinea pig granuloma tissue incubated with [^{14}C]proline or [^{14}C]hydroxyproline.

What conclusions can you draw from these results?

Figure 9.20 shows the incorporation of [^{14}C]proline into proline and hydroxyproline in a cell-free system from chick embryos.

What conclusions can you draw from these results?

Table 9.16 shows the incorporation of [^{3}H]proline into hydroxyproline in collagen formed by granuloma tissue from control and vitamin C deficient (scorbutic) guinea pigs, and Table 9.17 shows the effect of inhibiting protein synthesis on the stimulation by ascorbate of proline hydroxylation in mouse fibroblasts in culture.

Table 9.15 Incorporation of Radioactivity into Collagen from [^{14}C]Proline and [^{14}C]Hydroxyproline

	Tissue Incubated with	
Radioactivity (dpm/μmol)	[^{14}C]Proline	[^{14}C]Hydroxyproline
Free amino acids in tissue	2400	3500
Hydroxyproline in collagen	465	2.3[a]

[a] In samples maintained at 4°C, there was apparent incorporation of 2–2.5 dpm/μmol into hydroxyproline.

Source: Green, N.M. and Lowther, D.A., *Biochem. J.*, 71: 55–66, 1959.

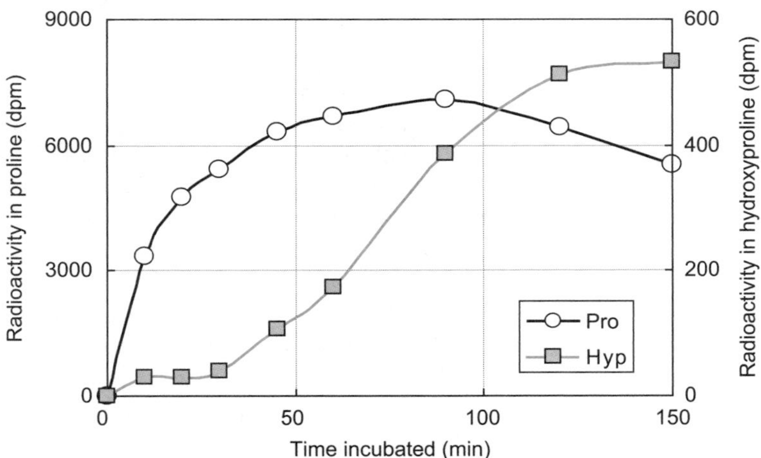

Figure 9.20 Incorporation of label from [^{14}C]proline into proline and hydroxyproline in proteins synthesized by a cell-free system. (From Peterkovsky, B. and Udenfriend, S., *J. Biol. Chem.*, 38: 3966–3977, 1963.)

Table 9.16 Incorporation of Radioactivity from [^{3}H]Proline into Hydroxyproline in Collagen Formed by Granuloma Tissue from Control and Vitamin C Deficient (Scorbutic) Guinea Pigs

	Radioactivity (dpm) in Hydroxyproline in Tissue from	
Time Incubated (min)	**Control Animals**	**Vitamin C Deficient Animals**
30	2400	100
60	5070	150
120	8700	360

Source: Stone, N. and Meister, A., *Nature*, 194: 555–557, 1962.

Table 9.17 The Effects of Inhibiting Protein Synthesis on the Stimulation by Ascorbate of Proline Hydroxylation in Mouse Fibroblasts in Culture

	Radioactivity in Hydroxyproline (dpm/mg protein)
No addition	27,700
+2.5 × 10^{-4} mol/L ascorbate	58,800
+Actinomycin D, then ascorbate 15 min later	58,700

Source: Stassen, F.L.H. et al., *Proc. Nat. Acad. Sci.*, 70: 1090–1093, 1973.

Table 9.18 The Disappearance of α-Ketoglutarate and Appearance of Hydroxyproline during Incubation of Purified Prolyl Hydroxylase

α-Ketoglutarate (nmol)			
Initial	**Remaining**	**Utilized**	**Proline Hydroxylated (nmol)**
15.1	1.3	?	13.7
31.6	3.2	?	28.2
46.0	8.0	?	40.1
64.6	16	?	47.7

Source: Rhoads, R.E. and Udenfriend, S., *Proc. Natl. Acad. Sci.*, 60: 1473–1478, 1968.

What conclusions can you draw from these results?

Prolyl hydroxylase has been purified. It requires ascorbate, molecular oxygen, and iron (Fe^{2+}) for activity. There is no change in the redox state of the iron during the reaction. In addition, with the purified enzyme there is an absolute requirement for α-ketoglutarate for activity. Table 9.18 shows the disappearance of ketoglutarate and appearance of hydroxyproline on incubation of purified prolyl hydroxylase.

What is the approximate ratio of ketoglutarate utilized to hydroxyproline formed? What conclusions can you draw from these results?

Studies with $^{18}O_2$ showed that one atom of oxygen is incorporated into hydroxyproline and the other into succinate formed by oxidative decarboxylation of ketoglutarate.

What conclusions can you draw from these results?

There is oxidation of ascorbate during the hydroxylation of proline, but much less than 1 mol of ascorbate is oxidized per mole of hydroxyproline or succinate formed, or of O_2 consumed. Figure 9.21 shows the hydroxylation of proline-containing peptides by purified prolyl hydroxylase in the presence and absence of ascorbate. The upper graph shows the results for incubation over 1 min; during the first 10 s, the enzyme catalyzes hydroxylation of ~30 mol of proline per mole of enzyme in the absence of ascorbate. The lower graph shows the results of incubation for 5 min, as well as the addition of ascorbate to the ascorbate-free incubation after 3 min. After 2 min of incubation without added ascorbate, the protein-bound iron had been oxidized from Fe^{2+} to Fe^{3+} and was reduced back to Fe^{2+} on addition of ascorbate.

What conclusions can you draw from these results? Can you explain the role of ascorbate in proline hydroxylation?

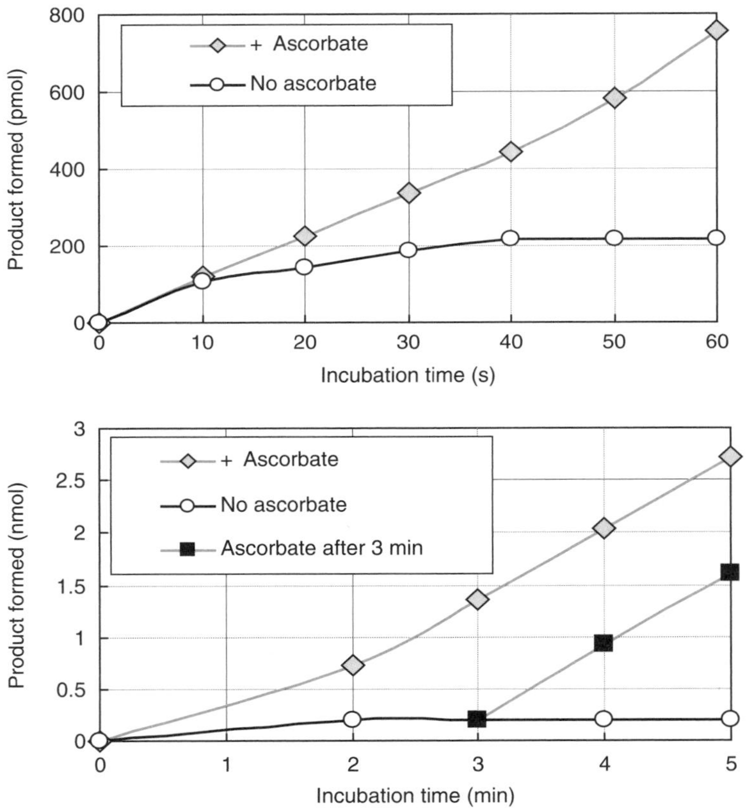

Figure 9.21 Activity of purified prolyl hydroxylase incubated with and without ascorbate. (From Myllylä, R. et al., *Biochem. Biophys. Res. Commun.*, 83: 441–448, 1978.)

Table 9.19 Recovery of Label in Urine after Intravenous Infusion of 20 mmol Urea Labeled with ^{13}C and ^{15}N

mmol/24 h	Initial Study	After Neomycin
Total urine N	609	613
Total urea	500	497
Total urine ^{15}N	34	39
Total urine ^{13}C	0.5	19.5
Urea ^{15}N	29	39
Urea ^{13}C	<0.1	19.5

Problem 9.4: An experiment with ^{13}C- and ^{15}N- labeled urea

The first enzyme to be crystallized (and hence the first evidence that enzymes are proteins) was urease, which catalyzes the hydrolysis of urea to ammonium and carbon dioxide. The original preparation of urease was from plant material, but the enzyme is also known to occur in a number of bacteria. In this study, a group of volunteers were given an intravenous infusion of 20 mmol urea labeled with both ^{13}C and ^{15}N and their urinary excretion of label measured over 24 h. Complete recovery of the label in urine would amount to 40 mmol ^{15}N and 20 mmol ^{13}C. The results are shown in the second column of Table 9.19. The experiment was repeated a week later after they had received the antibiotic neomycin for 4 days to sterilize the gut; these results are shown in the third column.

What conclusions can you draw from these results? What further experiments would you perform to confirm your hypothesis? Which compounds in the bloodstream (other than urea) would you expect to be labeled with ^{15}N in the first experiment? What is the nutritional significance of these observations?

Problem 9.5: Angela P

At the age of 28 weeks, Angela was admitted to the accident and emergency department of her local hospital in a coma, having suffered a convulsion after feeding. She had a mild infection and slight fever at the time. Since birth, she had been a sickly child and had frequently vomited and become drowsy after feeding. She was bottle-fed and at one time cow's milk allergy was suspected, although the problems persisted when she was fed on a soybean milk substitute.

On admission she was mildly hypoglycemic, ketotic, and with plasma pH 7.29. Analysis of a blood sample showed normal levels of insulin, but considerable hyperammonemia (plasma ammonium ion concentration 500 µmol/L; reference range 40–80 µmol/L). She responded well to intravenous glucose infusion and enteral administration of lactulose, regaining consciousness, although she showed poor muscle tone.

Table 9.20 Activity of Enzymes of the Urea Synthesis Cycle in Liver Biopsy Samples from Angela P on Admission and after 4 Days on a High Carbohydrate, Low Protein Diet, Compared with Activities in Postmortem Samples from Six Infants of the Same Age

	Product Formed (μmol/min /mg protein)		
	Angela P		
	On Admission	After 4 Days	Control
Carbamyl phosphate synthetase	0.337	1.45	1.30 ± 0.40
Ornithine carbamyltransferase	29.0	28.6	18.1 ± 4.9
Argininosuccinate synthetase	0.852	0.75	0.49 ± 0.09
Argininosuccinase	1.19	0.95	0.64 ± 0.15
Arginase	183	175	152 ± 56

A liver biopsy sample was taken and the activities of the enzymes of urea synthesis (Figure 9.16) determined and compared with activities in postmortem liver samples from six infants of the same age. The results are shown in Table 9.20. She remained well on a high carbohydrate, low protein diet for several days, although the poor muscle tone and muscle weakness persisted. A second liver biopsy sample was taken after 4 days and the activity of the enzymes determined again.

Her very low-protein diet was continued, but to ensure an adequate supply of essential amino acids for growth she was fed a mixture of the keto-acids of threonine, methionine, leucine, isoleucine, and valine. After each feed, she again became abnormally drowsy and markedly ketotic, with significant acidosis. Her plasma ammonium ion concentration was within the normal range and a glucose tolerance test was normal, with a normal increase in insulin secretion after glucose load.

High pressure liquid chromatography of her plasma revealed an abnormally high concentration of propionic acid (24 μmol/L; reference range 0.7–3.0 μmol/L). Urine analysis showed considerable excretion of methylcitrate (1.1 μmol/mg creatinine), which is not normally detectable. She was also excreting a significant amount of short-chain acyl carnitine (mainly propionyl carnitine)—28.6 μmol/24 h, compared with a reference range of 5.7 ± 3.5 μmol/24 h.

The metabolism of a test dose of [^{13}C]propionate given by intravenous infusion was determined in Angela, her parents, and a group of control subjects; skin fibroblasts were cultured and the activity of propionyl CoA carboxylase determined by incubation with propionate and $NaH^{14}CO_3$, followed by acidification and measurement of the radioactivity in products. The results are shown in Table 9.21.

Table 9.21 Metabolism of [^{13}C]Propionate

	Angela	Mother	Father	Controls
Percent recovered in $^{13}CO_2$ over 3 h	1.01	32.6	33.5	65 ± 5
dpm fixed per mg fibroblast protein per 30 min	5.0	230	265	561 ± 45

Table 9.22 Liver and Muscle Carnitine

	Liver		Muscle	
Wet Weight Tissue (μmol/g)	Angela P	Control	Angela P	Control
Total carnitine	0.23	0.83 ± 0.26	1.56	2.29 ± 0.75
Free carnitine	0.05	0.41 ± 0.17	0.29	1.62 ± 0.67
Short-chain acylcarnitine	0.16	0.37 ± 0.20	1.16	0.58 ± 0.32
Long-chain acylcarnitine	0.01	0.05 ± 0.02	0.11	0.09 ± 0.03

The results of measuring carnitine in the first liver biopsy sample and in a muscle biopsy sample gave the results shown in Table 9.22.

What conclusions can you draw from these results? Can you explain the biochemical basis of Angela's condition?

chapter ten

The integration and control of metabolism

There is an obvious need to regulate metabolic pathways within individual cells so as to ensure that catabolic and biosynthetic pathways do not attempt to operate at the same time. There is also a need to integrate and coordinate metabolism throughout the body so as to ensure a steady provision of metabolic fuels and control the extent to which different fuels are used by different tissues.

Objectives

After reading this chapter you, should be able to

- Explain what is meant by instantaneous, fast, and slow mechanisms of metabolic control
- Describe and explain allosteric regulation of enzyme activity
- Describe and explain the regulation of glycolysis, explain what is meant by substrate cycling and why it is important
- Describe and explain the hormonal control of glycogen synthesis and utilization
- Describe and explain the role of G-proteins and second messengers in signal transduction in response to fast-acting hormones and explain how there is amplification of the hormone signal
- Describe and explain the mechanisms involved in response to slow-acting hormones and explain how there is amplification of the hormone signal
- Describe and explain the role of insulin and the insulin receptor substrate in short- and long-term metabolic control
- Describe and explain hormonal control of the fed and fasting states; hormonal control of adipose tissue and liver metabolism
- Describe and explain the factors involved in the selection of fuels for muscle activity under different conditions
- Describe and explain the biochemical basis of the metabolic derangements in diabetes mellitus and the metabolic syndrome

10.1 Patterns of metabolic regulation

The rate at which different pathways operate is controlled by changes in the activity of key enzymes. In general, the first reaction unique to a given pathway or branch of a pathway will be most subject to regulation, although the activities of other enzymes are also regulated. The enzymes that exert the greatest control over flux (flow of metabolites) through a pathway are often those that catalyze essentially unidirectional reactions, that is, those for which the substrates and products are far from thermodynamic equilibrium.

Within any one cell, the activities of regulatory enzymes may be controlled by two mechanisms that act instantaneously:

- The availability of substrates
- Inhibition or activation by accumulation of precursors, end products, or intermediates of a pathway

On a whole-body basis, metabolic regulation is achieved by the actions of hormones. A hormone is released from the endocrine gland in which it is synthesized in response to a stimulus such as the blood concentration of metabolic fuels, circulates in the bloodstream, and acts only on target cells that have receptors for the hormone. In addition, there are locally acting hormones (sometimes called paracrine agents) that are secreted into the interstitial fluid (rather than the bloodstream) by cells that are close to target cells. There are also compounds that are secreted by cells that act on the secretory cells themselves—these are autocrine agents.

There are two types of response to hormones:

- Fast responses due to changes in the activity of existing enzymes, as a result of covalent modification of the enzyme protein. Fast-acting hormones activate cell-surface receptors, leading to the release of a second messenger inside the cell. The second messenger then acts directly or indirectly to activate an enzyme that catalyzes the covalent modification of the target enzymes.
- Slow responses due to changes in the rate of synthesis of enzymes. Slow-acting hormones activate intracellular receptors that bind to regulatory regions of DNA and increase or decrease the rate of transcription of one or more genes (Section 9.2.2.1).

Regardless of the mechanism by which a hormone acts to regulate a pathway, there are three key features of hormonal regulation:

- Tissue selectivity, determined by whether or not the tissue contains receptors for the hormone
- Amplification of the hormone signal
- A mechanism to terminate or reverse the hormone action as its secretion decreases

10.2 Intracellular regulation of enzyme activity

As discussed in Section 2.3.3, the rate at which an enzyme catalyzes a reaction increases with increasing concentration of substrate, until the enzyme is more or less saturated. This means that an enzyme that has a high K_m relative to the usual concentration of its substrate will be sensitive to changes in substrate availability. By contrast, an enzyme that has a low K_m relative to the usual concentration of its substrate will act at a more or less constant rate regardless of changes in substrate availability (see Problem 2.1).

The availability of substrate may be regulated by uptake from the bloodstream—for example, muscle and adipose tissue only take up glucose to any significant extent in response to insulin. In the absence of insulin, the glucose transporters are in intracellular vesicles; in response to insulin, these vesicles migrate to the cell surface and fuse with the cell membrane, revealing active glucose transporters.

10.2.1 Allosteric modification of the activity of regulatory enzymes

Allosteric regulation of enzyme activity is due to reversible, noncovalent binding of effectors to regulatory sites, leading to a change in the conformation of the active site. This may result in either increased catalytic activity (allosteric activation) or decreased catalytic activity (allosteric inhibition). Enzymes that are subject to allosteric regulation are usually multiple subunit proteins.

Many enzymes that are subject to allosteric regulation have two interconvertible conformations (Figure 10.1):

- A relaxed (R) form, which binds substrates well, and therefore has high catalytic activity. Allosteric activators bind to and stabilize the active R form of the enzyme.
- A tense (T) form, which binds substrates poorly, and therefore has low catalytic activity. Allosteric inhibitors bind to and stabilize the less active T form of the enzyme.

Compounds that act as allosteric inhibitors are often end products of the pathway, and this type of inhibition is known as end-product inhibition. The decreased rate of enzyme activity results in a lower rate of formation of a product that is present in adequate amounts.

Compounds that act as allosteric activators of enzymes are often precursors of the pathway, so this is a mechanism for feed-forward activation, increasing the activity of a controlling enzyme in anticipation of increased availability of substrate.

Enzymes that consist of multiple subunits frequently display cooperativity between the subunits, so that binding of substrate to the active site of one subunit leads to conformational changes that enhance the binding of substrate to the other active sites of the complex (Section 2.3.3.3). This again is allosteric activation of the enzyme, in this case by the substrate

Allosteric inhibition
The inhibitor stabilizes the T form of the enzyme, which binds substrate poorly
Inh
T
R
Substrate
Substrate

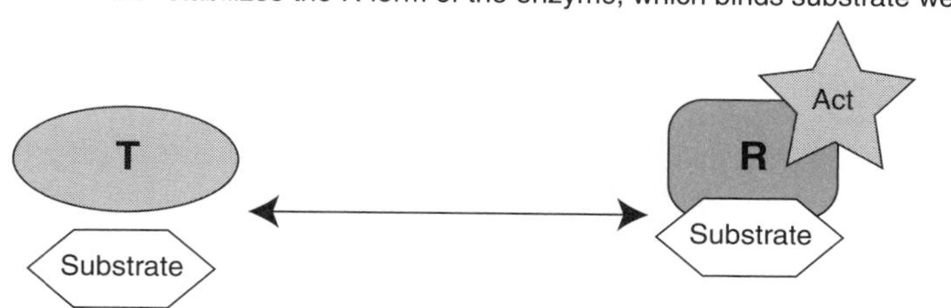

Figure 10.1 Allosteric inhibition and activation of enzymes.

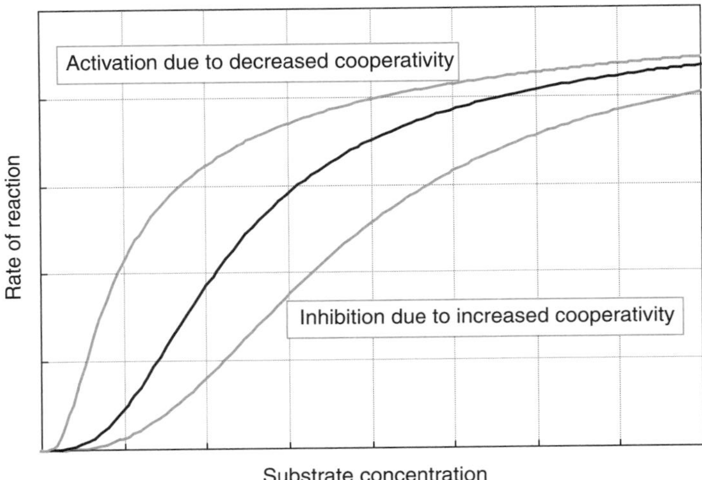

Figure 10.2 Allosteric inhibition and activation of an enzyme showing subunit cooperativity.

itself. The activity of such cooperative enzymes is more sharply dependent on the concentration of substrate than is the case for enzymes that do not show cooperativity.

As shown in Figure 10.2, an allosteric activator of an enzyme that shows substrate cooperativity acts by decreasing the cooperativity, so that the enzyme has a greater activity at a low concentration of the substrate than would otherwise be the case. Conversely, an allosteric inhibitor of a cooperative enzyme acts by increasing cooperativity, so that the enzyme has less activity at a low concentration of substrate than it would in the absence of the inhibitor.

10.2.2 Control of glycolysis—the allosteric regulation of phosphofructokinase

In glycolysis, most control is at the level of phosphofructokinase, which catalyzes the (irreversible) phosphorylation of fructose 6-phosphate to fructose 1,6-bisphosphate (Figure 5.10). In gluconeogenesis, the hydrolysis of fructose 1,6-bisphosphate is catalyzed by a separate enzyme, fructose bisphosphatase. Regulation of the activities of these two enzymes determines whether the overall metabolic flux is in the direction of glycolysis or gluconeogenesis.

Inhibition of phosphofructokinase leads to an accumulation of glucose 6-phosphate in the cell, and this results in inhibition of hexokinase, which has an inhibitory binding site for its product. The result of this is a decreased rate of entry of glucose into glycolysis. In addition to hexokinase, the liver also contains glucokinase, which is not inhibited by glucose 6-phosphate (Section 5.3.1). This means that despite inhibition of utilization of glucose as a metabolic fuel, the liver can take up glucose for glycogen synthesis (Section 5.6.3).

10.2.2.1 Feedback control of phosphofructokinase

ATP can be considered to be an end product of glycolysis, and phosphofructokinase is allosterically inhibited by ATP binding at a regulatory site that is distinct from the substrate-binding site for ATP. As shown in Figure 10.3, at physiological concentrations of ATP, phosphofructokinase has very low activity and a more markedly sigmoid dependency on the concentration of its substrate.

When there is a requirement for increased glycolysis, and hence increased ATP production, this inhibition is relieved and there may be a 100-fold or higher increase in

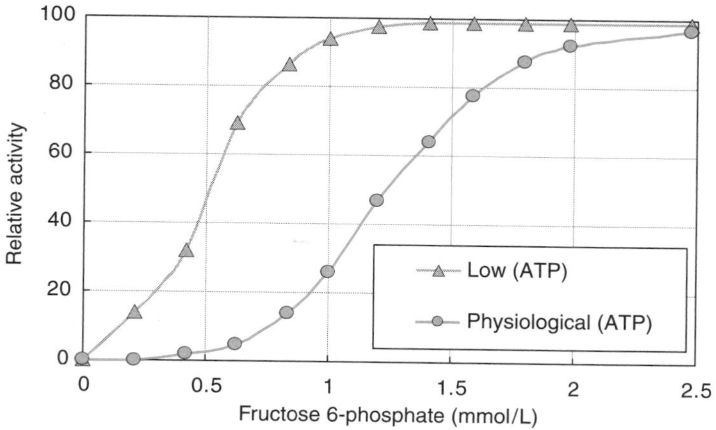

Figure 10.3 The substrate dependence of phosphofructokinase at low and physiological concentrations of ATP.

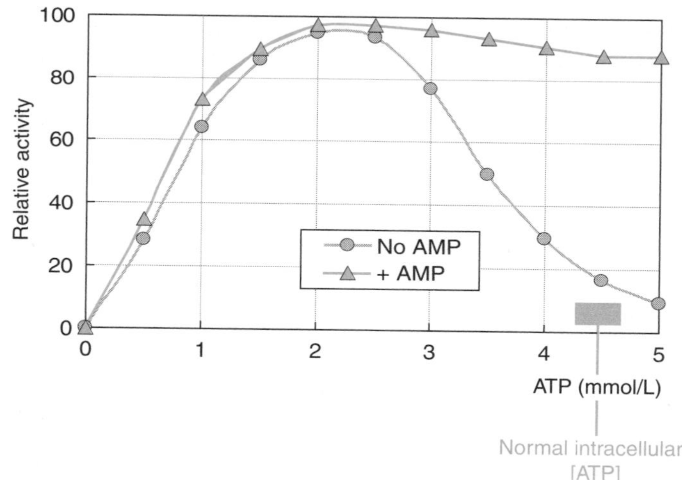

Figure 10.4 The inhibition of phosphofructokinase by ATP and relief of inhibition by 5′-AMP.

glycolytic flux in response to increased demand for ATP. However, there is less than a 10% change in the intracellular concentration of ATP. Figure 10.4 shows the inhibition of phosphofructokinase by ATP; a 10% change would not have a significant effect on the activity of the enzyme. As the concentration of ADP begins to increase, adenylate kinase catalyzes the reaction:

$$2 \times \text{ADP} \rightleftharpoons \text{ATP} + 5'\text{AMP}$$

5′AMP acts as a sensitive intracellular signal that energy reserves are low and ATP formation must be increased. It binds to phosphofructokinase and both reverses the inhibition caused by ATP and decreases the cooperativity between the subunits, so that the enzyme has greater affinity for fructose 6-phosphate. AMP also binds to fructose 1,6-bisphosphatase, reducing its activity.

In liver and adipose tissue, citrate in excess of requirements for citric acid cycle activity leaves mitochondria to provide a source of acetyl CoA for fatty acid synthesis (Section 5.6.1). As citrate accumulates in the cytosol in excess of the need for fatty acid synthesis, it inhibits phosphofructokinase, thereby reducing its own formation. In muscle, creatine phosphate (Section 3.2.3.1) has a similar effect.

Phosphoenolpyruvate is synthesized in the liver for gluconeogenesis (Section 5.7); under these conditions there is obviously a need to inhibit glycolysis, and phosphoenolpyruvate inhibits phosphofructokinase.

10.2.2.2 Feed-forward control of phosphofructokinase

High intracellular concentrations of fructose 6-phosphate activate a second enzyme, phosphofructokinase-2, which catalyzes the synthesis of fructose 2,6-bisphosphate from fructose 6-phosphate (Figure 10.5). Fructose 2,6-bisphosphate is an allosteric activator of phosphofructokinase and an allosteric inhibitor of fructose 1,6-bisphosphatase. It thus acts both to increase glycolysis and inhibit gluconeogenesis. This is feed-forward control—allosteric activation of phosphofructokinase because there is an increased concentration of substrate available.

Phosphofructokinase-2 is a bifunctional enzyme—a single protein with two catalytic sites. One site is the kinase that catalyzes the phosphorylation of fructose 6-phosphate to fructose 2,6-bisphosphate, while the other is the phosphatase that catalyzes hydrolysis of fructose 2,6-bisphosphate to fructose 6-phosphate and inorganic phosphate. A single regulatory site controls the activity of the two catalytic sites in opposite directions. In response to glucagon (which stimulates gluconeogenesis and inhibits glycolysis; Section 10.3), kinase activity is decreased and phosphatase activity increased. This results in a low concentration of fructose 2,6-bisphosphate, and hence decreased activity of phosphofructokinase and increased activity of fructose 1,6-bisphosphatase.

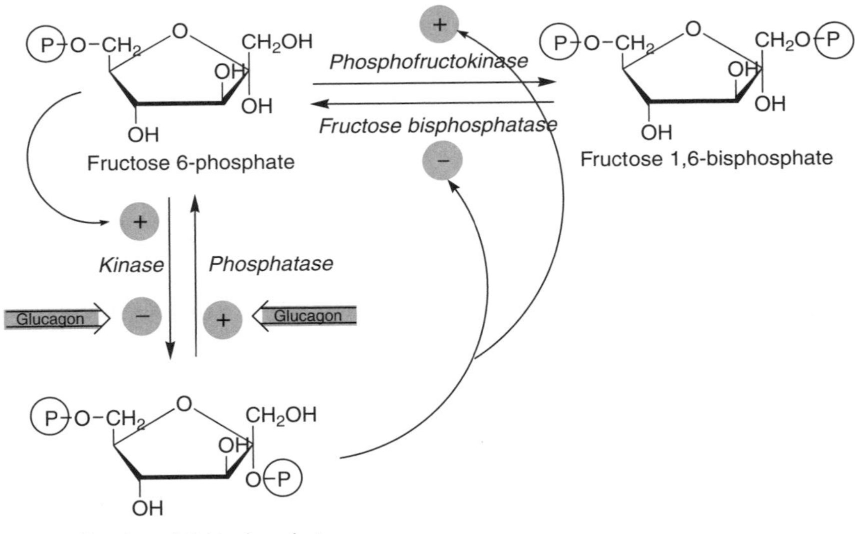

Figure 10.5 The role of 2,6-fructose bisphosphate in regulation of phosphofructokinase.

10.2.2.3 Substrate cycling

A priori, it would seem obvious that the activities of opposing enzymes such as phosphofructokinase and fructose 1,6-bisphosphatase should be regulated in such a way that one is active and the other inactive at any time. If both were active at the same time, then there would be cycling between fructose 6-phosphate and fructose 1,6-bisphosphate, with hydrolysis of ATP—a so-called futile cycle.

However, both enzymes are indeed active to some extent at the same time, although the activity of one is considerably greater than the other, so there is a net metabolic flux. A relatively small change in the activity of both enzymes (in opposite directions) will lead to a very large change in the rate of flux through the pathway. This permits rapid and sensitive control.

Another function of substrate cycling is thermogenesis—deliberate hydrolysis of ATP for heat production. It is not known to what extent substrate cycling can be increased to enhance thermogenesis (which is normally mediated by uncoupling of electron transport and oxidative phosphorylation; Section 3.3.1.4). However, it is noteworthy that the honey bee, which does not exhibit significant substrate cycling, cannot fly in cold weather, while the bumble bee, which has adaptive substrate cycling, can initiate thermogenesis and so fly in cold weather.

10.3 Responses to fast-acting hormones by covalent modification of enzyme proteins

A number of regulatory enzymes have a serine (or sometimes a tyrosine or threonine) residue at a regulatory site. This can undergo phosphorylation catalyzed by a protein kinase (Figure 10.6), which may increase or decrease the activity of the enzyme. Later, the phosphate group is removed from the enzyme by phosphoprotein phosphatase, thus restoring the enzyme to its original state. These responses are not instantaneous, but they are rapid, with a maximum response within a few seconds of hormone stimulation.

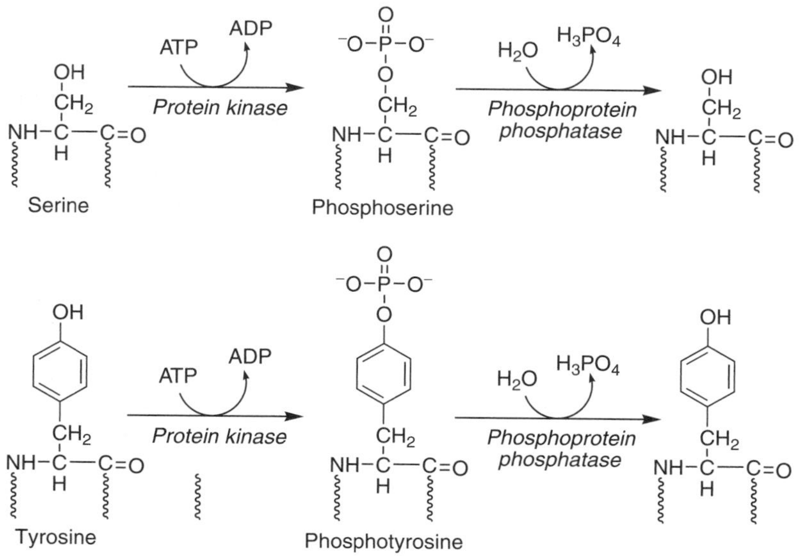

Figure 10.6 Regulation of enzyme activity by phosphorylation and dephosphorylation.

The reduction in activity of pyruvate dehydrogenase in response to increased concentrations of acetyl CoA and NADH (Section 10.5.2) is the result of phosphorylation. This control of enzyme phosphorylation by substrates is unusual. In most cases, the activities of protein kinases and phosphoprotein phosphatases are regulated by second messengers released intracellularly in response to fast-acting hormones binding to receptors at the cell surface. 5′-AMP, formed by the action of adenylate kinase (Section 10.2.2.1), also activates a protein kinase; in this case, it is acting as an intracellular messenger in response to changes in ATP availability, rather than in response to an external stimulus.

The hormonal regulation of glycogen synthesis and utilization is one of the best understood of such mechanisms. Two enzymes are involved, and obviously it is not desirable that both enzymes be active at the same time:

- Glycogen synthase catalyzes the synthesis of glycogen, adding glucose units from UDP-glucose (Section 5.6.3 and Figure 5.31).
- Glycogen phosphorylase catalyzes the removal of glucose units from glycogen as glucose 1-phosphate (Section 5.6.3.1 and Figure 5.9).

In response to insulin (secreted in the fed state), there is increased synthesis of glycogen and inactivation of glycogen phosphorylase. In response to glucagon (secreted in the fasting state) or adrenaline (secreted in response to fear or fright), there is inactivation of glycogen synthase and activation of glycogen phosphorylase, permitting mobilization of glucose from glycogen reserves. As shown in Figure 10.7, both effects are mediated by protein phosphorylation and dephosphorylation.

Protein kinase is activated in response to glucagon or adrenaline:

- Phosphorylation of glycogen synthase results in loss of activity.
- Phosphorylation of glycogen phosphorylase results in activation of the inactive enzyme.

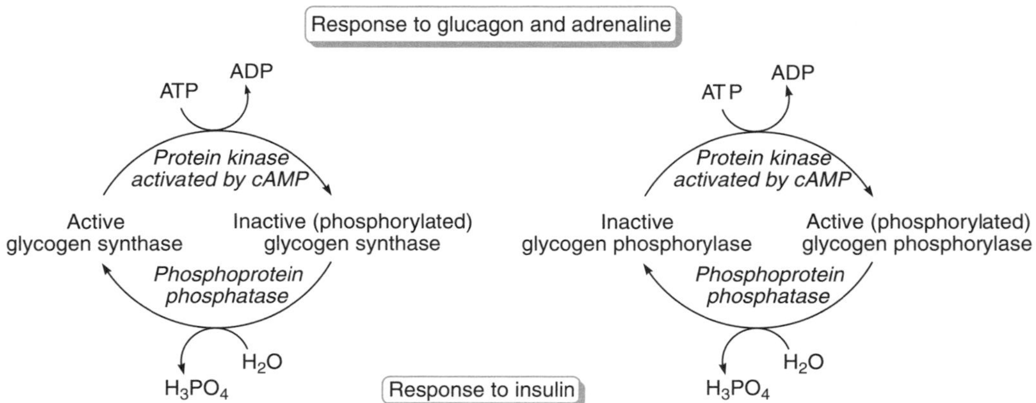

Figure 10.7 Hormonal regulation of glycogen synthase and glycogen phosphorylase: responses to glucagon or adrenaline and insulin.

Phosphoprotein phosphatase is activated in response to insulin:

- Dephosphorylation of phosphorylated glycogen synthase restores its activity.
- Dephosphorylation of phosphorylated glycogen phosphorylase results in loss of activity.

There is a further measure of instantaneous control by intracellular metabolites that can override this hormonal regulation:

- Inactive glycogen synthase is allosterically activated by high concentrations of glucose 6-phosphate.
- Active glycogen phosphorylase is allosterically inhibited by ATP, glucose, and glucose 6-phosphate.

10.3.1 Membrane receptors and G-proteins

A cell responds to a fast-acting hormone if it has cell-surface receptors for the hormone. The receptors are transmembrane proteins; at the outer face of the membrane, they have a site that binds the hormone in the same way as an enzyme binds its substrate, by noncovalent equilibrium binding.

When the receptor binds the hormone, it undergoes a conformational change that permits it to interact with proteins at the inner face of the membrane. These are known as G-proteins because they bind guanine nucleotides (GDP or GTP). They function to transmit information from an occupied membrane receptor protein to an intracellular effector, which in turn leads to the release into the cytosol of a second messenger, ultimately resulting in the activation of protein kinases.

The G-proteins that are important in hormone responses consist of three subunits, α, β, and γ (Figure 10.8). In the resting state, the α subunit has GDP bound and is separate from the βγ dimer. When the receptor is occupied by the hormone, it undergoes a conformational change and recruits the subunits to form a G-protein trimer–receptor complex. The complex then binds GTP, which displaces the bound GDP. Once GTP has been bound, the complex dissociates.

The α subunit of the G-protein with GTP bound then binds to and activates the effector, which may be adenylyl cyclase (Section 10.3.2), phospholipase C (Section 10.3.3), or an ion transport channel in a membrane, resulting in release of a second messenger.

The α subunit has relatively slow GTPase activity that catalyzes hydrolysis of the bound GTP to GDP. As this occurs, the α subunit–effector complex dissociates, and the effector loses its activity. The G-protein subunits are then available to be recruited by another receptor that has been activated by binding the hormone.

10.3.2 Cyclic AMP and cyclic GMP as second messengers

One of the intracellular effectors that is activated by the G-protein α subunit–GTP complex is adenylyl cyclase. This is an integral membrane protein that catalyzes the formation of cyclic AMP (cAMP) from ATP (Figure 10.9) as the second messenger in response to hormones such as glucagon and adrenaline. cAMP is an allosteric activator of protein kinases. It is also formed in the same way in response to a number of neurotransmitters.

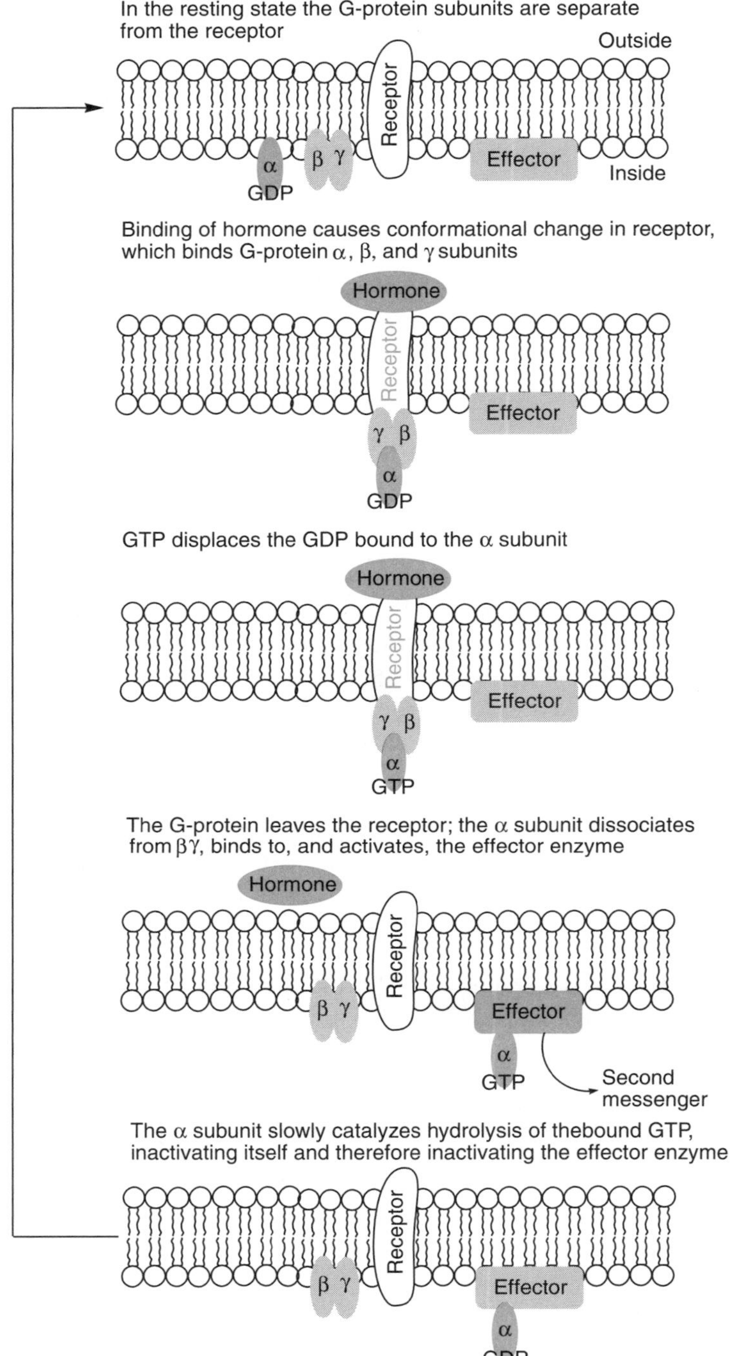

Figure 10.8 The role of G-proteins in the response to fast-acting (surface-acting) hormones.

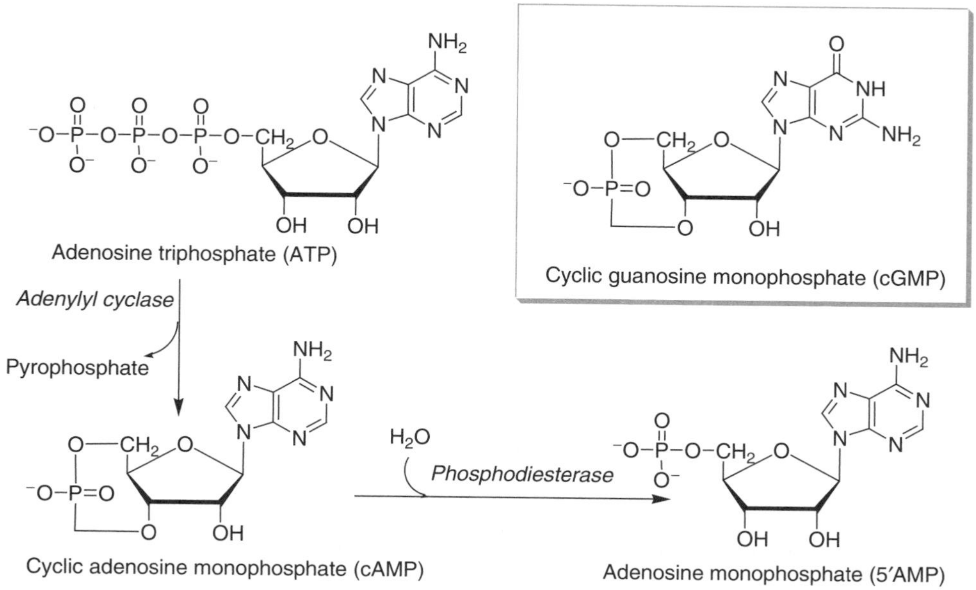

Figure 10.9 Adenylyl cyclase and the formation of cyclic AMP as an intracellular second messenger (the structure of cyclic GMP is shown in the box).

Phosphodiesterase catalyzes the hydrolysis of cAMP to yield 5′-AMP, thus providing a mechanism for termination of the intracellular response to the hormone. Under normal conditions, 5′-AMP is then phosphorylated to ADP by the reaction of adenylate kinase; it is only under conditions of relatively low ATP availability and relatively high ADP that adenylate kinase acts to form 5′-AMP as an intracellular signal of the energy state of the cell (Section 10.2.2.1).

Phosphodiesterase is activated in response to insulin action (which thus acts to terminate the actions of glucagon and adrenaline), and is inhibited by drugs such as caffeine and theophylline, which therefore potentiate hormone and neurotransmitter action.

In the same way that cAMP is formed from ATP by adenylyl cyclase, the guanine analog, cGMP, can be formed from GTP by guanylyl cyclase. This may either be an integral membrane protein, like adenylyl cyclase, or a cytosolic protein. cGMP is produced in response to a number of neurotransmitters and also nitric oxide, the endothelium-derived relaxation factor that is important in vasodilatation.

10.3.2.1 Amplification of the hormone signal

In response to fear or fright, adrenaline is secreted by the adrenal glands; its plasma concentration is in the nanomolar range (10^{-9} mol/L). Within a few seconds, as a result of activation of glycogen phosphorylase in the liver, the blood concentration of glucose rises by several millimoles per liter—an approximately 10^6-fold amplification of the hormone signal.

As shown in Figure 10.10, the active (G-protein α subunit) GTP released in response to binding of 1 mol of hormone to the surface receptor will activate adenylyl cyclase for as long as it contains GTP. The hydrolysis to yield inactive (G-protein α subunit)-GDP occurs relatively slowly; a single molecule of (G-protein α subunit)-GTP will lead to the production of about 40 mol of cAMP as second messenger.

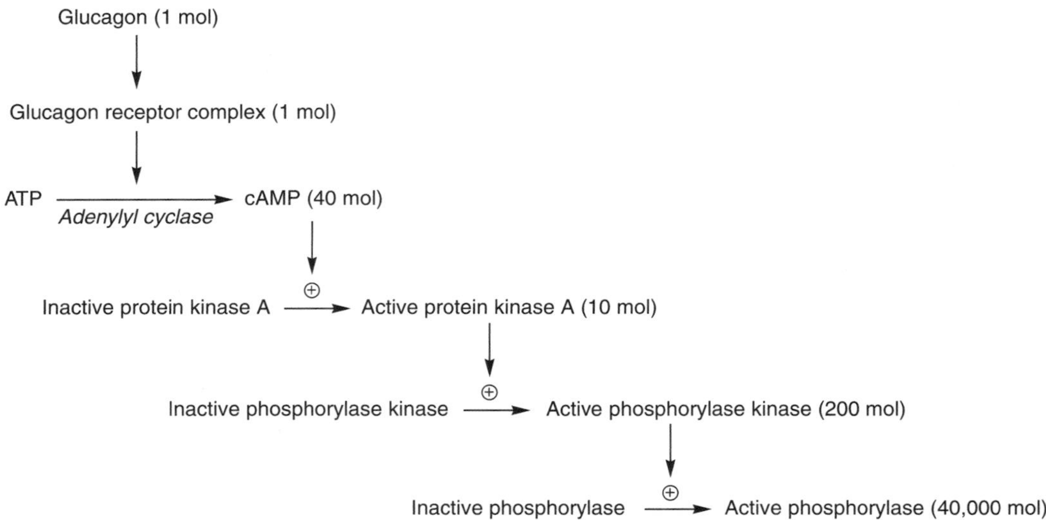

Figure 10.10 Amplification of the hormone signal through a phosphorylation cascade.

There is an equilibrium between cAMP bound to protein kinase and that in free solution in the cytosol, and therefore accessible to phosphodiesterase for inactivation. Each molecule of cAMP activates a molecule of protein kinase for as long as it remains bound, resulting in the phosphorylation of about 20 molecules of phosphorylase kinase.

Phosphorylase kinase remains active until it is dephosphorylated in response to insulin or another counterregulatory hormone, and so phosphorylates some 200 molecules of glycogen phosphorylase. Similarly, glycogen phosphorylase remains active until it is dephosphorylated in response to a counteracting hormone and will catalyze the release of several thousand molecules of glucose 6-phosphate per second.

10.3.3 Inositol trisphosphate and diacylglycerol as second messengers

The other response to G-protein activation involves phosphatidylinositol, one of the phospholipids in cell membranes (Section 4.3.1.2). Phosphatidylinositol can undergo two phosphorylations, catalyzed by phosphatidylinositol kinase, to yield phosphatidylinositol bisphosphate (PIP_2). PIP_2 is a substrate for phospholipase C inside the membrane, which is activated by the binding of a G-protein α subunit with GTP bound. The products of phospholipase C action are inositol trisphosphate (IP_3) and diacylglycerol (Figure 10.11), both of which act as intracellular second messengers.

Inositol trisphosphate opens a calcium transport channel in the membrane of the endoplasmic reticulum. This leads to an influx of calcium from storage in the endoplasmic reticulum and a 10-fold increase in the cytosolic concentration of calcium ions. A number of enzymes are directly sensitive to this increased intracellular calcium, including protein kinase C, which phosphorylates target proteins in the same way as does protein kinase A activated by cAMP (Section 10.3.2).

Calmodulin is a small calcium-binding protein found in all cells. Its affinity for calcium is such that at the resting concentration of calcium in the cytosol (of the order of 0.1 μmol/L), little or none is bound to calmodulin. When the cytosolic concentration of calcium rises to about 1 μmol/L in response to opening of the endoplasmic reticulum calcium transport

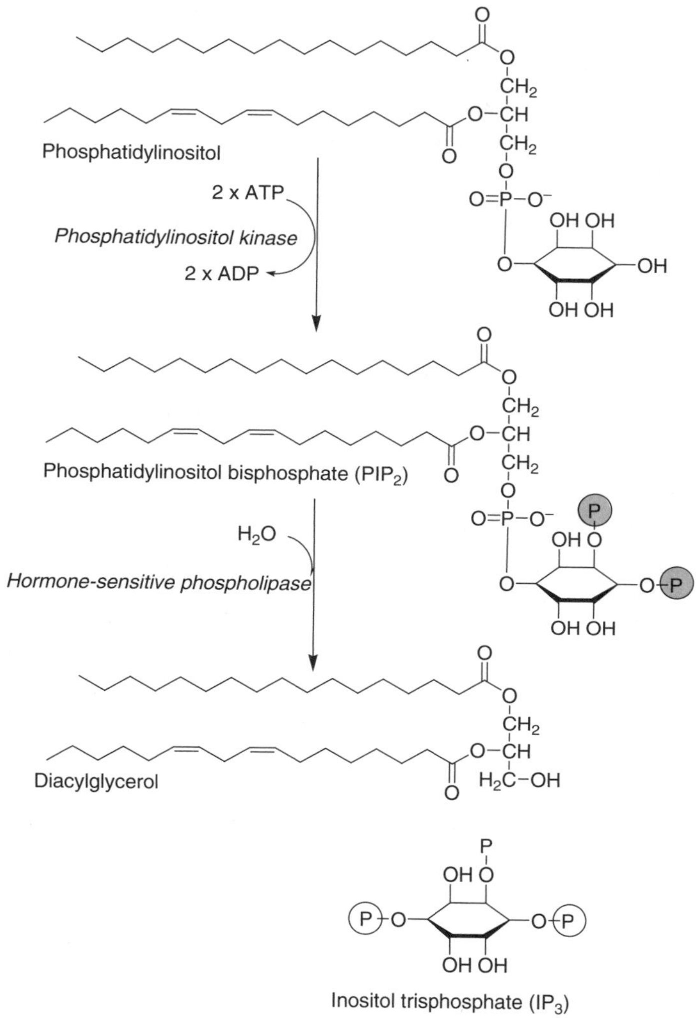

Figure 10.11 Phospholipase and the formation of inositol trisphosphate and diacylglycerol as intracellular messengers.

channel, calmodulin binds 4 mol of calcium per mole of protein. When this occurs, it undergoes a conformational change, and calcium–calmodulin binds to and activates cytosolic protein kinases, which in turn phosphorylate target enzymes.

Some of the diacylglycerol released by phospholipase C action remains in the membrane, where it activates a membrane-bound protein kinase. It also diffuses into the cytosol, where it enhances the binding of calcium–calmodulin to cytosolic protein kinases.

Inositol trisphosphate is inactivated by further phosphorylation to inositol tetrakisphosphate (IP_4), and the diacylglycerol is inactivated by hydrolysis to glycerol and fatty acids.

10.3.3.1 Amplification of the hormone signal

The active (G-protein α subunit) GTP released in response to binding of 1 mol of hormone to the cell-surface receptor will activate phospholipase C for as long as it contains GTP, and therefore a single molecule of (G-protein α subunit) GTP complex will lead to the production of many moles of IP_3 and diacylglycerol as second messengers.

Each molecule of diacylglycerol will activate the membrane-bound protein kinase until it is hydrolyzed (relatively slowly) by lipase, so resulting in the phosphorylation of many molecules of target protein, each of which will catalyze the metabolism of many thousands of moles of substrate per second, until it is dephosphorylated by phosphoprotein phosphatase.

Similarly, each molecule of IP_3 will continue to keep the endoplasmic reticulum calcium channel open until it is phosphorylated to inactive inositol tetrakisphosphate, thus maintaining a flow of calcium ions into the cytosol. Each molecule of calcium–calmodulin will bind to and activate a molecule of protein kinase for as long as the cytosol calcium concentration remains high. It is only as the calcium is pumped back into the endoplasmic reticulum that the calcium concentration falls low enough for calmodulin to lose its bound calcium and be inactivated. Again, each molecule of phosphorylated enzyme will catalyze the metabolism of many thousands of moles of substrate per second, until it is dephosphorylated by phosphoprotein phosphatase.

10.3.4 The insulin receptor

The insulin receptor consists of two α subunits at the outer face of the membrane, which bind insulin, and two β subunits that span the membrane. In response to insulin binding to the α subunit dimer, there is a conformational change in the receptor, leading to activation of the protein kinase activity of the cytosolic region of the β subunits, and autophosphorylation of tyrosine residues on the β subunits. The phosphorylated β subunits then bind and phosphorylate the insulin receptor substrate protein (Figure 10.12).

Phosphorylated insulin receptor substrate can bind to either of two protein kinases:

- Protein kinase B is responsible for initiating the cascade of actions leading to the rapid metabolic responses to insulin—stimulation of glucose transport, glycogen and fatty acid synthesis, inhibition of lipolysis and glycogenolysis, and stimulation of protein synthesis by increasing translation.
- The mitogen-activated protein kinases (MAP kinases) are responsible for initiating a cascade of actions leading to increased gene expression and cell division.

A number of growth-factor receptors act in the same way as the insulin receptor to activate MAP kinases; a mutant of the epidermal growth factor (EGF) receptor is permanently activated, even when not occupied. This results in continuous signaling for cell division and is one of the underlying mechanisms in cancer.

10.4 Slow-acting hormones: changes in enzyme synthesis

There is continual turnover of proteins in the cell, and not all proteins are broken down and replaced at the same rate. Some are relatively stable, while others, and especially enzymes that are important in metabolic regulation, have short half-lives—of the order of minutes or hours (Section 9.1.1). This rapid turnover means that it is possible to control metabolic pathways by changing the rate at which a key enzyme is synthesized, and hence the total amount of that enzyme in the tissue. An increase in the rate of synthesis of an enzyme is induction, while the reverse, a decrease in the rate of synthesis of the enzyme by a metabolite, is repression. A number of key enzymes in metabolic pathways are induced by their substrates, and similarly many are repressed by high concentrations of the end products of the pathways they control.

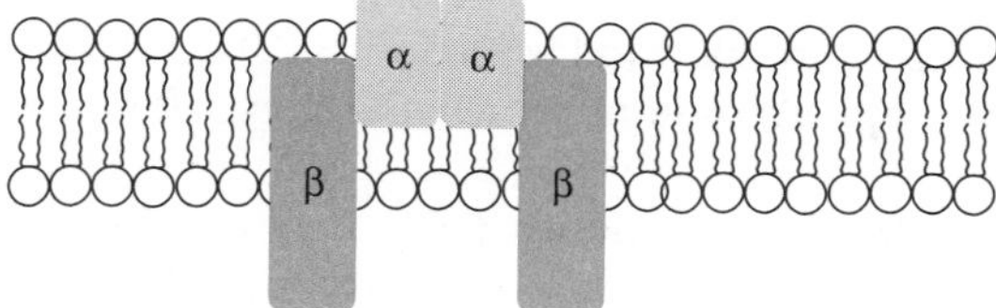

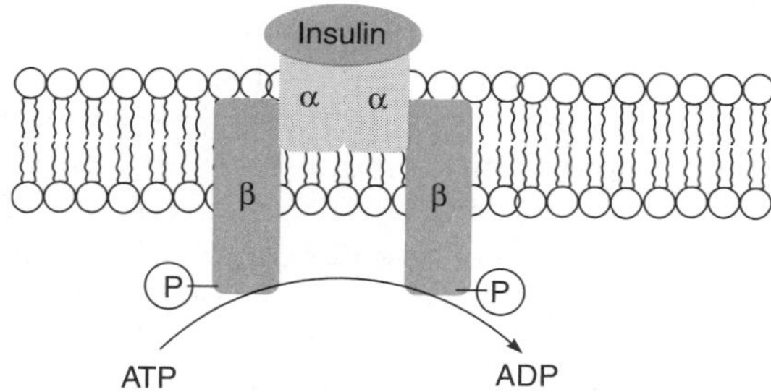

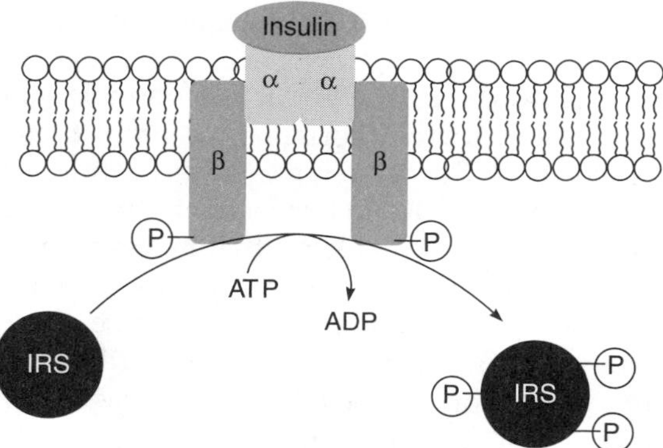

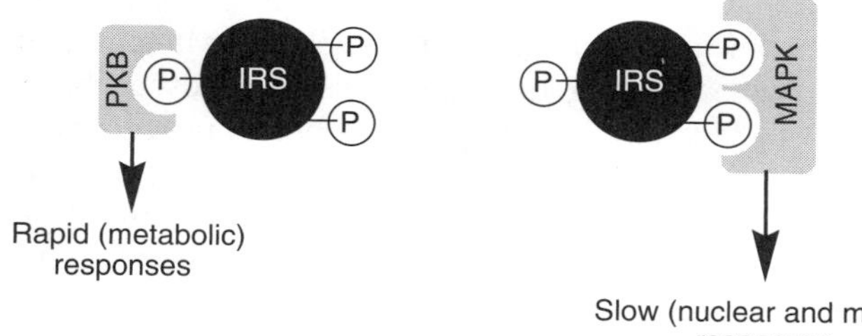

Figure 10.12 Signaling in response to stimulation of the insulin receptor.

Slow-acting hormones—including the steroid hormones such as cortisol and the sex steroids (androgens, estrogens, and progesterone), retinoic acid derived from vitamin A (Section 11.2.3.2), calcitriol derived from vitamin D (Section 11.3.3), and the thyroid hormones (Section 11.15.3.3)—act by changing the rate at which the genes for specific enzymes are expressed.

The responses are slower than for hormones that increase the activity of existing enzyme molecules, because of the need for an adequate amount of new enzyme protein to be synthesized. Similarly, the response is prolonged, because after the hormone has ceased to act there is still an increased amount of enzyme protein in the cell, and the effect will only diminish as the newly synthesized enzyme is catabolized. The time scale of action of slow-acting hormones ranges between a few hours to several days.

The hormone diffuses into the cell and binds to an intracellular receptor protein. Binding of the hormone causes a conformational change in the receptor protein, and loss of a chaperone protein that is bound to the unoccupied receptor. Loss of the chaperone protein reveals a dimerization site on the receptor. The hormone–receptor complex dimerizes and undergoes phosphorylation that enables it to bind to a hormone response element on DNA (Figure 10.13). Binding of the activated hormone–receptor complex to the hormone response element acts as a signal to recruit the various transcription factors required for transcription of the gene, leading to increased synthesis of mRNA (Section 9.2.2.1). Increased synthesis of mRNA results in increased synthesis of the protein (Section 9.2.3).

While some slow-acting hormone receptors form homodimers (two identical receptor proteins, each with hormone bound), others form heterodimers with the vitamin A RXR receptor, which binds 9-*cis*-retinoic acid (Section 11.2.3.2). This means that vitamin A is important in the actions of a number of hormones. Vitamin A deficiency will lead to a lack of occupied RXR to form active heterodimers. However, RXR without 9-*cis*-retinoic acid bound can also form heterodimers with vitamin D and thyroid hormone receptors; these bind to, but do not activate, hormone response elements. Conversely, excessive vitamin A may also impair hormone responses, because the occupied RXR can form a homodimer, meaning that less is available to form heterodimers. There is some evidence that excessive intake of vitamin A impairs vitamin D responsiveness and may be a factor in bone disease (Section 11.3.4).

A cell will only respond to a slow-acting hormone if it synthesizes the receptor protein. The response to the same hormone in different tissues, and at different stages in development, may well be different, because only genes that are expressed in the cell will be induced. The control of gene expression by slow-acting hormones is not a matter of switching on a gene that is otherwise silent; the hormone increases the expression of a gene that is anyway being transcribed at a low rate. Similarly, the secretion of steroid hormones is not a strictly on/off affair, but a matter of changes in the amount being secreted.

Although there is a great deal of information about the molecular mechanisms involved in initiating the responses to nuclear-acting hormones, less is known about the termination of their action. Vitamin B_6 (Section 11.9.2) displaces hormone–receptor complexes from DNA binding, and there is evidence that the responsiveness of target tissues to slow-acting hormones is increased in vitamin B_6 deficiency. As hormone stimulation decreases, the newly synthesized enzymes are catabolized as discussed in Section 9.1.1.1.

10.4.1 *Amplification of the hormone signal*

The amplification of the hormone signal in response to a slow-acting hormone is the result of increased synthesis of mRNA—there is increased transcription for as long as the hormone-receptor complex remains bound to the hormone-response element on DNA.

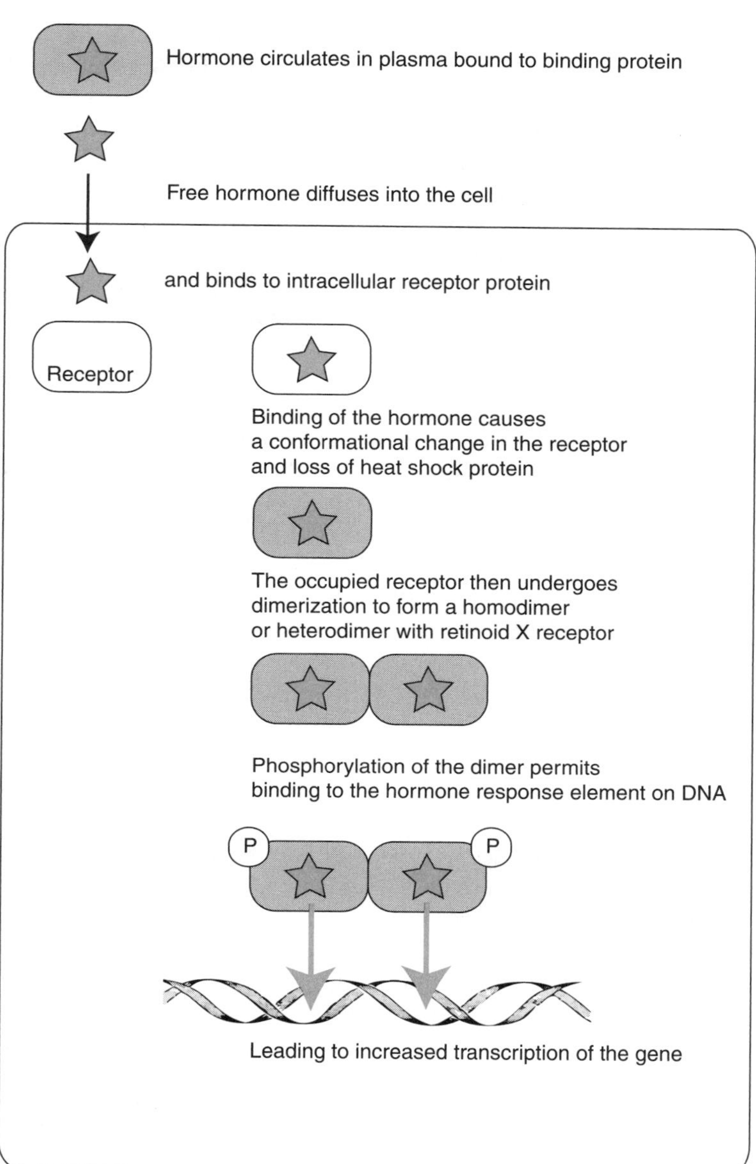

Figure 10.13 The action of steroid hormones.

Each molecule of mRNA is translated many times over, leading to a considerable albeit (relatively) slow increase in the amount of enzyme protein in the cell. Each molecule of enzyme will then catalyze the metabolism of many thousands of moles of substrate per second, until it is catabolized.

10.5 Hormonal control in the fed and fasting states

In the fed state (Figure 5.6), when there is an ample supply of metabolic fuels from the gut, the main processes occurring are synthesis of reserves of triacylglycerol and glycogen;

glucose is in plentiful supply and is the main fuel for most tissues. At the same time, there is an increase in protein synthesis to replace that lost in the fasting state (Section 9.1.1).

In the fasting state (Figure 5.7), the reserves of triacylglycerol and glycogen are mobilized for use; glucose, which is now scarce, must be spared for use by the brain and red blood cells, and protein synthesis slows down, so that there is net protein catabolism, releasing amino acids for gluconeogenesis (Section 5.7).

The principal hormones involved are insulin in the fed state, and glucagon in the fasting state. Adrenaline and noradrenaline share many of the actions of glucagon and act to provide an increased supply of metabolic fuels from triacylglycerol and glycogen reserves in response to fear or fright, regardless of whether or not fuels are being absorbed from the gut.

In liver and muscle, insulin and glucagon act to regulate the synthesis and breakdown of glycogen as shown in Figure 10.7. They also regulate glycolysis (stimulated by insulin and inhibited by glucagon) and gluconeogenesis (inhibited by insulin and stimulated by glucagon). The result of this is that in the fed state, the liver takes up and utilizes glucose to form either glycogen, which is stored in the liver, or triacylglycerol, which is exported to other tissues in very low density lipoproteins (VLDL). By contrast, in the fasting state the liver exports glucose arising from both the breakdown of glycogen and gluconeogenesis. It also oxidizes fatty acids and exports ketone bodies for use by other tissues (Section 5.5.3).

10.5.1 Hormonal control of adipose tissue metabolism

Insulin has three actions in adipose tissue in the fed state (Figure 10.14) described below:

Stimulation of glucose uptake. In the absence of insulin, glucose transporters in adipose tissue are in intracellular vesicles. An early response to insulin is migration of these vesicles to the cell surface, where they fuse with the cell membrane, exposing glucose transporters. This results in an increased rate of glucose uptake, and hence increased glycolysis (Section 5.4.1) and increased availability of acetyl CoA for fatty acid synthesis (Section 5.6.1). In the fasting state, when insulin secretion is low, little or no glucose is taken up into adipose tissue cells.

Induction of lipoprotein lipase. Lipoprotein lipase has a half-life of about 1 h (Table 9.2). It is induced in response to insulin action, and the newly synthesized enzyme migrates to the surface of the blood vessel endothelial walls, where it binds chylomicrons or VLDL (Section 5.6.2) and catalyzes the hydrolysis of triacylglycerol. The nonesterified fatty acids are mainly taken up by adipose tissue and used for synthesis of triacylglycerol reserves.

Inhibition of intracellular lipase (hormone-sensitive lipase). This reduces the hydrolysis of triacylglycerol reserves and halts the release of nonesterified fatty acids into the bloodstream.

cAMP, produced in response to adrenaline and noradrenaline, stimulates protein kinase, which activates intracellular hormone-sensitive lipase and represses the synthesis of lipoprotein lipase. Hormone-sensitive lipase catalyzes the hydrolysis of the triacylglycerol stored in adipose tissue cells, leading to release into the bloodstream of free fatty acids, which are transported bound to albumin, and glycerol, which is a substrate for gluconeogenesis in the liver.

Even in the fed state, there is some release of nonesterified fatty acids into the bloodstream as a result of the extracellular action of lipoprotein lipase—not all the fatty acid released

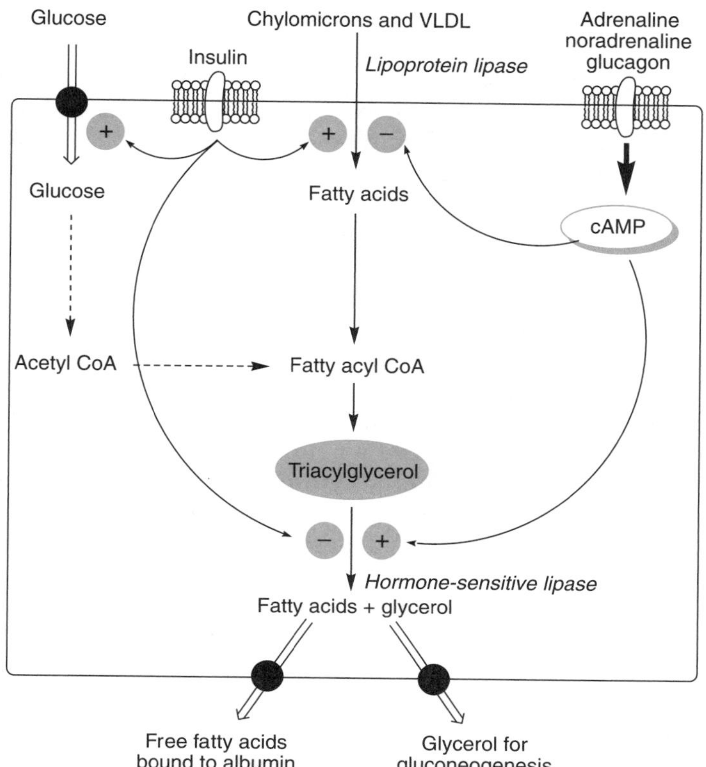

Figure 10.14 Hormonal control of the synthesis and hydrolysis of triacylglycerol in adipose tissue.

enters the adipocytes. In the fed state most of this fatty acid is taken up by the liver, re-esterified to form triacylglycerol, and exported in VLDL (Section 5.6.2.2). This ATP-expensive cycling between lipolysis in adipose tissue and re-esterification in the liver provides a continual supply of nonesterified fatty acid for muscle. The extent to which muscle utilizes fatty acids is determined more by the intensity of physical activity than by their availability (Section 10.6.1), and muscle has a requirement for fatty acids that is independent of the relative concentrations of insulin and glucagon.

10.5.2 Control of lipid metabolism in the liver

The liver synthesizes fatty acids in the fed state and oxidizes them in the fasting state. The direction of metabolic flux (lipogenesis or lipolysis) is controlled in response to insulin and glucagon and also by intracellular concentrations of substrates.

In the fed state, insulin stimulates glycolysis (and inhibits gluconeogenesis), leading to increased formation of pyruvate, which results in increased formation of acetyl CoA and hence increased formation of citrate, which is exported to the cytosol for fatty acid synthesis (Section 5.6.1). Insulin also stimulates the activity of acetyl CoA carboxylase, leading to increased formation of malonyl CoA for fatty acid synthesis (Figure 5.28).

In the fasting state, glucagon has the opposite actions, decreasing glycolysis (and thus reducing the availability of pyruvate, acetyl CoA, and hence citrate for fatty acid synthesis), increasing gluconeogenesis, and decreasing the activity of acetyl CoA carboxylase.

Pyruvate dehydrogenase is inhibited in response to increased acetyl CoA and also an increase in the NADH:NAD$^+$ ratio in the mitochondrion. The concentration of acetyl CoA will be high when β-oxidation of fatty acids is occurring, and there is no need to utilize pyruvate as a metabolic fuel. Similarly, the NADH:NAD$^+$ ratio will be high when there is an adequate amount of metabolic fuel being oxidized in the mitochondrion, so that again pyruvate is not required as a source of acetyl CoA. Under these conditions, pyruvate will mainly be carboxylated to oxaloacetate for gluconeogenesis (Section 5.7).

The regulation of pyruvate dehydrogenase is the result of phosphorylation of the enzyme (Figure 10.6). Pyruvate dehydrogenase kinase is allosterically activated by acetyl CoA and NADH, and catalyzes the phosphorylation of pyruvate dehydrogenase to an inactive form. Pyruvate dehydrogenase phosphatase acts constantly to dephosphorylate the inactive enzyme, thus restoring its activity and maintaining sensitivity to changes in the concentrations of acetyl CoA and NADH.

Citrate only leaves the mitochondria to provide a source of acetyl CoA for fatty acid synthesis when there is an adequate amount to maintain citric acid cycle activity (Section 5.6.1). As citrate accumulates in the cytosol, it acts as a feed-forward activator of acetyl CoA carboxylase, increasing the formation of malonyl CoA. If citrate in the cytosol is not used as a source of acetyl CoA for fatty acid synthesis, it inhibits phosphofructokinase, thus inhibiting its own formation (Section 10.2.2.1).

Fatty acyl CoA in the cytosol implies a high rate of fatty acid uptake from the bloodstream; fatty acyl CoA inhibits acetyl CoA carboxylase, and so reduces the rate of malonyl CoA synthesis and fatty acid synthesis.

Besides being the substrate for fatty acid synthesis, malonyl CoA is important in controlling the β-oxidation of fatty acids. Malonyl CoA is a potent inhibitor of carnitine acyl transferase 1, the mitochondrial outer membrane enzyme that regulates uptake of fatty acyl CoA into the mitochondria (Section 5.5.1). This means that under conditions when fatty acids are being synthesized in the cytosol, they will not be taken up into the mitochondria for β-oxidation (see also Section 10.6.2.1 for a discussion on the role of malonyl CoA in regulating muscle fuel selection).

10.6 Selection of fuel for muscle activity

Muscle can use a variety of fuels:

- Plasma glucose
- Its own reserves of glycogen
- Triacylglycerol from plasma lipoproteins
- Plasma nonesterified fatty acids
- Plasma ketone bodies
- Triacylglycerol from adipose tissue reserves within the muscle

The selection of metabolic fuel depends on the intensity of work being performed, the duration of the exercise, and whether the individual is in the fed or fasting state.

10.6.1 The effect of work intensity on muscle fuel selection

Skeletal muscle contains two types of fibers:

Type I (red muscle) fibers. These are also known as slow-twitch muscle fibers. They are relatively rich in mitochondria and myoglobin (hence their color), and have a high rate of citric acid cycle metabolism, with a low rate of glycolysis. They metabolize mainly fatty acids. These are the fibers used mainly in prolonged, relatively moderate work.

Type II (white muscle) fibers. These are also known as fast-twitch fibers. They are relatively poor in mitochondria and myoglobin and have a high rate of glycolysis. Type IIA fibers also have a high rate of aerobic (citric acid cycle) metabolism, while type IIB have a low rate of citric acid cycle activity and are mainly glycolytic. White muscle fibers are used mainly in high-intensity work of short duration (e.g., sprinting and weight lifting).

Intense physical activity requires rapid production of ATP usually for a relatively short time. Under these conditions, substrates and oxygen cannot enter the muscle at an adequate rate to meet the demand, and muscle depends on anaerobic glycolysis of its glycogen reserves. This leads to the release of lactate into the bloodstream, which is used as a substrate for gluconeogenesis in the liver (Section 5.7). Less intense physical activity is often referred to as aerobic exercise, because it involves mainly red muscle fibers (and type IIA white fibers) and there is less accumulation of lactate.

Resting muscle is relatively poorly perfused with blood and resting muscle tone is largely maintained by anaerobic glycolysis, producing lactate. In response to stimulation, blood flow through the muscle increases, and in moderate exercise there is mainly aerobic metabolism.

The increased rate of glycolysis for exercise is achieved in three ways:

- As ADP begins to accumulate in muscle, it undergoes the reaction catalyzed by adenylate kinase: $2 \times \text{ADP} \rightleftharpoons \text{ATP} + 5'\text{AMP}$. 5′AMP is a potent activator of phosphofructokinase, reversing the inhibition of this key regulatory enzyme by ATP, thus increasing the rate of glycolysis (Section 10.2.2.1).
- Nerve stimulation of muscle results in an increased cytosolic concentration of calcium ions, and hence activation of calmodulin (Section 10.3.3). Calcium–calmodulin activates glycogen phosphorylase, thus increasing the rate of formation of glucose 1-phosphate and providing an increased amount of substrate for glycolysis.
- Adrenaline released from the adrenal glands in response to fear or fright acts on cell-surface receptors, leading to the formation of cAMP, which leads to increased activity of protein kinase and increased activity of glycogen phosphorylase (Figure 10.7).

In prolonged aerobic exercise at a relatively high intensity (e.g., cross-country or marathon running), muscle glycogen and endogenous triacylglycerol are the major fuels initially, with a modest contribution from plasma nonesterified fatty acids and glucose (Figure 10.15). As the exercise continues, and muscle glycogen and triacylglycerol begin to be depleted, plasma nonesterified fatty acids become more important.

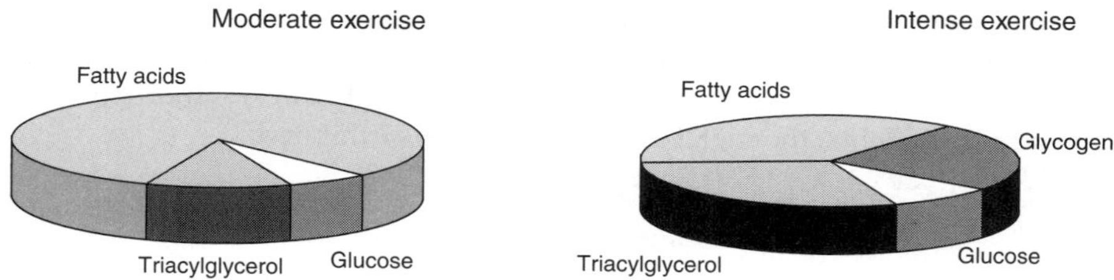

Figure 10.15 Utilization of different metabolic fuels in muscle in moderate and intense exercise.

At more moderate levels of exercise (e.g., gentle jogging or walking briskly), plasma nonesterified fatty acids provide the major fuel. This means that for weight reduction, where the aim is to reduce adipose tissue reserves (Section 7.3), relatively prolonged exercise of moderate intensity is more desirable than shorter periods of more intense exercise. More importantly for overweight people, most of the nonesterified fatty acids that are metabolized in moderate exercise are derived from abdominal rather than subcutaneous adipose tissue (Section 7.2.3).

At rest, triacylglycerol from plasma lipoproteins is a significant fuel for muscle, providing 5%–10% of the fatty acids for oxidation, but nonesterified fatty acids are more important in exercise.

10.6.2 Muscle fuel utilization in the fed and fasting states

Glucose is the main fuel for muscle in the fed state, but in the fasting state glucose is spared for use by the brain and red blood cells; glycogen, fatty acids, and ketone bodies are now the main fuels for muscle.

There are five mechanisms involved in the control of glucose utilization by muscle (Figure 10.16):

- Glucose transport into muscle is dependent on insulin, as it is in adipose tissue (Section 10.5.1), so that in the fasting state, when insulin secretion is low, there will be little uptake of glucose.
- Hexokinase is inhibited by its product, glucose 6-phosphate, which may arise either as a result of the action of hexokinase on glucose or by isomerization of glucose 1-phosphate from glycogen breakdown (Figure 5.9). Activation of glycogen phosphorylase leads to increased glucose 6-phosphate, which inhibits the utilization of glucose that has entered the cell, and so reduces glucose uptake further.
- The activity of pyruvate dehydrogenase is reduced in response to increasing concentrations of both NADH and acetyl CoA (Section 10.5.2). This means that the oxidation of fatty acids and ketone bodies will inhibit the decarboxylation of pyruvate. Under these conditions, the pyruvate that is formed from muscle glycogen by glycolysis will undergo transamination (Section 9.3.1.2) to form alanine. Alanine is exported from muscle and used for gluconeogenesis in the liver (Section 5.7 and Problem 9.1). Thus, although muscle cannot directly release glucose from its glycogen reserves (because it lacks glucose 6-phosphatase), muscle glycogen is an indirect source of blood glucose in the fasting state.
- If alanine accumulates in muscle, it acts as an allosteric inhibitor of pyruvate kinase, thus reducing the rate at which pyruvate is formed. This end-product inhibition of pyruvate kinase by alanine is overridden by high concentrations of fructose bisphosphate, which acts as a feed-forward activator of pyruvate kinase.
- ATP is an inhibitor of pyruvate kinase and phosphofructokinase (Section 10.2.2.1). This means that under conditions where the supply of ATP (which can be regarded as the end-product of all energy-yielding metabolic pathways) is more than adequate to meet requirements, the metabolism of glucose is inhibited.

10.6.2.1 Regulation of fatty acid metabolism in muscle

β-Oxidation of fatty acids is controlled by the uptake of fatty acids into the mitochondria; in turn, this is controlled by the activity of carnitine acyl transferase on the outer

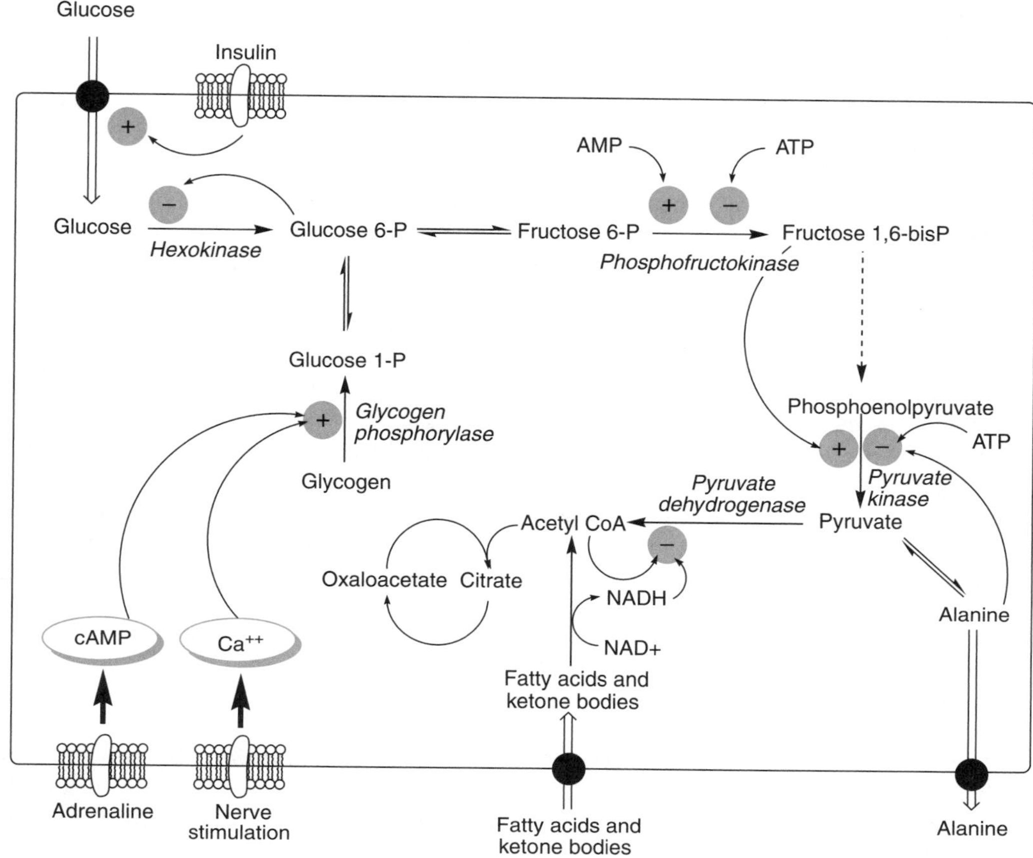

Figure 10.16 Control of the utilization of metabolic fuels in muscle.

mitochondrial membrane, and the countertransport of acyl-carnitine and free carnitine across the inner mitochondrial membrane (Section 5.5.1).

Carnitine acyl transferase activity is regulated by malonyl CoA. In liver and adipose tissue, this serves to inhibit mitochondrial uptake and β-oxidation of fatty acids when fatty acids are being synthesized in the cytosol (Section 10.5.2). Muscle also has an active acetyl CoA carboxylase and synthesizes malonyl CoA, although it does not synthesize fatty acids. Muscle carnitine acyl transferase is more sensitive to inhibition by malonyl CoA than is the enzyme in liver and adipose tissue.

Muscle also has malonyl CoA decarboxylase, which acts to decarboxylate malonyl CoA back to acetyl CoA. Acetyl CoA carboxylase and malonyl CoA decarboxylase are regulated in opposite directions by phosphorylation catalyzed by a 5′AMP-dependent protein kinase (which thus reflects the state of ATP reserves in the cell; Section 10.2.2.1). Phosphorylation in response to an increase in intracellular 5′AMP results in inactivation of acetyl CoA carboxylase and activation of malonyl CoA decarboxylase. This results in a rapid fall in the concentration of malonyl CoA, thus relieving the inhibition of carnitine acyl transferase and permitting mitochondrial uptake and β-oxidation of fatty acids in response to a fall in ATP, signaling a need for increased energy-yielding metabolism.

In the fed state, there is decreased oxidation of fatty acids in muscle as a result of increased activity of acetyl CoA carboxylase in response to insulin action.

10.7 Diabetes mellitus—a failure of regulation of blood glucose concentration

Diabetes mellitus is an impaired ability to regulate the concentration of blood glucose, as a result of a failure of the normal control by insulin. Therefore, the plasma glucose concentration is considerably higher than normal, both in the fasting state and after a meal. When it rises above the capacity of the kidney to reabsorb it from the glomerular filtrate (the renal threshold, approximately 11 mmol/L), the result is glucosuria—excretion of glucose in the urine. As a result of glucosuria, there is increased excretion of urine because of osmotic diuresis; one of the common presenting signs of diabetes is frequent urination, accompanied by excessive thirst.

Diabetes mellitus is diagnosed by elevated fasting glucose, followed by measurement of plasma glucose after an oral dose of 1 g/kg body weight—an oral glucose tolerance test. The normal response is a modest increase in plasma glucose, followed by a return to the initial level as it is taken up into liver, muscle, and adipose tissue for synthesis of glycogen and fatty acids (Section 5.6). In a diabetic subject, fasting plasma glucose is higher than normal, and in response to the test dose it rises considerably higher (possibly above the renal threshold), and remains elevated for a considerable time (Figure 10.17).

There are two main types of diabetes mellitus:

Type I diabetes (insulin-dependent diabetes mellitus, IDDM) is due to a failure to secrete insulin, as a result of damage to the β-cells of the pancreatic islets resulting from viral infection or autoimmune disease. There is a genetic susceptibility; the concordance of IDDM in monozygotic (identical) twins is about 50%. IDDM commonly develops in childhood and is sometimes known as juvenile-onset diabetes. Injection of insulin and strict control of carbohydrate intake are essential for control of blood glucose.

Type II diabetes (non-insulin-dependent diabetes mellitus, NIDDM) is due to failure of responsiveness to insulin (insulin resistance), as a result of decreased sensitivity of insulin receptors. There is a genetic susceptibility to type II diabetes, which usually develops in middle age, with a gradual onset, and is sometimes known as maturity-onset diabetes, although it is increasingly common in obese young adults and adolescents (Section 7.2.3.1).

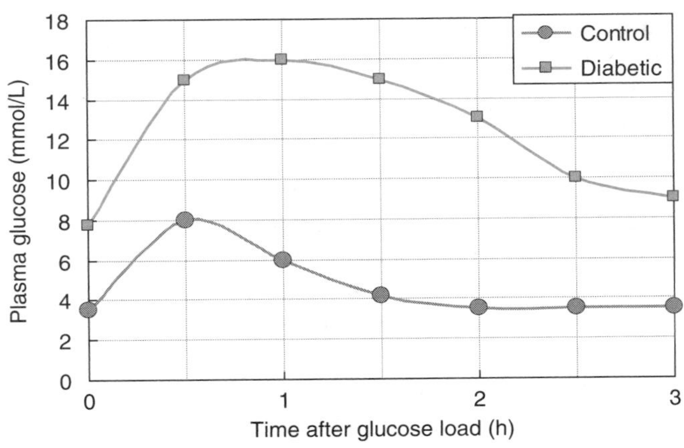

Figure 10.17 The oral glucose tolerance test in control and diabetic subjects.

Initially, insulin secretion in response to glucose is normal or higher than normal in people with insulin resistance and they can maintain adequate glycemic control, although they have an impaired response to a glucose tolerance test. When the demand for insulin exceeds the synthetic capacity of the β-islet cells of the pancreas, overt diabetes is the result.

NIDDM is more common in obese people, and especially those with abdominal rather than subcutaneous obesity. Significant weight loss can often restore normal glycemic control without the need for any other treatment. The metabolic syndrome (Section 7.2.3) is the simultaneous development of insulin resistance, hypertension, and hypertriglyceridemia, all associated with (abdominal) obesity.

At least in the early stages of NIDDM, control of glucose metabolism can be achieved by using oral hypoglycemic agents, which stimulate increased insulin secretion and also enhance insulin receptor function. Increasingly, as biosynthetic human insulin has become widely available, treatment of NIDDM includes insulin injection to maintain better glycemic control.

10.7.1 Adverse effects of poor glycemic control

Acutely, diabetics are liable to coma as a result of hypo- or hyperglycemia. Hypoglycemic coma occurs if the plasma concentration of glucose falls below about 2 mmol/L, as a result of administration of insulin or oral hypoglycemic agents without an adequate intake of carbohydrate. Strenuous exercise without additional food intake can also cause hypoglycemia. In such cases, oral or intravenous glucose is required.

Hyperglycemic coma develops in people with insulin-dependent diabetes because despite an abnormally high plasma concentration of glucose, tissues are unable to utilize it in the absence of insulin. The high plasma concentration of glucose leads to elevated plasma osmolarity, which results in coma. Because glucose cannot be utilized, ketone bodies are synthesized in the liver (Section 5.5.3). However, when the metabolism of glucose is impaired, there is little pyruvate available for synthesis of oxaloacetate to maintain citric acid cycle activity (Section 5.4.4). The result is keto-acidosis together with a very high plasma concentration of glucose. In such cases insulin injection is required, as well as intravenous bicarbonate if the acidosis is severe.

In the long term, failure of glycemic control and a persistently high plasma glucose concentration results in damage to capillary blood vessels (especially in the retina, leading to a risk of blindness), kidneys, peripheral nerves (leading to loss of sensation), and the development of cataracts in the lens of the eye and abnormal metabolism of plasma lipoproteins (which increases the risks of atherosclerosis and ischemic heart disease). At high concentrations, glucose can be reduced to sorbitol by aldose reductase. In tissues such as the lens of the eye and nerves, which cannot metabolize sorbitol, it accumulates, causing osmotic damage.

Glucose can react nonenzymically with free amino groups on proteins, resulting in glycation of the proteins (Figure 10.18). Glycated proteins include the following:

- Collagen, leading to the thickening of basement membranes in blood capillaries, resulting in kidney damage and blindness because of retinopathy. Glycated collagen in joints also explains the increased risk of osteoarthritis.
- Apolipoprotein B, leading to increased risk of atherosclerosis and ischemic heart disease.
- α-Crystallin in the lens, leading to the development of cataracts.
- Hemoglobin A, leading to reduced oxygen carrying capacity of the blood.

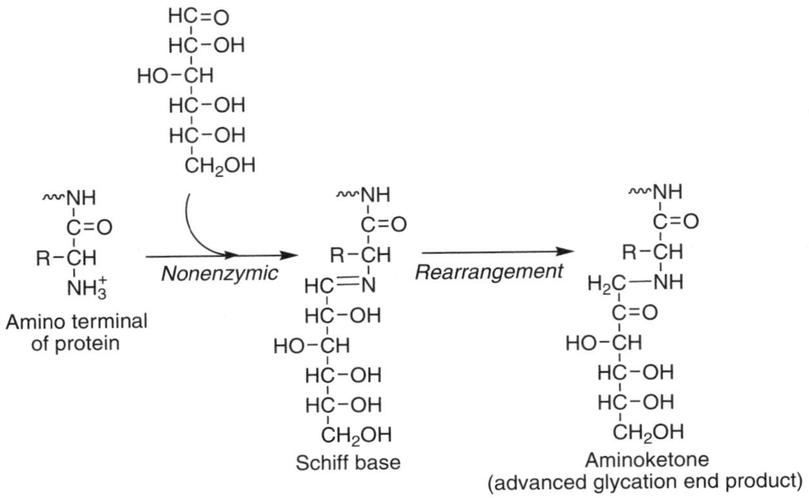

$$\text{Amino terminal of protein: } {\sim}NH{-}C(=O){-}CH(R){-}NH_3^+ \;+\; \text{glucose } (HC{=}O{-}HC{-}OH{-}HO{-}CH{-}HC{-}OH{-}HC{-}OH{-}CH_2OH) \xrightarrow{\text{Nonenzymic}} \text{Schiff base} \xrightarrow{\text{Rearrangement}} \text{Aminoketone (advanced glycation end product)}$$

Schiff base: ~NH–C=O–R–CH–HC=N–HC–OH–HO–CH–HC–OH–HC–OH–CH₂OH

Aminoketone (advanced glycation end product): ~NH–C=O–R–CH–H_2C—NH–C=O–HO–CH–HC–OH–HC–OH–CH_2OH

Figure 10.18 Nonenzymic glycation of proteins by high concentrations of glucose in poorly controlled diabetes mellitus.

Glycation of hemoglobin A (with the formation of what can be measured as hemoglobin A_{1c}) provides a sensitive means of assessing glycemic control over the preceding 4–6 weeks. It provides a better index of compliance with dietary restriction than a simple spot test of plasma glucose.

Key points

- Within any one cell, metabolism can be regulated instantaneously in response to changes in concentrations of substrates, as well as in response to precursors and end-products that act as allosteric regulators of key enzymes.
- Phosphofructokinase is a key regulatory enzyme of glycolysis and is inhibited by ATP and citrate. The inhibition by physiological concentrations of ATP is relieved by 5′AMP, which acts as a signal of the energy state of the cell.
- Substrate cycling permits rapid and sensitive control over pathways, and may also be important in thermogenesis.
- Fast-acting hormones act by changing the activity of existing enzyme protein by covalent modification. They bind to cell-surface receptors, activating G-proteins that lead to the synthesis of intracellular second messengers. These initiate cascades of intracellular responses, resulting in considerable amplification of the hormone signal.
- Slow-acting hormones act by changing the rate of gene expression. They bind to and activate intracellular receptors that bind to hormone response elements on DNA.
- In adipose tissue and liver, lipolysis and lipogenesis are controlled in opposite directions in response to insulin, glucagon, and adrenaline.
- Muscle can use a variety of fuels; the selection of fuel to be metabolized depends on the intensity and duration of exercise, and whether the subject is in the fed or fasting state.
- Diabetes mellitus is impaired ability to regulate the concentration of blood glucose; it may be due to failure of insulin synthesis and secretion (type I diabetes) or loss of insulin receptors sensitivity (type II diabetes).

Problem 10.1: Louis C

Louis was born in 1967 at term after an uneventful pregnancy. He was a sickly infant and did not grow well. On a number of occasions his mother noted that he appeared drowsy, or even comatose, and said that there was a "chemical, alcohol-like" smell on his breath, and in his urine. The GP suspected diabetes mellitus, and sent him to the Middlesex Hospital for a glucose tolerance test, which showed clearly that he was diabetic (Figure 10.17).

Samples were also taken for measurement of insulin at zero time and 1 h after the glucose load. At this time a new method of measuring insulin was being developed, radioimmunoassay, and therefore both this and the conventional biological assay were used. The biological method of measuring insulin is by its ability to stimulate the uptake and metabolism of glucose in rat muscle *in vitro*; this can be performed relatively simply by measuring the radioactivity in $^{14}CO_2$ after incubating duplicate samples of the muscle with [^{14}C]glucose, with and without the sample containing insulin. The then newly developed method of measuring insulin is by its ability to bind to anti-insulin antibodies, in competition with radioactively labeled insulin—this is radioimmunoassay and is generally preferred because it is possible to assay a large number of samples at the same time. The antibody recognizes and binds to the surface of the tertiary structure of the protein. The results are shown in Table 10.1.

As a part of their studies of the new radioimmunoassay for insulin, the team at the Middlesex Hospital performed gel exclusion chromatography of a pooled sample of normal serum, and determined insulin in the fractions eluted from the columns both by radioimmunoassay (graph A in Figure 10.19) and by stimulation of glucose oxidation (graph B). Gel exclusion chromatography separates compounds by their molecular mass, so that larger molecules flow through the column faster and are eluted earlier than smaller molecules. Three molecular mass markers were used; they eluted as follows: M_r 9000 in fraction 10, M_r 6000 in fraction 23, and M_r 4500 in fraction 27.

The investigators also measured insulin in the fractions eluted from the chromatography column after treatment of each fraction with trypsin. The results are shown in graph C.

After seeing the results of these studies, they subjected the same pooled serum sample to brief treatment with trypsin, and

Table 10.1 Serum Insulin by Biological Assay and Radioimmunoassay

	Fasting		1 h after Glucose	
	Louis C	Control Subjects	Louis C	Control Subjects
Biological assay	0.8	6 ± 2	5	40 ± 11
Radioimmunoassay	10	6 ± 2	50	40 ± 11

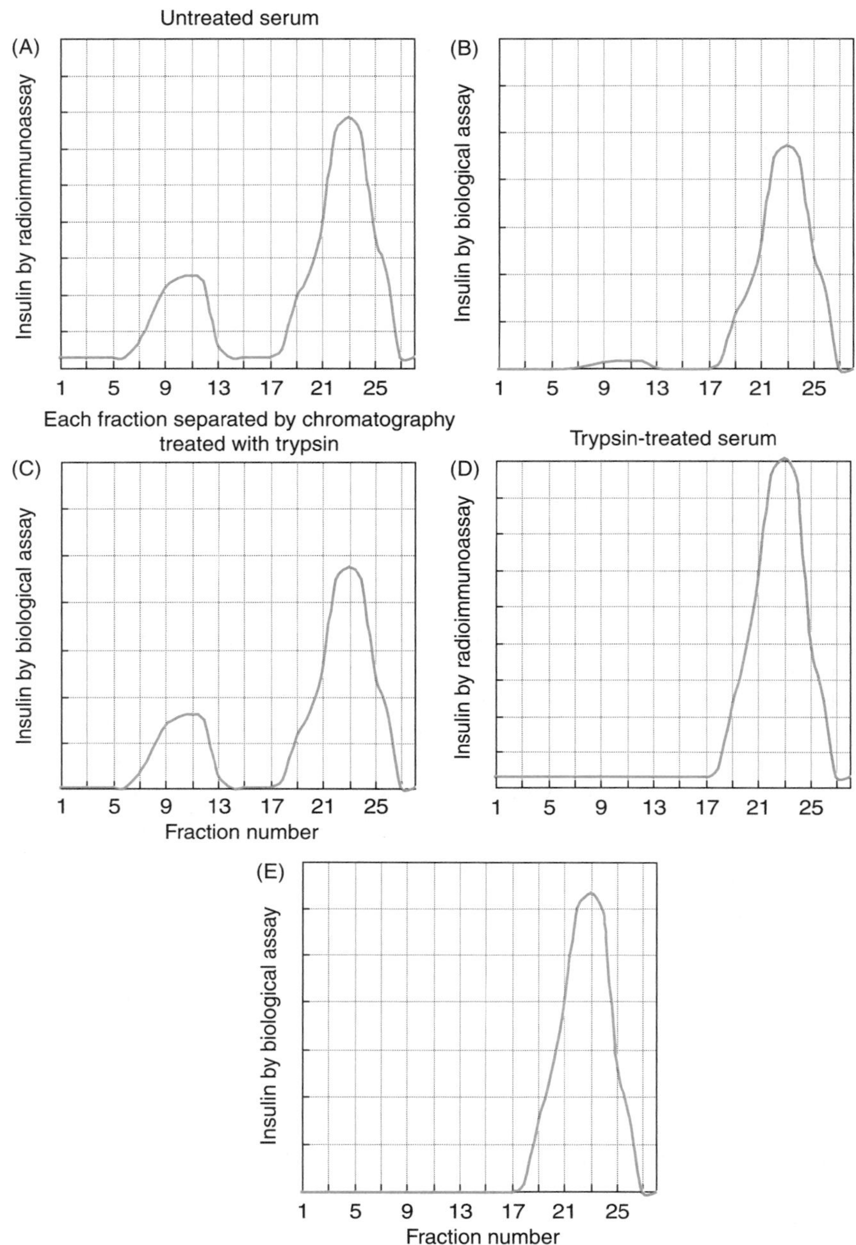

Figure 10.19 Gel filtration of serum insulin and measurement by radioimmunoassay and biological assay.

performed gel exclusion chromatography on the product. Again they measured insulin by radioimmunoassay (graph D) and biological assay (graph E).

What conclusions can you draw from these results?

More recently, the gene for human insulin has been cloned. Although insulin consists of two peptide chains, 21 and 30 amino acids long respectively, these are coded for by a single gene, which has a total of 330 base pairs between the initiator and stop codons. As you would expect for a secreted protein, there is a signal sequence coding for 24 amino acids at the 5′ end of the gene.

What does this information suggest about the processes that occur in the synthesis of insulin?

What is likely to be the underlying biochemical basis of Louis' problem?

Problem 10.2: Lucinda K

Lucinda is the second child of unrelated parents. She was born at term after an uneventful pregnancy, weighing 3.4 kg and was breast-fed, with gradual introduction of solids from 3 months of age onward. Her mother reported that while Lucinda liked cheese, meat, and fish, she frequently became irritable and grizzly after meals, and became lethargic, drowsy, and "floppy" after eating relatively large amounts of protein-rich foods. Her urine had a curious odor, described by her mother as being "cat-like" on such occasions.

At 9 months of age, she was admitted to the accident and emergency department of University College Hospital in a coma, and suffering convulsions. She had been unwell for three days, with a slight fever, and for the past 12 h had been refusing all food and drink. At this time she weighed 8.8 kg, and her body length was 70.5 cm.

Emergency blood tests revealed moderate acidosis (pH 7.25) and severe hypoglycemia (glucose < 1 mmol/L); a dipstick test for plasma ketone bodies was negative. A blood sample was taken for full clinical chemistry tests, and she was given intravenous glucose. Within a short time she recovered consciousness. The results of the blood tests are shown in Table 10.2.

Lucinda remained in hospital for several weeks, while further tests were performed. She was generally well through this time, but

Table 10.2 Clinical Chemistry Results for a Plasma Sample from Lucinda K on Admission and Reference Range for 24 h Fasting

	Lucinda K	Reference Range
Glucose, mmol/L	0.22	4–5
pH	7.25	7.35–7.45
Bicarbonate, mmol/L	11	21–29
Ammonium, μmol/L	120	<50
Ketone bodies, mmol/L	Undetectable	2.5–3.5
Nonesterified fatty acids, mmol/L	2	1.0–1.2
Insulin, mU/L	5	5–35
Glucagon, ng/mL	140	130–160

became drowsy and severely hypoglycemic, and hyperventilated, if she was deprived of food for more than about 8–9 h. Her muscle tone was poor, and she was very weak, with considerably less strength (e.g., in pushing her arms or legs against the pediatrician's hand) than would be expected for a girl of her age.

On one occasion, her blood glucose was monitored at 30 min intervals over 3 h from waking without being fed; it fell from 3.4 mmol/L on waking to 1.3 mmol/L 3 h later. She was deprived of breakfast again the next day, and again blood glucose was measured at 30 min intervals for 3 h during which she received an intravenous infusion of β-hydroxybutyrate (50 μmol/min/kg body weight). During the infusion of β-hydroxybutyrate, her plasma glucose remained between 3.3 and 3.5 mmol/L.

At no time were ketone bodies detected in her urine, and there was no evidence of any abnormal excretion of amino acids. However, a number of abnormal organic acids were detected in her urine, including relatively large amounts of 3-hydroxy-3-methylglutaric and 3-hydroxy-3-methylglutaconic acids. The excretion of these two acids increased considerably under two conditions:

- When she was fed a relatively high protein meal (she became grizzly, lethargic, and irritable). A blood sample taken after such a meal showed significant hyperammonemia (130 μmol/L), but normal glucose (5.5 mmol/L).
- When she was fasted for more than the normal overnight fast, with or without the infusion of β-hydroxybutyrate.

One obvious metabolic precursor of 3-hydroxy-3-methylglutaric acid is 3-hydroxy-3-methylglutaryl CoA (HMG-CoA), which is normally cleaved to yield acetoacetate and acetyl CoA by the enzyme hydroxymethyglutaryl CoA lyase (Figure 5.25). Therefore, the activity of this enzyme was determined in leukocytes from blood samples from Lucinda and her parents. The results are shown in Table 10.3.

Analysis of Lucinda's urine also revealed considerable excretion of carnitine as shown in Table 10.4.

What is the likely biochemical basis of Lucinda's problem? To what extent can you account for her various metabolic problems from the information you are given?

What dietary manipulation(s) would be likely to maintain her in good health and prevent further emergency hospital admissions?

Table 10.3 Leukocyte HMG CoA Lyase Activity (nmol Product Formed/min/g Protein)

Lucinda K	1.7
Mother	10.2
Father	11.4
Control subjects	19.7 ± 2.0

Table 10.4 Urinary Excretion of Carnitine (nmol/mg Creatinine)

	Lucinda K	Reference Range
Total carnitine	680	125 ± 75
Free carnitine	31	51 ± 40
Acyl carnitine	649	74 ± 40

Table 10.5 Clinical Chemistry Results for a Plasma Sample from Barry B on Admission and Reference Range for 24 h Fasting

	Barry B	Reference Range
Glucose, mmol/L	3.3	3.5–5.5
pH	6.9	7.35–7.45
Bicarbonate, mmol/L	2.0	21–25
Ketone bodies, mmol/L	21	1–2.5
Lactate, mmol/L	7.3	0.5–2.2
Pyruvate, mmol/L	0.31	<0.15

Problem 10.3: Barry B

Barry is the second child of unrelated parents; his brother is 5 years old, fit, and healthy. He was born at full term after an uneventful pregnancy, weighing 3.4 kg (the 50th centile), and developed normally until he was 6 months old, after when he showed some retardation of development. He also developed a fine scaly skin rash about this time, and his hair, which had been normal, became thin and sparse.

At 9 months of age, he was admitted to the Royal Free Hospital in a coma; the results of clinical chemistry tests on a plasma sample are shown in Table 10.5.

The acidosis was treated by intravenous infusion of bicarbonate, and he recovered consciousness. Over the next few days he continued to show signs of acidosis (rapid respiration), and even after a meal ketone bodies were present in his urine. His plasma lactate, pyruvate, and ketone bodies remained high; plasma glucose was in the low normal range, and his plasma insulin was normal both in the fasting state and after an oral glucose load.

Urine analysis revealed the presence of significant amounts of a number of organic acids that are not normally excreted in the urine:

- Lactate, pyruvate, and alanine
- Propionate, hydroxypropionate, and propionylglycine
- Methyl citrate
- Tiglate and tiglylglycine
- 3-Methylcrotonate, 3-methylcrotonylglycine, and 3-hydroxy-isovalerate

His skin rash and hair loss were reminiscent of the signs of biotin deficiency, as caused by excessive consumption of uncooked egg white (Section 11.12.3). However, his mother said that Barry did not eat raw or undercooked eggs at all, although he was fond of hard-boiled eggs and yeast extract (which are rich sources of biotin). His plasma biotin was 0.2 nmol/L, (normal > 0.8 nmol/L), and he excreted a significant amount of biotin in the form of biocytin and small biocytin-containing peptides (Figure 11.24), which are not normally detectable in urine.

He was treated with 5 mg of biotin per day. After 3 days, the abnormal organic acids were no longer detectable in his urine and his plasma lactate, pyruvate, and ketone bodies had returned to normal, although his excretion of biocytin and biocytin-containing peptides increased. At this stage, he was discharged from hospital with a supply of biotin tablets. After 3 weeks his skin rash began to clear and his hair loss ceased.

Three months later, at a regular outpatient visit, it was decided to cease the biotin supplements. Within a week the abnormal organic acids were again detected in his urine, and he was treated with varying doses of biotin until the organic aciduria ceased. This was achieved at an intake of 150 µg/day (compared with the reference intake of 10–20 µg/day for an infant under 2 years of age).

He has continued to take 150 µg of biotin daily and has remained in good health for the last 4 years.

Can you account for the biochemical basis of Barry's problem?

Problem 10.4: Amelia Q

Amelia is the only child of nonconsanguineous parents, born at term after an uneventful pregnancy. At 14 months of age she was admitted to hospital with a 1 day history of persistent vomiting, rapid shallow respiration, and dehydration. On admission, her respiration rate was 60/min and her pulse 178/min. The first column in Table 10.6 shows the results of clinical chemistry tests at that time. She responded rapidly to intravenous bicarbonate and a single intramuscular injection of insulin.

The results of a glucose tolerance test 3 days after admission were normal, and her plasma insulin response to an oral glucose load was within the normal range. She was discharged from hospital 7 days after admission, apparently fit and well. The second column in Table 10.6 shows the results of clinical chemistry tests taken shortly before her discharge.

Amelia was readmitted to hospital at 16, 25, 31, and 48 months of age, suffering from restlessness, unsteady gait, rapid shallow respiration, persistent vomiting, and dehydration. Each time the crisis was preceded by a common childhood illness and decreased appetite, and she responded well to intravenous fluids and

Table 10.6 Clinical Chemistry Results for Plasma and Urine Samples from Amelia Q on Admission and Again 1 Week Later

	Acute Admission	1 Week Later	Reference Range
Plasma			
Glucose, mmol/L	14	5.1	3.5–5.5
Sodium, mmol/L	132	137	135–145
Chloride, mmol/L	111	105	100–106
Bicarbonate, mmol/L	1.5	20	21–25
Urea, mmol/L	4.1	4.9	2.9–8.9
Lactate, mmol/L	7.3	5.5	0.5–2.2
Pyruvate, mmol/L	0.31	0.25	<0.15
Alanine, mmol/L	–	852	99–313
Aspartate, mmol/L	–	Undetectable	3–11
pH	6.89	7.36	7.35–7.45
Urine			
Lactate, mg/g creatinine	–	1.48	<0.1
Ketone bodies, using Ketostix	Very high	Negative	Negative

Table 10.7 Activities of Mitochondrial Enzymes from Cultured Skin Fibroblasts (nmol Product Formed/min/mg Protein)

	Amelia Q	Control Subjects
Citrate synthase	32.8	76.3 ± 15.1
Cytochrome c reduction by NADH	11.6	16.7 ± 4.6
Cytochrome c reduction by succinate	9.43	12.3 ± 3.2
Cytochrome oxidase	37.7	50.3 ± 11.6
NADH dehydrogenase	633	910 ± 169
Pyruvate carboxylase	0.03	1.62 ± 0.39
Pyruvate dehydrogenase	1.86	1.72 ± 0.35
Succinate oxidase	190	210 ± 30

bicarbonate. A number of milder episodes were treated at home by oral fluid and bicarbonate.

During her admission at age 25 months, a skin biopsy was taken, fibroblasts were cultured, and the mitochondrial enzyme activities shown in Table 10.7 were determined.

Can you explain the biochemical basis of Amelia's condition?

chapter eleven

Micronutrients—the vitamins and minerals

In addition to an adequate source of metabolic fuels (carbohydrates, fats, and proteins; Chapter 5) and protein (Chapter 9), there is a requirement for very much smaller amounts of other nutrients: the vitamins and minerals. Collectively, these are referred to as micronutrients because of the small amounts that are required.

Vitamins are organic compounds that are required for the maintenance of normal health and metabolic integrity. They cannot be synthesized in the body but must be provided in the diet. They are required in very small amounts, of the order of milligrams or micrograms per day, and thus can be distinguished from the essential fatty acids (Sections 4.3.1.1 and 5.6.1.1) and the essential amino acids (Section 9.1.3), which are required in amounts of grams per day.

The essential minerals are those inorganic elements that have a physiological function in the body. Obviously, since they are elements, they must be provided in the diet, because elements cannot be interconverted. The amounts required vary from grams per day for sodium and calcium, through milligrams per day (e.g., iron) to micrograms per day for the trace elements (so called because they are required in such small amounts).

Objectives

After reading this chapter, you should be able to

- Describe and explain the way in which micronutrient requirements are determined and how reference intakes are calculated; explain how it is that different national and international authorities have different reference intakes for some nutrients
- Describe and explain the chemistry, metabolic functions, and deficiency signs associated with each of the vitamins and important minerals

11.1 The determination of requirements and reference intakes

For any nutrient, there is a range of intakes between that which is clearly inadequate, leading to clinical deficiency disease, and that which is so much in excess of the body's metabolic capacity that there may be signs of toxicity. Between these two extremes is a level of intake that is adequate for normal health and the maintenance of metabolic integrity, and a series of more precisely definable levels of intake that are adequate to meet specific criterion and may be used to determine requirements and appropriate levels of intake:

- Clinical deficiency disease, with clear anatomical and functional lesions, and severe metabolic disturbances, possibly proving fatal. Prevention of deficiency disease is a minimal goal in determining requirements.
- Covert deficiency, where there are no signs of deficiency under normal conditions but any trauma or stress reveals the precarious state of the body reserves and may

precipitate clinical signs. For example, an intake of 10 mg of vitamin C per day is adequate to prevent clinical deficiency, but at least 20 mg/day is required for healing of wounds (Section 11.14.2).

- Metabolic abnormalities under normal conditions, such as impaired carbohydrate metabolism in thiamin deficiency (Section 11.6.3), or excretion of methylmalonic acid in vitamin B_{12} deficiency (Section 11.10.4).
- Abnormal response to a metabolic load, such as the inability to metabolize a test dose of histidine in folate deficiency (Section 11.11.6.1) or tryptophan in vitamin B_6 deficiency (Section 11.9.5.1), although at normal levels of intake there may be no metabolic impairment.
- Inadequate saturation of enzymes with (vitamin-derived) coenzymes. This can be tested for three vitamins, using red blood cell enzymes: thiamin (Section 11.6), riboflavin (Section 11.7), and vitamin B_6 (Section 11.9).
- Low plasma concentration of the nutrient, indicating that there is an inadequate amount in tissue reserves to permit normal transport between tissues. For some nutrients, this may reflect the failure to synthesize a transport protein rather than primary deficiency of the nutrient itself.
- Low urinary excretion of the nutrient, reflecting low intake and changes in metabolic turnover.
- Incomplete saturation of body reserves.
- Adequate body reserves and normal metabolic integrity.
- Possibly beneficial effects of intakes more than adequate to meet requirements—the promotion of optimum health and life expectancy.
- Pharmacological (drug-like) actions at very high levels of intake.
- Abnormal accumulation in tissues and overloading of normal metabolic pathways, leading to signs of toxicity and possibly irreversible lesions. Iron (Section 11.15.2.3); selenium (Section 11.15.2.5); niacin (Section 11.8.5.1); and vitamins A (Section 11.2.5.2), D (Section 11.3.5.1), and B_6 (Section 11.9.6.1) are all known to be toxic in excess.

Having decided on an appropriate criterion of adequacy, requirements are determined by feeding volunteers an otherwise adequate diet, but lacking the nutrient under investigation, until there is a detectable metabolic or other abnormality. They are then repleted with graded intakes of the nutrient until the abnormality is just corrected.

Problems arise in interpreting the results, and therefore defining requirements, when different markers of adequacy respond to different levels of intake. This explains the difference in the tables of reference intakes published by different national and international authorities (see Tables 11.1 through 11.4).

11.1.1 Dietary reference values

All individuals do not have the same requirement for nutrients even when calculated on the basis of body size or energy expenditure. There is a range of individual requirements of up to 25% around the average. Therefore, to set population goals and assess the adequacy of diets, it is necessary to set a reference level of intake that is high enough to ensure that no one will either suffer from deficiency or be at risk of toxicity.

As shown in the upper graph in Figure 11.1, if it is assumed that individual requirements are normally distributed around the observed mean requirement, then a range of ± 2 standard deviations (SD) around the mean will include the requirements of 95% of the population. This 95% range is conventionally used as the "normal" or reference range

Table 11.1 Reference Nutrient Intakes of Vitamins and Minerals, United Kingdom, 1991

Age	Vitamin B_1 (mg)	Vitamin B_2 (mg)	Niacin (mg)	Vitamin B_6 (mg)	Vitamin B_{12} (μg)	Folate (μg)	Vitamin C (mg)	Vitamin A (μg)	Vitamin D (μg)	Ca (mg)	P (mg)	Mg (mg)	Fe (mg)	Zn (mg)	Cu (mg)	Se (μg)	I (μg)
0–3 months	0.2	0.4	3	0.2	0.3	50	25	350	8.5	525	400	55	1.7	4.0	0.2	10	50
4–6 months	0.2	0.4	3	0.2	0.3	50	25	350	8.5	525	400	60	4.3	4.0	0.3	13	60
7–9 months	0.2	0.4	4	0.3	0.4	50	25	350	7	525	400	75	7.8	5.0	0.3	10	60
10–12 months	0.3	0.4	5	0.4	0.4	50	25	350	7	525	400	80	7.8	5.0	0.3	10	60
1–3 years	0.5	0.6	8	0.7	0.5	70	30	400	7	350	270	85	6.9	5.0	0.4	15	70
4–6 years	0.7	0.8	11	0.9	0.8	100	30	500	–	450	350	120	6.1	6.5	0.6	20	100
7–10 years	0.7	1.0	12	1.0	1.0	150	30	500	–	550	450	200	8.7	7.0	0.7	30	110
Males																	
11–14 years	0.9	1.2	15	1.2	1.2	200	35	600	–	1000	775	280	11.3	9.0	0.8	45	130
15–18 years	1.1	1.3	18	1.5	1.5	200	40	700	–	1000	775	300	11.3	9.5	1.0	70	140
19–50 years	1.0	1.3	17	1.4	1.5	200	40	700	–	700	550	300	8.7	9.5	1.2	75	140
50+years	0.9	1.3	16	1.4	1.5	200	40	700	10	700	550	300	8.7	9.5	1.2	75	140
Females																	
11–14 years	0.7	1.1	12	1.0	1.2	200	35	600	–	800	625	280	14.8	9.0	0.8	45	130
15–18 years	0.8	1.1	14	1.2	1.5	200	40	600	–	800	6254	300	14.8	7.0	1.0	60	140
19–50 years	0.8	1.1	13	1.2	1.5	200	40	600	–	700	550	270	14.8	7.0	1.2	60	140
50+years	0.8	1.1	12	1.2	1.5	200	40	600	10	700	550	270	8.7	7.0	1.2	60	140
Pregnant	+0.1	+0.3	–	–	–	+100	+10	+100	10	–	–	–					
Lactating	+0.1	+0.5	+2	–	+0.5	+60	+30	+350	10	+550	+440	+50		+6.0	+0.3	+15	

Source: Department of Health, Dietary Reference Values for Food Energy and Nutrients for the United Kingdom, HMSO, London, 1991.

Table 11.2 Population Reference Intakes of Vitamins and Minerals, European Union, 1993

Age	Vitamin A (μg)	Vitamin B_1 (mg)	Vitamin B_2 (mg)	Niacin (mg)	Vitamin B_6 (mg)	Folate (μg)	Vitamin B_{12} (μg)	Vitamin C (mg)	Ca (mg)	P (mg)	Fe (mg)	Zn (mg)	Cu (mg)	Se (μg)	I (μg)
6–12 months	350	0.3	0.4	5	0.4	50	0.5	20	400	300	6	4	0.3	8	50
1–3 years	400	0.5	0.8	9	0.7	100	0.7	25	400	300	4	4	0.4	10	70
4–6 years	400	0.7	1.0	11	0.9	130	0.9	25	450	350	4	6	0.6	15	90
7–10 years	500	0.8	1.2	13	1.1	150	1.0	30	550	450	6	7	0.7	25	100
Males															
11–14 years	600	1.0	1.4	15	1.3	180	1.3	35	1000	775	10	9	0.8	35	120
15–17 years	700	1.2	1.6	18	1.5	200	1.4	40	1000	775	13	9	1.0	45	130
18+years	700	1.1	1.6	18	1.5	200	1.4	45	700	550	9	9.5	1.1	55	130
Females															
11–14 years	600	0.9	1.2	14	1.1	180	1.3	35	800	625	18	9	0.8	35	120
15–17 years	600	0.9	1.3	14	1.1	200	1.4	40	800	625	17	7	1.0	45	130
18+years	600	0.9	1.3	14	1.1	200	1.4	45	700	550	16*	7	1.1	55	130
Pregnant	700	1.0	1.6	14	1.3	400	1.6	55	700	550	*	7	1.1	55	130
Lactating	950	1.1	1.7	16	1.4	350	1.9	70	1200	950	16	12	1.4	70	160

*8 mg Fe postmenopausally; supplements required in latter half of pregnancy.
Source: Scientific Committee for Food, *Nutrient and Energy Intakes for the European Community*, Commission of the European Communities, Luxembourg, 1993.

Table 11.3 Recommended Dietary Allowances and Acceptable Intakes for Vitamins and Minerals, United States and Canada, 1997–2001

Age	Vitamin A (µg)	Vitamin D (µg)	Vitamin E (mg)	Vitamin K (µg)	Vitamin B_1 (mg)	Vitamin B_2 (mg)	Niacin (mg)	Vitamin B_6 (mg)	Folate (µg)	Vitamin B_{12} (µg)	Vitamin C (mg)	Ca (mg)	P (mg)	Fe (mg)	Zn (mg)	Cu (mg)	Se (µg)	I (µg)
0–6 months	400	5	4	2.0	0.2	0.3	2	0.1	65	0.4	40	210	100	–	2.0	200	15	110
7–12 months	500	5	5	2.5	0.3	0.4	4	0.3	80	0.5	50	270	275	11	3	220	20	130
1–3 years	300	5	6	30	0.5	0.5	6	0.5	150	0.9	15	500	460	7	3	340	20	90
4–8 years	400	5	7	55	0.5	0.6	8	0.6	200	1.2	25	800	500	10	5	440	30	90
Males																		
9–13 years	600	5	11	60	0.9	0.9	12	1.0	300	1.8	45	1300	1250	8	8	700	40	120
14–18 years	900	5	15	75	1.2	1.3	16	1.3	400	2.4	75	1300	1250	11	11	890	55	150
19–30 years	900	5	15	120	1.2	1.3	16	1.3	400	2.4	90	1000	700	8	11	900	55	150
31–50 years	900	5	15	120	1.2	1.3	16	1.3	400	2.4	90	1000	700	8	11	900	55	150
51–70 years	900	10	15	120	1.2	1.3	16	1.7	400	2.4	90	1200	700	8	11	900	55	150
>70 years	900	15	15	120	1.2	1.3	16	1.7	400	2.4	90	1200	700	8	11	900	55	150
Females																		
9–13 years	600	5	11	60	0.9	0.9	12	1.0	300	1.8	45	1300	1250	8	8	700	40	120
14–18 years	700	5	15	75	1.0	1.0	14	1.2	400	2.4	65	1300	1250	15	9	890	55	150
19–30 years	700	5	15	90	1.1	1.1	14	1.3	400	2.4	75	1000	700	18	8	900	55	150
31–50 years	700	5	15	90	1.1	1.1	14	1.3	400	2.4	75	1000	700	18	8	900	55	150
51–70 years	700	10	15	90	1.1	1.1	14	1.5	400	2.4	75	1200	700	8	8	900	55	150
>70 years	700	15	15	90	1.1	1.1	14	1.5	400	2.4	75	1200	700	8	8	900	55	150
Pregnant	770	5	15	90	1.4	1.4	18	1.9	600	2.6	85	1000	700	27	11	1000	60	220
Lactating	900	5	16	90	1.4	1.6	17	2.0	500	2.8	120	1000	700	9	12	1300	70	290

Note: Figures for infants under 12 months are adequate intakes based on the observed mean intake of infants fed principally on breast milk; for nutrients other than vitamin K figures are RDA, based on estimated average requirement + 2SD; figures for vitamin K are adequate intakes based on observed average intakes.

Sources: Standing Committee on the Scientific Evaluation of Dietary Reference Intakes, Food and Nutrition Board, Institute of Medicine. Dietary Reference Intakes for calcium, phosphorus, magnesium, vitamin D and fluoride, 1997; Dietary Reference Intakes for thiamin, riboflavin, niacin, vitamin B_6, folate, vitamin B_{12}, pantothenic acid, biotin and choline, 1998; Dietary Reference Intakes for vitamin C, vitamin E, selenium and carotenoids, 2000; Dietary Reference Intakes for vitamin A, vitamin K, arsenic, boron, chromium, copper, iodine, iron, manganese, molybdenum, nickel, silicon, vanadium and zinc, 2001, National Academy Press, Washington, DC.

Table 11.4 Recommended Nutrient Intakes for Vitamins, FAO, 2001

Age	Vitamin A (μg)	Vitamin D (μg)	Vitamin K (μg)	Vitamin B_1 (mg)	Vitamin B_2 (mg)	Niacin (mg)	Vitamin B_6 (mg)	Folate (μg)	Vitamin B_{12} (μg)	Vitamin C (mg)	Panto (mg)	Biotin (μg)
0–6 months	375	5	5	0.2	0.3	2	0.1	80	0.4	25	1.7	5
7–12 months	400	5	10	0.3	0.4	4	0.3	80	0.5	30	1.8	6
1–3 years	400	5	15	0.5	0.5	6	0.5	160	0.9	30	2.0	8
4–6 years	450	5	20	0.6	0.6	8	0.6	200	1.2	30	3.0	12
7–9 years	500	5	25	0.9	0.9	12	1.0	300	1.8	35	4.0	20
Males												
10–18 years	600	5	35–55	1.2	1.3	16	1.3	400	2.4	40	5.0	30
19–50 years	600	5	65	1.2	1.3	16	1.3	400	2.4	45	5.0	30
50–65 years	600	10	65	1.2	1.3	16	1.7	400	2.4	45	5.0	30
>65 years	600	15	65	1.2	1.3	16	1.7	400	2.4	45	5.0	30
Females												
10–18 years	600	5	35–55	1.1	1.0	16	1.2	400	2.4	40	5.0	25
19–50 years	600	5	55	1.1	1.1	14	1.3	400	2.4	45	5.0	30
50–65 years	600	10	55	1.1	1.1	14	1.5	400	2.4	45	5.0	30
>65 years	600	15	55	1.1	1.1	14	1.5	400	2.4	45	5.0	30
Pregnant	800	5	55	1.4	1.4	18	1.9	600	2.6	55	6.0	30
Lactating	850	5	55	1.5	1.6	17	2.0	500	2.8	70	7.0	35

Source: Food and Agriculture Organization of the United Nations and World Health Organization, *Human Vitamin and Mineral Requirements*, FAO, Rome, 2001.

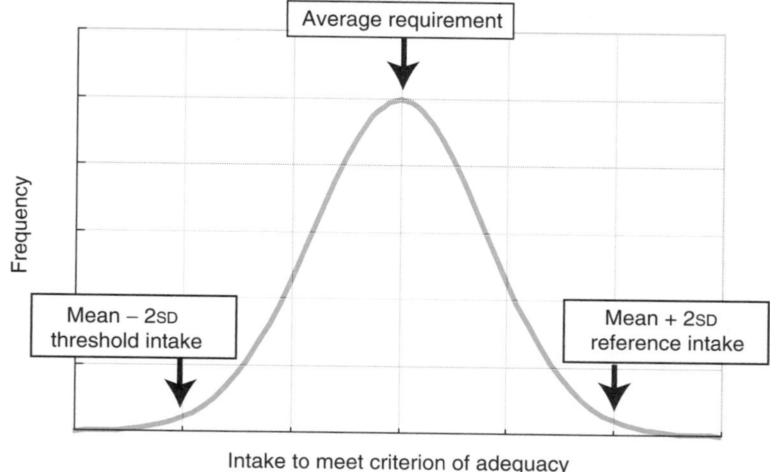

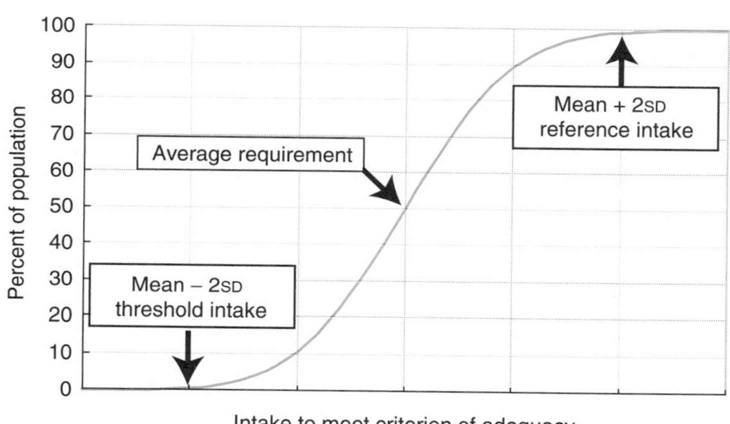

Figure 11.1 The derivation of reference intakes of nutrients from the distribution around the observed mean requirement; plotted below as a cumulative distribution curve, permitting estimation of the probability that a given level of intake is adequate to meet an individual's requirement.

(e.g., in clinical chemistry to assess the normality or otherwise of a test result) and is used to define three levels of nutrient intake:

- *The estimated average requirement (EAR).* This is the observed mean requirement to meet the chosen criterion of adequacy in experimental studies.
- *The reference nutrient intake (RNI).* This is two standard deviations above the observed mean requirement and is therefore more than adequate to meet the individual requirements of 97.5% of the population. This is the goal for planning diets, for example, in institutional feeding and the standard against which the intake of a population can be assessed. In the European Union tables (Table 11.2), this is called the population reference intake (PRI); in the United States it is called the recommended dietary allowance (RDA; Table 11.3);

- *The lower reference nutrient intake (LNRI).* This is two standard deviations below the observed mean requirement and is therefore adequate to meet the requirements of only 2.5% of the population. In the European Union tables, this is called the "lower threshold intake" to stress that it is a level of intake at or below which it is extremely unlikely that normal metabolic integrity could be maintained.

The lower graph in Figure 11.1 shows the distribution of requirements plotted as the cumulative percentage of the population whose requirements have been met at each level of intake. This can therefore be used to estimate the probability that a given level of intake is adequate to meet an individual's requirements.

For some nutrients, deficiency is unknown except under experimental conditions, and there are no estimates of average requirements and therefore no reference intakes. Since deficiency does not occur, average levels of intake are more than adequate to meet requirements, and for these nutrients there is a range of intakes that is defined as safe and adequate, based on the observed range of intakes.

The reference intakes of vitamins and minerals shown in Tables 11.1 through 11.4 are age and gender specific. Apart from foods for infants and children, the highest requirement for any population group is used to provide the basis for nutritional labeling of foods.

11.1.1.1 Supplements and safe levels of intake

In general, the amounts of micronutrients in foods pose no health hazards, although liver may contain undesirably high levels of vitamin A for pregnant women (Section 11.2.5.2). However, the amounts that may be consumed in supplements may be hazardous. Table 11.5 shows the tolerable upper levels of habitual intake for those nutrients where there is adequate evidence to set a level of intake at or below which there is no evidence of any hazard.

11.1.2 The vitamins

Vitamins are organic compounds that are required in small amounts for the maintenance of normal metabolic function. Deficiency causes a specific disease, which is cured or prevented only by restoring the vitamin to the diet. This is important; it is not enough just to show that a compound has effects, since these may be pharmacological actions not related to the maintenance of normal health and metabolic integrity.

As can be seen from Table 11.6, the vitamins are named in a curious way. This is a historical accident and results from the way in which they were discovered. Studies at the beginning of the twentieth century showed that there was something in milk that was essential, in very small amounts, for the growth of animals fed on a diet consisting of purified fat, carbohydrate, protein, and mineral salts. Two factors were found to be essential: one was found in the cream and the other in the watery part of milk. Logically, they were called factor A (fat soluble, in the cream) and factor B (water soluble, in the watery part of the milk). Factor B was identified chemically as an amine, and in 1913 the name "vitamin" was coined for these "vital amines."

Further studies showed that vitamin B was a mixture of a number of compounds with different functions, and so they were given numbers as well: vitamin B_1, vitamin B_2, and so on. There are gaps in the numerical order of the B vitamins. When what might have been called vitamin B_3 was discovered, it was found to be a chemical compound that was already known, nicotinic acid. It was therefore not given a number. Other gaps are because compounds that were believed to be vitamins were later shown either not to be dietary essentials, or to be vitamins that had already been described by other researchers and given other names.

Table 11.5 Safe Upper Levels of Supplement Consumption for Adults

Supplement	Tolerable Upper Intake Level
Vitamin A	3000 μg
Vitamin D	50 μg
Vitamin E	1000 mg
Niacin	35 mg
Vitamin B_6	100 mg
Folate	1000 μg
Vitamin C	2000 mg
Choline	3.5 g
Boron	20 mg
Calcium	2.5 g
Copper	10 mg
Fluoride	10 mg
Iodine	1100 μg
Iron	45 mg
Magnesium	350 mg
Manganese	11 mg
Molybdenum	2 mg
Nickel	1.0 mg
Phosphorus	4 g
Selenium	400 μg
Vanadium	1.8 g
Zinc	40 mg
Sodium	2.3 g
Chloride	3.6 g

As the chemistry of the vitamins was elucidated, they were given names as well. When only one chemical compound has the biological activity of the vitamin, this is quite easy. Thus, vitamin B_1 is thiamin, vitamin B_2 is riboflavin, etc. With several vitamins, a number of chemically related compounds found in foods can be interconverted in the body, and all show the same biological activity. Such chemically related compounds are called vitamers, and a generic descriptor is used to include all compounds that display the same biological activity. Thus, niacin is the generic descriptor for two compounds, nicotinic acid and nicotinamide, which have the same biological activity. Vitamin B_6 is used to describe the six compounds that have vitamin B_6 activity.

Correctly, for a compound to be classified as a vitamin, it should be a dietary essential that cannot be synthesized in the body. By this strict definition, two vitamins should not really be included, since they can be made in the body. However, both were discovered as a result of investigations of deficiency diseases, and they are usually considered as vitamins:

- Vitamin D is made in the skin after exposure to sunlight (Section 11.3.2.1) and should really be regarded as a steroid hormone rather than a vitamin. It is only when sunlight exposure is inadequate that a dietary source is required.
- Niacin can be formed from the essential amino acid, tryptophan (Section 11.8.2). Indeed, synthesis from tryptophan is probably more important than a dietary intake of preformed niacin.

Table 11.6 The Vitamins

Vitamin		Functions	Deficiency Disease
A	Retinol β-Carotene	Visual pigments in the retina; regulation of gene expression and cell differentiation (β-carotene is an antioxidant)	Night blindness, xerophthalmia; keratinization of skin
D	Calciferol	Maintenance of calcium balance; enhances intestinal absorption of Ca^{2+} and mobilizes bone mineral	Rickets—poor mineralization of bone; osteomalacia—bone demineralization
E	Tocopherols Tocotrienols	Antioxidant, especially in cell membranes	Extremely rare—serious neurological dysfunction
K	Phylloquinone Menaquinones	Coenzyme in formation of γ-carboxyglutamate in proteins of blood clotting and bone matrix	Impaired blood clotting, hemorrhagic disease
B_1	Thiamin	Coenzyme in pyruvate and α-ketoglutarate dehydrogenases and transketolase; role in nerve conduction	Peripheral nerve damage (beriberi) or central nervous system lesions (Wernicke–Korsakoff syndrome)
B_2	Riboflavin	Coenzyme in oxidation and reduction reactions; prosthetic group of flavoproteins	Lesions of corner of mouth, lips, and tongue; sebhorreic dermatitis
Niacin	Nicotinic acid Nicotinamide	Coenzyme in oxidation and reduction reactions, functional part of NAD and NADP	Pellagra—photosensitive dermatitis, depressive psychosis
B_6	Pyridoxine Pyridoxal Pyridoxamine	Coenzyme in transamination and decarboxylation of amino acids, and glycogen phosphorylase; role in steroid hormone action	Disorders of amino acid metabolism, convulsions
	Folic acid	Coenzyme in transfer of one-carbon fragments	Megaloblastic anemia
B_{12}	Cobalamin	Coenzyme in transfer of one-carbon fragments and metabolism of folate	Pernicious anemia—megaloblastic anemia with degeneration of the spinal cord
	Pantothenic acid	Functional part of CoA and acyl carrier protein in fatty acid synthesis and metabolism	Peripheral nerve damage (burning foot syndrome)
H	Biotin	Coenzyme in carboxylation reactions in gluconeogenesis and fatty acid synthesis	Impaired fat and carbohydrate metabolism, dermatitis
C	Ascorbic acid	Coenzyme in hydroxylation of proline and lysine in collagen synthesis; antioxidant; enhances absorption of iron	Scurvy—impaired wound healing, loss of dental cement, subcutaneous hemorrhage

11.2 Vitamin A

Vitamin A was the first vitamin to be discovered, initially as an essential dietary factor for growth. It has roles in vision (as the prosthetic group of the light-sensitive proteins in the retina) and the regulation of gene expression and tissue differentiation. Deficiency is a major problem of public health in large areas of the world.

11.2.1 Vitamin A vitamers and international units

Two groups of compounds (Figure 11.2) have vitamin A activity: retinol, retinaldehyde, and retinoic acid (preformed vitamin A); and a variety of carotenes and related compounds (collectively known as carotenoids), which can be cleaved oxidatively to yield retinaldehyde, and hence retinol and retinoic acid. Those carotenoids that can be cleaved to yield retinaldehyde are known as are known as provitamin A carotenoids.

Retinol and retinoic acids are found only in foods of animal origin, and a small number of bacteria, mainly as the ester retinyl palmitate. The oxidation of retinaldehyde to retinoic acid is irreversible; retinoic acid cannot be converted to retinol *in vivo* and does not support either vision or fertility in deficient animals.

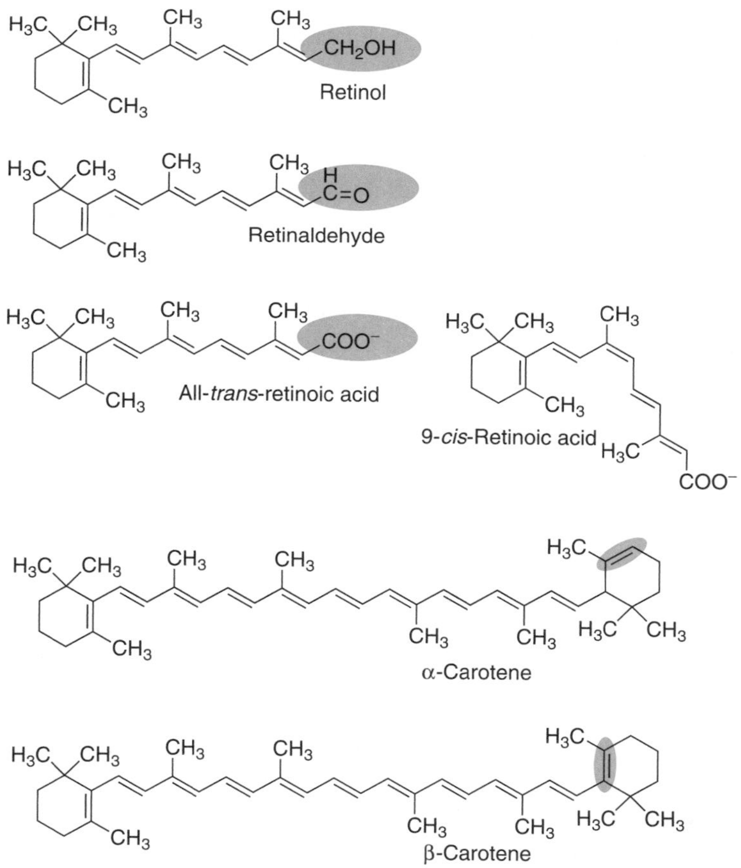

Figure 11.2 Vitamin A: retinoids and major provitamin A carotenoids.

Some 50 or more dietary carotenoids are potential sources of vitamin A: α-, β-, and γ-carotenes, and cryptoxanthin are quantitatively the most important. Although it would appear from its structure that one molecule of β-carotene will yield two of retinol, this is not so in practice (Section 11.2.2.1); 6 μg of β-carotene is equivalent to 1 μg of preformed retinol. For other carotenes with vitamin A activity, 12 μg is equivalent to 1 μg of preformed retinol.

The total amount of vitamin A in foods is expressed as microgram retinol equivalents, calculated from the sum:

1 μg preformed vitamin A + 1/6 × β-carotene (μg) + 1/12 × other provitamin A carotenoids (μg).

Before pure vitamin A was available for chemical analysis, the vitamin A content of foods was determined by biological assay, and the results expressed in international units (iu): 1 iu = 0.3 μg retinol, or 1 μg of retinol = 3.33 iu. Although obsolete, iu is sometimes still used in food labeling.

11.2.2 Metabolism of vitamin A and provitamin A carotenoids

Retinol and carotene are absorbed from the small intestine dissolved in lipid, so that with diets providing less than about 10% of energy from fat, absorption is impaired, and very low fat diets are associated with vitamin A deficiency. About 70%–90% of dietary retinol is normally absorbed, and even at high levels of intake this falls only slightly. Between 5 and 60% of dietary carotene is absorbed depending on the nature of the food and whether it is cooked or raw.

Retinyl esters formed in the intestinal mucosa enter the lymphatic circulation in chylomicrons (Section 4.3.2.2) together with dietary lipid and carotenoids. Tissues can take up retinyl esters from chylomicrons, but most remain in the chylomicron remnants that are taken up by the liver. Here, the esters are hydrolyzed and the vitamin may either be secreted from the liver bound to retinol binding protein or be transferred to stellate cells in the liver, where it is stored as esters in intracellular lipid droplets.

At normal levels of intake, most retinol is catabolized by oxidation to retinoic acid and excreted in the bile as retinoyl glucuronide. As the liver concentration of retinol rises above 70 μmol/kg, microsomal cytochrome P_{450}-dependent oxidation occurs, leading to polar metabolites that are excreted in urine and bile. At high intakes, this pathway becomes saturated, and excess retinol is toxic because there is no further capacity for its catabolism and excretion.

11.2.2.1 Carotene dioxygenase and the formation of retinol from carotenes

As shown in Figure 11.3, β-carotene and other provitamin A carotenoids are cleaved in the intestinal mucosa by carotene dioxygenase, yielding retinaldehyde, which is reduced to retinol, esterified, and secreted in chylomicrons together with esters formed from dietary retinol.

Only a proportion of carotene is oxidized in the intestinal mucosa, and a significant amount enters the circulation in chylomicrons. Carotene in the chylomicron remnants is cleared by the liver, where some is cleaved by hepatic carotene dioxygenase and the remainder is secreted in very low density lipoprotein.

Central oxidative cleavage of β-carotene as shown in Figure 11.3 should yield two molecules of retinaldehyde, which can be reduced to retinol. However, the biological activity of β-carotene, on a molar basis, is considerably lower than that of retinol, not twofold higher

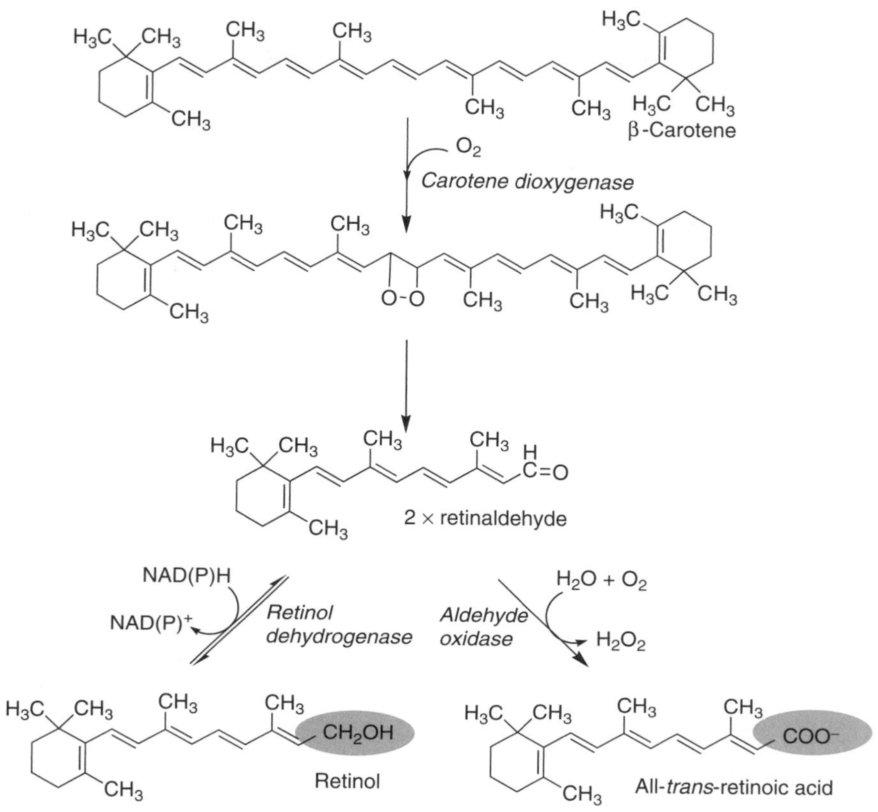

Figure 11.3 The reaction of carotene dioxygenase.

as might be expected. In addition to the relatively poor absorption of carotene from the diet, three factors may account for this:

- The intestinal activity of carotene dioxygenase is relatively low, so a significant proportion of ingested β-carotene may appear in the circulation unchanged.
- Other carotenoids in the diet are not substrates and may inhibit carotene dioxygenase and reduce the proportion that is converted to retinol.
- The principal site of carotene dioxygenase attack is the central bond of β-carotene, but asymmetric cleavage also occurs, leading to the formation of 8′-, 10′-, and 12′-apocarotenals, which are oxidized to retinoic acid, but are not precursors of retinol or retinaldehyde.

11.2.2.2 Plasma retinol-binding protein (RBP)

Retinol is released from the liver bound to an α-globulin, retinol binding protein (RBP); this serves to maintain the vitamin in aqueous solution, protects it against oxidation, and also delivers the vitamin to target tissues. RBP is secreted from the liver as a 1:1 complex with the thyroxine-binding prealbumin, transthyretin. This is important to prevent urinary loss of retinol since RBP alone is small enough to be filtered by the kidney, with a considerable loss of vitamin A from the body.

Cell-surface receptors on target tissues take up retinol from the RBP–transthyretin complex. The cell-surface receptors also remove the carboxyl terminal arginine residue from RBP, thus inactivating it by reducing its affinity for both transthyretin and retinol. The apoprotein is not recycled; it is filtered at the glomerulus, reabsorbed in the proximal renal tubules, and then hydrolyzed.

11.2.3 Metabolic functions of vitamin A

Vitamin A has two major functions: in vision and (as retinoic acids) in regulation of gene expression and tissue differentiation. In addition to their role as vitamin A precursors, carotenes can act as radical-trapping antioxidants (Section 6.5.3.4).

11.2.3.1 Vitamin A in vision

In the retina, retinaldehyde functions as the prosthetic group of the light-sensitive opsin proteins, forming rhodopsin (in rods) and iodopsin (in cones). Any one cone cell contains only one type of opsin and is sensitive to only one color of light. Color blindness results from loss or mutation of one or other of the cone opsins.

In the pigment epithelium of the retina, all-*trans*-retinol is isomerized to 11-*cis*-retinol and oxidized to 11-*cis*-retinaldehyde. This reacts with a lysine residue in opsin, forming the holoprotein rhodopsin. Opsins are cell-type specific; they shift the absorption of 11-*cis*-retinaldehyde from the ultraviolet (UV) into what we call, in consequence, the visible range—either a relatively broad spectrum of sensitivity for vision in dim light (in the rods) or more defined spectral peaks for differentiation of colors in bright light (in the cones).

As shown in Figure 11.4, the absorption of light by rhodopsin causes isomerization of the retinaldehyde bound to opsin from 11-*cis* to all-*trans*, and a conformational change in opsin. This results in the release of retinaldehyde from the protein and the initiation of a nerve impulse. The overall process is known as bleaching since it results in the loss of the color of rhodopsin.

The all-*trans*-retinaldehyde released from rhodopsin is reduced to all-*trans*-retinol, and joins the pool of retinol in the pigment epithelium for isomerization to 11-*cis*-retinol and regeneration of rhodopsin. The key to initiation of the visual cycle is the availability of 11-*cis*-retinaldehyde, and hence vitamin A. In deficiency, both the time taken to adapt to darkness and the ability to see in poor light are impaired.

The formation of the initial excited form of rhodopsin, bathorhodopsin, occurs within picoseconds of illumination and is the only light-dependent step in the visual cycle. Thereafter there is a series of conformational changes leading to the formation of metarhodopsin II. The conversion of metarhodopsin II to metarhodopsin III is relatively slow, with a time course of minutes. The final step is hydrolysis to release all-*trans*-retinaldehyde and opsin.

Metarhodopsin II is the excited form of rhodopsin that initiates a G-protein cascade (Section 10.3.1), leading to a nerve impulse.

11.2.3.2 Retinoic acid and the regulation of gene expression

The most important function of vitamin A is in the control of cell differentiation and turnover. All-*trans*-retinoic acid and 9-*cis*-retinoic acid (Figure 11.3) act in the regulation of growth, development, and tissue differentiation; they have different actions in different tissues. Like the steroid hormones (Section 10.4) and vitamin D (Section 11.3.3), retinoic

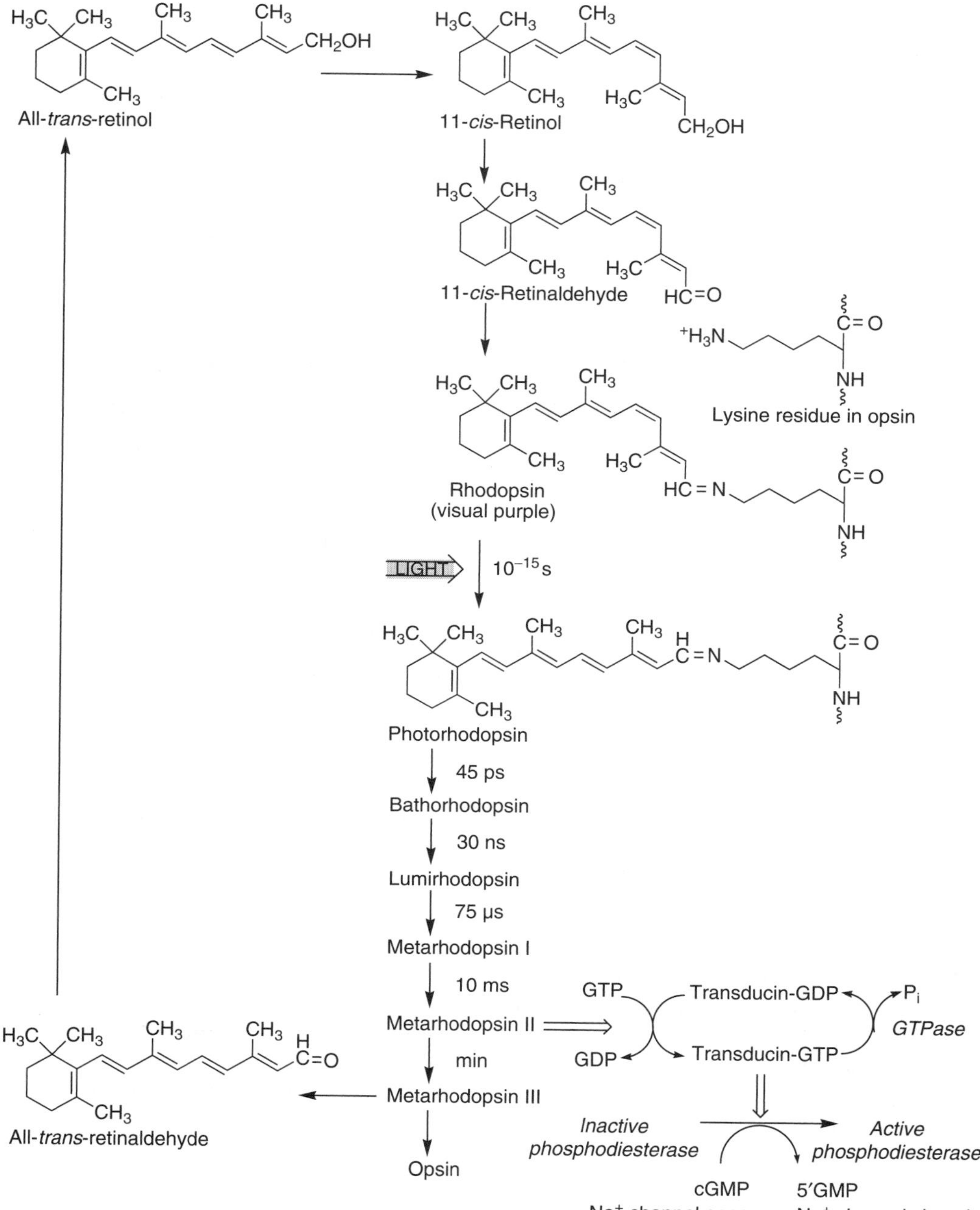

Figure 11.4 The role of retinaldehyde in the visual cycle.

acid binds to nuclear receptors that bind to response elements (control regions) of DNA and regulate the transcription of specific genes.

There are two families of nuclear retinoid receptors: the retinoic acid receptors (RAR) bind all-*trans*-retinoic acid or 9-*cis*-retinoic acid, and the retinoid X receptors (RXR) bind

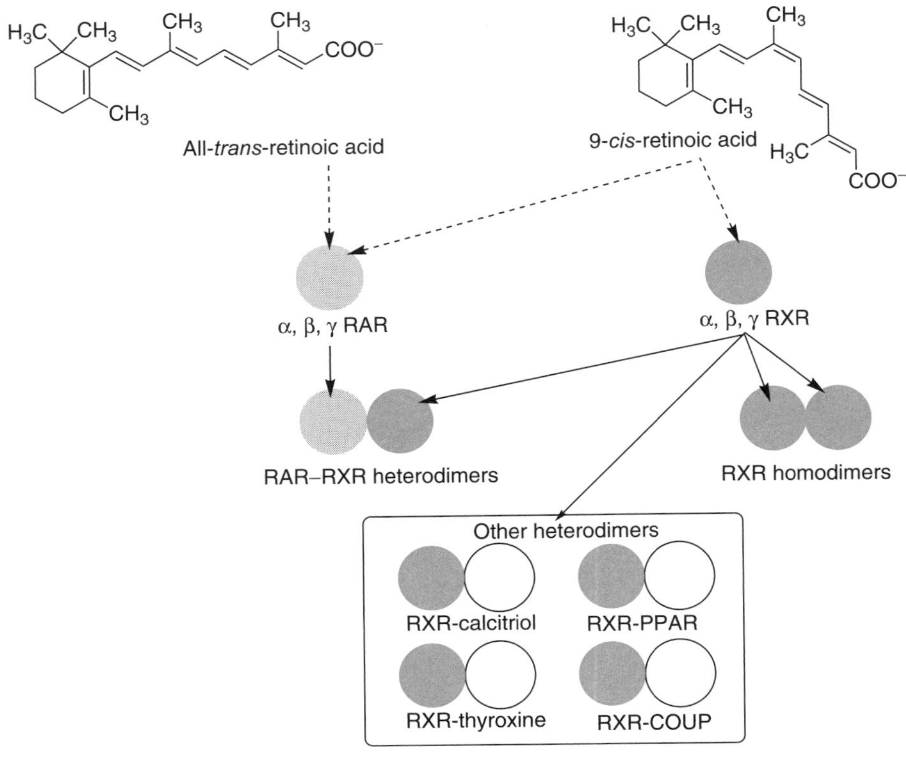

Figure 11.5 Retinoic acid and retinoid receptors.

9-*cis*-retinoic acid (Figure 11.5). Retinoic acid is involved in the regulation of a wide variety of genes; there are three types of activated retinoid receptor dimers, which bind to different response elements on DNA:

- RXR can form homodimers (i.e., RXR–RXR dimers).
- RAR and RXR can form RAR–RXR heterodimers.
- RXR can form heterodimers with a wide variety of other nuclear acting receptors, including those for vitamin D (Section 11.3.3), thyroid hormone (Section 11.15.3.3), long-chain polyunsaturated fatty acid derivatives (the PPAR receptors), and one for which the physiological ligand has not yet been identified (the COUP receptor).

11.2.4 *Vitamin A deficiency—night blindness and xerophthalmia*

Worldwide, vitamin A deficiency is a major public health problem and the most important preventable cause of blindness. The earliest signs of deficiency are connected with vision. Initially, there is a loss of sensitivity to green light; this is followed by impairment of the ability to adapt to dim light, followed by inability to see at all in dim light: night blindness. More prolonged or severe deficiency leads to the condition called xerophthalmia: keratinization of the cornea, followed by ulceration—irreversible damage to the eye that causes blindness. At the same time there are changes in the skin, again with excessive keratinization.

Vitamin A also has an important role in the differentiation of immune system cells, and mild deficiency, not severe enough to cause any disturbance of vision, leads to increased susceptibility to infectious diseases. At the same time, the synthesis of RBP is reduced in response to infection (it is a negative acute phase protein), so that there is a reduction in the circulating concentration of the vitamin and further impairment of immune responses.

Signs of vitamin A deficiency also occur in protein-energy malnutrition (Section 8.2), even when the intake of vitamin A is adequate. This is due to reduced synthesis of plasma RBP, so that despite adequate liver reserves, there is functional vitamin A deficiency. In this case, there is severely impaired immunity to infection as a result of both the functional vitamin A deficiency and also the impairment of immune responses associated with undernutrition.

11.2.5 Vitamin A requirements and reference intakes

There have been relatively few studies of vitamin A requirements in which subjects have been depleted of the vitamin for long enough to permit the development of clear deficiency signs. Current estimates of requirements are based on the intakes required to maintain a concentration of 70 μmol of retinol/kg in the liver, as determined by measurement of the rate of metabolism of isotopically labeled vitamin A. This is adequate to maintain normal plasma concentrations of the vitamin, and people with this level of liver reserves can be maintained on a vitamin A free diet for many months before they develop any signs of deficiency.

The average requirement to maintain a concentration of 70 μmol/kg of liver is 6.7 μg retinol equivalents per kilogram body weight, and this is the basis for calculation of reference intakes.

11.2.5.1 Assessment of vitamin A status

In field surveys to identify those suffering from vitamin A deficiency, the earliest signs of corneal damage are detected by conjunctival impression cytology; abnormalities develop only when liver reserves are seriously depleted. The ability to adapt to dim light is impaired early in deficiency, and dark adaptation time is sometimes used to assess vitamin A status. The test is not suitable for use on children (the group most at risk of deficiency) and the apparatus is not suited to use in the field.

The plasma concentration of vitamin A falls only when the liver reserves are nearly depleted. In deficiency there is accumulation of apo-RBP in the liver, which can be secreted only when vitamin A is available. This provides the basis for the relative dose-response test for vitamin A status—the ability of a dose of retinol to raise the plasma concentration several hours later after chylomicrons have been cleared from the circulation.

11.2.5.2 Toxicity of vitamin A

Although there is an increase in the rate of metabolism and excretion of retinol as the concentration in the liver rises above 70 μmol/kg, there is only a limited capacity to metabolize the vitamin. Excessively high intakes lead to accumulation in the liver and other tissues, above the capacity of binding proteins, so that free, unbound vitamin A is present, leading to tissue damage.

Single doses of 60 mg of retinol are given to children in developing countries as prophylaxis against vitamin A deficiency—an amount adequate to meet the child's needs for 4–6 months. About 1% of children so treated show transient signs of toxicity, but this is

Table 11.7 Recommended Upper Limits of Habitual Intake of Preformed Retinol

	Upper Limit of Intake (μg/day)	RNI (μg/day)
Infants	900	350
1–3 y	1800	400
4–6 y	3000	500
6–12 y	4500	500
13–20 y	6000	600–700
Adult men	9000	700
Adult women	7500	600
Pregnant women	3300	700

considered an acceptable risk in view of the high prevalence and devastating effects of deficiency.

The chronic toxicity of vitamin A is a more general cause for concern; prolonged habitual intake of more than about 7.5–9 mg/day by adults (and significantly less for children, Table 11.7) causes signs and symptoms of toxicity affecting:

- The central nervous system: headache, nausea, ataxia, and anorexia, all associated with increased cerebrospinal fluid pressure
- The liver: hepatomegaly with histological changes in the liver, increased collagen formation, and hyperlipidemia
- Bones: joint pains, thickening of the long bones, hypercalcemia, and calcification of soft tissues
- The skin: excessive dryness, scaling and chapping of the skin, desquamation, and alopecia (hair loss)

The synthetic retinoids, 13-*cis*-retinoic acid and etretinate, used to treat dermatological problems are highly teratogenic. After women have been treated with them, it is recommended that contraceptive precautions be continued for 12 months, because of their retention in the body. By extrapolation, it has been assumed that retinol is also teratogenic, and pregnant women are advised not to consume more than 3000–3300 μg of preformed vitamin A per day.

High intakes of carotene are not known to have any adverse effects apart from giving an orange–yellow color to the skin. However, in two intervention studies in the 1990s with supplements of β-carotene, there was increased mortality from lung cancer in those receiving the supplements. It is likely that under conditions of high oxygen availability, β-carotene (and presumably also other carotenoids) has a more marked pro-oxidant action than an antioxidant action (Section 6.5.3.4).

11.3 Vitamin D

Vitamin D is not strictly a vitamin since it can be synthesized in the skin, and indeed under most conditions endogenous synthesis is the major source of the vitamin—it is only when sunlight exposure is inadequate that a dietary source is required. It is important in the regulation of calcium absorption and homeostasis, and has a wide range of other actions mediated by nuclear receptors that regulate gene expression and cell differentiation. Deficiency, leading to rickets in children and osteomalacia in adults, continues to be a problem in northern latitudes, where sunlight exposure is poor, and there is increasing evidence that higher levels of intake or increased sunlight exposure may provide protection against various chronic diseases.

11.3.1 Vitamers and international units

The normal dietary form of vitamin D is cholecalciferol (also known as calciol). This is also the compound that is formed in the skin by UV irradiation of 7-dehydrocholesterol. Some foods are enriched with the synthetic compound ergocalciferol, which is synthesized by UV irradiation of the steroid ergosterol. Ergocalciferol is metabolized in the same way as cholecalciferol and has the same biological activity. Early studies assigned the name vitamin D_1 to an impure mixture of products derived from the irradiation of ergosterol; when ergocalciferol was identified, it was called vitamin D_2; and when the physiological compound was identified as cholecalciferol, it was called vitamin D_3.

Like vitamin A, vitamin D was measured in international units of biological activity before the pure compound was isolated: 1 iu = 25 ng of cholecalciferol; 1 μg of cholecalciferol = 40 iu.

11.3.2 Absorption and metabolism of vitamin D

There are a few dietary sources of vitamin D, mainly oily fish; while eggs, liver, and butter provide modest amounts. It is absorbed in lipid micelles and incorporated into chylomicrons, so that people with a low fat diet will absorb little of such dietary vitamin D as is available. For most people, endogenous synthesis in the skin is the major source of the vitamin.

11.3.2.1 Synthesis of vitamin D in the skin

7-Dehydrocholesterol is an intermediate in the synthesis of cholesterol, which accumulates in the skin but not other tissues. It undergoes a nonenzymic reaction on exposure to UV light, yielding previtamin D (Figure 11.6). This undergoes a further reaction over a period

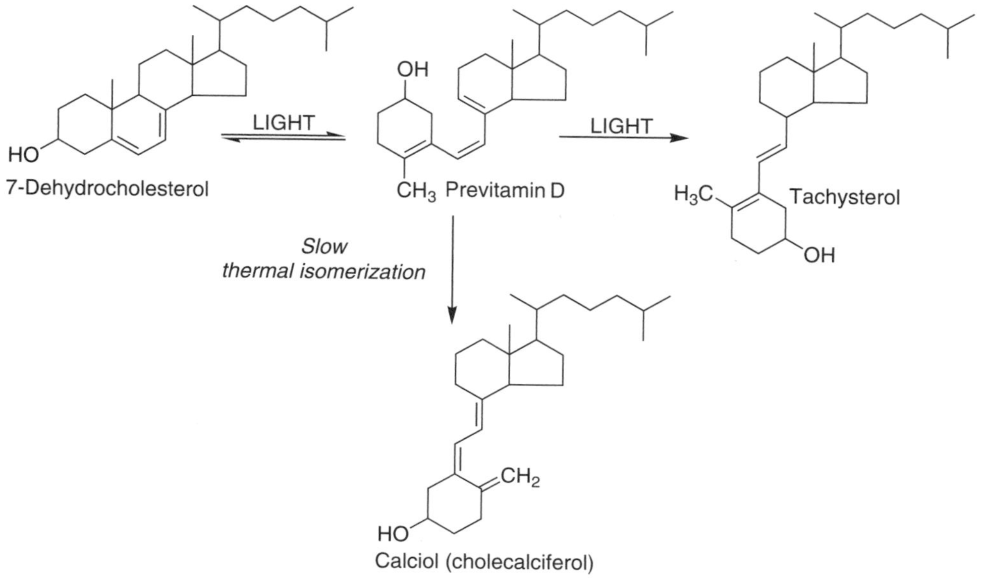

Figure 11.6 The synthesis of vitamin D in the skin.

of hours to form cholecalciferol, which is absorbed into the bloodstream. The photolytic reaction occurs with radiation in the UV-B range, between 290 and 310 nm, with a relatively sharp peak at 296.5 nm.

In temperate climates, there is a marked seasonal variation in the plasma concentration of vitamin D; it is highest at the end of summer and lowest at the end of winter. Although there may be bright sunlight in winter, beyond about 40°N or S there is very little UV radiation of the appropriate wavelength for cholecalciferol synthesis when the sun is low in the sky. By contrast, during summer, when the sun is more or less overhead, there is a considerable amount of UV light even on a moderately cloudy day and enough can penetrate thin clothes to result in significant formation of vitamin D.

11.3.2.2 Metabolism to the active metabolite, calcitriol

Cholecalciferol, either synthesized in the skin or taken in from foods, undergoes two hydroxylations to yield the active metabolite, 1,25-dihydroxyvitamin D or calcitriol (Figure 11.7).

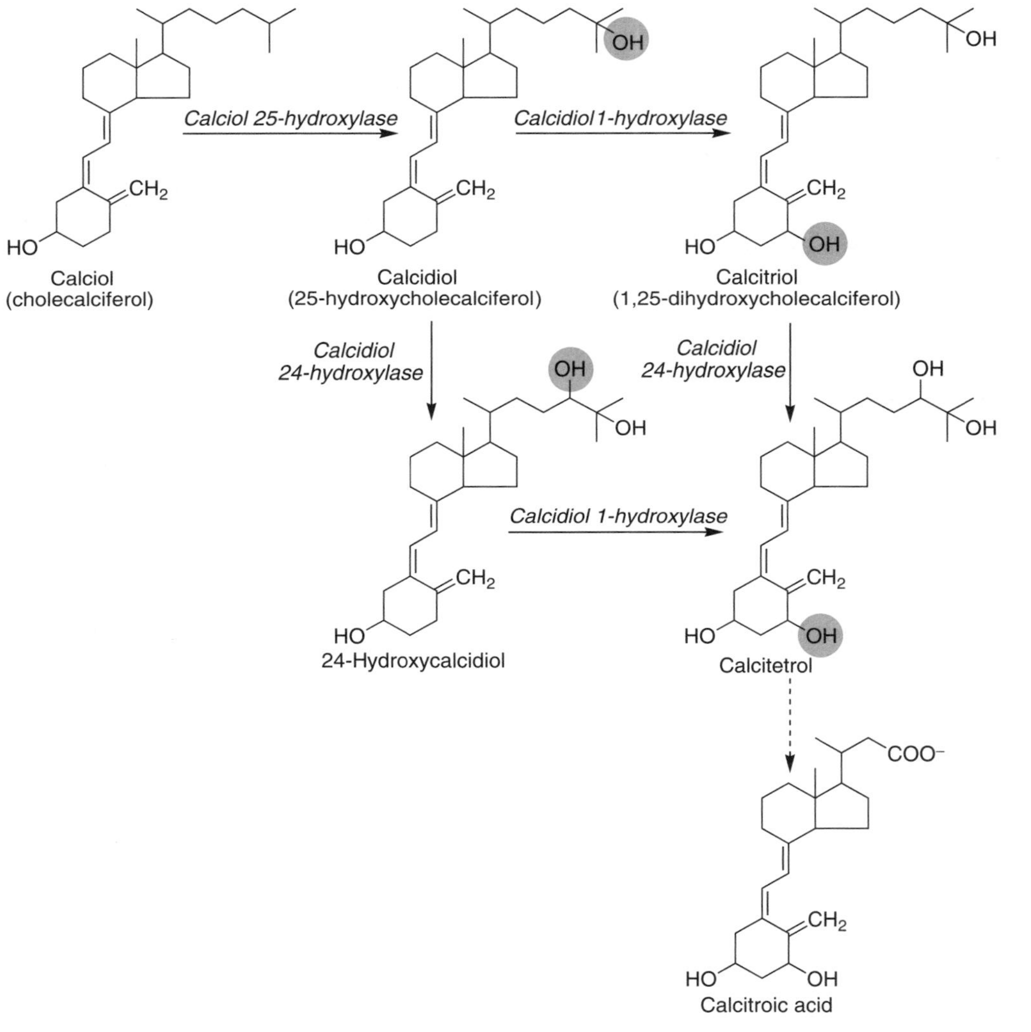

Figure 11.7 Metabolism of vitamin D.

Table 11.8 Nomenclature of Vitamin D Metabolites

Trivial Name	Recommended Name	Abbreviation
Vitamin D_3		
Cholecalciferol	Calciol	–
25-Hydroxycholecalciferol	Calcidiol	$25(OH)D_3$
1α-Hydroxycholecalciferol	1(*S*)-hydroxycalciol	$1\alpha(OH)D_3$
24,25-Dihydroxycholecalciferol	24(*R*)-hydroxycalcidiol	$24,25(OH)_2D_3$
1,25-Dihydroxycholecalciferol	Calcitriol	$1,25(OH)_2D_3$
1,24,25-Trihydroxycholecalciferol	Calcitetrol	$1,24,25(OH)_3D_3$
Vitamin D_2		
Ergocalciferol	Ercalciol	–
25-Hydroxyergocalciferol	Ercalcidiol	$25(OH)D_2$
24,25-Dihydroxyergocalciferol	24(*R*)-hydroxyercalcidiol	$24,25(OH)_2D_2$
1,25-Dihydroxyergocalciferol	Ercalcitriol	$1,25(OH)_2 D_2$
1,24,25-Trihydroxyergocalciferol	Ercalcitetrol	$1,24,25(OH)_3D_2$

Note: The abbreviations shown in column 3 are not recommended, but are frequently used in the literature.

Ergocalciferol from fortified foods undergoes similar hydroxylation to yield ercalcitriol. The nomenclature of the vitamin D metabolites is shown in Table 11.8.

The first hydroxylation occurs in the liver to form the 25-hydroxy-derivative, calcidiol. This is released into the circulation bound to a vitamin D binding globulin. There is no tissue storage of vitamin D; plasma calcidiol is the main reserve of the vitamin and it is plasma calcidiol that shows the most significant seasonal variation in temperate climates.

The second hydroxylation occurs in the kidney, where calcidiol undergoes either 1-hydroxylation to yield the active metabolite 1,25-dihydroxyvitamin D (calcitriol) or 24-hydroxylation to yield an apparently inactive metabolite, 24,25-dihydroxyvitamin D (24-hydroxycalcidiol).

The main function of vitamin D is in the control of calcium homeostasis (Section 11.15.1), and in turn vitamin D metabolism is regulated at the level of 1- or 24-hydroxylation by factors that respond to plasma concentrations of calcium and phosphate:

- Calcitriol acts to reduce its own synthesis. It induces the 24-hydroxylase and represses the synthesis of 1-hydroxylase in the kidney, acting on gene expression through calcitriol receptors.
- Parathyroid hormone is secreted in response to a fall in plasma calcium. In the kidney, it acts to increase the activity of calcidiol 1-hydroxylase and decrease that of the 24-hydroxylase. This is not an effect on protein synthesis but the result of changes in the activity of existing enzyme protein, mediated by cAMP (Section 10.3.2). In turn, both calcitriol and high concentrations of calcium repress the synthesis of parathyroid hormone.
- Calcium exerts its main effect on the synthesis and secretion of parathyroid hormone. However, calcium ions also have a direct effect on the kidney, reducing the activity of calcidiol 1-hydroxylase (but with no effect on the activity of 24-hydroxylase).

11.3.3 Metabolic functions of vitamin D

Calcitriol acts like a steroid hormone, binding to a nuclear receptor protein (Section 10.4), and forming a heterodimer with the vitamin A (RXR) receptor (Section 11.2.3.2). The active receptor complex binds to the enhancer site of the gene coding for a calcium binding protein, increasing its transcription and thus increasing the amount of calcium binding protein in the cell.

The principal function of vitamin D is to maintain the plasma concentration of calcium; calcitriol achieves this in three ways:

- Increased intestinal absorption of calcium
- Reduced excretion of calcium (by stimulating reabsorption in the distal renal tubules)
- Mobilization of bone mineral

In addition, calcitriol has a variety of permissive or modulatory effects; it is a necessary but not sufficient factor in

- Insulin secretion
- Synthesis and secretion of parathyroid and thyroid hormones
- Inhibition of production of interleukin by activated T-lymphocytes and of immunoglobulin by activated B-lymphocytes
- Differentiation of monocyte precursor cells in the immune system
- Modulation of cell proliferation

The best studied actions of vitamin D are in the intestinal mucosa where the intracellular calcium binding protein is essential for the absorption of calcium from the diet. Here the vitamin has another action as well, to increase the transport of calcium across the mucosal membrane. The increase in calcium transport is seen immediately after feeding vitamin D, whereas the increase in absorption is slower since it depends on new synthesis of the binding protein. The rapid response to vitamin D does not involve new protein synthesis, but reflects an effect on preformed calcium transport proteins in the cell membrane.

11.3.3.1 *The role of calcitriol in bone metabolism*

The maintenance of bone structure is due to the balanced activity of osteoclasts, which erode existing bone mineral and organic matrix; and osteoblasts, which synthesize and secrete the proteins of bone matrix. Mineralization of the organic matrix is largely controlled by the availability of calcium and phosphate.

Calcitriol raises plasma calcium by activating osteoclasts to stimulate the mobilization of calcium from bone. It acts later to stimulate the laying down of new bone to replace the loss by stimulating the differentiation and recruitment of osteoblast cells.

11.3.4 *Vitamin D deficiency: rickets and osteomalacia*

Historically, rickets is a disease of toddlers, especially in northern industrial cities. Their bones are undermineralized, as a result of poor absorption of calcium in the absence of adequate amounts of calcitriol. When the child begins to walk, the long bones of the legs are deformed, leading to bowlegs or knock-knees. More seriously, rickets can also lead to collapse of the rib cage and deformities of the bones of the pelvis. Similar problems may also occur in adolescents who are deficient in vitamin D during the adolescent growth spurt, when there is again a high demand for calcium for new bone formation.

Osteomalacia is the adult equivalent of rickets. It results from the demineralization of bone, rather than the failure to mineralize it in the first place, as is the case with rickets. Women who have little exposure to sunlight are especially at risk from osteomalacia after several pregnancies, because of the strain that pregnancy places on their marginal reserve of calcium.

Osteomalacia also occurs in the elderly. Here again the problem may be inadequate exposure to sunlight, but there is also evidence that the capacity to form 7-dehydrocholesterol in the skin decreases with advancing age, so that the elderly are more reliant on the few dietary sources of vitamin D.

11.3.5 Vitamin D requirements and reference intakes

It is difficult to determine requirements for dietary vitamin D since the major source is synthesis in the skin. The main criterion of adequacy is the plasma concentration of calcidiol. In elderly subjects with little sunlight exposure, a dietary intake of 10 μg of vitamin D per day results in a plasma calcidiol concentration of 20 nmol/L, the lower end of the reference range for younger adults at the end of winter. Therefore, the U.K. reference intake for the elderly is 10 μg/day; the same figure is used for younger adults in the U.S., with an RDA of 15 μg/day for older people. Average intakes of vitamin D are less than 4 μg/day, so to achieve an intake of 10–15 μg/day will almost certainly require either fortification of foods or the use of vitamin D supplements.

Evidence is accumulating that the functions of vitamin D in regulation of gene expression and cell differentiation suggest that higher levels of intake are desirable, with reference intakes of the order of 15–20 μg/day or higher. This level of intake certainly could not be achieved from unfortified foods, but would be achievable by increased sunlight exposure. The problem is that excessive sunlight exposure is associated with increased risk of skin cancer.

11.3.5.1 Vitamin D toxicity

During the 1950s, rickets was more or less totally eradicated in Britain and other temperate countries. This was due to enrichment of a large number of infant foods with vitamin D. However, a small number of infants suffered from vitamin D poisoning, the most serious effect of which is an elevated plasma concentration of calcium. This can lead to contraction of blood vessels, and hence dangerously high blood pressure, and calcinosis—the calcification of soft tissues, including the kidney, heart, lungs, and blood vessel walls.

Some infants are sensitive to intakes of vitamin D as low as 50 μg/day. To avoid the serious problem of vitamin D poisoning in these susceptible infants, the fortification of infant foods with vitamin D was reduced considerably. Unfortunately, this means that a small proportion of infants, who have relatively high requirements, are at risk of developing rickets. The problem is to identify those who have high requirements and provide them with supplements.

The toxic threshold in adults is not known, but patients suffering from vitamin D intoxication who have been investigated were taking more than 250 μg of vitamin D/day.

Although excess dietary vitamin D is toxic, excessive exposure to sunlight does not lead to vitamin D poisoning. There is a limited capacity to form the precursor, 7-dehydrocholesterol, in the skin, and a limited capacity to take up cholecalciferol from the skin. Furthermore, prolonged exposure of previtamin D to UV light results in further reactions to yield biologically inactive compounds.

11.4 Vitamin E

Although vitamin E was identified as a dietary essential for animals in the 1920s, it was not until 1983 that it was clearly demonstrated to be a dietary essential for humans. Vitamin E acts as a lipid-soluble antioxidant in cell membranes and plasma lipoproteins, and has a number of other membrane-specific functions, including roles in cell signaling

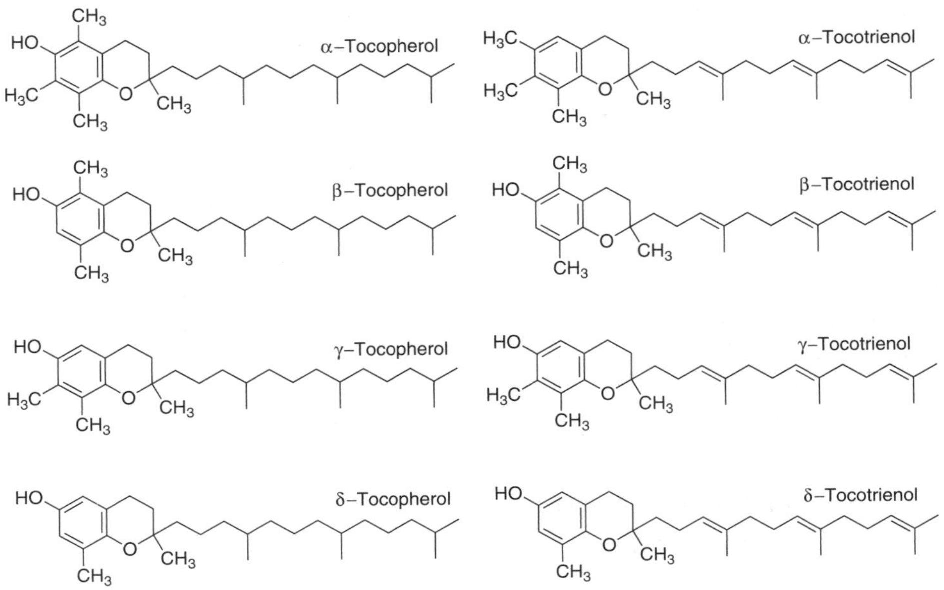

Figure 11.8 Vitamin E vitamers.

and platelet aggregation. There is epidemiological evidence that high intakes of vitamin E are associated with lower incidence of cardiovascular disease (Section 6.5.3.3).

11.4.1 Vitamers and units of activity

Vitamin E is the generic descriptor for two families of compounds, the tocopherols and the tocotrienols (Figure 11.8). The different vitamers have different biological potency as shown in Table 11.9. The most active is α-tocopherol, and it is usual to express vitamin E intake in terms of milligram α-tocopherol equivalents. This is the sum of:

$$\text{mg } \alpha\text{-tocopherol} + 0.5 \text{ mg } \beta\text{-tocopherol} + 0.1 \text{ mg } \gamma\text{-tocopherol} \\ + 0.3 \text{ mg } \alpha\text{-tocotrienol}$$

The other vitamers either occur in negligible amounts in foods or have negligible vitamin activity.

The obsolete international unit of vitamin E activity is still sometimes used: 1 iu = 0.67 mg α-tocopherol equivalent; 1 mg α-tocopherol = 1.49 iu.

Synthetic α-tocopherol does not have the same biological potency as the naturally occurring compound, because the side chain of tocopherol has three centers of asymmetry (Figure 11.9), and when it is synthesized chemically the product is a mixture of the various isomers. In the naturally occurring compound, all three centers of asymmetry have the *R* configuration, and naturally occurring α-tocopherol is all -*R*, or *RRR*-α-tocopherol.

11.4.2 Absorption and metabolism of vitamin E

Tocopherols and tocotrienols are absorbed in lipid micelles, incorporated into chylomicrons (Section 4.3.2.2), then secreted by the liver in very low density lipoproteins (VLDL).

Table 11.9 Relative Biological Activity of the Vitamin E Vitamers

	iu/mg	Relative Activity
D-α-tocopherol (*RRR*)	1.49	1.0
D-β-tocopherol (*RRR*)	0.75	0.49
D-γ-tocopherol (*RRR*)	0.15	0.10
D-δ-tocopherol (*RRR*)	0.05	0.03
D-α-tocotrienol	0.45	0.29
D-β-tocotrienol	0.08	0.05
D-γ-tocotrienol	–	–
D-δ-tocotrienol	–	–
L-α-tocopherol (*SRR*)	0.46	0.31
RRS-α-tocopherol	1.34	0.90
SRS-α-tocopherol	0.55	0.37
RSS-α-tocopherol	1.09	0.73
SSR-α-tocopherol	0.31	0.21
RSR-α-tocopherol	0.85	0.57
SSS-α-tocopherol	1.10	0.74

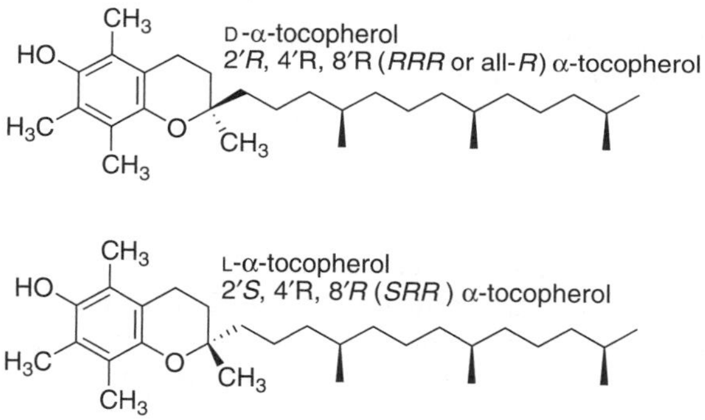

Figure 11.9 Asymmetric centers in α-tocopherol.

The major route of excretion is in the bile as a variety of metabolites. There may also be significant excretion of the vitamin through the skin.

There are two mechanisms for tissue uptake of vitamin E. Lipoprotein lipase releases the vitamin by hydrolyzing the triacylglycerol in chylomicrons and VLDL, while separately there is uptake of low density lipoprotein (LDL) bound vitamin E by means of LDL receptors. Retention within tissues depends on intracellular binding proteins, and the differences in biological activity of the vitamers are due to differential protein binding. γ-Tocopherol and α-tocotrienol bind relatively poorly, while *SRR*-α-tocopherol and *RRR*-α-tocopherol acetate do not bind to liver tocopherol binding protein to any significant extent.

11.4.3 *Metabolic functions of vitamin E*

The main function of vitamin E is as a radical-trapping antioxidant in cell membranes and plasma lipoproteins. It is especially important in limiting radical damage resulting from oxidation of polyunsaturated fatty acids, by reacting with the lipid peroxide radicals before they can establish a chain reaction (Section 6.5). The radical formed from vitamin E is relatively unreactive and persists long enough to undergo reaction to yield nonradical products. Commonly, the vitamin E radical in a membrane or a lipoprotein is reduced back to tocopherol by reaction with vitamin C in plasma (Figure 6.17). The resultant monodehydroascorbate radical then undergoes enzymic or nonenzymic reaction to yield ascorbate and dehydroascorbate (Figure 6.18), neither of which is a radical.

The antioxidant function of vitamin E is dependent on the stability of the tocopheroxyl radical, which means that it survives long enough to undergo reaction to yield nonradical products. However, this stability also means that the tocopheroxyl radical can also penetrate further into cells or deeper into plasma lipoproteins and potentially propagate a chain reaction. Therefore, although it is regarded as an antioxidant, vitamin E may, like other antioxidants, also have pro-oxidant actions, especially at high concentrations. This may explain why although epidemiological studies have shown a clear association between high blood concentrations of vitamin E and lower incidence of atherosclerosis, the results of intervention studies with relatively high doses of vitamin E have generally been disappointing (Section 6.5.3.3).

There is a considerable overlap between the functions of vitamin E and selenium (Section 11.15.2.5). Vitamin E reduces lipid peroxides to unreactive fatty acids (Figure 6.17); the selenium dependent enzyme glutathione peroxidase reduces hydrogen peroxide to water (Figure 5.15), thus lowering the intracellular concentration of potentially lipid-damaging peroxide. Glutathione peroxidase will also reduce the tocopheroxyl radical back to tocopherol. Thus, vitamin E acts to remove the products of lipid peroxidation, while selenium acts both to remove the cause of lipid peroxidation and also to recycle vitamin E. In vitamin E-deficient animals, selenium will prevent many of the signs of deficiency, but not central nervous system necrosis (Section 11.4.4).

11.4.3.1 Hypocholesterolemic actions of tocotrienols

Tocotrienols have lower biological activity than tocopherols, and indeed it is conventional to consider only γ-tocotrienol as a significant part of vitamin E intake. However, the tocotrienols have a hypocholesterolemic action not shared by the tocopherols. In plants, tocotrienols are synthesized from hydroxymethylglutaryl CoA (HMG CoA), which is also the precursor for cholesterol synthesis (Figure 6.19). High levels of tocotrienols repress the synthesis of HMG CoA reductase, the rate-limiting enzyme in the pathway for synthesis of both cholesterol and tocotrienols.

11.4.4 Vitamin E deficiency

In experimental animals, vitamin E deficiency results in a number of different conditions:

- Deficient female animals suffer the death and resorption of the fetuses. This provided the basis of the original biological assay of vitamin E.
- Deficient male animals suffer testicular atrophy and degeneration of the germinal epithelium of the seminiferous tubules.
- Both skeletal and cardiac muscle are affected in deficiency. This is sometimes called nutritional muscular dystrophy, an unfortunate term, since there is no evidence that human muscular dystrophy is related to vitamin E deficiency and the condition is better called necrotizing myopathy.

- The integrity of blood vessel walls is affected, with leakage of blood plasma into subcutaneous tissues, and accumulation under the skin of a green-colored fluid—exudative diathesis.
- The nervous system is affected with the development of central nervous system necrosis and axonal dystrophy. This is exacerbated by feeding diets rich in polyunsaturated fatty acids.

Dietary deficiency of vitamin E in humans is unknown, although patients with severe fat malabsorption, cystic fibrosis, some forms of chronic liver disease, or (very rare) congenital lack of plasma β-lipoprotein or intracellular vitamin E-binding proteins suffer deficiency because they are unable to absorb the vitamin or transport it around the body. They suffer from severe damage to nerve and muscle membranes.

Premature infants are at risk of vitamin E deficiency since they are often born with inadequate reserves of the vitamin. The red blood cell membranes of deficient infants are abnormally fragile as a result of unchecked oxidative radical attack. This may lead to hemolytic anemia if they are not given supplements of the vitamin.

Experimental animals that are depleted of vitamin E become sterile. However, there is no evidence that vitamin E nutritional status is in any way associated with human fertility and there is certainly no evidence that vitamin E supplements increase sexual potency, prowess, or vigor.

11.4.5 Vitamin E requirements

It is difficult to establish vitamin E requirements, partly because deficiency is more or less unknown and also because the requirement depends on the intake of polyunsaturated fatty acids. It is generally accepted that an acceptable intake of vitamin E is 0.4 mg α-tocopherol equivalent per gram dietary polyunsaturated fatty acid. The plant oils that are rich sources of polyunsaturated fatty acids are also rich sources of vitamin E.

11.4.5.1 Indices of vitamin E status

Erythrocytes are incapable of *de novo* lipid synthesis, so peroxidative damage resulting from oxygen stress has a serious effect, shortening red-cell life and possibly precipitating hemolytic anemia in vitamin E deficiency. This can be used as a method of assessing status (although unrelated factors affect the results) by measuring the hemolysis of red cells induced by dilute hydrogen peroxide.

An alternative method of assessing functional antioxidant status, again one that is affected by both vitamin E and other antioxidants, is by measuring the exhalation of pentane arising from the metabolism of the peroxides ω6 polyunsaturated fatty acids or ethane from peroxides of ω3 polyunsaturated fatty acids.

11.5 Vitamin K

Vitamin K was discovered as a result of investigations into the cause of a bleeding disorder (hemorrhagic disease) of cattle fed on silage made from sweet clover and of chickens fed on a fat-free diet. The missing factor in the diet of the chickens was identified as vitamin K, while the problem in the cattle was that the feed contained dicumarol, an antagonist of the vitamin. Because of its importance in blood coagulation, it was called the *koagulations-vitamine* (vitamin K) when the original results were reported (in German).

Since the effect of an excessive intake of dicumarol was severely impaired blood clotting, it was isolated and tested in low doses as an anticoagulant for use in patients at risk of thrombosis. Although it was effective, it had unwanted side effects and synthetic vitamin K antagonists were developed for clinical use as anticoagulants. The most commonly used of these is Warfarin, which is also used, in larger amounts, to kill rodents.

11.5.1 Vitamers of vitamin K

Three compounds have the biological activity of vitamin K (Figure 11.10):

- Phylloquinone, the normal dietary source, found in green leafy vegetables
- Menaquinones, a family of related compounds synthesized by intestinal bacteria, with differing lengths of side chain
- Menadione and menadiol diacetate, synthetic compounds that can be metabolized to phylloquinone

Phylloquinone is found in all green leafy vegetables; the richest sources are spring (collard) greens, spinach, and brussels sprouts. In addition, soybean, rapeseed, cottonseed, and olive oils are relatively rich in vitamin K, although other oils are not.

About 80% of dietary phylloquinone is normally absorbed into the lymphatic system in chylomicrons and is then taken up by the liver from chylomicron remnants and released into the circulation in VLDL.

Intestinal bacteria synthesize a variety of menaquinones, which are absorbed to a limited extent from the large intestine, again into the lymphatic system, cleared by the

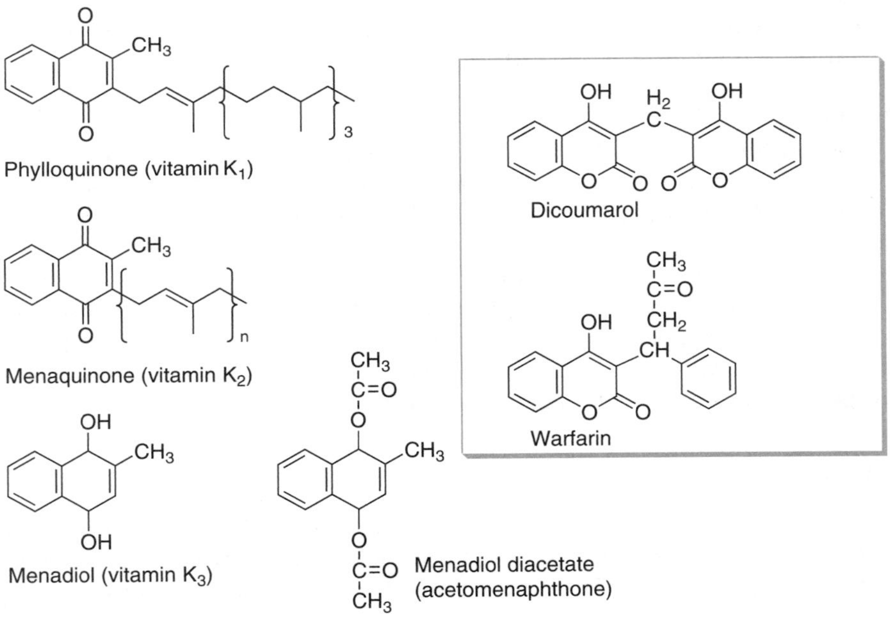

Figure 11.10 Vitamin K vitamers; the vitamin K antagonists dicoumarol and Warfarin are shown in the box. Menadione and menadiol diacetate are synthetic compounds that are converted to menaquinone in the liver.

liver, and released in VLDL. It is often suggested that about half the requirement for vitamin K is met by intestinal bacterial synthesis, but there is little evidence for this, other than the fact that about half the vitamin K in liver is phylloquinone and the remainder a variety of menaquinones. It is not clear to what extent the menaquinones are biologically active—it is possible to induce signs of vitamin K deficiency simply by feeding a phylloquinone-deficient diet, without inhibiting intestinal bacterial action.

11.5.2 Metabolic functions of vitamin K

Vitamin K is the cofactor for the carboxylation of glutamate residues in the postsynthetic modification of proteins to form the unusual amino acid γ-carboxyglutamate, abbreviated to Gla (Figure 11.11; see Problem 9.2).

The first step in the reaction is oxidation of vitamin K hydroquinone to the epoxide. This epoxide then activates a glutamate residue in the protein substrate to a carbanion that reacts nonenzymically with carbon dioxide to form γ-carboxyglutamate. Vitamin K epoxide is then reduced to the quinone by a Warfarin-sensitive reductase, and the quinone is reduced to the active hydroquinone by either the same Warfarin-sensitive reductase or a Warfarin-insensitive quinone reductase.

In the presence of Warfarin, vitamin K epoxide cannot be reduced back to the active hydroquinone, but accumulates and is conjugated and excreted. If enough vitamin K is provided in the diet, the quinone can be reduced to the active hydroquinone by the Warfarin-insensitive enzyme, and carboxylation can continue with stoichiometric utilization of vitamin K and excretion of the epoxide. High doses of vitamin K are used to treat patients who have received an overdose of Warfarin, and at least part of the resistance

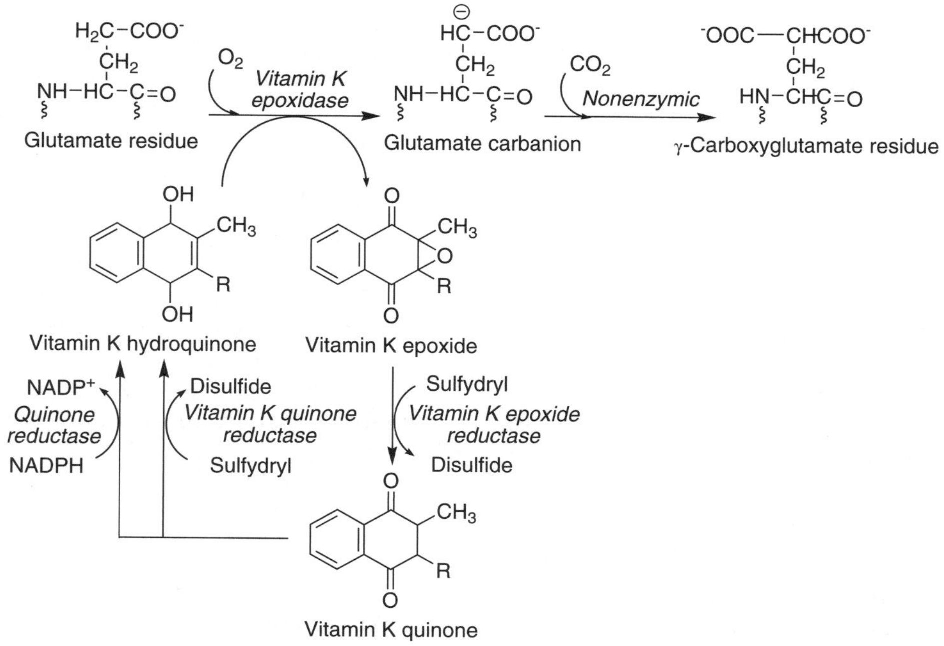

Figure 11.11 The role of vitamin K in γ-carboxyglutamate synthesis.

of some populations of rats to the action of Warfarin is due to a high consumption of vitamin K from maram grass, although there are also genetically resistant populations of rodents.

Prothrombin and several other proteins of the blood clotting system (factors VII, IX, and X, and proteins C and S) each contain between 4 and 6 γ-carboxyglutamate residues per mole. γ-Carboxyglutamate chelates calcium ions and so permits the binding of the blood clotting proteins to membranes. In vitamin K deficiency or in the presence of an antagonist such as Warfarin, an abnormal precursor of prothrombin (preprothrombin) containing little or no γ-carboxyglutamate is released into the circulation. Preprothrombin cannot chelate calcium or bind to phospholipid membranes, and so is unable to initiate blood clotting. Preprothrombin is sometimes known as PIVKA—the protein induced by vitamin K absence.

11.5.2.1 Vitamin K dependent proteins in bone

Treatment of pregnant women with Warfarin can lead to bone abnormalities in the child—the fetal Warfarin syndrome. Two proteins in the bone matrix contain γ-carboxyglutamate: osteocalcin and the bone matrix Gla protein. Osteocalcin is interesting in that besides γ-carboxyglutamate, it also contains hydroxyproline, so its synthesis is dependent not only on vitamin K but also on vitamin C (Section 11.14.2.2); in addition, its synthesis is induced by vitamin D, and the release into the circulation of osteocalcin provides a sensitive index of vitamin D action (Section 11.3.3.1). Osteocalcin comprises some 1%–2% of total bone protein, and it functions as a calcium binding protein, modifying the crystallization of bone mineral. The matrix Gla protein is found in a variety of tissues, where it functions to maintain calcium in solution and prevent mineralization.

11.5.3 Vitamin K deficiency and requirements

Apart from experimental depletion, vitamin K deficiency is unknown, and determination of requirements is complicated by a lack of data on the importance of menaquinones synthesized by intestinal bacteria.

The main way of determining vitamin K status and monitoring the efficacy of anticoagulant therapy is by measuring the time required for the formation of a fibrin clot in citrated blood plasma after the addition of calcium ions and thromboplastin—the prothrombin time. A more sensitive index is provided by direct measurement of preprothrombin in plasma, most commonly by immunoassay using antisera against preprothrombin that do not react with prothrombin. Such studies suggest that an intake of 1 μg per kilogram body weight per day is adequate, leading reference intakes between 65 and 80 μg/day for adults.

A small number of newborn infants have very low reserves of vitamin K and are at risk of potentially fatal hemorrhagic disease. It is therefore generally recommended that all neonates be given a single prophylactic dose of vitamin K.

11.6 Vitamin B_1 (thiamin)

Historically, thiamin deficiency affecting the peripheral nervous system (beriberi) was a major public health problem in Southeast Asia following the introduction of the steam-powered mill that made highly polished (thiamin depleted) rice widely available. There are still sporadic outbreaks of deficiency among people whose diet is rich

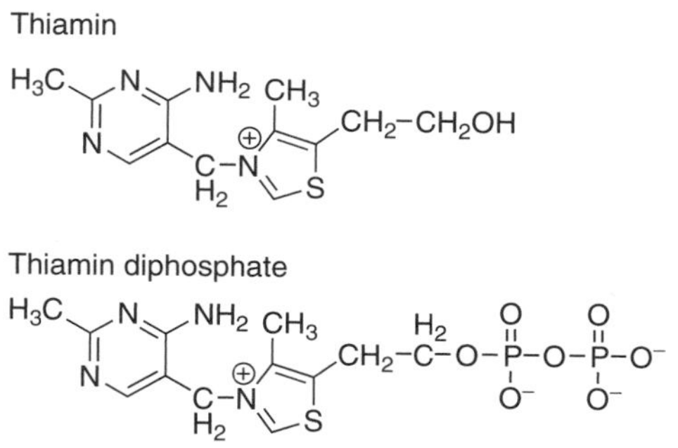

Thiamin

Thiamin diphosphate

Figure 11.12 Thiamin (vitamin B_1) and the coenzyme thiamin diphosphate.

in carbohydrate and poor in thiamin. More commonly, thiamin deficiency affecting the heart and central nervous system is a problem in people with an excessive consumption of alcohol.

The structures of thiamin and the coenzyme thiamin diphosphate are shown in Figure 11.12. Thiamin is unstable to light, and although bread and flour contain significant amounts of thiamin, much or all of this can be lost when baked goods are exposed to sunlight in a shop window.

Thiamin is also destroyed by sulfites, and in potato products that have been blanched by immersion in sulfite solution there is little or no thiamin remaining. Polyphenols, including tannic acid in tea and betel nuts, also destroy thiamin and have been associated with thiamin deficiency. Fermented raw fish is also devoid of thiamin because of the action of thiaminases that cleave the vitamin.

11.6.1 *Absorption and metabolism of thiamin*

Most dietary thiamin is present as phosphates, which are readily hydrolyzed by intestinal phosphatases, and free thiamin is readily absorbed in the duodenum and proximal jejunum, and then transferred to the portal circulation as free thiamin or thiamin monophosphate. This is an active transport process and is inhibited by alcohol, which explains why alcoholics are especially susceptible to thiamin deficiency.

Tissues take up both free thiamin and thiamin monophosphate, then phosphorylate them further to yield thiamin diphosphate (the active coenzyme) and thiamin triphosphate. Some free thiamin is excreted in the urine, increasing with diuresis, and a significant amount may also be lost in sweat. Most urinary excretion is as thiochrome, the result of nonenzymic cyclization, as well as a variety of products of side-chain oxidation and ring cleavage.

There is little storage of thiamin in the body, and biochemical signs of deficiency can be observed within a few days of initiating a thiamin free diet.

11.6.2 *Metabolic functions of thiamin*

Thiamin has a central role in energy-yielding metabolism, and especially the metabolism of carbohydrates. Thiamin diphosphate (also known as thiamin pyrophosphate; Figure 11.12) is the coenzyme for three multienzyme complexes that catalyze oxidative decarboxylation of the substrate linked to reduction of enzyme-bound lipoamide, and eventually reduction of NAD^+ to NADH:

- Pyruvate dehydrogenase in carbohydrate metabolism (Section 5.4.3.1 and Figure 5.16)
- α-Ketoglutarate dehydrogenase in the citric acid cycle (Section 5.4.4)
- The branched-chain keto-acid dehydrogenase involved in the metabolism of leucine, isoleucine, and valine

It is also the coenzyme for transketolase, in the pentose phosphate pathway of carbohydrate metabolism (Section 5.4.2). Thiamin triphosphate has a role in nerve conduction as the phosphate donor for phosphorylation of a nerve membrane sodium transport channel.

11.6.3 Thiamin deficiency

Thiamin deficiency can result in three distinct syndromes:

- A chronic peripheral neuritis, beriberi, which may or may not be associated with heart failure and edema
- Acute pernicious (fulminating) beriberi (shoshin beriberi), in which heart failure and metabolic abnormalities predominate, with little evidence of peripheral neuritis
- Wernicke's encephalopathy with Korsakoff's psychosis, a thiamin-responsive condition associated especially with alcohol and narcotic abuse

In general, a relatively acute deficiency is involved in the central nervous system lesions of the Wernicke–Korsakoff syndrome, and a high energy intake, as in alcoholics, is also a predisposing factor. Dry beriberi is associated with a more prolonged, less severe, deficiency, with a generally low food intake, while higher carbohydrate intake and physical activity predispose to wet beriberi.

The role of thiamin diphosphate in pyruvate dehydrogenase means that in deficiency there is impaired conversion of pyruvate to acetyl CoA, and hence impaired entry of pyruvate into the citric acid cycle (Section 5.4.3.1). Especially in subjects on a relatively high carbohydrate diet, this results in increased plasma concentrations of lactate and pyruvate, which may lead to life-threatening lactic acidosis (see Problem 5.2).

11.6.3.1 Dry beriberi

Chronic deficiency of thiamin, especially associated with a high carbohydrate diet, results in beriberi, which is a symmetrical ascending peripheral neuritis. Initially the patient complains of weakness, stiffness and cramps in the legs, and is unable to walk more than a short distance. There may be numbness of the feet and ankles, and vibration sense may be diminished. As the disease progresses, the ankle jerk reflex is lost, and the muscular weakness spreads upward, involving first the extensor muscles of the foot, then the muscles of the calf, and finally the extensors and flexors of the thigh. At this stage, there is pronounced toe and foot drop—the patient is unable to keep either the toe or the whole foot extended off the ground. When the arms are affected, there is a similar inability to keep the hand extended—wrist drop.

The affected muscles become tender, numb, and hyperesthetic. The hyperesthesia extends in the form of a band around the limb, the so-called stocking and glove distribution, and is followed by anesthesia. There is deep muscle pain, and in the terminal stages, when the patient is bedridden, even slight pressure, as from bed clothes, causes considerable pain.

11.6.3.2 Wet beriberi

The heart may also be affected in beriberi, with dilatation of arterioles, rapid blood flow and increased pulse rate and pressure, and increased jugular venous pressure leading to right-sided heart failure and edema—so-called wet beriberi. The signs of chronic heart failure may be seen without peripheral neuritis. The arteriolar dilatation, and possibly also the edema, probably result from high circulating concentrations of lactate and pyruvate as a result of impaired activity of pyruvate dehydrogenase.

11.6.3.3 Acute pernicious (fulminating) beriberi—shoshin beriberi

Heart failure without increased cardiac output, and no peripheral edema, may also occur acutely associated with severe lactic acidosis. This was a common presentation of deficiency in Japan, where it was called shoshin (acute) beriberi; in the 1920s, some 26,000 deaths a year were recorded.

With improved knowledge of the cause, and improved nutritional status, the disease had become more or less unknown, although in the 1980s it reappeared among Japanese adolescents consuming a diet based largely on high-carbohydrate, low-nutrient foods such as sweet carbonated drinks, "instant" noodles, and polished rice. It also occurs among alcoholics, when the lactic acidosis may be life threatening, without clear signs of heart failure. Acute beriberi has also been reported when previously starved subjects are given intravenous glucose.

11.6.3.4 The Wernicke–Korsakoff syndrome

While peripheral neuritis and acute cardiac beriberi with lactic acidosis occur in thiamin deficiency associated with alcohol abuse, the more usual presentation is the Wernicke–Korsakoff syndrome, due to central nervous system lesions. Initially there is a confused state, Korsakoff's psychosis, which is characterized by confabulation and loss of recent memory, although memory for past events may be unimpaired. Later, neurological signs develop, Wernicke's encephalopathy, characterized by nystagmus and extraocular palsy. Postmortem examination shows characteristic brain lesions.

Like shoshin beriberi, Wernicke's encephalopathy can develop acutely, without the more gradual development of Korsakoff's psychosis, among previously starved patients given intravenous glucose and seriously ill patients given parenteral hyperalimentation.

11.6.4 Thiamin requirements

Because thiamin has a central role in energy-yielding, and especially carbohydrate, metabolism, requirements depend mainly on carbohydrate intake and have been related to non-fat energy. In practice, requirements and reference intakes are calculated on the basis of total energy intake, assuming that the average diet provides 40% of energy from fat. For diets that are lower in fat content, and hence higher in carbohydrate and protein, thiamin requirements may be somewhat higher.

The activation of apotransketolase in erythrocyte lysate by thiamin diphosphate added *in vitro* has become the most widely used and accepted index of thiamin nutritional status (Section 2.7.3). An activation coefficient >1.25 is indicative of deficiency, and <1.15 is considered to reflect adequate thiamin nutrition. The reference intake of 0.5 mg/1000 kcal (100 μg/MJ) is based on the amount to maintain a normal transketolase activation; for people with a low energy intake, a minimum intake of 0.8–1.0 mg/day allows for metabolism of endogenous substrates.

11.7 Vitamin B_2 (riboflavin)

Riboflavin deficiency is a significant public health problem in many areas of the world. The vitamin has a central role as a coenzyme in energy-yielding metabolism, yet deficiency is rarely, if ever, fatal—there is very efficient conservation and recycling of riboflavin in deficiency. The structures of riboflavin and the riboflavin-derived coenzymes (also known as flavin coenzymes) are shown in Figures 2.18 and 2.19.

The main dietary sources of riboflavin are milk and dairy products, providing 25% or more of the total intake in most diets, and to a considerable extent average riboflavin status in different countries reflects milk consumption. In addition, because of its intense yellow color, riboflavin is widely used as a food color.

Photolysis of riboflavin leads to the formation of lumiflavin (in alkaline solution) and lumichrome (in acidic or neutral solution), both of which are biologically inactive. Exposure of milk in clear glass bottles to sunlight or fluorescent light (with a peak wavelength of 400–550 nm) can result in the loss of nutritionally important amounts of riboflavin. Lumiflavin and lumichrome catalyze oxidation of lipids (to peroxides) and methionine (to methional), resulting in the development of an unpleasant flavor—the so-called sunlight flavor. Light of 400–550 nm can penetrate both clear glass bottles and cardboard cartons; cartons for milk include a protective lining that is opaque at this wavelength.

11.7.1 Absorption and metabolism of riboflavin

Apart from milk and eggs, which contain relatively large amounts of free riboflavin, most of the vitamin in foods is as flavin coenzymes bound to enzymes, which are released when the protein is hydrolyzed. Intestinal phosphatases then hydrolyze the coenzymes to riboflavin, which is absorbed in the upper small intestine. Much of the absorbed riboflavin is phosphorylated in the intestinal mucosa by flavokinase and enters the bloodstream as riboflavin phosphate.

Tissues contain very little free riboflavin; most is present as FAD and riboflavin phosphate bound to enzymes. Uptake into tissues is by passive carrier-mediated transport of free riboflavin, followed by metabolic trapping (Section 3.2.2.2) by phosphorylation to riboflavin phosphate, then onward metabolism to FAD.

FAD that is not protein bound is rapidly hydrolyzed to riboflavin phosphate by nucleotide pyrophosphatase; unbound riboflavin phosphate is hydrolyzed to riboflavin by nonspecific phosphatases, and free riboflavin diffuses out of tissues into the bloodstream.

Riboflavin and riboflavin phosphate that are not bound to plasma proteins are filtered at the glomerulus. Renal tubular reabsorption of riboflavin is saturated at normal plasma concentrations. There is also active tubular secretion of the vitamin; urinary excretion of riboflavin after high doses can be two- to threefold greater than the glomerular filtration rate.

There is no significant storage of riboflavin; any surplus intake is excreted rapidly, so that once metabolic requirements have been met urinary excretion of riboflavin and its metabolites reflects intake until intestinal absorption is saturated. In depleted animals, the maximum growth response is achieved with intakes that give about 75% saturation of tissues, and the intake to achieve tissue saturation is that at which there is quantitative excretion of the vitamin.

There is very efficient conservation of tissue riboflavin in deficiency, with only a fourfold difference between the minimum concentration of flavins in the liver in deficiency and the level at which saturation occurs. In deficiency, almost the only loss of riboflavin from tissues will be the small amount that is covalently bound to enzymes; the noncovalently bound coenzymes are recycled when proteins are catabolized.

11.7.2 *Metabolic functions of the flavin coenzymes*

The metabolic function of the flavin coenzymes is as electron carriers in a wide variety of oxidation and reduction reactions central to all metabolic processes (Figure 2.19), including the mitochondrial electron transport chain (Section 3.3.1.2), and key enzymes in fatty acid (Section 5.5.2) and amino acid (Section 9.3.1.1) oxidation, and the citric acid cycle (Section 5.4.4). Flavin coenzymes remain bound to the enzyme throughout the catalytic cycle. The majority of flavoproteins have FAD as the prosthetic group; some have both flavin coenzymes, and some have other prosthetic groups as well.

Reoxidation of the reduced flavin in oxygenases and mixed-function oxidases proceeds by way of formation of the flavin radical and flavin hydroperoxide, with the intermediate generation of superoxide and perhydroxyl radicals and hydrogen peroxide. Because of this, flavin oxidases make a significant contribution to the total oxidative stress in the body (Section 6.5.2.1).

11.7.3 *Riboflavin deficiency*

Although riboflavin is involved in all areas of metabolism, and deficiency is widespread on a global scale, deficiency is not fatal. There seem to be two reasons for this:

- Although deficiency is common, the vitamin is widespread in foods, and most diets will provide minimally adequate amounts to permit maintenance of central metabolic pathways.
- There is efficient reutilization of the riboflavin that is released by the turnover of flavoproteins, so that only a very small amount is metabolized or excreted.

Riboflavin deficiency is characterized by lesions of the margin of the lips (cheilosis) and corners of the mouth (angular stomatitis), a painful desquamation of the tongue, so that it is red, dry, and atrophic (magenta tongue) and a sebhorreic dermatitis, with filiform excrescences.

The main metabolic effect of riboflavin deficiency is on lipid metabolism. Riboflavin deficient animals have a lower metabolic rate than controls and require a 15%–20% higher food intake to maintain body weight. Feeding a high fat diet leads to more marked impairment of growth and a higher requirement for riboflavin to restore growth.

11.7.3.1 *Resistance to malaria in riboflavin deficiency*

A number of studies have noted that in areas where malaria is endemic, riboflavin deficient people are relatively resistant and have a lower parasite burden than adequately nourished people. The biochemical basis of this resistance to malaria in riboflavin deficiency is not known, but two possible mechanisms have been proposed:

- Malarial parasites may have a particularly high requirement for riboflavin—a number of flavin analogs have antimalarial action.
- As a result of impaired antioxidant activity in erythrocytes, there may be increased fragility of erythrocyte membranes. As in sickle cell trait, which also protects against malaria, this may result in exposure of the parasites to the host's immune system at a vulnerable stage in their development, resulting in the production of protective antibodies.

11.7.4 Riboflavin requirements

Glutathione reductase is especially sensitive to riboflavin depletion, and the usual way of assessing riboflavin status is by measurement of the activation of red blood cell glutathione reductase by FAD added *in vitro* (Section 2.7.3). An activation coefficient >1.7 indicates deficiency. Normal values of the activation coefficient are seen in subjects whose habitual intake of riboflavin is between 1.2 and 1.5 mg/day.

11.8 Niacin

Niacin is not strictly a vitamin since it can be synthesized in the body from the essential amino acid tryptophan. Indeed, it is only when tryptophan metabolism is deranged that dietary preformed niacin becomes important. Nevertheless, niacin was discovered as a nutrient during studies of the deficiency disease pellagra, associated with diets based largely on maize, which was a major public health problem in the southern United States throughout the first half of the twentieth century, and continued to be a problem in parts of India and sub-Saharan Africa until the 1990s.

Two compounds, nicotinic acid and nicotinamide, have the biological activity of niacin. When nicotinic acid was discovered to be a curative and a preventive factor for pellagra, it was already known as a chemical compound and was therefore never assigned a number among the B vitamins. The name niacin was coined in the United States when it was decided to enrich maize meal with the vitamin to prevent pellagra—it was considered that the name nicotinic acid was not desirable because of the similarity to nicotine. In the United States, the term niacin is commonly used to mean specifically nicotinic acid, and nicotinamide is known as niacinamide; elsewhere niacin is used as a generic descriptor for both vitamers. Figure 2.20 shows the structures of nicotinic acid, nicotinamide, and the nicotinamide nucleotide coenzymes—NAD and NADP.

11.8.1 Metabolism of niacin

The nicotinamide ring of NAD can be synthesized in the body from the essential amino acid tryptophan (Figure 11.13). In adults, an amount of tryptophan equivalent to almost all the dietary intake is metabolized by this pathway and hence is potentially available for NAD synthesis. A number of studies have investigated the equivalence of dietary tryptophan and preformed niacin as precursors of the nicotinamide nucleotides, generally by determining the excretion of niacin metabolites in response to test doses of the precursors, in subjects maintained on deficient diets. There is a considerable variation between subjects in the response to tryptophan and niacin, and to allow for this it is generally assumed that 60 mg of tryptophan is equivalent to 1 mg of preformed niacin.

Changes in hormonal status may result in considerable changes in this ratio, with between 7 and 30 mg of dietary tryptophan equivalent to 1 mg of preformed niacin in late pregnancy. The intake of tryptophan also affects the ratio, and at low intakes 1 mg of tryptophan may be equivalent to only 1/125 mg preformed niacin.

The niacin content of foods is generally expressed as milligram niacin equivalents:

$$1 \text{ mg niacin equivalent} = 1 \text{ mg preformed niacin} + 1/60 \text{ mg tryptophan}$$

Because most of the niacin in cereals is biologically unavailable (Section 11.8.1.1), it is conventional to ignore preformed niacin in cereal products.

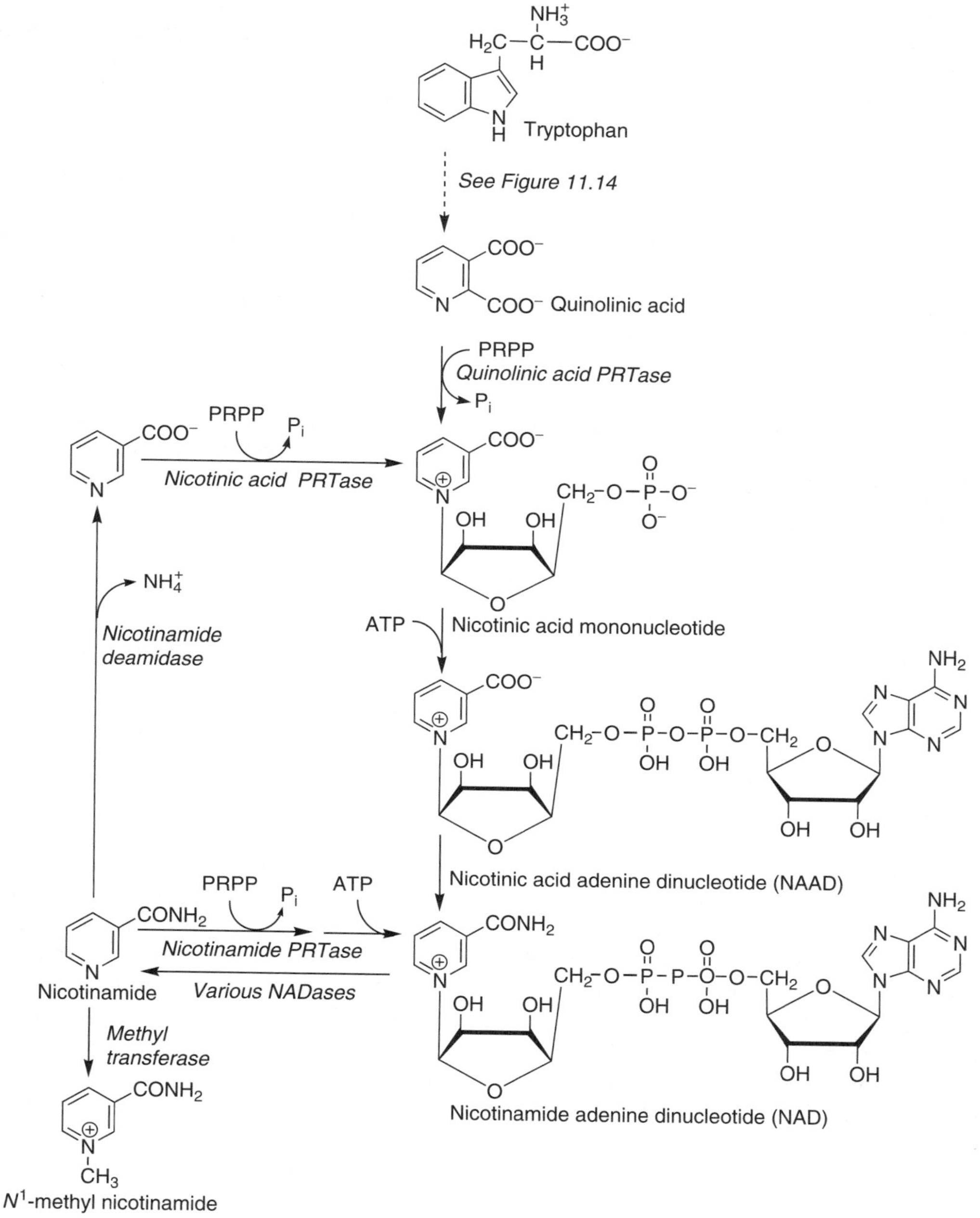

Figure 11.13 The metabolism of the nicotinamide nucleotide coenzymes. (PRPP = phosphoribosyl pyrophosphate; PRTase = phosphosibosyltransferase).

11.8.1.1 *Unavailable niacin in cereals*

Chemical analysis reveals niacin in cereals (largely in the bran), but this is biologically unavailable since it is bound as niacytin–nicotinoyl esters to polysaccharides, polypeptides, and glycopeptides.

Treatment of cereals with alkali (e.g., soaking overnight in calcium hydroxide solution, the traditional method for the preparation of tortillas in Mexico) releases much of the nicotinic acid. This may explain why pellagra has always been rare in Mexico, despite the fact that maize is the dietary staple. Up to 10% of the niacin in niacytin may be biologically available as a result of hydrolysis by gastric acid.

11.8.1.2 Absorption and metabolism of niacin

Niacin is present in tissues, and therefore in foods, mainly as the nicotinamide nucleotides. The postmortem hydrolysis of NAD(P) is extremely rapid in animal tissues, so it is likely that much of the niacin in meat (a major dietary source of the vitamin) is free nicotinamide. Both nicotinic acid and nicotinamide are absorbed from the small intestine by a sodium dependent saturable process.

11.8.1.3 Metabolism of the nicotinamide nucleotide coenzymes

The nicotinamide nucleotide coenzymes can be synthesized from either of the niacin vitamers, and from quinolinic acid, an intermediate in the metabolism of tryptophan (Figure 11.13). In the liver, oxidation of tryptophan results in a considerably greater synthesis of NAD than is required, and this is catabolized to release nicotinic acid and nicotinamide, which are taken up and used by other tissues for synthesis of the coenzymes.

The catabolism of NAD^+ is catalyzed by four enzymes:

- NAD glycohydrolase, which releases nicotinamide and ADP-ribose.
- NAD pyrophosphatase, which releases nicotinamide mononucleotide. This can either be hydrolyzed by NAD glycohydrolase to release nicotinamide, or can be reutilized to form NAD.
- ADP-ribosyltransferases.
- Poly(ADP-ribose) polymerase.

The activation of ADP-ribosyltransferase and poly(ADP-ribose) polymerase by toxins that cause DNA damage (Section 11.8.3.1) may result in considerable depletion of intracellular NAD(P) and may indeed provide a suicide mechanism to ensure that cells that have suffered very severe damage die as a result of NAD(P) depletion. The administration of DNA-breaking carcinogens to experimental animals results in the excretion of large amounts of nicotinamide metabolites and depletion of tissue NAD(P). Chronic exposure to such carcinogens and mycotoxins may be a contributory factor in the etiology of pellagra when dietary intakes of tryptophan and niacin are marginal.

Under normal conditions, there is little or no urinary excretion of either nicotinamide or nicotinic acid. This is because both vitamers are actively reabsorbed from the glomerular filtrate. It is only when the concentration is so high that the transporter is saturated that there is any significant excretion. The main urinary metabolites of niacin are N^1-methyl nicotinamide and onward metabolic products, methyl pyridone-2-carboxamide and methyl pyridone-4-carboxamide.

11.8.2 The synthesis of nicotinamide nucleotides from tryptophan

Under normal conditions, almost all the dietary intake of tryptophan, apart from the small amounts that are used for net new protein synthesis and synthesis of 5-hydroxytryptophan, is metabolized by the oxidative pathway (Figure 11.14), and hence is potentially available for NAD synthesis.

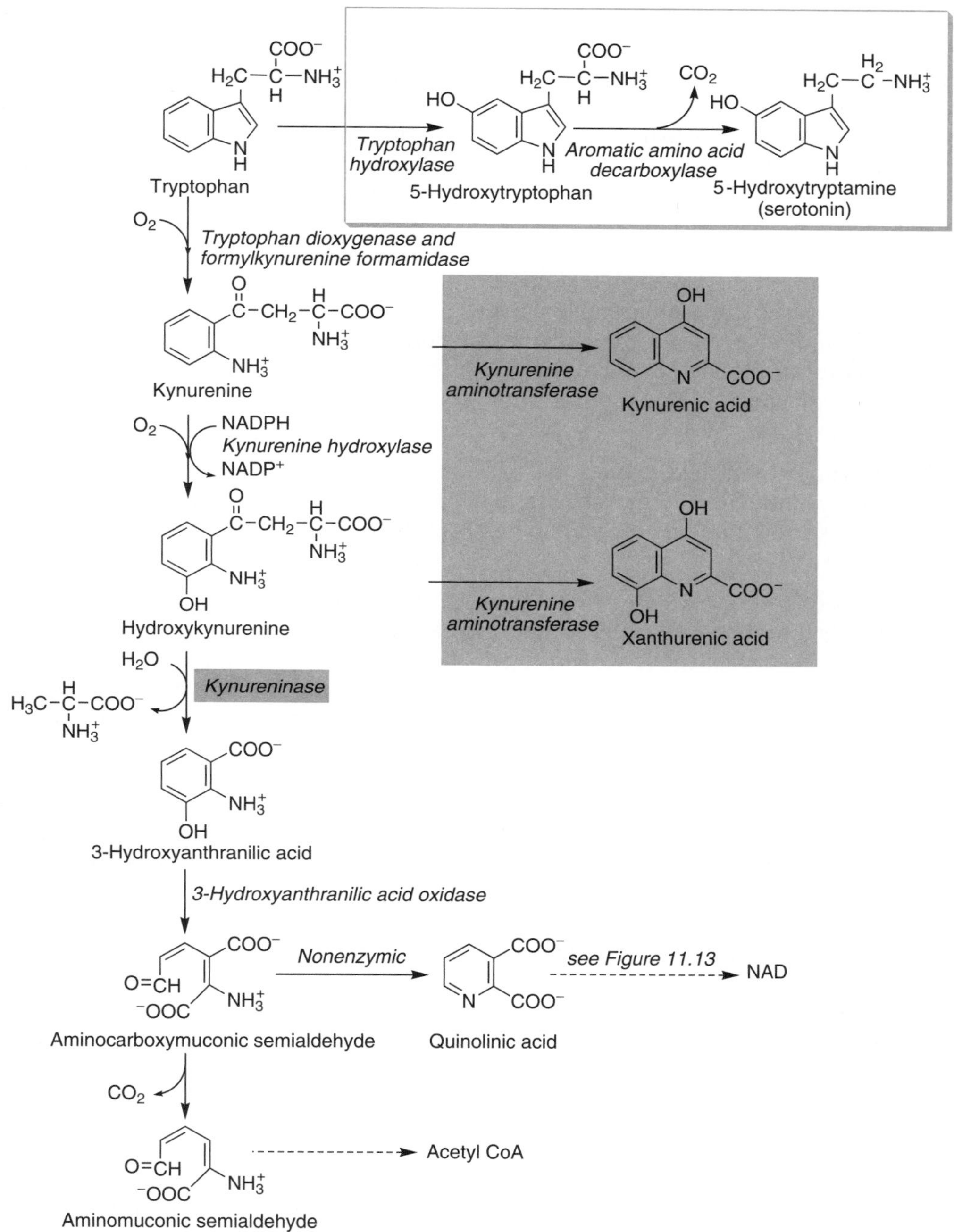

Figure 11.14 Tryptophan metabolism.

The synthesis of NAD from tryptophan involves the nonenzymic cyclization of aminocarboxymuconic semialdehyde to quinolinic acid. The alternative metabolic fate of aminocarboxymuconic semialdehyde is decarboxylation, catalyzed by picolinate carboxylase, leading to acetyl CoA and total oxidation. There is thus competition between an enzyme-catalyzed reaction, which has hyperbolic, saturable kinetics, and a nonenzymic reaction with linear kinetics. At low rates of flux through the pathway, most metabolism will be by way of the enzyme-catalyzed pathway, leading to oxidation. As the rate of formation of aminocarboxymuconic semialdehyde increases and picolinate carboxylase nears saturation, an increasing proportion will be available to undergo cyclization to quinolinic acid and onward metabolism to NAD. There is thus no simple stoichiometric relationship between tryptophan and niacin, and the equivalence of the coenzyme precursors will depend on the amount of tryptophan to be metabolized and the rate of its metabolism.

The activities of three enzymes, tryptophan dioxygenase, kynurenine hydroxylase, and kynureninase, affect the rate of formation of aminocarboxymuconic semialdehyde, as may the rate of uptake of tryptophan into the liver.

Tryptophan dioxygenase is the enzyme that controls the entry of tryptophan into the oxidative pathway. It has a short half-life (of the order of 2 h) and is subject to regulation by three mechanisms:

- Stabilization by its heme cofactor
- Hormonal induction by glucocorticoid hormones and glucagon (Section 9.1.2.2)
- Feedback inhibition and repression by NAD(P)

The activities of both kynurenine hydroxylase and kynureninase are only slightly higher than that of tryptophan dioxygenase, and increased tryptophan dioxygenase activity in response to glucocorticoid action is accompanied by increased accumulation and excretion of kynurenine, hydroxykynurenine and their transamination products, kynurenic and xanthurenic acids. Impairment of the activity of either enzyme may impair the onward metabolism of kynurenine, and thus reduce the accumulation of aminocarboxymuconic semialdehyde and hence the synthesis of NAD.

Kynurenine hydroxylase is FAD dependent, and the activity of kynurenine hydroxylase in the liver of riboflavin deficient rats is only 30%–50% of that in control animals. Riboflavin deficiency (Section 11.7.3) may thus be a contributory factor in the etiology of pellagra when intakes of tryptophan and niacin are marginal.

Kynureninase is a pyridoxal phosphate (vitamin B_6) dependent enzyme, and its activity is extremely sensitive to vitamin B_6 depletion. Indeed, the ability to metabolize a test dose of tryptophan has been used to assess vitamin B_6 nutritional status (Section 11.9.5.1). Deficiency of vitamin B_6 will lead to severe impairment of NAD synthesis from tryptophan. Kynureninase is also inhibited by estrogen metabolites.

11.8.3 Metabolic functions of niacin

The best defined role of niacin is in oxidation and reduction reactions as the functional nicotinamide part of the coenzymes NAD and NADP (Section 2.4.1.3). In general, NAD^+ is involved as an electron acceptor in energy-yielding metabolism, being oxidized by the mitochondrial electron transport chain (Section 3.3.1.2), while the major coenzyme for reductive synthetic reactions is NADPH. An exception to this general rule is the pentose phosphate pathway of glucose metabolism (Section 5.4.2), which results in the reduction of $NADP^+$ to NADPH, and is the source of half the NADPH required for fatty acid synthesis (Section 5.6.1).

11.8.3.1 The role of NAD in ADP-ribosylation

In addition to its coenzyme role, NAD^+ is the source of ADP-ribose for:

- ADP-ribosyltransferases, which modify the activities of enzymes by catalyzing reversible ADP-ribosylation
- Poly(ADP-ribose) polymerase, which is activated by binding to breakage points in DNA, and activates the DNA repair mechanism

11.8.4 Pellagra—a disease of tryptophan and niacin deficiency

Pellagra became common in Europe when maize was introduced from the New World as a convenient high-yielding dietary staple, and by the late nineteenth century it was widespread throughout southern Europe, north and south Africa, and the southern United States. The proteins of maize are particularly lacking in tryptophan, and as with other cereals little or none of the preformed niacin is biologically available (Section 11.8.1.1).

Pellagra is characterized by a photosensitive dermatitis, like severe sunburn, affecting all parts of the skin that are exposed to sunlight. Similar skin lesions may also occur in areas not exposed to sunlight, but subject to pressure, such as the knees, elbows, wrists, and ankles. Advanced pellagra is also accompanied by dementia (more correctly a depressive psychosis), and there may be diarrhea. Untreated pellagra is fatal. The depressive psychosis is due to reduced synthesis of the neurotransmitter serotonin as a result of lack of the essential amino acid tryptophan, and not to a deficiency of niacin *per se*.

Although the nutritional etiology of pellagra is well established, and tryptophan or niacin will prevent or cure the disease, additional factors, including deficiency of riboflavin (and hence impaired activity of kynurenine hydroxylase) or vitamin B_6 (and hence impaired activity of kynureninase), may be important when intakes of tryptophan and niacin are only marginally adequate.

During the first half of the twentieth century, of the 87,000 people who died from pellagra in the United States, there were twice as many women as men. Reports of individual outbreaks of pellagra, both in the United States and more recently elsewhere, show a similar sex ratio. This may well be the result of inhibition of kynureninase, and impairment of the activity of kynurenine hydroxylase, by estrogen metabolites, and hence reduced synthesis of NAD from tryptophan.

11.8.5 Niacin requirements

Although the nicotinamide nucleotide coenzymes function in a large number of oxidation and reduction reactions, this cannot be exploited as a means of assessing niacin status, because the coenzymes are not tightly bound to their apoenzymes but act as cosubstrates of the reactions, binding to and leaving the enzyme as the reaction proceeds. No specific metabolic lesions associated with NAD(P) depletion have been identified.

The two methods of assessing niacin nutritional status are measurement of the ratio of NAD to NADP in red blood cells and the urinary excretion of niacin metabolites, neither of which is wholly satisfactory.

On the basis of depletion/repletion studies in which the urinary excretion of niacin metabolites was measured after feeding tryptophan or preformed niacin, the average requirement for niacin is 1.3 mg (niacin equivalents)/MJ energy expenditure, and reference intakes are based on 1.6 mg/MJ. Average intakes of tryptophan in Western diets will more than meet requirements without the need for a dietary source of preformed niacin.

11.8.5.1 Niacin toxicity

Nicotinic acid has been used to lower blood triacylglycerol and cholesterol in patients with hyperlipidemia. However, relatively large amounts are required (of the order of 1–3 g/day, compared with reference intakes of 18–20 mg/day). At this level of intake, nicotinic acid causes dilatation of blood vessels and flushing, with skin irritation, itching, and a burning sensation. This effect wears off after a few days.

High intakes of both nicotinic acid and nicotinamide, in excess of 1 g/day, also cause liver damage, and prolonged use can result in liver failure. This is especially a problem with sustained release preparations of niacin, which permit a high blood level to be maintained for a relatively long time.

11.9 Vitamin B_6

Apart from a single outbreak in the 1950s due to overheated infant milk formula, vitamin B_6 deficiency is unknown except under experimental conditions. Nevertheless, there is a considerable body of evidence that marginal status and biochemical deficiency may be relatively widespread.

The generic descriptor vitamin B_6 includes six vitamers (Figure 11.15): the alcohol pyridoxine, the aldehyde pyridoxal, the amine pyridoxamine, and their 5′-phosphates. The vitamers are metabolically interconvertible and have equal biological activity; they are all

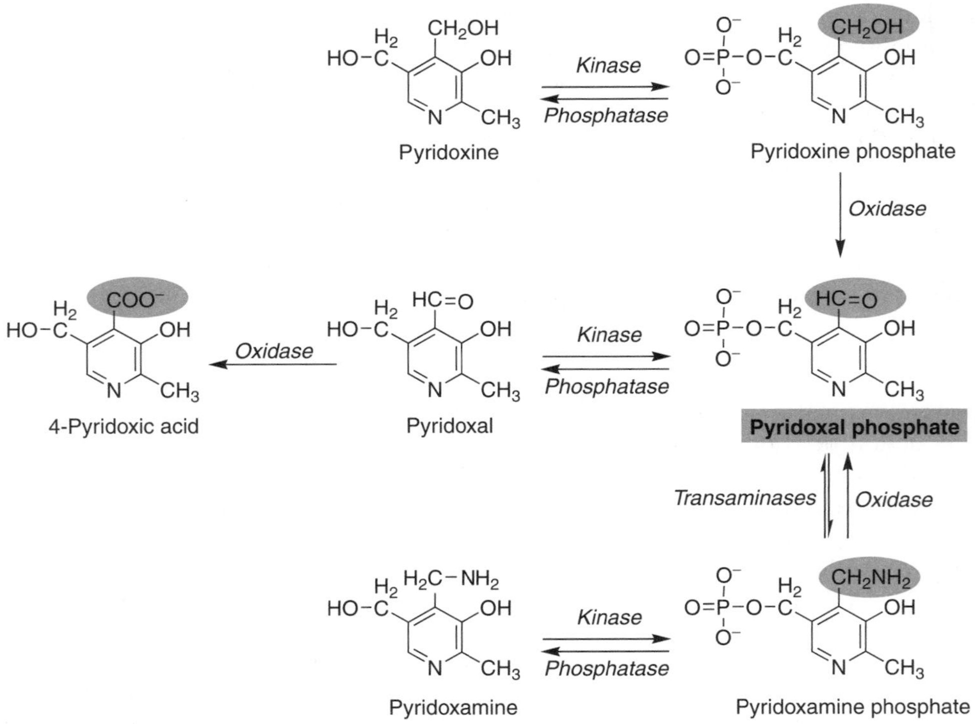

Pyridoxine ⇌ (Kinase / Phosphatase) Pyridoxine phosphate

Pyridoxine phosphate → (Oxidase) Pyridoxal phosphate

4-Pyridoxic acid ← (Oxidase) Pyridoxal ⇌ (Kinase / Phosphatase) **Pyridoxal phosphate**

Pyridoxal phosphate ⇌ (Transaminases) Pyridoxamine phosphate; Pyridoxamine phosphate → (Oxidase) Pyridoxal phosphate

Pyridoxamine ⇌ (Kinase / Phosphatase) Pyridoxamine phosphate

Figure 11.15 Interconversion of the vitamin B_6 vitamers.

converted in the body to the metabolically active form, pyridoxal phosphate. 4-Pyridoxic acid is a biologically inactive end-product of vitamin B_6 metabolism.

When foods are heated, pyridoxal and pyridoxal phosphate can react with the ε-amino groups of lysine to form a Schiff base (aldimine). This renders both the vitamin B_6 and the lysine biologically unavailable (Section 9.1.3.2); more importantly, the pyridoxyl-lysine released during digestion is absorbed and has antivitamin B_6 antimetabolite activity.

11.9.1 Absorption and metabolism of vitamin B_6

The phosphorylated vitamers are hydrolyzed by alkaline phosphatase in the intestinal mucosa; the dephosphorylated vitamers absorbed rapidly by diffusion, then phosphorylated, and pyridoxine and pyridoxamine phosphates are oxidized to pyridoxal phosphate. Much of the ingested vitamin is released into the portal circulation as pyridoxal after dephosphorylation at the serosal surface.

Most of the absorbed vitamin enters the liver by diffusion, followed by metabolic trapping as the phosphate. Pyridoxal phosphate and some pyridoxal are exported from the liver bound to albumin. Free pyridoxal remaining in the liver is rapidly oxidized to 4-pyridoxic acid and excreted.

Extrahepatic tissues take up both pyridoxal and pyridoxal phosphate from the plasma. The phosphate is hydrolyzed to pyridoxal, which can cross cell membranes, by extracellular alkaline phosphatase, then trapped intracellularly by phosphorylation.

Some 80% of the body's total vitamin B_6 is pyridoxal phosphate in muscle, mostly associated with glycogen phosphorylase (Section 5.6.3.1). This does not function as a reserve of the vitamin and is not released from muscle in times of deficiency; it is released into the circulation (as pyridoxal) in starvation, when glycogen reserves are exhausted and there is less requirement for phosphorylase activity. Under these conditions, it is available for redistribution to other tissues and especially liver and kidney, to meet the increased requirement for gluconeogenesis from amino acids (Section 5.7).

11.9.2 Metabolic functions of vitamin B_6

Pyridoxal phosphate is a coenzyme in three main areas of metabolism:

- Various reactions of amino acids, especially transamination, in which it functions as the intermediate carrier of the amino group (Section 9.3.1.2), and decarboxylation to form amines.
- As the cofactor of glycogen phosphorylase (Section 5.6.3.1) in muscle and liver, where it is the phosphate group that is catalytically important.
- In the regulation of the action of steroid hormones (Section 10.4). Pyridoxal phosphate acts to remove the hormone–receptor complex from DNA binding, and so terminates the action of the hormones.

11.9.3 Vitamin B_6 deficiency

Deficiency of vitamin B_6 severe enough to lead to clinical signs is extremely rare, and clear deficiency has only been reported in one outbreak during the 1950s when babies were fed on a milk preparation that had been severely overheated during manufacture. Many of the affected infants suffered convulsions, which ceased rapidly following the administration of vitamin B_6.

Moderate vitamin B_6 deficiency results in a number of abnormalities of amino acid metabolism, and especially of tryptophan (Section 11.9.5.1) and methionine (Section 11.9.5.2). In experimental animals, it also leads to increased sensitivity of target tissues to steroid hormone action. This may be important in the development of hormone-dependent cancer of the breast, uterus, and prostate, and vitamin B_6 status may therefore affect the prognosis.

11.9.4 *Vitamin B_6 requirements*

Most studies of vitamin B_6 requirements have followed the development of abnormalities of tryptophan and methionine metabolism during depletion and normalization during repletion with graded intakes of the vitamin. Adults maintained on vitamin B_6 deficient diets develop abnormalities of tryptophan and methionine metabolism faster and their blood vitamin B_6 falls more rapidly when their protein intake is relatively high (80–160 g/day in various studies) than on low protein intakes (30–50 g/day). Similarly, during repletion of deficient subjects, tryptophan and methionine metabolism and blood vitamin B_6 are normalized faster at low than at high levels of protein intake.

From such studies, the mean requirement for vitamin B_6 is estimated to be 13 μg/g dietary protein, and reference intakes are based on 15–16 μg/g dietary protein.

11.9.5 *Assessment of vitamin B_6 status*

Fasting plasma total vitamin B_6, or more specifically pyridoxal phosphate, is widely used as an index of vitamin B_6 nutritional status. Urinary excretion of 4-pyridoxic acid is also used, but it reflects recent intake of the vitamin rather than underlying nutritional status.

The most widely used method of assessing vitamin B_6 status is by the activation of erythrocyte transaminases by pyridoxal phosphate added *in vitro* (Section 2.7.3). The ability to metabolize test doses of tryptophan (Section 11.9.5.1) or methionine (Section 11.9.5.2) has also been used.

11.9.5.1 *The tryptophan load test*

The tryptophan load test for vitamin B_6 nutritional status (the ability to metabolize a test dose of tryptophan) is one of the oldest metabolic tests for functional vitamin nutritional status. It was developed as a result of observation of the excretion of an abnormal colored compound, later identified as the tryptophan metabolite xanthurenic acid, in the urine of deficient animals.

Kynureninase (Figure 11.14) is a pyridoxal phosphate dependent enzyme, and its activity falls markedly in vitamin B_6 deficiency, at least partly because it undergoes a slow mechanism-dependent inactivation that leaves catalytically inactive pyridoxamine phosphate at the active site. The enzyme can only be reactivated if there is an adequate supply of pyridoxal phosphate. This means that in vitamin B_6 deficiency, there is a considerable accumulation of both hydroxykynurenine and kynurenine, sufficient to permit greater metabolic flux than usual through kynurenine transaminase, resulting in increased formation of kynurenic and xanthurenic acids.

Xanthurenic and kynurenic acids and kynurenine and hydroxykynurenine are easy to measure in urine, so the tryptophan load test (the ability to metabolize a test dose of 2–5 g of tryptophan) has been widely adopted as a convenient and sensitive index of vitamin B_6 nutritional status. However, because glucocorticoid hormones increase tryptophan dioxygenase activity, abnormal results of the tryptophan load test must be regarded with caution and cannot necessarily be interpreted as indicating vitamin B_6 deficiency. Increased entry of tryptophan into the pathway will overwhelm the capacity of kynureninase, leading to increased formation of xanthurenic and kynurenic acids. Similarly, estrogen metabolites inhibit kynureninase, leading to results that have been misinterpreted as vitamin B_6 deficiency.

11.9.5.2 The methionine load test

The metabolism of methionine (Figure 11.21) includes two pyridoxal phosphate dependent steps: cystathionine synthetase and cystathionase. Cystathionase activity falls markedly in vitamin B_6 deficiency, and as a result there is an increase in the urinary excretion of homocysteine and cystathionine, especially after a loading dose of methionine. However, homocysteine metabolism is more affected by folate status than vitamin B_6 status (Section 11.11.3.3) and like the tryptophan load test, the methionine load test is probably not a reliable index of vitamin B_6 status in field studies.

11.9.6 Non-nutritional uses of vitamin B_6

A number of studies have suggested that oral contraceptives cause vitamin B_6 deficiency. As a result of this, supplements of vitamin B_6 of between 50 and 100 mg/day, and sometimes higher, have been used to overcome the side effects of oral contraceptives. Similar supplements have also been recommended for the treatment of the premenstrual syndrome, although there is little evidence of efficacy from placebo-controlled trials.

All the studies that suggested that oral contraceptives cause vitamin B_6 deficiency used the tryptophan load test (Section 11.9.5.1). When other biochemical markers of status were also assessed, they were not affected by oral contraceptive use. Furthermore, most of these studies were performed using the now obsolete high-dose contraceptive pills. Oral contraceptives do not cause vitamin B_6 deficiency. The problem is that estrogen metabolites inhibit kynureninase and reduce the activity of kynurenine hydroxylase. This results in the excretion of abnormal amounts of tryptophan metabolites similar to what is seen in vitamin B_6 deficiency, but for quite a different reason.

Doses of 50–200 mg of vitamin B_6 per day have an antiemetic effect, and the vitamin is widely used, alone or in conjunction with other antiemetics, to minimize the nausea associated with radiotherapy and to treat pregnancy sickness. There is no evidence that vitamin B_6 has any beneficial effect in pregnancy sickness, or that women who suffer from morning sickness have lower vitamin B_6 nutritional status than other pregnant women.

11.9.6.1 Vitamin B_6 toxicity

In experimental animals, doses of vitamin B_6 of 50 mg/kg body weight cause histological damage to dorsal nerve roots, and doses of 200 mg/kg body weight lead to the development of signs of peripheral neuropathy, with ataxia, muscle weakness, and loss of balance. Sensory neuropathy has been reported in seven patients taking 2–7 g of pyridoxine per day. Although there was some residual damage, withdrawal of these extremely high doses resulted in a considerable recovery of sensory nerve function.

11.10 Vitamin B_{12}

Dietary deficiency of vitamin B_{12} occurs only in strict Vegans, since the vitamin is found almost exclusively in animal foods. However, functional deficiency (pernicious anemia, with spinal cord degeneration) as a result of impaired absorption is relatively common,

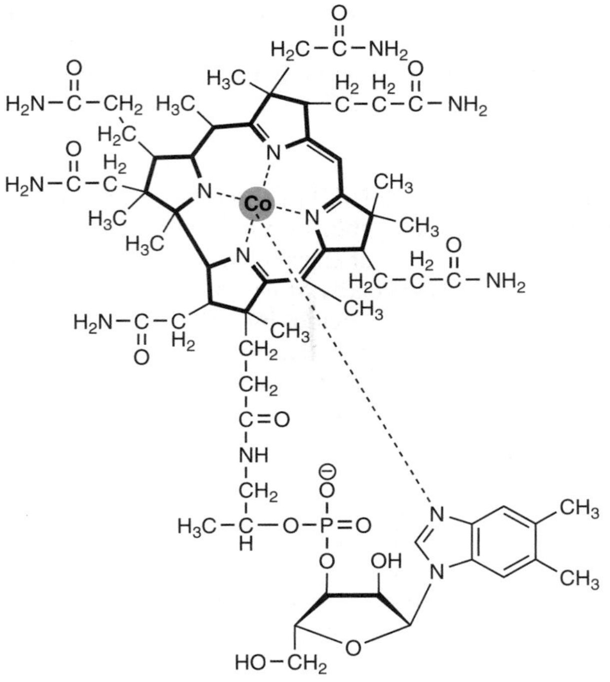

Figure 11.16 Vitamin B_{12}. Four coordination sites on the central cobalt atom are chelated by the nitrogen atoms of the corrin ring, and one by the nitrogen of the dimethylbenzimidazole nucleotide. The sixth coordination site may be occupied by CN^- (cyanocobalamin), OH^- (hydroxocobalamin), H_2O (aquocobalamin), $-CH_3$ (methyl cobalamin), or 5′-deoxyadenosine (adenosylcobalamin).

especially in elderly people with atrophic gastritis. The absorption of vitamin B_{12} is discussed in Section 4.5.2.1.

The structure of vitamin B_{12} is shown in Figure 11.16. The term corrinoid is used as a generic descriptor for cobalt-containing compounds of this general structure, which, depending on the substituents in the pyrrole rings, may or may not have vitamin activity. Some of the corrinoids that are growth factors for microorganisms not only have no vitamin B_{12} activity but may be antimetabolites of the vitamin.

Vitamin B_{12} is found only in foods of animal origin. There are no plant sources of this vitamin, although it is also formed by some bacteria. This means that strict vegetarians (Vegans), who eat no foods of animal origin are at risk of dietary vitamin B_{12} deficiency. Preparations of vitamin B_{12} made by bacterial fermentation that are ethically acceptable to Vegans are readily available.

There are claims that some plants (especially algae) contain vitamin B_{12}. This seems to be incorrect. The problem is that the officially recognized and legally required method of determining vitamin B_{12} in food analysis depends on the growth of microorganisms for which vitamin B_{12} is an essential growth factor. However, these organisms can also use some corrinoids that have no vitamin activity. Therefore, analysis reveals the presence of something that appears to be vitamin B_{12} but in fact is not the active vitamin and is useless in human nutrition. Where biologically active vitamin B_{12} has been identified in algae, it is almost certainly the result of bacterial contamination of the lakes from which the algae were harvested.

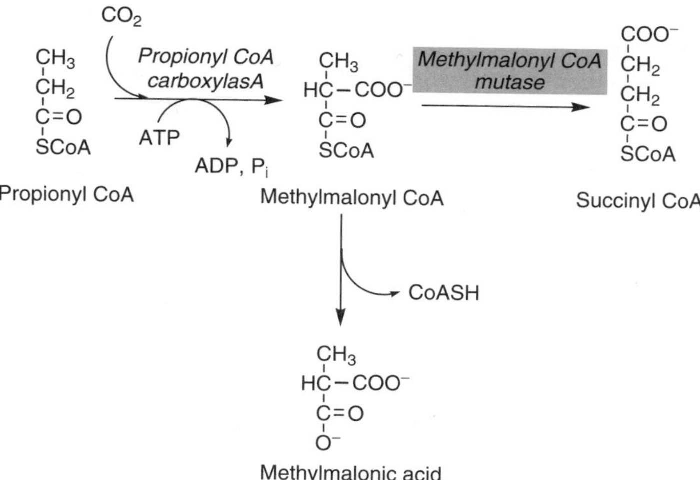

Figure 11.17 The reaction of methyl malonyl CoA mutase and formation of methylmalonic acid in vitamin B_{12} deficiency.

11.10.1 Metabolic functions of vitamin B_{12}

There are three vitamin B_{12} dependent enzymes in human tissues: methylmalonyl CoA mutase, leucine aminomutase, and methionine synthetase. Methionine synthetase is discussed in Section 11.11.3.2.

Methylmalonyl CoA is formed as an intermediate in the catabolism of valine and by the carboxylation of propionyl CoA arising in the catabolism of isoleucine, cholesterol, and (rare) fatty acids with an odd number of carbon atoms. It undergoes vitamin B_{12} dependent rearrangement to succinyl CoA, catalyzed by methylmalonyl CoA mutase (Figure 11.17). The activity of this enzyme is greatly reduced in vitamin B_{12} deficiency, leading to an accumulation of methylmalonyl CoA, some of which is hydrolyzed to yield methylmalonic acid, which is excreted in the urine; urinary excretion of methylmalonic acid provides a means of assessing vitamin B_{12} nutritional status and monitoring therapy in patients with pernicious anemia (Section 11.10.4).

11.10.2 Vitamin B_{12} deficiency: pernicious anemia

Vitamin B_{12} deficiency causes pernicious anemia—the release into the bloodstream of immature precursors of red blood cells (megaloblastic anemia), because deficiency impairs the metabolism of folate (Section 11.11.3.2) and causes functional folate deficiency. This disrupts the normal proliferation of red blood cells, causing immature precursors to be released into the circulation.

The other clinical feature of vitamin B_{12} deficiency, which is very rarely seen in folate deficiency, is degeneration of the spinal cord—hence the name "pernicious" for the anemia of vitamin B_{12} deficiency. The spinal cord degeneration is due to a failure of the methylation of one arginine residue in myelin basic protein and occurs in about one-third of people with megaloblastic anemia due to vitamin B_{12} deficiency, and in about one-third of deficient people who do not show signs of anemia.

The usual cause of pernicious anemia is failure of the absorption of vitamin B_{12} (Section 4.5.2.1) rather than dietary deficiency. Failure of intrinsic factor secretion is commonly due to autoimmune disease; 90% of patients with pernicious anemia have antibodies to the gastric parietal cells. Similar auto-antibodies are found in 30% of the relatives of pernicious anemia patients, suggesting that there is a genetic basis for the condition.

About 70% of patients also have anti-intrinsic factor antibodies in plasma, saliva, and gastric juice. Although the oral administration of partially purified preparations of intrinsic factor will restore the absorption of vitamin B_{12} in many patients with pernicious anemia, this can result eventually in the production of anti-intrinsic factor antibodies, so parenteral administration of vitamin B_{12} is the preferred means of treatment. For patients who secrete anti-intrinsic factor antibodies in the saliva or gastric juice, oral intrinsic factor will be useless.

11.10.3 Vitamin B_{12} requirements

The total body pool of vitamin B_{12} is of the order of 2.5 mg, with a minimum desirable body pool of about 1 mg. The daily loss is about 0.1% of the body pool in subjects with normal enterohepatic circulation of the vitamin (Section 4.5.2.1); on this basis requirements are about 1–2.5 µg/day, and reference intakes for adults range between 1.4 and 2.0 µg.

11.10.4 Assessment of vitamin B_{12} status

A number of reliable radioligand binding assays have been developed for measurement of plasma concentrations of vitamin B_{12}. They may give falsely high values if the binding protein is cobalophilin, which binds a number of metabolically inactive corrinoids; more precise determination of true vitamin B_{12} comes from assays in which the binding protein is purified intrinsic factor.

A serum concentration of vitamin B_{12} below 110 pmol/L is associated with megaloblastic bone marrow, incipient anemia, and myelin damage. Below 150 pmol/L, there are early bone marrow changes, abnormalities of the deoxyuridine monophosphate (dUMP) suppression test (Section 11.11.6.2), and methylmalonic aciduria after a valine load (Section 11.10.1)

11.10.4.1 The Schilling test for vitamin B_{12} absorption

The absorption of vitamin B_{12} can be determined by the Schilling test. An oral dose of [^{57}Co] or [^{58}Co]vitamin B_{12} is given together with a parenteral flushing dose of 1 mg of non-radioactive vitamin to saturate body reserves, and the urinary excretion of radioactivity is followed as an index of absorption of the oral material. Normal subjects excrete 16%–45% of the radioactivity over 24 h, while patients lacking intrinsic factor excrete less than 5%.

The test can be repeated, giving intrinsic factor orally together with the radioactive vitamin B_{12}; if the impaired absorption was due to a simple lack of intrinsic factor and not to anti-intrinsic factor antibodies in saliva or gastric juice, then a normal amount of the radioactive material should be absorbed and excreted.

11.11 Folic acid

Folate functions in the transfer of one-carbon fragments in a wide variety of biosynthetic and catabolic reactions; it is therefore metabolically related to vitamin B_{12}. Deficiency of either vitamin has similar clinical effects, and the main effects of vitamin B_{12} deficiency are exerted by effects on folate metabolism.

Although folate is widely distributed in foods, dietary deficiency is not uncommon and a number of commonly used drugs can cause folate depletion. More importantly, there is good evidence that intakes of folate considerably higher than normal dietary levels reduce the risk of neural tube defects, and pregnant women are recommended to take supplements. There is also evidence that high intakes of folate may also be effective in reducing plasma homocysteine in subjects genetically at risk of hyperhomocystinemia (some 10%–20% of the population), and hence reducing the risk of ischemic heart disease and stroke.

11.11.1 Folate vitamers and dietary equivalence

The structure of folic acid (pteroylglutamate) is shown in Figure 11.18. The folate coenzymes may have up to seven additional glutamate residues linked by γ-peptide bonds, forming pteroyldiglutamate ($PteGlu_2$), pteroyltriglutamate ($PteGlu_3$), etc., collectively known as folate or pteroyl polyglutamate conjugates ($PteGlu_n$).

Folate is the preferred trivial name for pteroylglutamate, although both folate and folic acid may also be used as a generic descriptor to include various polyglutamates. $PteGlu_2$ is sometimes referred to as folic acid diglutamate, $PteGlu_3$ as folic acid triglutamate, etc.

Tetrahydrofolate can carry one-carbon fragments attached to N-5 (formyl, formimino, or methyl groups), N-10 (formyl), or bridging N-5–N-10 (methylene or methenyl groups). 5-Formyl-tetrahydrofolate is more stable to atmospheric oxidation than folate itself and is usually used in pharmaceutical preparations; it is also known as folinic acid, and the synthetic (racemic) compound as leucovorin.

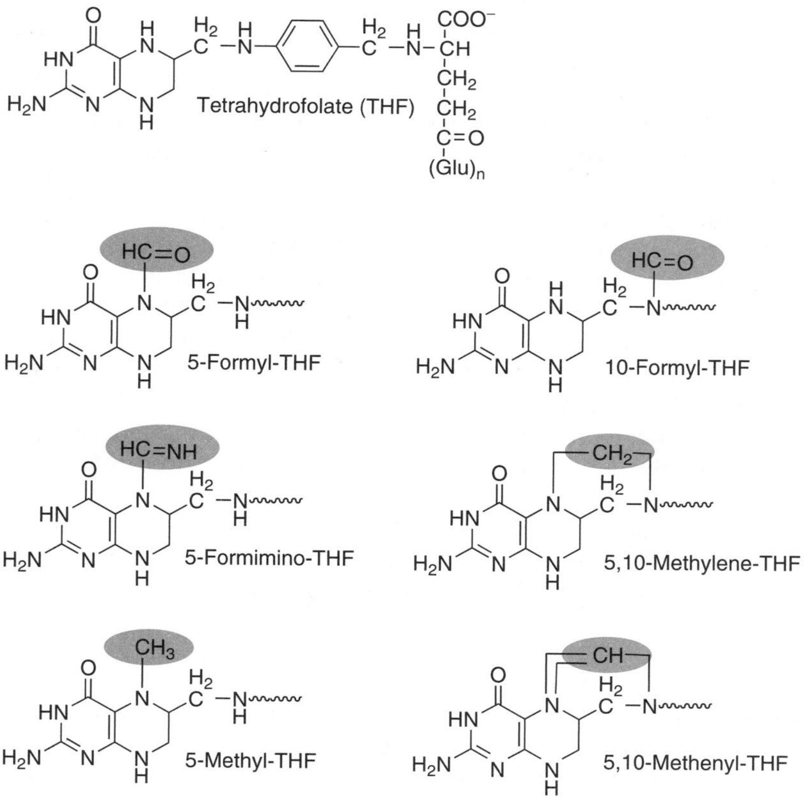

Figure 11.18 Folic acid and the various one-carbon substituted folates.

The extent to which the different forms of folate can be absorbed varies; to permit calculation of folate intakes, the dietary folate equivalent has been defined as 1 μg mixed food folates or 0.6 μg free folic acid. On this basis

total dietary folate equivalents = μg food folate + 1.7 × synthetic (free) folic acid

11.11.2 Absorption and metabolism of folate

About 80% of food folate consists of polyglutamates; a variable amount may be substituted with various one-carbon units or be present as dihydrofolate derivatives. Folate conjugates are hydrolyzed in the small intestine by conjugase (pteroylpolyglutamate hydrolase), a zinc-dependent enzyme of the pancreatic juice, bile, and mucosal brush border; zinc deficiency can impair folate absorption. Free folate, released by conjugase action, is absorbed by active transport in the jejunum.

The folate in milk is mainly bound to a specific binding protein; the complex is absorbed intact, mainly in the ileum, by a mechanism that is distinct from the active transport system for the absorption of free folate. The biological availability of folate from milk or of folate from diets to which milk has been added is greater than that of unbound folate.

Much of the dietary folate undergoes methylation and reduction within the intestinal mucosa, so that what enters the portal bloodstream is largely 5-methyltetrahydrofolate (Figure 11.18). Other substituted and unsubstituted folate monoglutamates and dihydrofolate are also absorbed; they are reduced and methylated in the liver, then secreted in the bile. The liver also takes up various folates released by tissues; again these are reduced, methylated, and secreted in the bile.

The total daily enterohepatic circulation of folate is equivalent to about one-third of the dietary intake. Despite this, there is very little fecal loss of folate; jejunal absorption of methyltetrahydrofolate is a very efficient process, and the fecal excretion of some 200 μg (450 nmol) of folates per day represents synthesis by intestinal flora and does not reflect intake to any significant extent.

Methyltetrahydrofolate circulates bound to albumin and is available for uptake by extrahepatic tissues. Small amounts of other one-carbon substituted folate also circulate and will enter cells by the same carrier-mediated process, where they are trapped by formation of polyglutamates, which do not cross cell membranes.

The main circulating folate is methyltetrahydrofolate, which is a poor substrate for polyglutamylation, demethylation by the action of methionine synthetase (Section 11.11.3.2) is required for effective metabolic trapping of folate. In vitamin B_{12} deficiency, when methionine synthetase activity is impaired, there is therefore impaired retention of folate in tissues.

The catabolism of folate is largely by cleavage of the C-9–N-10 bond, catalyzed by carboxypeptidase G. The *p*-aminobenzoic acid moiety is amidated and excreted in the urine as conjugates; pterin is excreted either unchanged or as biologically inactive metabolites.

11.11.3 Metabolic functions of folate

The metabolic role of folate is as a carrier of one-carbon units in both catabolism and biosynthetic reactions. These may be carried as formyl, formimino, methyl, methylene, or methylene residues (Figure 11.18). The major sources of these one-carbon units and their major uses, as well as the interconversions of the substituted folates, are shown in Figure 11.19.

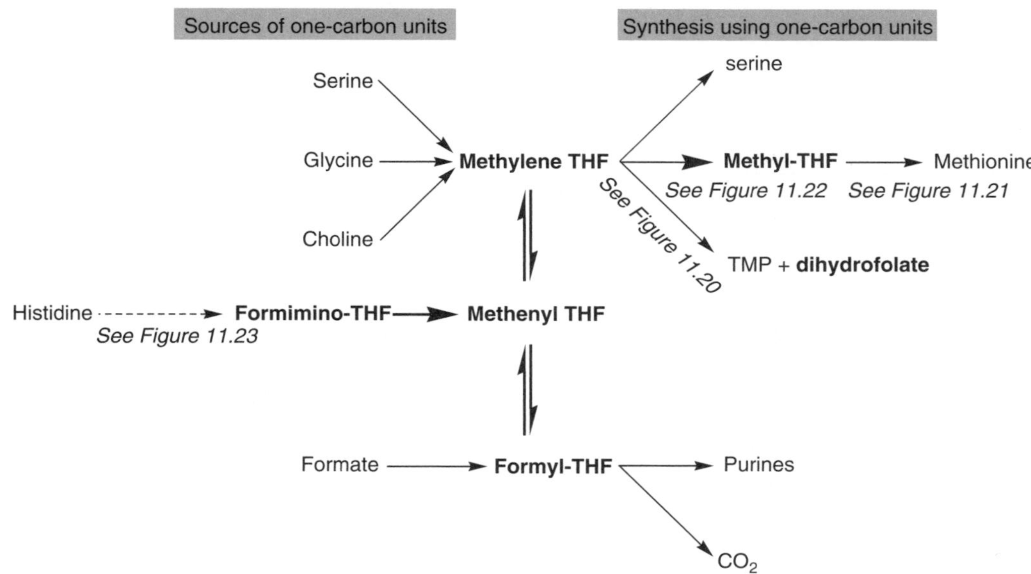

Figure 11.19 Sources and utilization of folate derivatives carrying one-carbon fragments and interconversion of the one-carbon-substituted folates.

The major point of entry for one-carbon fragments into substituted folates is methylenetetrahydrofolate, which is formed by the catabolism of glycine, serine, and choline.

Serine hydroxymethyltransferase is a pyridoxal phosphate dependent enzyme that catalyzes the cleavage of serine to glycine and methylenetetrahydrofolate. While folate is required for the catabolism of a number of compounds, serine is the most important source of substituted folates for biosynthetic reactions, and the activity of serine hydroxymethyltransferase is regulated by the availability of folate. The reaction is freely reversible, and under appropriate conditions in the liver it functions to form serine from glycine as a substrate for gluconeogenesis (Section 5.7).

The catabolism of histidine leads to the formation of formiminoglutamate (FIGLU; Section 11.11.6.1). The formimino group is transferred onto tetrahydrofolate to form formiminotetrahydrofolate, which is subsequently deaminated to form methenyltetrahydrofolate.

Methylene-, methenyl-, and 10-formyl tetrahydrofolates are freely interconvertible. This means that when one-carbon folates are not required for synthetic reactions, the oxidation of the formyl group of formyltetrahydrofolate to carbon dioxide provides a means of maintaining an adequate tissue pool of free folate.

By contrast, the reduction of methylenetetrahydrofolate to methyltetrahydrofolate is irreversible, and the only way in which free folate can be formed from methyltetrahydrofolate is by the reaction of methionine synthetase (Section 11.11.3.2).

10-Formyl and methylenetetrahydrofolate are donors of one-carbon fragments in a number of biosynthetic reactions, including especially the synthesis of purines, pyrimidines, and porphyrins. In most cases, the reaction is a simple transfer of the one-carbon group from substituted folate onto the acceptor substrate. Two reactions are of special interest: thymidylate synthetase and methionine synthetase.

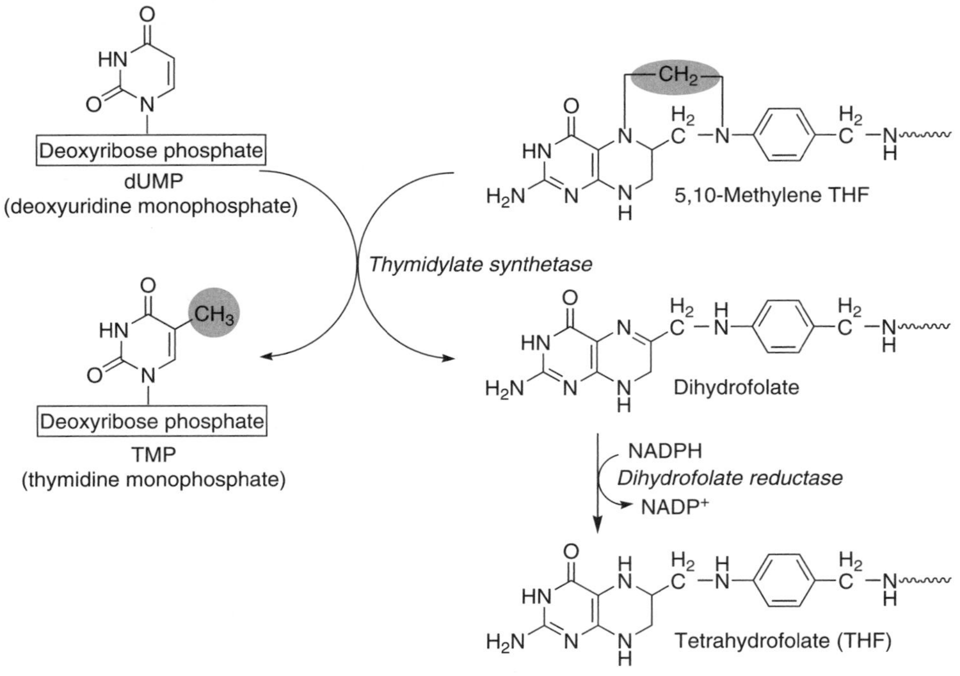

Figure 11.20 The reaction of thymidylate synthetase and dihydrofolate reductase.

11.11.3.1 Thymidylate synthetase and dihydrofolate reductase

The methylation of dUMP to thymidine monophosphate (TMP), catalyzed by thymidylate synthetase (Figure 11.20), is essential for the synthesis of DNA, although preformed TMP can be reutilized by salvage from the catabolism of DNA.

The methyl donor is methylenetetrahydrofolate; the reaction involves reduction of the one-carbon fragment to a methyl group at the expense of the folate, which is oxidized to dihydrofolate. Dihydrofolate is then reduced to tetrahydrofolate by dihydrofolate reductase.

Thymidylate synthase and dihydrofolate reductase are especially active in tissues with a high rate of cell division, and hence a high rate of DNA replication and a high requirement for thymidylate. Because of this, inhibitors of dihydrofolate reductase have been exploited as anticancer drugs. The most successful of these is methotrexate, an analog of 10-methyltetrahydrofolate. Chemotherapy consists of alternating periods of administration of methotrexate and folate (normally as 5-formyltetrahydrofolate, leucovorin) to replete the normal tissues and avoid folate deficiency—so-called leucovorin rescue.

The dihydrofolate reductase of some bacteria and parasites differs significantly from the human enzyme, so that inhibitors of the enzyme can be used as antibacterial drugs (e.g., trimethoprim) and antimalarial drugs (e.g., pyrimethamine).

11.11.3.2 Methionine synthetase and the methyl-folate trap

In addition to its role in the synthesis of proteins, methionine, as the *S*-adenosyl derivative, acts as a methyl donor in a wide variety of biosynthetic reactions; the resultant homocysteine may either be metabolized to yield cysteine or be remethylated to yield methionine (Figure 11.21).

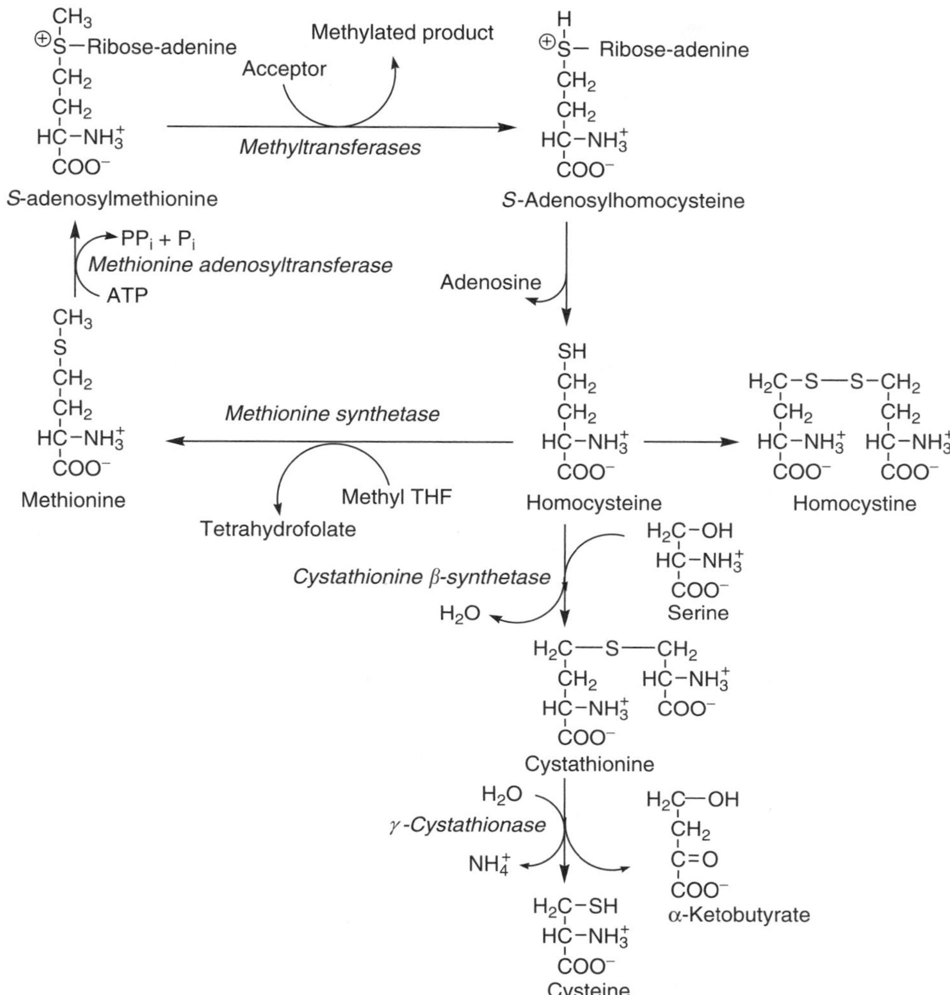

Figure 11.21 Methionine metabolism and the reaction of methionine synthetase.

Two enzymes catalyze the methylation of homocysteine to methionine:

- Methionine synthetase is a vitamin B_{12} dependent enzyme, for which the methyl donor is methyltetrahydrofolate.
- Homocysteine methyltransferase utilizes betaine (an intermediate in the catabolism of choline) as the methyl donor and is not vitamin B_{12} dependent.

Both enzymes are found in most tissues, but only the vitamin B_{12} dependent methionine synthetase occurs in the central nervous system.

The reduction of methylenetetrahydrofolate to methyltetrahydrofolate is irreversible, and the major source of folate for tissues is methyltetrahydrofolate. The only metabolic role of methyltetrahydrofolate is the methylation of homocysteine to methionine, and this is the only way in which methyltetrahydrofolate can be demethylated to yield free folate in tissues. Methionine synthetase thus provides the link between the physiological functions of folate

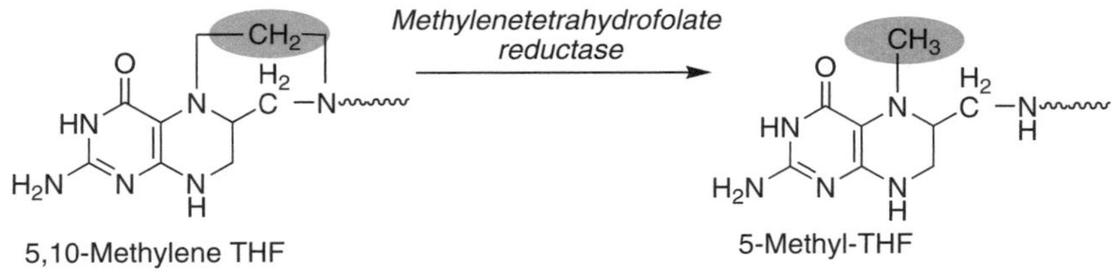

Figure 11.22 The reaction of methylenetetrahydrofolate reductase.

and vitamin B_{12}. Impairment of methionine synthetase activity in vitamin B_{12} deficiency will result in the accumulation of methyltetrahydrofolate, which can neither be utilized for any other one-carbon transfer reactions nor be demethylated to provide free folate. There is therefore functional deficiency of folate, secondary to the deficiency of vitamin B_{12}.

11.11.3.3 Methylenetetrahydrofolate reductase and hyperhomocysteinemia

Elevated blood homocysteine is a significant risk factor for atherosclerosis, thrombosis, and hypertension, independent of factors such as dietary lipids and plasma lipoproteins (Section 6.3.2). Between 5% and 10% of the population, and almost 20% of people with ischemic heart disease have an abnormal variant of methylenetetrahydrofolate reductase (Figure 11.22), which is unstable and loses activity faster than normal.

The result of this is that people with the abnormal form of the enzyme have an impaired ability to form methyltetrahydrofolate (the main form in which folate is taken up by tissues), and suffer from functional folate deficiency. Therefore, they are unable to remethylate homocysteine to methionine adequately and develop hyperhomocysteinemia.

People with the abnormal variant of methylenetetrahydrofolate reductase do not develop hyperhomocysteinemia if they have a relatively high intake of folate. This seems to be due to the methylation of folate in the intestinal mucosa during absorption; intestinal mucosal cells have a rapid turnover (Section 4.1), and therefore it is not important that methylene tetrahydrofolate reductase is less stable than normal—there is still an adequate activity of the enzyme in the intestinal mucosa to maintain absorption of methyltetrahydrofolate. Equally, the unstable enzyme may be stabilized by the presence of a relatively high concentration of its substrate.

This has led to the suggestion that higher intakes of folate will reduce the incidence of cardiovascular disease; to date there is no evidence from intervention studies or from countries where there has been mandatory enrichment of flour with folate for some years, that the lowering of plasma homocysteine by folate supplements does reduce the risk. Although there are sound biochemical reasons why elevated homocysteine may increase the risk of cardiovascular disease, is it also possible the elevated plasma homocysteine is the result of damage to the kidney in the early stages of atherosclerosis, rather than a cause of atherosclerosis.

11.11.4 Folate deficiency: megaloblastic anemia

Dietary deficiency of folate is not uncommon, and as noted above deficiency of vitamin B_{12} also leads to functional folate deficiency. In either case, it is cells that are dividing rapidly, and therefore have a large requirement for thymidine for DNA synthesis, that are most severely affected. These are the cells of the bone marrow that form red blood cells, the cells of the intestinal mucosa, and the hair follicles. Clinically, folate deficiency leads to megaloblastic anemia, the release into the circulation of immature precursors of red blood cells.

11.11.5 Folate requirements

Depletion or repletion studies to determine folate requirements using folic acid monoglutamate suggest a requirement of the order of 80–100 µg (170–220 nmol)/day. The total body pool of folate in adults is some 17 µmol (7.5 mg), with a biological half-life of 101 days. This suggests a minimum requirement for replacement of 85 nmol (37 µg)/day. Studies of the urinary excretion of folate metabolites in subjects maintained on folate-free diets suggest that there is catabolism of some 80 µg (folate)/day.

Because of the problems of determining the biological availability of the various folate polyglutamate conjugates found in foods, reference intakes allow a wide margin of safety and are based on an allowance of 3 µg (6.8 nmol)/kg body weight.

11.11.5.1 Folate in pregnancy

During the 1980s, a considerable body of evidence accumulated that *spina bifida* and other neural tube defects (which occur in about 0.75%–1% of pregnancies) were associated with low intakes of folate, and that increased intake during pregnancy might be protective. It is now established that supplements of folate begun periconceptually result in a significant reduction in the incidence of neural tube defects, and it is recommended that intakes be increased by 400 µg/day before conception. The studies were conducted using folate monoglutamate, and it is unlikely that an equivalent increase in intake could be achieved from unfortified foods; supplements are recommended. Closure of the neural tube occurs by day 28 of pregnancy, which is before the woman knows that she is pregnant. The advice therefore is that all women who are or may be about to become pregnant should take folate supplements.

11.11.5.2 Higher levels of folate intake

Marginal folate status leads to reduced methylation of key regulatory areas of DNA involved in regulating gene expression (Section 6.4.1), and higher intakes of folate are associated with lower incidence of colorectal (and possibly other) cancer. There is some evidence that supplements of folate may be protective against some cancers.

Folate supplements of 400 µg/day reduce the incidence of *spina bifida* and neural tube defect; about 1% of pregnant women are at risk (Section 11.11.5.1). Similar supplements lower plasma homocysteine in people with the unstable variant of methylenetetrahydrofolate reductase (Section 11.11.3.3).

Folate supplements in excess of 350 µg/day may impair zinc absorption. More importantly, there are two potential problems that have to be considered when advocating either widespread use of folate supplements or widespread enrichment of foods with folate:

- High levels of folate intake mask the megaloblastic anemia of vitamin B_{12} deficiency (Section 11.10.2), so that the presenting sign is irreversible nerve damage. This is especially a problem for the elderly, who may have impaired absorption of vitamin B_{12} as a result of gastric atrophy. It has been suggested that the addition of crystalline vitamin B_{12} as well as folate to foods would permit absorption of adequate amounts of vitamin B_{12} to prevent deficiency developing.
- Antagonism between folate and the anticonvulsants used in the treatment of epilepsy is part of their mechanism of action; about 2% of the population have (drug-controlled) epilepsy. Relatively large supplements of folic acid (in excess of 1000 µg/day) may antagonize the anticonvulsants and lead to an increase in the frequency of epileptic attacks.

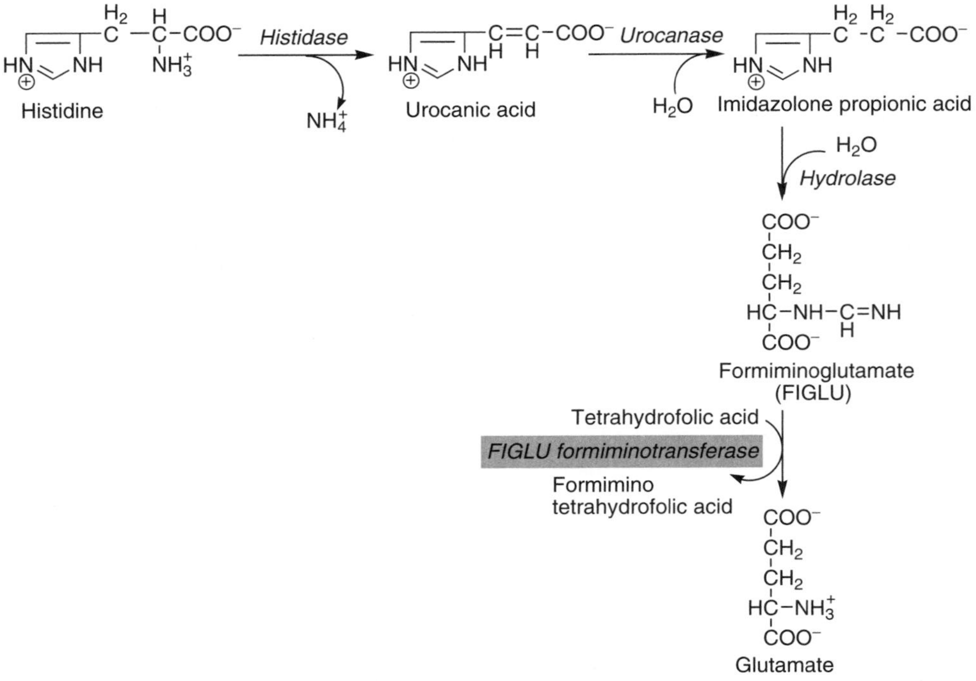

Histidine → (Histidase, −NH_4^+) → Urocanic acid → (Urocanase, +H_2O) → Imidazolone propionic acid → (Hydrolase, +H_2O) → Formiminoglutamate (FIGLU) → (FIGLU formiminotransferase; Tetrahydrofolic acid → Formimino tetrahydrofolic acid) → Glutamate

Figure 11.23 Metabolism of histidine—the FIGLU test for folate status.

11.11.6 Assessment of folate status

The serum or red blood cell concentration of folate can be measured by radioligand binding assays, but there are a number of problems and in some centers microbiological determination is preferred. In addition, there are two tests for functional folate status, the FIGLU test and the dUMP suppression test.

11.11.6.1 Histidine metabolism—the FIGLU test

The ability to metabolize a test dose of histidine provides a sensitive functional test of folate nutritional status; FIGLU is an intermediate in histidine catabolism (Figure 11.23) and is metabolized by a folate dependent enzyme. In deficiency, the activity of this enzyme is impaired and FIGLU accumulates and is excreted in the urine, especially after a test dose of histidine—the so-called FIGLU test.

Although the FIGLU test depends on folate nutritional status, the metabolism of histidine will also be impaired, and hence a positive result obtained, in vitamin B_{12} deficiency, because of the secondary deficiency of free folate. About 60% of vitamin B_{12} deficient subjects show increased FIGLU excretion after a histidine load.

11.11.6.2 The dUMP suppression test

Rapidly dividing cells can either use preformed TMP for DNA synthesis or can synthesize it *de novo* from dUMP (Section 11.11.3.1). Isolated bone marrow cells or stimulated lymphocytes incubated with [^{3}H]TMP will incorporate label into DNA. In the presence of adequate amounts of methylenetetrahydrofolate, the addition of dUMP as a substrate for thymidylate synthetase reduces the incorporation of [^{3}H]TMP as a result of dilution of the pool of labeled material by newly synthesized TMP and inhibition of thymidylate kinase by thymidine triphosphate.

This suppression of ability of the incorporation of [^{3}H]thymidine into DNA in rapidly dividing cells by added deoxyuridine provides an index of folate status. In normal cells, the incorporation of [^{3}H]thymidine into DNA after preincubation with dUMP is 1.4%–1.8% of that without preincubation. By contrast, cells that are deficient in folate form little or no thymidine from dUMP and hence incorporate nearly as much of the [^{3}H]thymidine after incubation with dUMP as they do without preincubation.

Either a primary deficiency of folate or a functional deficiency secondary to vitamin B_{12} deficiency will have the same effect. In folate deficiency, addition of any biologically active form of folate, but not vitamin B_{12}, will normalize the dUMP suppression of [^{3}H]thymidine incorporation. In vitamin B_{12} deficiency, addition of vitamin B_{12} or methylenetetrahydrofolate, but not methyltetrahydrofolate, will normalize dUMP suppression.

11.12 Biotin

Biotin was originally discovered as part of the complex called *bios*, which promoted the growth of yeast, and separately as vitamin H, the protective or curative factor in "egg white injury"—the disease caused experimentally by feeding diets containing large amounts of uncooked egg white.

Biotin is widely distributed in many foods. It is synthesized by intestinal flora, and in balance studies the total output of biotin in urine plus feces is three- to sixfold greater than the intake, reflecting bacterial synthesis. It is not known to what extent this is available to the host.

11.12.1 Absorption and metabolism of biotin

Most biotin in foods is present as biocytin (ε-amino-biotinyllysine; Figure 11.24), which is released on proteolysis, then hydrolyzed by biotinidase in the pancreatic juice and intestinal mucosal secretions to yield free biotin. The extent to which bound biotin in foods is biologically available is not known.

Free biotin is absorbed from the small intestine by active transport and circulates in the bloodstream both free and bound to a serum glycoprotein that has biotinidase activity, catalyzing the hydrolysis of biocytin.

Biotin enters tissues by a saturable transport system and is then incorporated into biotin dependent enzymes as the ε-amino-lysine peptide, biocytin. Unlike other B vitamins where concentrative uptake into tissues can be achieved by facilitated diffusion followed by metabolic trapping, the incorporation of biotin into enzymes is relatively slow and cannot be considered part of the uptake process. On catabolism of the enzymes, biocytin is hydrolyzed by biotinidase, permitting reutilization (see Problem 10.4).

11.12.2 Metabolic functions of biotin

Biotin functions to transfer carbon dioxide in a small number of carboxylation reactions. The reactive intermediate is 1-*N*-carboxy-biocytin (Figure 11.24), formed from bicarbonate in an ATP-dependent reaction. A single holocarboxylase synthetase acts on the apoenzymes of acetyl CoA carboxylase (a key enzyme in fatty acid synthesis;

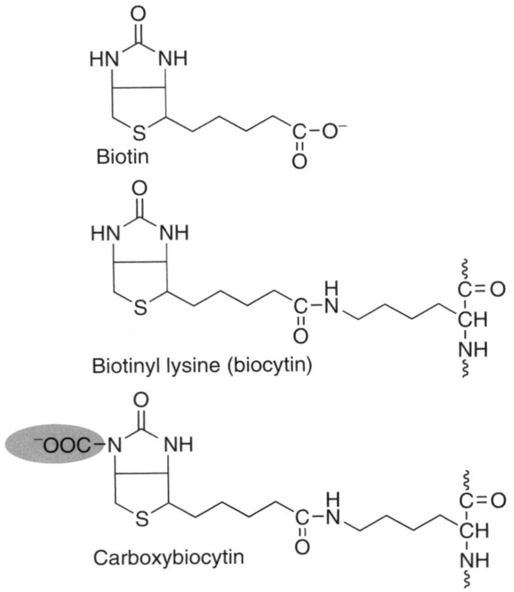

Figure 11.24 Biotin, biocytin (ε-amino biotinyllysine), and carboxy-biocytin.

Section 5.6.1), pyruvate carboxylase (a key enzyme in gluconeogenesis; Section 5.7), propionyl CoA carboxylase (Figure 11.17), and methylcrotonyl CoA carboxylase to form the active holoenzymes from (inactive) apoenzymes and free biotin.

11.12.3 Biotin deficiency and requirements

Biotin is widely distributed in foods, and deficiency is unknown except among people maintained for many months on total parenteral nutrition and a very small number of people who eat abnormally large amounts of uncooked egg. Avidin, a protein in egg white, binds biotin extremely tightly and renders it unavailable for absorption. It is denatured by cooking and loses its ability to bind biotin. The amount of avidin in uncooked egg white is relatively small, and problems of biotin deficiency have only occurred in people eating abnormally large amounts—a dozen or more raw eggs a day for some years.

The few early reports of human biotin deficiency concerned people who consumed large amounts of uncooked eggs. They developed a fine scaly dermatitis and hair loss (alopecia). Histology of the skin showed an absence of sebaceous glands and atrophy of the hair follicles. Provision of biotin supplements of between 200 and 1000 μg/day resulted in cure of the skin lesions, and regrowth of hair despite continuing their abnormal diet. There have been no studies of provision of smaller doses of biotin to such people. More recently, similar signs of biotin deficiency have been observed in patients receiving total parenteral nutrition for prolonged periods, after major resection of the gut. The signs resolve following the provision of biotin, but again there have been no studies of the amounts of biotin required; intakes have ranged between 60 and 200 μg/day.

There is no evidence on which to estimate requirements for biotin. Average intakes are between 10 and 200 μg/day. Since dietary deficiency does not occur, such intakes are obviously more than adequate to meet requirements.

11.13 Pantothenic acid

Pantothenic acid (sometimes known as vitamin B_5) has a central role in energy-yielding metabolism as the functional moiety of coenzyme A (Figure 5.23) and in the biosynthesis of fatty acids as the prosthetic group of acyl carrier protein (Section 5.6.1).

Pantothenic acid is widely distributed in all foodstuffs; the name derives from the Greek for "from everywhere," as opposed to other vitamins, which were originally isolated from individual especially rich sources. As a result, deficiency has not been unequivocally reported in humans except in specific depletion studies, which have generally used the antagonist ω-methyl pantothenic acid.

11.13.1 Absorption, metabolism, and metabolic functions of pantothenic acid

About 85% of dietary pantothenic acid is as coenzyme A or phosphopantetheine, which is hydrolyzed to pantothenic acid. The intestinal absorption of pantothenic acid is by diffusion and occurs at a constant rate throughout the length of the small intestine; intestinal bacterial synthesis may contribute to pantothenic acid nutrition.

The first step in pantothenic acid utilization is phosphorylation. Pantothenate kinase is rate limiting, so that unlike vitamins that are accumulated by metabolic trapping, there can be significant accumulation of free pantothenic acid in tissues.

11.13.1.1 Coenzyme A and acyl carrier protein

All tissues are capable of forming coenzyme A from pantothenic acid. CoA functions as the carrier of fatty acids, as thioesters, in mitochondrial β-oxidation (Section 5.5.2). The resultant two-carbon fragments, as acetyl CoA, then undergo oxidation in the citric acid cycle (Section 5.4.4). CoA also functions as a carrier in the transfer of acetyl (and other fatty acyl) moieties in a variety of biosynthetic and catabolic reactions, including:

- Cholesterol and steroid hormone synthesis
- Synthesis of long-chain fatty acids from palmitate and elongation of polyunsaturated fatty acids in mitochondria
- Acylation of serine, threonine, and cysteine residues on proteolipids and acetylation of neuraminic acid

Fatty acid synthesis (Section 5.6.1) is catalyzed by a cytosolic multienzyme complex in which the growing fatty acyl chain is bound by thioester linkage to an enzyme-bound 4′-phospho-pantetheine residue, rather than to free CoA as in β-oxidation. This component of the fatty acid synthetase complex is the acyl carrier protein.

11.13.2 Pantothenic acid deficiency; safe and adequate levels of intake

Prisoners of war in the Far East in the 1940s, who were severely malnourished, showed, among other signs and symptoms of vitamin deficiency diseases, a new condition of paresthesia and severe pain in the feet and toes, which was called the "burning foot syndrome" or nutritional melalgia. Although it was tentatively attributed to pantothenic acid deficiency, no specific trials of pantothenic acid were carried out, rather the subjects were given yeast extract and other rich sources of all vitamins as part of an urgent program of nutritional rehabilitation.

Experimental pantothenic acid depletion, commonly together with the administration of ω-methyl pantothenic acid, results in the following signs and symptoms after 2–3 weeks:

- Neuromotor disorders, including paresthesia of the hands and feet, hyperactive deep tendon reflexes, and muscle weakness. These can be explained by the role of acetyl CoA in the synthesis of the neurotransmitter acetylcholine, and impaired formation of threonine acyl esters in myelin. Dysmyelination may explain the persistence and recurrence of neurological problems many years after nutritional rehabilitation in people who had suffered from burning foot syndrome.
- Mental depression, which again may be related to either acetyl choline deficit or impaired myelin synthesis.
- Gastrointestinal complaints, including severe vomiting and pain with depressed gastric acid secretion in response to gastrin.
- Decreased serum cholesterol and decreased urinary excretion of 17-ketosteroids, reflecting the impairment of steroidogenesis.
- Decreased acetylation of *p*-aminobenzoic acid, sulfonamides, and other drugs, reflecting reduced availability of acetyl CoA for these reactions.

There is no evidence on which to estimate pantothenic acid requirements. Average intakes are between 3 and 7 mg/day, and since deficiency does not occur, such intakes are obviously more than adequate to meet requirements.

11.14 Vitamin C (ascorbic acid)

Vitamin C is a vitamin for only a limited number of vertebrate species: humans and other primates, the guinea pig, bats, the passeriform birds, and most fishes. Ascorbate is synthesized as an intermediate in the gulonolactone pathway of glucose metabolism; in those vertebrate species for which it is a vitamin, one enzyme of the pathway, gulonolactone oxidase, is absent.

The vitamin C deficiency disease, scurvy, has been known for many centuries and was described in the Ebers papyrus of 1500 BC and by Hippocrates. The Crusaders are said to have lost more men through scurvy than were killed in battle, while in some of the long voyages of exploration of the fourteenth and fifteenth centuries up to 90% of the crew died from scurvy. Cartier's expedition to Quebec in 1535 was struck by scurvy; local native Americans taught him to use an infusion of swamp spruce leaves to prevent or cure the condition.

Recognition that scurvy was due to a dietary deficiency came relatively early. James Lind demonstrated in 1757 that orange and lemon juice were protective, and Cook maintained his crew in good health during his circumnavigation of the globe (1772–1775) by stopping

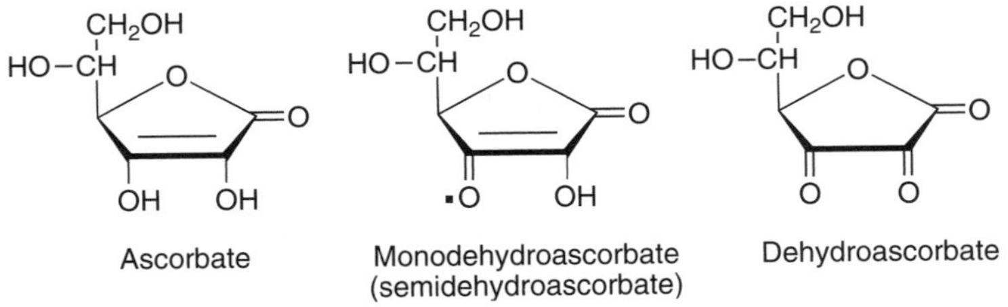

Ascorbate

Monodehydroascorbate (semidehydroascorbate)

Dehydroascorbate

Figure 11.25 Vitamin C.

frequently to take on fresh fruits and vegetables. In 1804, the British Navy decreed a daily ration of lemon or lime juice for all ratings, a requirement that was extended to the merchant navy in 1865.

Both ascorbic acid and dehydroascorbic acid have vitamin C activity (Figure 11.25).

Vitamin C is found in fruits and vegetables. Very significant losses of vitamin C occur as vegetables wilt, or when they are cut, as a result of release of ascorbate oxidase from the plant tissue. Significant losses of the vitamin also occur in cooking, both through leaching into the cooking water, and atmospheric oxidation, which continues when foods are left to stand before serving.

11.14.1 *Absorption and metabolism of vitamin C*

At intakes of about 100 mg/day, between 80% and 95% of dietary ascorbate is absorbed by active transport at the intestinal mucosal brush border membrane. As the transporter becomes saturated, a lower proportion of high intakes is absorbed.

About 70% of blood ascorbate is in plasma and erythrocytes (which do not concentrate the vitamin from plasma). The remainder is in white cells, which have a marked ability to concentrate it (Section 11.14.5). There is no specific storage organ for ascorbate; apart from leukocytes (which account for only 10% of total blood ascorbate), the only tissues showing a significant concentration of the vitamin are the adrenal and pituitary glands.

Ascorbic acid is excreted in the urine, either unchanged or as dehydroascorbate and diketogulonate. Both ascorbate and dehydroascorbate are filtered at the glomerulus, then reabsorbed. When glomerular filtration of ascorbate and dehydroascorbate exceeds the capacity of the transport systems, at a plasma concentration of ascorbate between 70 and 85 μmol/L, the vitamin is excreted in the urine in amounts proportional to intake.

11.14.2 *Metabolic functions of vitamin C*

Ascorbic acid has specific roles in two groups of enzymes: the copper-containing hydroxylases and the α-ketoglutarate-linked iron-containing hydroxylases. It also increases the activity of a number of other enzymes *in vitro,* although this is a nonspecific reducing action rather than reflecting any metabolic function of the vitamin. In addition, it has a number of nonenzymic effects due to its action as a reducing agent and oxygen radical quencher (Section 6.5.3.5).

11.14.2.1 *Copper-containing hydroxylases*

Dopamine β-hydroxylase is a copper-containing enzyme involved in the synthesis of the catecholamines noradrenaline and adrenaline from tyrosine in the adrenal medulla and central nervous system. The enzyme contains Cu^{+}, which is oxidized to Cu^{2+} during the hydroxylation of the substrate; reduction back to Cu^{+} specifically requires ascorbate, which is oxidized to monodehydroascorbate.

A number of peptide hormones have a carboxyl terminal amide that is essential for biological activity. The amide group is derived from a glycine residue on the carboxyl side of the amino acid that will become the amidated terminal of the mature peptide. This glycine is hydroxylated on the α-carbon by a copper-containing enzyme, peptidylglycine hydroxylase. The α-hydroxyglycine residue then decomposes nonenzymically to yield the amidated peptide and glyoxylate. The copper prosthetic group is oxidized in the reaction, and as in dopamine β-hydroxylase, ascorbate is specifically required for reduction back to Cu^{+}.

11.14.2.2 α-Ketoglutarate-linked iron-containing hydroxylases

A number of iron-containing hydroxylases share a common reaction mechanism, in which hydroxylation of the substrate is linked to decarboxylation of α-ketoglutarate. Many of these enzymes are involved in the modification of precursor proteins to yield the final, mature, protein. This is a process of postsynthetic modification—modification of an amino acid residue after it has been incorporated into the protein during synthesis on the ribosome (see Problem 9.3 and Section 9.2.3.4):

- Proline and lysine hydroxylases are required for the postsynthetic modification of procollagen in the formation of mature, insoluble, collagen, and proline hydroxylase is also required for the postsynthetic modification of the precursor proteins of osteocalcin and the C1q component of complement.
- Aspartate β-hydroxylase is required for the postsynthetic modification of the precursor of protein C, the vitamin K dependent protease that hydrolyzes activated factor V in the blood-clotting cascade.
- Trimethyllysine and γ-butyrobetaine hydroxylases are required for the synthesis of carnitine (Section 5.5.1).

Ascorbate is oxidized during the reaction of these enzymes, but not stoichiometrically with the decarboxylation of α-ketoglutarate and hydroxylation of the substrate. The purified enzyme is active in the absence of ascorbate, but after some 5–10 s (about 15–30 cycles of enzyme action), the rate of reaction begins to fall. At this stage the iron in the catalytic site has been oxidized to Fe^{3+}, which is catalytically inactive; activity is restored only by ascorbate, which reduces it back to Fe^{2+}. The oxidation of Fe^{2+} is the consequence of accidental oxidation by the bound oxygen, rather than the main reaction of the enzyme, which explains why the enzyme can remain active for several seconds in the absence of ascorbate, and why the consumption of ascorbate is not stoichiometric.

11.14.3 Vitamin C deficiency: scurvy

The vitamin C deficiency disease, scurvy, was formerly a common problem at the end of winter, when there had been no fresh fruits and vegetables for many months.

Although there is no specific organ for storage of vitamin C in the body, signs of deficiency do not develop in previously adequately nourished subjects until they have been deprived of the vitamin for 4–6 months, by which time plasma and tissue concentrations have fallen considerably. The earliest signs in volunteers maintained on a vitamin C free diet are skin changes, beginning with plugging of hair follicles by horny material, followed by enlargement of the hyperkeratotic follicles, and petechial hemorrhage as a result of increased fragility of blood capillaries.

At a later stage, there is also hemorrhage of the gums. This is frequently accompanied by secondary bacterial infection and considerable withdrawal of the gum from the necks of the teeth. As the condition progresses, there is loss of dental cement, and the teeth become loose in the alveolar bone, and may be lost.

Wounds show only superficial healing in scurvy, with little or no formation of (collagen-rich) scar tissue, so that healing is delayed and wounds can readily be reopened (see Problem 9.3). Scorbutic scar tissue has only about half the tensile strength of that normally formed.

Advanced scurvy is accompanied by intense pain in the bones, which can be attributed to changes in bone mineralization as a result of abnormal collagen synthesis. Bone formation ceases and the existing bone becomes rarefied, so that the bones fracture with minimal trauma.

The name scurvy is derived from the Italian *scorbutico*, meaning an irritable, neurotic, discontented, whining, and cranky person. The disease is associated with listlessness and general malaise, and sometimes changes in personality and psychomotor performance and a lowering of the general level of arousal. These behavioral effects can be attributed to impaired synthesis of catecholamine neurotransmitters, as a result of low activity of dopamine β-hydroxylase.

Most of the other clinical signs of scurvy can be accounted for by the effects of ascorbate deficiency on collagen synthesis, as a result of impaired proline and lysine hydroxylase activity. Depletion of muscle carnitine (Section 5.5.1), as a result of impaired activity of trimethyllysine and γ-butyrobetaine hydroxylases, may account for the lassitude and fatigue that precede clinical signs of scurvy.

11.14.3.1 Anemia in scurvy

Anemia is frequently associated with scurvy and may be either macrocytic, indicative of folate deficiency (Section 11.11.4) or hypochromic, indicative of iron deficiency (Section 11.15.2.3).

Folate deficiency may be epiphenomenal since the major dietary sources of folate are the same as those of ascorbate. However, some patients with clear megaloblastic anemia respond to the administration of vitamin C alone, suggesting that there may be a role of ascorbate in the maintenance of normal pools of reduced folates, although there is no evidence that any of the reactions of folate is ascorbate dependent.

Iron deficiency in scurvy may well be secondary to reduced absorption of inorganic iron and impaired mobilization of tissue iron reserves (Section 11.15.2.3). At the same time, the hemorrhages of advanced scurvy will cause a significant loss of blood.

There is also evidence that erythrocytes have a shorter half-life than normal in scurvy, possibly as a result of oxidative damage to membrane lipids due to impairment of the reduction of tocopheroxyl radical by ascorbate (Section 6.5.3.3).

11.14.4 Vitamin C requirements

Vitamin C illustrates extremely well how different criterion of adequacy and different interpretations of experimental evidence (Section 11.1), can lead to different estimates of requirements, and reference intakes ranging between 30 and 90 mg/day for adults.

The requirement for vitamin C to prevent clinical scurvy is less than 10 mg/day. However, at this level of intake wounds do not heal properly, and an intake of 20 mg/day is required for optimum wound healing. Allowing for individual variation in requirements, this gives a reference intake for adults of 30 mg/day, which was the U.K. RDA until 1991.

The 1991 British Reference Nutrient Intake (RNI) for vitamin C is based on the level of intake at which the plasma concentration rises sharply, showing that requirements have now been met, tissues are saturated, and there is spare vitamin being transported between tissues available for excretion. This criterion of adequacy gives an RNI of 40 mg/day for adults.

The alternative approach to determining requirements is to estimate the total body content of vitamin C, then measure the rate at which it is metabolized, by giving a test dose of isotopically labeled vitamin. This was the basis of both the 1989 U.S. RDA of 60 mg/day for adults and the Netherlands RDA of 80 mg/day. Indeed, it also provides an alternative basis for the RNI of 40 mg/day adopted in Britain in 1991.

The problem lies in deciding what is an appropriate body content of vitamin C. The American studies were performed on subjects whose total body vitamin C was estimated to be 1500 mg at the beginning of a depletion study. However, there is no evidence that this is a necessary, or even a desirable, body content of the vitamin. It is simply the body content of the vitamin among a small group of young people eating a self-selected diet rich in fruit. There is good evidence that body pool of 900 mg is more than adequate. It is three times larger than that at which the first signs of deficiency are observed and will protect against the development of any signs of deficiency for several months on a completely vitamin C free diet.

There is a further problem in interpreting the results of this kind of study. The rate at which vitamin C is metabolized varies with the intake and body pool. This means that as the experimental subjects become depleted, the rate at which they metabolize the vitamin decreases. Thus, calculation of the amount required to maintain the body content depends on the way in which results obtained during depletion studies are extrapolated to the rate in subjects consuming a normal diet, and on the amount of vitamin C in that diet.

An intake of 40 mg/day is more than adequate to maintain a total body content of 900 mg of vitamin C—the same as the U.K. RNI. At a higher level of habitual intake, 60 mg/day is adequate to maintain a total body content of 1500 mg (the 1989 U.S. RDA). Making allowances for changes in the rate of metabolism with different levels of intake, and allowing for incomplete absorption of the vitamin, gives the Netherlands RDA of 80 mg/day.

The 2000 U.S. RDA for vitamin C, shown in Table 11.3, is based achieving near complete saturation of neutrophils with the vitamin, with minimal urinary loss, giving an RDA of 90 mg/day for men and an extrapolated RDA of 75 mg/day for women.

11.14.4.1 *Possible benefits of high intakes of vitamin C*

At intakes above about 100 mg/day, the body's capacity to metabolize vitamin C is saturated, and any further intake is excreted in the urine unchanged. Therefore, it would not seem justifiable to recommend higher levels of intake. However, vitamin C enhances the intestinal absorption of inorganic iron (Section 4.5.3.1), both by maintaining it in the Fe^{2+} state and also by chelating it. A dose of 25 mg of vitamin C taken together with a meal increases the absorption of iron some 65%, while a 1 g dose gives a ninefold increase. This occurs only when ascorbic acid is present together with the test meal; neither intravenous administration of vitamin C nor intake several hours before the test meal has any effect on iron absorption. Optimum iron absorption may therefore require significantly more than 100 mg of vitamin C/day.

The safety of nitrates and nitrites used in curing meat, a traditional method of preservation, has been questioned because of the formation of nitrosamines by reaction between nitrite and amines naturally present in foods under the acid conditions in the stomach. In experimental animals, nitrosamines are potent carcinogens, and some authorities have limited the amounts of these salts that are permitted, although there is little evidence of any hazard to humans from endogenous nitrosamine formation. Ascorbate can prevent the formation of nitrosamines by reacting nonenzymically with nitrite and other nitrosating reagents, forming NO, NO_2, and N_2. Again, this is an effect of ascorbate present in the stomach at the same time as the dietary nitrites and amines, rather than an effect of vitamin C nutritional status.

11.14.4.2 *Pharmacological uses of vitamin C*

A number of studies have reported low ascorbate status in patients with advanced cancer—perhaps an unsurprising finding in seriously ill patients. With very little experimental evidence, it has been suggested that very high intakes of vitamin C (of the order of

10 g/day or more) may be beneficial in enhancing host resistance to cancer, and preventing the development of AIDS in people who are HIV positive. Controlled studies with patients matched for age, sex, site, stage of primary tumors and metastases, and for previous chemotherapy have not shown any beneficial effect of high dose ascorbic acid in the treatment of advanced cancer.

High doses of vitamin C have been recommended for the prevention and treatment of the common cold, with some evidence that the vitamin reduces the duration and severity of symptoms.

11.14.4.3 *Toxicity of vitamin C*

Regardless of whether or not high intakes of ascorbate have any beneficial effects, large numbers of people habitually take between 1 and 5 g/day of vitamin C supplements (compared with reference intakes of 30–100 mg/day), and some take considerably more. There is little evidence of any significant toxicity. Once the plasma concentration of ascorbate reaches the renal threshold, it is excreted more or less quantitatively with increasing intake, and there is no evidence that higher intakes increase the body pool above 1500 mg/kg body weight. Unabsorbed ascorbate in the intestinal lumen is a substrate for bacterial fermentation, and may cause diarrhea and intestinal discomfort.

Up to 5% of the population are at risk from the development of renal oxalate stones. The risk is from both ingested oxalate and that formed endogenously, mainly from the metabolism of glycine. A number of reports have suggested that people consuming high intakes of vitamin C excrete more oxalate in the urine. However, no pathway for the formation of oxalate from ascorbate is known, and it seems that the oxalate is formed nonenzymically under alkaline conditions either in the bladder or after collection, and high vitamin C intake is probably not a risk factor for renal stone formation.

11.14.5 *Assessment of vitamin C status*

It is relatively easy to assess the state of body reserves of vitamin C by measuring the excretion after a test dose. A subject whose tissue reserves are saturated will excrete more or less the whole of a test dose of 500 mg of ascorbate over 6 h.

The plasma concentration of vitamin C falls relatively rapidly during experimental depletion studies to undetectably low levels within 4 weeks of initiating a vitamin C free diet, although clinical signs of scurvy may not develop for a further 3–4 months, and tissue concentrations of the vitamin may be as high as 50% of saturation.

The concentration of ascorbate in leukocytes is well correlated with the concentrations in other tissues and falls more slowly than the plasma concentration in depletion studies. The reference range of leukocyte ascorbate is 1.1–2.8 mol/10^6 cells; a significant loss of leukocyte ascorbate coincides with the development of clear clinical signs of scurvy.

Without a differential white cell count, leukocyte ascorbate concentration does not give a meaningful index of vitamin C status. The different types of leukocyte have different capacities to accumulate ascorbate. This means that a change in the proportion of granulocytes, platelets, and mononuclear leukocytes will result in a change in the total concentration of ascorbate per 10^6 cells, although there may well be no change in vitamin nutritional status. Stress, myocardial infarction, infection, burns, and surgical trauma all result in changes in leukocyte distribution with an increase in the proportion of granulocytes (which are saturated at a lower concentration of ascorbate than other leukocytes), and hence an apparent change in leukocyte ascorbate. This has been widely misinterpreted to indicate an increased requirement for vitamin C in these conditions.

11.15 Minerals

Those inorganic minerals that have a function in the body must obviously be provided in the diet, since elements cannot be interconverted. Many of the essential minerals are of little practical nutritional importance, since they are widely distributed in foods, and most people eating a normal mixed diet are likely to receive adequate intakes.

In general, mineral deficiencies are a problem when people live largely on foods grown in one region, where the soil may be deficient in some minerals. Iodine deficiency is a major problem in many areas of the world (Section 11.15.3.3). For people whose diet consists of foods grown in a variety of different regions, mineral deficiencies are unlikely. Iron deficiency is a problem in most parts of the world, because if iron losses from the body are relatively high (e.g., from heavy menstrual blood loss), it is difficult to achieve an adequate intake to replace the losses (Section 11.15.2.3).

Mineral deficiency is unlikely among people eating an adequate mixed diet. More importantly, many of the minerals, including those that are dietary essentials, are toxic in even fairly modest excess. This is unlikely to be a problem with high mineral content of foods, although crops grown in regions where the soil content of selenium is especially high may provide dangerously high levels of intake of this mineral (Section 11.15.2.5). The problem arises when people take inappropriate supplements of minerals or are exposed to contamination of food and water supplies.

11.15.1 Calcium

The most obvious requirement for calcium in the body is in the mineral of bones and teeth—a complex mixture of calcium carbonates and phosphates (hydroxyapatite) together with magnesium salts and fluorides. An adult has about 1.2 kg of calcium in the body, 99% of which is in the skeleton and teeth. This means that calcium requirements are especially high in times of rapid growth—during infancy and adolescence, and in pregnancy and lactation.

Although the major part of the body's calcium is in bones, the most important functions of calcium are in the maintenance of muscle contractility, and responses to hormones and neurotransmitters. To maintain these essential regulatory functions, bone calcium is mobilized in deficiency, so as to ensure that the plasma and intracellular concentrations are kept within a strictly controlled range. If the plasma concentration of calcium falls, neuromuscular regulation is lost, leading to tetany.

The main sources of calcium are milk and cheese; dietary calcium is absorbed by an active process in the mucosal cells of the small intestine, and is dependent on vitamin D. Calcitriol, the active metabolite of vitamin D, induces the synthesis of a calcium binding protein, which permits the mucosal cells to accumulate calcium from the intestinal lumen, and in vitamin D deficiency the absorption of calcium is seriously impaired (Section 11.3.3.1).

Although the effect of vitamin D deficiency is impairment of the absorption and utilization of calcium, rickets (Section 11.3.4) is not simply the result of calcium deficiency. Calcium deficient children with adequate vitamin D nutritional status do not develop rickets but have a much reduced rate of growth. Nevertheless, calcium deficiency may be a contributory factor in the development of rickets when vitamin D status is marginal.

11.15.1.1 Osteoporosis

Osteoporosis is a progressive loss of bone with increasing age, after the peak bone mass has been achieved at the age of about 30. The cause is the normal process of bone turnover with reduced replacement of the tissue that has been broken down (Section 11.3.3.1). Both mineral and the organic matrix of bone are lost in osteoporosis, unlike osteomalacia (Section 11.3.4), where there is loss of bone mineral but the organic matrix is unaffected.

Osteoporosis can occur in relatively young people, as a result of prolonged bed rest (or weightlessness in space flight); bone continues to be degraded, but without physical activity there is less stimulus for replacement of the lost tissue. More importantly, it occurs as an apparently unavoidable part of the aging process. Here, the main problem is the reduced secretion of estrogens (in women) and androgens (in men) with increasing age; among other actions, the sex steroids are required for the differentiation of osteoblasts for new bone formation. The problem is especially serious in women, since there is a much more abrupt fall in estrogen secretion at the menopause than the more gradual (and less severe) fall in androgen secretion in men with increasing age. As a result, many more elderly women than men suffer from osteoporosis. Postmenopausal hormone replacement therapy with estrogens has a protective effect.

People with higher peak bone mass are less at risk from osteoporosis, since they can tolerate more loss of bone before there are serious effects. Therefore, adequate calcium and vitamin D nutrition through adolescence and young adulthood is likely to provide protection against osteoporosis in old age. High intakes of calcium have less effect once peak bone mass has been achieved. However, there are no adverse effects either because of the close regulation of calcium homeostasis; problems of hypercalcemia and calcinosis (the calcification of soft tissues) occur as a result of vitamin D intoxication (Section 11.3.5.1), or other disturbances of calcium homeostasis, not as a result of high intakes of calcium.

11.15.2 Minerals that function as prosthetic groups in enzymes

11.15.2.1 Cobalt

In addition to its role in vitamin B_{12} (Section 11.10), cobalt provides the prosthetic group of a small number of enzymes. It is therefore a dietary essential, despite the fact that vitamin B_{12} cannot be synthesized in the body. However, no clinical signs of cobalt deficiency are known, except in ruminant animals whose intestinal bacteria synthesize vitamin B_{12}.

11.15.2.2 Copper

Copper provides the essential functional part of a number of enzymes involved in oxidation and reduction reactions, including dopamine β-hydroxylase in the synthesis of noradrenaline and adrenaline (Section 11.14.2.1), cytochrome oxidase in the electron transport chain (Section 3.3.1.2), and superoxide dismutase, one of the enzymes involved in protection against oxygen radicals (Section 6.5.3.1). Copper is also important in the oxidation of lysine to form the cross links in collagen and elastin. In copper deficiency, the bones are abnormally fragile because the abnormal collagen does not permit the normal flexibility of the bone matrix. More importantly, elastin is less elastic than normal and copper deficiency can lead to death following rupture of the aorta (see Problem 4.4).

11.15.2.3 Iron

The most obvious function of iron is in the heme of hemoglobin, the oxygen-carrying protein in red blood cells, and myoglobin in muscles. Heme is also important as the coenzyme for oxidation and reduction reactions in a variety of enzymes, including the cytochromes

(Section 3.3.1.2). A number of enzymes also contain nonheme iron (i.e., iron bound to the enzyme other than in heme), which is essential to their function.

Deficiency of iron leads to reduced synthesis of hemoglobin, and hence a lower than normal amount of hemoglobin in red blood cells. Iron deficiency anemia is a major problem worldwide, especially among women. The problem is due to a loss of blood greater than can be replaced by absorption of dietary iron. In developing countries intestinal parasites (especially hookworm), which cause large losses of blood in the feces, are a common cause of anemia in both men and women. In developed countries, it is mainly women who are at risk of iron deficiency, as a result of heavy menstrual losses of blood. Probably 10%–15% of women have menstrual losses of iron greater than can be met from a normal dietary intake, and are therefore at risk of developing anemia unless they take iron supplements.

Iron in foods occurs in two forms: heme in meat and meat products, and inorganic iron salts in plant foods. The absorption of heme iron is better than that of inorganic iron salts; as discussed in Section 4.5.3.1, only about 10% of the inorganic iron of the diet is absorbed, although this is increased by vitamin C (Section 11.14.4.1).

11.15.2.4 Molybdenum

Molybdenum functions as the prosthetic group of a small number of enzymes, including xanthine oxidase (which is involved in the metabolism of purines to uric acid for excretion) and pyridoxal oxidase (which metabolizes vitamin B_6 to the inactive excretory product pyridoxic acid; Section 11.9.1). It occurs in an organic complex, molybdopterin, which is chemically similar to folate (Section 11.11.1) but can be synthesized in the body as long as adequate amounts of molybdenum are available.

Molybdenum deficiency has been associated with increased incidence of cancer of the esophagus, but this seems to be an indirect association. The problem occurs among people living largely on maize grown on soil that is poor in molybdenum. For reasons that are not altogether clear, molybdenum deficient maize is more susceptible to attack by fungi that produce carcinogenic toxins. Thus, while the people living on this diet are at risk of molybdenum deficiency, the main problem is not one of molybdenum deficiency in the people, but rather of fungal spoilage of their food.

11.15.2.5 Selenium

Selenium functions in a number of enzymes, including glutathione peroxidase (Section 6.5.3.2) and thyroxine deiodinase, which forms the active thyroid hormone, tri-iodothyronine, from thyroxine secreted by the thyroid gland (Figure 11.26). It is present as the selenium analog of the amino acid cysteine, selenocysteine.

Selenium deficiency is widespread in parts of China, and in some parts of the United States and Finland the soil is so poor in selenium that it is added to fertilizers to increase the selenium intake of the population and prevent deficiency. In New Zealand, despite the low selenium content of the soil, it was decided not to use selenium-rich fertilizers, because of the hazards of selenium toxicity.

Selenium is extremely toxic even in modest excess. The RNI for selenium for adults is 75 μg/day; signs of poisoning can be seen at intakes above 450 μg/day and the World Health Organization recommends that selenium intakes should not exceed 200 μg/day. In some parts of the world, the soil is so rich in selenium that locally grown crops would provide more than this recommended upper limit of selenium intake if they were the main source of food, and it is not possible to graze cattle safely on the pastures in these regions.

11.15.2.6 Zinc

Zinc is the prosthetic group of more than a hundred enzymes with a wide variety of functions. It is also involved in the receptor proteins for steroid and thyroid hormones, calcitriol, and vitamin A. In these proteins, zinc forms an integral part of the region of the protein that interacts with the promoter site on DNA to initiate gene transcription in response to hormone action (Section 10.4).

Overt zinc deficiency occurs only among people living in tropical or subtropical areas whose diet is very largely based on unleavened wholemeal bread. The problem is seen mainly as delayed puberty, so that young men aged 18–20 are still prepubertal. This is a result of reduced sensitivity of target tissues to androgens because of the role of zinc in steroid hormone receptors. Two separate factors contribute to the deficiency:

- Wheat flour provides very little zinc, and in unleavened wholemeal bread much of the zinc that is present is not available for absorption because it is bound to phytate and dietary fiber.
- Sweat contains a relatively high concentration of zinc, and in tropical conditions there can be a considerable loss of zinc in sweat.

Marginal zinc deficiency is associated with poor wound healing, increased susceptibility to infection, and impairment of the senses of taste and smell.

11.15.3 Minerals that have a regulatory role in neurotransmission, as enzyme activators or in hormones

11.15.3.1 Calcium

In addition to its role in bone mineral, calcium has a major function in metabolic regulation (Section 10.3.3), nerve conduction, and muscle contraction. Calcium nutrition is discussed in Section 11.15.1.

11.15.3.2 Chromium

Chromium is involved as an organic complex, the glucose tolerance factor, in the interaction between insulin and its cell-surface receptor (Section 10.3.4) and deficiency is associated with impaired glucose tolerance. There is no evidence that increased intakes of chromium have any beneficial effect in diabetes, and while there is no evidence of harm from organic chromium complexes, inorganic chromium salts are highly toxic.

11.15.3.3 Iodine

Iodine is required for the synthesis of the thyroid hormones, thyroxine and tri-iodothyronine. Deficiency, leading to goiter (a visible enlargement of the thyroid gland), is widespread in inland upland areas over limestone soil. This is because the soil over limestone is thin, and minerals, including iodine, readily leach out, so that locally grown plants are deficient in iodine. Near the coast, sea spray contains enough iodine to replace these losses. Worldwide, many millions of people are at risk of deficiency, and in parts of central Brazil, the Himalayas, and central Africa goiter may affect more than 90% of the population.

Thyroid hormones regulate metabolic activity, and people with thyroid deficiency have a low metabolic rate (Section 5.1.3.1) and hence gain weight readily. They tend to be lethargic and have a dull mental apathy. Children born to iodine deficient mothers are especially at risk, and more so if they are then weaned onto an iodine-deficient diet. They may suffer from very severe mental retardation (goitrous cretinism) and congenital deafness.

By contrast, overactivity of the thyroid gland, and hence overproduction of thyroid hormones, leads to a greatly increased metabolic rate, possibly leading to very considerable weight loss, despite an apparently adequate intake of food. Hyperthyroid people are lean and have a tense nervous energy.

Iodide is accumulated in the thyroid gland, where specific tyrosine residues in the protein thyroglobulin are iodinated to yield di-iodotyrosine (Figure 11.26). The next stage is the transfer of the di-iodophenol residue of one di-iodotyrosine onto another, yielding protein-bound thyroxine, which is stored in the colloid of the thyroid gland. In response to stimulation by thyrotropin, thyroglobulin is hydrolyzed, releasing thyroxine into the circulation. The active hormone is tri-iodothyronine, which is formed from thyroxine by a selenium dependent de-iodinase, both in the thyroid gland and, more importantly, in target tissues. Because of the role of selenium in the metabolism of the thyroid hormones, the effects of iodine deficiency will be exacerbated by selenium deficiency.

In developed countries where there is a risk of iodine deficiency, supplementation of foods is common. Iodized salt may be available, or bread may be baked using iodized salt. In remote regions of developing countries this is rarely possible, and the treatment and prevention of iodine deficiency depends on periodic visits by medical teams who give relatively large doses of iodized oil by intramuscular injection.

The problem of widespread iodization of foods in areas of deficiency is that adults whose thyroid glands have enlarged, in an attempt to secrete an adequate amount of

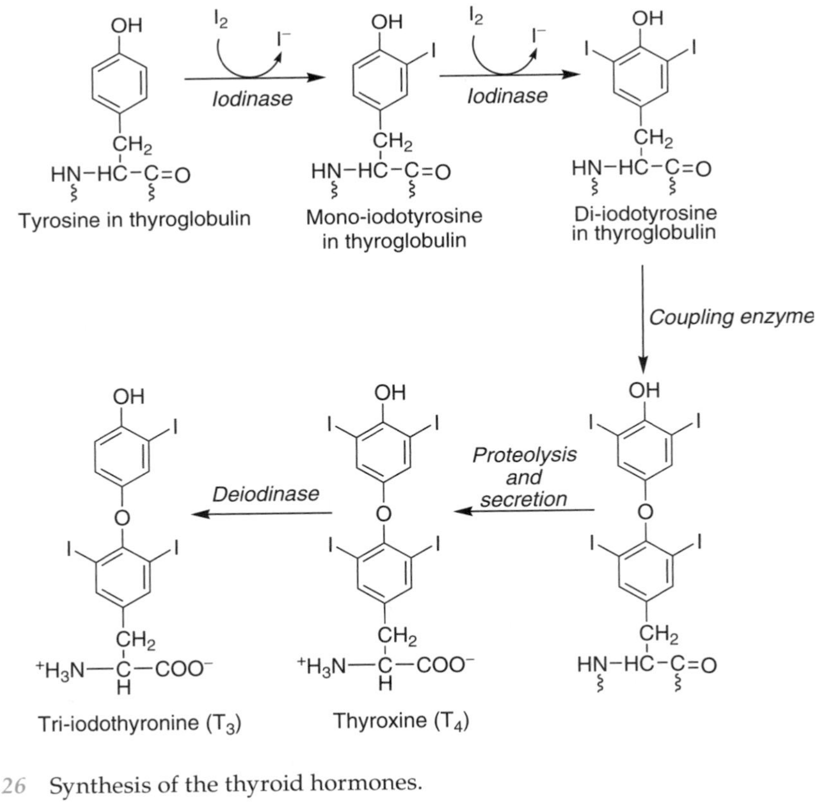

Figure 11.26 Synthesis of the thyroid hormones.

thyroid hormone despite iodine deficiency, now become hyperthyroid. This is considered an acceptable risk to prevent the much more serious problems of goitrous cretinism among the young.

11.15.3.4 Magnesium

Magnesium is a cofactor for enzymes that utilize ATP and also several of the enzymes involved in DNA replication and transcription (Sections 9.2.1.1 and 9.2.2.1). It is not clear whether or not magnesium deficiency is an important nutritional problem since there are no clear signs of deficiency. However, it has been established that intravenous administration of magnesium salts is beneficial immediately after a heart attack.

11.15.3.5 Manganese

Manganese functions as the prosthetic group of a variety of enzymes, including superoxide dismutase, a part of the body's antioxidant defense system (Section 6.5.3.1), pyruvate carboxylase in gluconeogenesis (Section 5.7), and arginase in urea synthesis (Section 9.3.1.4). Deficiency has only been observed in deliberate depletion studies.

11.15.3.6 Sodium and potassium

The maintenance of the normal composition of intracellular and extracellular fluids, and osmotic homeostasis, depends largely on the maintenance of relatively high concentrations of potassium inside cells and sodium outside. The gradient of sodium and potassium across cell membranes is maintained by active (ATP-dependent) pumping (Section 3.2.2.3). Nerve conduction depends on the rapid reversal of this transmembrane gradient to create and propagate the electrical impulse, followed by a more gradual restoration of the normal ion gradient.

There is little or no problem in meeting sodium requirements; indeed, the main problem with sodium is an excessive intake rather than deficiency (Section 6.3.4).

11.15.4 Minerals known to be essential, but whose function is unknown

11.15.4.1 Silicon

Silicon is known to be essential for the development of connective tissue and the bones, although its function in these processes is not known. The silicon content of blood vessel walls decreases with age, and with the development of atherosclerosis. It has been suggested, although the evidence is not convincing, that silicon deficiency may be a factor in the development of atherosclerosis.

11.15.4.2 Vanadium

Experimental animals maintained under very strictly controlled conditions show a requirement of vanadium for normal growth. There is some evidence that vanadium has a role in regulation of the activity of sodium/potassium pumps (Section 3.2.2.3), although this has not been proven.

11.15.4.3 Nickel and tin

There is some evidence from experimental animals maintained under strictly controlled conditions that a dietary intake of nickel and tin is required for optimum growth and development. No metabolic function has been established for either mineral.

11.15.5 Minerals that have effects in the body, but whose essentiality is not established

11.15.5.1 Fluoride

Fluoride has clear beneficial effects in modifying the structure of bone mineral and dental enamel, strengthening the bones, and protecting teeth against decay. The use of fluoride toothpaste and the addition of fluoride to drinking water in many regions, has resulted in a very dramatic decrease in the incidence of dental decay despite high consumption of sucrose and other extrinsic sugars (Section 6.3.3.1). These benefits are seen at levels of fluoride of the order of 1 ppm in drinking water. Such concentrations occur naturally in many parts of the world, and this is the concentration at which fluoride is added to water in many areas.

Excessive intake of fluoride leads to brown discoloration of the teeth (dental fluorosis). A concentration above about 12 ppm in drinking water, as occurs naturally in some parts of the world, is associated with excessive deposition of fluoride in the bones, leading to increased fragility (skeletal fluorosis).

Although fluoride has beneficial effects, there is no evidence that it is a dietary essential. Fluoride prevents dental decay, but it is probably not correct to call dental decay a fluoride deficiency disease.

11.15.5.2 Lithium

Lithium salts are used in the treatment of bipolar manic-depressive disease; they act by altering the responsiveness of some neurons to stimulation. However, this seems to be a purely pharmacological effect, and there is no evidence that lithium has any essential function in the body, or that it provides any benefits for healthy people.

11.15.5.3 Other minerals

In addition to minerals that are known to be dietary essentials, there a number that may be consumed in relatively large amounts, but which have, as far as is known, no function in the body. Indeed, excessive accumulation of these minerals may be dangerous, and a number of them are well known as poisons. Such elements include aluminum, arsenic, antimony, boron, cadmium, cesium, germanium, lead, mercury, silver, and strontium.

Key points

- Vitamins are organic nutrients with essential metabolic functions, generally required in small amounts in the diet, which cannot be synthesized by the body. The lipid-soluble vitamins (A, D, E, and K) are hydrophobic molecules requiring normal fat absorption for their absorption and the avoidance of deficiency symptoms.
- Vitamin A (retinol) present in meat and the provitamin (β-carotene) found in plants form retinaldehyde, utilized in vision, and retinoic acid, which acts in the control of gene expression.
- Vitamin D is a prohormone yielding the active derivative, calcitriol, which regulates calcium and phosphate metabolism; deficiency leads to rickets and osteomalacia.
- Vitamin E (tocopherol) is the most important antioxidant in the body, acting in the lipid phase of membranes to protect against the effects of free radicals.
- Vitamin K is the cofactor for a carboxylase that acts on glutamate residues of precursor proteins of clotting factors and bone proteins to enable them to chelate calcium.

- Thiamin is the cofactor in oxidative decarboxylation of α-keto acids and of transketolase in the pentose phosphate pathway.
- Riboflavin and niacin are cofactors in oxidation and reduction reactions.
- Pantothenic acid is present in coenzyme A and acyl carrier protein, which act as carriers for acyl groups in metabolic reactions.
- Vitamin B_6, as pyridoxal phosphate, is the coenzyme for enzymes of amino acid metabolism and of glycogen phosphorylase; it also acts to terminate the actions of nuclear-acting hormones.
- Biotin is the coenzyme for carboxylation reactions.
- Vitamin B_{12} and folate are involved in metabolism of one-carbon units.
- Vitamin C is a water-soluble antioxidant that maintains vitamin E and many metal cofactors in the reduced state, and is the cofactor for a number of hydroxylation reactions.
- Inorganic mineral elements that have a function in the body must be provided in the diet. When intake is insufficient deficiency may develop, and excessive intakes may be toxic.

Appendix

Table A1 Units of Physical Quantities

Physical Quantity	Unit	Symbol	Definition
Amount of substance	mole	mol	SI base unit
Electric current	ampere	A	SI base unit
Electric potential difference	volt	V	$JA^{-1}s^{-1}$
Energy	joule	J	m^2kgs^{-2}
	calorie	cal	4.186 J
Force	newton	N	Jm^{-1}
Frequency	hertz	Hz	S^{-1}
Length	meter	m	SI base unit
	ångström	Å	10^{-10} m
Mass	kilogram	kg	SI base unit
Power	watt	W	Js^{-1}
Pressure	pascal	Pa	Nm^{-2}
	bar	bar	10^5 Pa
Radiation dose absorbed	gray	Gy	Jkg^{-1}
Radioactivity	becquerel	Bq	S^{-1}
Temperature	degree Celsius	°C	–273.15 K
	kelvin	K	SI base unit
Time	second	s	SI base unit

Table A2 Multiples and Submultiples of Units

	Name	Symbol
10^{21}	zetta	Z
10^{18}	exa	E
10^{15}	peta	P
10^{12}	tera	T
10^{9}	giga	G
10^{6}	mega	M
10^{3}	kilo	k
10^{2}	centa	ca
10	deca	da
10^{-1}	deci	d
10^{-2}	centi	c
10^{-3}	milli	m
10^{-6}	micro	μ (or mc)
10^{-9}	nano	n
10^{-12}	pico	p
10^{-15}	femto	f
10^{-18}	atto	a
10^{-21}	zepto	z

Glossary

In addition to the brief glossary here, the following small and reasonably priced reference books will be useful:

Bender, D.A., *A Dictionary of Food and Nutrition*, Oxford Paperback Reference, 2005.
Daintith, J., *A Dictionary of Chemistry*, Oxford Paperback Reference, 2004.
Martin, E., *A Dictionary of Biology*, Oxford Paperback Reference, 2004.
Martin, E., *Concise Medical Dictionary*, Oxford Paperback Reference, 2003.
Sharp, D.W.A., *Penguin Dictionary of Chemistry*, Penguin Reference, 2003.
Thain, M., Hickman, M., Abercrombie, M. and Hickman, C.J., *Penguin Dictionary of Biology*, Penguin Reference, 2004.

acid: A compound that, when dissolved in water, dissociates to yield hydrogen ions (H^+).

acidosis: A condition in which the pH of blood plasma falls below the normal value of 7.4; a fall to pH 7.2 is life threatening.

acyl group: In an ester or other compound, the part derived from a fatty acid is called an acyl group.

ADP: Adenosine diphosphate.

alcohol: A compound with an −OH group attached to an aliphatic carbon chain. Also used generally to mean ethanol (ethyl alcohol), the commonly consumed alcohol in beverages.

aldehyde: A compound with an HC=O group attached to a carbon atom.

aliphatic: A compound with chains of carbon atoms (straight or branched) rather than rings. Aliphatic compounds may be saturated or unsaturated.

alkali: A compound that gives an alkaline solution when dissolved in water—one with a pH above 7.

alkalosis: A condition in which the pH of blood plasma rises above the normal value of 7.4.

amide: The product of a condensation reaction between a carboxylic acid and ammonia, a $-CONH_2$ group.

amine: A compound with an amino ($-NH_2$) group attached to a carbon atom.

amino acid: A compound with both an amino ($-NH_2$) and a carboxylic acid ($-COOH$) group attached to the α-carbon.

AMP: Adenosine monophosphate.

amylopectin: The branched chain structure of starch.

amylose: The straight chain structure of starch.

anabolism: Metabolic reactions resulting in the synthesis of more complex compounds from simple precursors. Commonly linked to the hydrolysis of ATP to ADP and phosphate.

anaerobic: Occurring in the absence of oxygen.

anion: An ion that has a negative electric charge and therefore migrates to the anode (positive pole) in an electric field. The ions of nonmetallic elements are anions.

antibiotic: Substance produced by one organism to prevent the growth of another. Many are clinically useful to treat bacterial infections, while others are too toxic.

anticodon: The three-base region of transfer RNA that recognizes, and binds to, the codon on messenger RNA.

apoptosis: Programmed cell death.

aromatic: A cyclic compound in which the ring consists of alternating single and double bonds.

atom: The smallest particle of an element that can exist as an entity. The atom consists of a nucleus containing protons, neutrons, and other uncharged particles, surrounded by a cloud of electrons.

atomic mass: The mass of the atom of any element, relative to that of carbon 12; 1 unit of atomic mass = 1.660×10^{-27} kg.

atomic number: The number of protons in the nucleus of an atom (and hence the number of electrons surrounding the nucleus) determines the atomic number of that element.

ATP: Adenosine triphosphate.

autocrine: Produced and secreted by a cell and acting on the cell that secreted it.

basal metabolic rate (BMR): The energy expenditure by the body at complete rest, but not asleep; in the postprandial state.

base: Chemically, an alkali. Also used as a general term for the purines and pyrimidines in DNA and RNA.

BMI: Body mass index.

BMR: Basal metabolic rate.

body mass index (BMI): The ratio of body weight (in kilogram) to square of the height (in meter). A BMI over 25 is considered overweight and over 30 is obesity.

buffer: A solution of a weak acid and its salt that can prevent changes in pH as the concentration of hydrogen ions changes, by shifting the equilibrium between the dissociated and undissociated acid. Any buffer system only acts around the pH at which the acid is half dissociated.

calorie: A (obsolete) unit of heat or energy. The amount of heat required to raise 1 g of water through 1°C. Nutritionally, the kcal is used; 1 kcal = 1000 cal, 1 cal = 4.186 J, 1 J = 0.239 cal.

calorimetry: The measurement of energy expenditure by heat output; indirect calorimetry estimates heat output from oxygen consumption.

carbohydrate: Compounds of carbon, hydrogen, and oxygen in the ratio $C_nH_{2n}O_n$. The dietary carbohydrates are sugars, starches, and nonstarch polysaccharides.

carboxylic acid: A compound with a −COOH group attached to a carbon atom.

catabolism: Metabolic reactions resulting in the breakdown of complex molecules to simpler products, commonly oxidation to carbon dioxide and water, linked to the phosphorylation of ADP to ATP.

catalyst: Something that increases the rate at which a chemical reaction achieves equilibrium without itself being consumed in or altered by the reaction.

cation: A positively charged ion that migrates to the cathode (negative pole) in an electric field. The ions of metallic elements are cations.

cellulose: A polymer of glucose linked by $\beta 1 \rightarrow 4$ glycoside links, which are not digested by human enzymes.

codon: A sequence of three nucleic acid bases in DNA or mRNA, which specify an individual amino acid.

coenzyme: A nonprotein organic compound that is required for an enzyme reaction. Coenzymes may be loosely or tightly associated with the enzyme protein and may be covalently bound to the enzyme, in which case they are known as prosthetic groups.

condensation: A chemical reaction in which water is eliminated from two compounds to result in the formation of a new compound. The formation of esters, peptides, and amides is a condensation reaction.

covalent bond: A bond between two atoms in which electrons are shared between the atoms.

deoxyribose: A pentose (five-carbon) sugar in which one hydroxyl (−OH) group has been replaced by hydrogen. The sugar of DNA.

dietary fiber: The residue of plant cell walls after extraction and treatment with digestive enzymes. Chemically, a mixture of lignin and a variety of nonstarch polysaccharides, including cellulose, hemicellulose, pectin, gums, and mucilages.

disaccharide: A sugar consisting of two monosaccharides linked by a glycoside bond. The common dietary disaccharides are sucrose (cane or beet sugar), lactose, maltose, and isomaltose.

dissociation: The process whereby a molecule separates into ions on solution in water.

DNA: Deoxyribonucleic acid.

double bond: A covalent bond in which two pairs of electrons are shared between the participating atoms.

electrolyte: A compound that undergoes partial or complete dissociation into ions when dissolved, and so is capable of transporting an electric current. In clinical chemistry, electrolyte is normally used to mean the major inorganic ions in body fluids.

electron: The smallest unit of negative electric charge. The fundamental particles that surround the nucleus of an atom.

electronegative: An electronegative atom exerts greater attraction for the shared electrons in a covalent bond than does its partner, thus developing a partial negative charge.

electropositive: An electropositive atom exerts less attraction for the shared electrons in a covalent bond than does its partner, thus developing a partial positive charge.

element: A substance that cannot be further divided or modified by chemical means. The basic substances from which compounds are formed.

endergonic: A chemical reaction that will only proceed with an input of energy, usually as heat.

endocrine: A substance produced by one organ that circulates in the bloodstream and acts on distant organs and tissues.

endonuclease: An enzyme that hydrolyzes a polynucleotide at a specific sequence within the chain, as opposed to an exonuclease.

endopeptidase: An enzyme that hydrolyzes a peptide adjacent to a specific amino acid within the sequence, as opposed to an exopeptidase.

endothermic: A chemical reaction that will only proceed with an input of heat.

enzyme: A protein that acts as a catalyst in a metabolic reaction.

enzyme unit: The activity of an enzyme expressed as micromoles of product formed per minute at 30°C.

essential amino acid: Nine of the amino acids that are required for protein synthesis and cannot be synthesized in the body but must be provided in the diet.

essential fatty acids: Those polyunsaturated fatty acids that cannot be synthesized in the body and must be provided in the diet. Linoleic and linolenic acids are the only two that are dietary essentials, since the other polyunsaturated fatty acids can be synthesized from them.

ester: The product of a condensation reaction between an alcohol and a carboxylic acid.

exergonic: A chemical reaction that proceeds with an output of energy, usually as heat.

exon: A region of DNA that codes for a gene (as opposed to intron).

exonuclease: An enzyme that removes a terminal nucleotide from a polynucleotide, as opposed to an endonuclease.

exopeptidase: An enzyme that removes a terminal amino acid from a polypeptide, as opposed to an endopeptidase.

exothermic: A chemical reaction that proceeds with an output of heat.

fat: Triacylglycerols, esters of glycerol with three fatty acids; fats are generally considered to be those triacylglycerols that are solid at room temperature, while oils are triacylglycerols that are liquid at room temperature.

fatty acid: Aliphatic carboxylic acids (i.e., with a –COOH group). The metabolically important fatty acids have between 2 and 24 carbon atoms (always an even number) and may be completely saturated or have one (monounsaturated) or more (polyunsaturated) C=C double bonds in the carbon chain.

galactose: A hexose (six-carbon) monosaccharide.

gene: A region of DNA, which carries the information for a single protein or polypeptide chain.

genetic code: The sequence of triplets of the nucleic acid bases (purines and pyrimidines), which specifies the individual amino acids.

genome: The complete genetic sequence of an organism; hence, the science of genomics.

gluconeogenesis: The process of synthesis of glucose from noncarbohydrate precursors.

glucose: A monosaccharide; a hexose (six-carbon) sugar of empirical formula $C_6H_{12}O_6$.

glycerol: A trihydric alcohol to which three fatty acid molecules are esterified in the formation of triacylglycerols (fats and oils). Glycerol has a sweet taste and is hygroscopic (attracts water); it is commonly used as a humectant in food processing.

glycogen: A branched-chain polymer of glucose, linked by a 1–4 bonds, with branch points provided by 1–6 bonds; the storage carbohydrate of mammalian liver and muscle.

glycolysis: The metabolic pathway by which glucose is oxidized to pyruvate.

hexose: A monosaccharide with six carbon atoms and hence the empirical formula $C_6H_{12}O_6$. The nutritionally important hexoses are glucose, galactose, and fructose.

hydrocarbon: A compound of carbon and hydrogen only. Hydrocarbons may have linear, branched, or cyclic structures and may be saturated or unsaturated.

hydrogen bond: The attraction between a partial positive charge on a hydrogen atom attached to an electronegative atom and a partial negative charge associated with an electronegative atom in another molecule or region of the same macromolecule.

hydrolysis: The process of splitting a chemical bond between two atoms by the introduction of water, usually adding −H to one side of the bond and −OH to the other, resulting in the formation of two separate product molecules. The digestion of proteins to amino acids, polysaccharides and disaccharides to monosaccharides, and triacylglycerols to glycerol and fatty acids is a hydrolysis reaction.

hydrophilic: A compound that is soluble in water or a region of a macromolecule that can interact with water molecules.

hydrophobic: A compound that is insoluble in water but soluble in lipids, or a region of a macromolecule that cannot interact with water although it does interact with lipids.

induction: The initiation of new synthesis of an enzyme or other protein by activation of the transcription of the gene for the protein. Inducers are commonly metabolic intermediates or hormones. Induction results in an increase in the amount of enzyme protein in the cell.

inhibition: Decrease in the activity of an enzyme, with no effect on the amount of enzyme protein present in the cell.

inorganic: Any chemical compound other than those carbon compounds that are considered to be organic.

insoluble fiber: Lignin and nonstarch polysaccharides in plant cell walls (cellulose and hemicellulose).

international units (iu): Before vitamins and other substances were purified, their potency was expressed in arbitrary, but standardized, units of biological activity. Now obsolete, but vitamins A, D and E are still sometimes quoted in iu.

intron: A region of DNA in between regions that code for a gene (these are exons).

ion: An atom or group of atoms that has lost or gained one or more electrons and thus has an electric charge.

isomers: Forms of the same chemical compound, but with a different spatial arrangement of atoms or groups in the molecule. D and L isomerism refers to the arrangement of four different substituents around a carbon atom relative to the arrangement in the triose sugar D-glyceraldehyde. *R* and *S* isomerism refers to the arrangement of four different substituents around a carbon atom according to a set of systematic chemical rules. *Cis* and *trans* isomerism refers to the arrangement of groups adjacent to a carbon–carbon double bond.

isotope: Different forms of the same chemical element (i.e., having the same number of protons in the nucleus and the same number of electrons surrounding the nucleus as each other) differing in the number of neutrons in the nucleus, and hence in the relative atomic mass.

iu: International unit.

joule: The SI unit of energy. One joule is the work done when the point of application of a force of 1 newton moves 1 meter in the direction of the force. 1 J = 0.239 cal, 1 cal = 4.186 J.

ketone: A compound with a carbonyl (C=O) group attached to two aliphatic groups.

ketone bodies: Acetoacetate and β-hydroxybutyrate (not chemically a ketone) formed in the liver from fatty acids in the fasting state and released into the circulation as metabolic fuels for use by other tissues. Acetone, also formed nonenzymically from acetoacetate, circulates in the blood but cannot be metabolized as a metabolic fuel.

ketosis: An elevation of the plasma concentrations of acetoacetate, hydroxybutyrate, and acetone, as occurs in the fasting state.

kwashiorkor: A disease of protein-energy malnutrition in which there is edema masking the severe muscle wastage, fatty infiltration of the liver, and abnormalities of hair structure, and hair and skin pigmentation.

lactose: The sugar of milk. A disaccharide composed of glucose and galactose.

lipid: A general term, including fats and oils (triacylglycerols), phospholipids, and steroids.

lipogenesis: The metabolic pathway for synthesis of fatty acids from acetyl CoA, then the synthesis of triacylglycerols by esterification of glycerol with fatty acids.

lipolysis: The hydrolysis of triacylglycerols to yield fatty acids and glycerol.

lower reference nutrient intake (LRNI): An intake of a nutrient below which it is unlikely that physiological needs will be met or metabolic integrity be maintained.

macromolecule: A term used to describe the large molecules of, for example, proteins, nucleic acids, and polysaccharides.

macronutrients: The metabolic fuels, those nutrients required in large amounts—fats, proteins, and carbohydrates.

maltose: A disaccharide composed of two molecules of glucose linked by a 1–4 glycoside bond.

marasmus: A disease of protein-energy malnutrition in which there is extreme emaciation as a result of catabolism of adipose tissue and protein reserves.

metabolic fuel: Those dietary components that are oxidized as a source of metabolic energy—fats, carbohydrates, proteins, and alcohol.

metabolism: The processes of interconversion of chemical compounds in the body.

metabolomics: Measurement of all the small molecules (metabolites) present in the organism, representing the interactions between the genome, transcriptome, and proteome.

micronutrients: Those nutrients required in milligram or microgram amounts—vitamins and minerals.

mineral: Inorganic salts, so called because they can be obtained by mining.

mitochondrion: A subcellular organelle that contains the enzymes of the citric acid cycle, fatty acid oxidation, and the electron transport chain for oxidative phosphorylation of ADP to ATP.

mol: Abbreviation for mole—the SI unit for the amount of material. The relative molecular mass of a compound expressed in grams. One mole of any compound contains 6.0223×10^{23} molecules.

molar: Concentration of a compound expressed in mol/L, sometimes abbreviated to M.

molecular mass: The mass of a molecule of a compound, relative to that of carbon 12; the sum of the relative atomic masses of the atoms that comprise the molecule.

molecule: The smallest particle of a compound that can exist in a free state.

monosaccharide: A simple sugar, the basic units from which disaccharides and polysaccharides are composed. The nutritionally important monosaccharides are the pentoses (five-carbon sugars) ribose and deoxyribose, and the hexose (six-carbon sugars) glucose, galactose, and fructose.

neutron: One of the fundamental particles in the nucleus of an atom. Neutrons have no electric charge and a mass approximately equal to that of a proton. Differences in the number of neutrons in atoms of the same element account for the occurrence of isotopes.

nitrogen balance: The difference between the intake of nitrogenous compounds (mainly protein) and the output of nitrogenous products from the body. Positive nitrogen balance occurs in growth when there is a net increase in the body content of protein; negative nitrogen balance means that there is a loss of protein from the body.

nonessential amino acid: Those amino acids that are required for protein synthesis but can be synthesized in the body in adequate amounts to meet requirements, and therefore do not have to be provided in the diet.

nonstarch polysaccharides: A group of polysaccharides other than starch, which occur in plant foods. They are not digested by human enzymes, although they may be fermented by intestinal bacteria. They provide the major part of dietary fiber. The main nonstarch polysaccharides are cellulose, hemicellulose (insoluble nonstarch polysaccharides) and pectin and the plant gums and mucilages (soluble nonstarch polysaccharides).

nucleic acid: DNA and RNA—polymers of nucleotides that carry the genetic information of the cell (DNA in the nucleus) and information from DNA for protein synthesis (RNA).

nucleotides: Phosphate esters of purine or pyrimidine bases with ribose (ribonucleotides) or deoxyribose (deoxyribonucleotides).

nucleus: Chemically, the central part of an atom containing protons, neutrons, and a variety of other subatomic particles. Biologically, the subcellular organelle that contains the genetic information, as DNA, arranged in chromosomes.

obesity: Excessive body weight due to accumulation of adipose tissue. Obesity is generally considered to be a body mass index greater than 30; between 25 and 30 is overweight.

oil: Triacylglycerols, esters of glycerol with three fatty acids; oils are those triacylglycerols that are liquid at room temperature, while fats are solid. Mineral oil and lubricating oil are chemically completely different and are mainly long-chain hydrocarbons.

oligopeptide: A chain of 2–10 amino acids linked by peptide bonds. Longer chains of amino acids are known as polypeptides (up to about 50 amino acids) or proteins.

oligosaccharide: A general term for polymers containing about 3–10 monosaccharides.

orbital: An allowed energy level for an electron around the nucleus of an atom or of two atoms in a molecule.

organic: Chemically, all compounds of carbon other than simple carbonate and bicarbonate salts. These are called organic since they were originally discovered in living matter. Also used to describe foods grown under specified conditions without the use of fertilizers, pesticides, etc.

osmolality: The concentration of osmotically active ions or molecules per kilogram of solution (important in physiology because the density of water, and hence the volume of a solution, is different at 37°C from that at room temperature).

osmolarity: The concentration of osmotically active ions or molecules per liter of solution.

overweight: Body weight relative to height greater than is considered desirable (on the basis of life expectancy), but not so much as to be considered obese.

oxidation: A chemical reaction in which the number of electrons in a compound is decreased. In organic compounds, this is generally seen as a decrease in the proportion of hydrogen, an increase in the number of carbon–carbon double bonds, or an increase in the proportion of oxygen in the molecule.

oxidative phosphorylation: The phosphorylation of ADP to ATP, linked to the oxidation of metabolic fuels in the mitochondrial membrane.

PAL: Physical activity level.

PAR: Physical activity ratio.

paracrine: Substance produced by one cell and acting on nearby cells (cf. endocrine, autocrine).

pentose: A monosaccharide sugar with five carbon atoms and hence the empirical formula $C_5H_{10}O_5$. The most important pentose sugars are ribose and deoxyribose (in which one hydroxyl group has been replaced by hydrogen).

peptide bond: The link between amino acids in a protein formed by condensation between the carboxylic acid group (–COOH) of one amino acid and the amino group ($-NH_2$) of another to give a –CO–NH– link between the amino acids.

pH: A measure of the acidity (or alkalinity) of a solution. A neutral solution has pH = 7.0; lower values are acid, higher values are alkaline. pH stands for potential hydrogen and is the negative logarithm of the concentration of hydrogen ions (H^+) in the solution.

phospholipid: A lipid in which glycerol is esterified to two fatty acids but the third hydroxyl group is esterified to phosphate, and through the phosphate to one of a variety of other compounds. Phospholipids are both hydrophilic and hydrophobic, and have a central role in the structure of cell membranes.

phosphorolysis: The cleavage of a bond between two parts of a molecule by the introduction of phosphate, yielding two product molecules. The breakdown of glycogen, to yield glucose 1-phosphate, proceeds by way of sequential phosphorolysis reactions.

phosphorylation: The addition of a phosphate group to a compound.

physical activity level (PAL): Energy expenditure, averaged over 24 h, expressed as a ratio of the basal metabolic rate. The sum of the PAR multiplied by the time spent for each activity during the day.

physical activity ratio (PAR): Energy expenditure in a given activity, expressed as a ratio of the basal metabolic rate.

polypeptide: A chain of amino acids linked by peptide bonds. Generally, up to about 50 amino acids constitute a polypeptide, while a larger polypeptide would be called a protein.

polysaccharide: A polymer of monosaccharide units linked by glycoside bonds. The nutritionally important polysaccharides can be divided into starch, and nonstarch polysaccharides.

polyunsaturated: Fatty acids with two or more carbon–carbon bonds in the molecule.

PRI: Population reference intake of a nutrient, a term introduced in the 1993 EU Tables of Nutrient Requirements. See RDA.

prosthetic group: A nonprotein part of an enzyme, which is essential for the catalytic activity of the enzyme, and which is covalently bound to the protein.

protein: A polymer of amino acids joined by peptide bonds.

proteome: The ensemble of proteins present in an organism, representing the interactions between the genome and transcriptome; hence, the science of proteomics.

proton: The positively charged subatomic particle in the nucleus of atoms. The number of protons in the nucleus determines the atomic number of the element. The hydrogen ion (H^+) is a proton.

purine: Two of the bases in nucleic acids (DNA and RNA) are purines: adenine and guanine.

pyrimidine: Three of the bases in nucleic acids are pyrimidines: cytidine and uracil in DNA; cytidine and thymidine in RNA.

radical: A free radical is a highly reactive molecule with an unpaired electron.

RDA: Recommended daily (or dietary) allowance (or amount) of a nutrient. An intake of the nutrient two standard deviations above the observed mean requirement, and hence greater than the requirements of 97.5% of the population.

RDI: Recommended daily (or dietary) intake of a nutrient. See RDA.

reducing sugar: A sugar that has a free aldehyde (−HC=O) group, which can therefore act as a chemical reducing agent. Glucose, galactose, maltose, and lactose are all reducing sugars.

reduction: A chemical reaction in which the number of electrons in a compound is increased. In organic compounds, this is generally seen as an increase in the proportion of hydrogen, a decrease in the number of carbon–carbon double bonds, or a decrease in the proportion of oxygen in the molecule. The opposite of oxidation.

repression: Decreased synthesis of an enzyme or other protein as a result of blocking the transcription of the gene for that enzyme. Metabolic intermediates, end products of pathways, and hormones may act as repressors.

respiratory quotient (RQ): The ratio of carbon dioxide produced to oxygen consumed in the metabolism of metabolic fuels. The RQ for carbohydrates is 1.0; for fats, 0.71; for proteins, 0.8.

resting metabolic rate (RMR): The energy expenditure of the body at rest, but not measured under the strict conditions required for determination of basal metabolic rate.

ribose: A pentose (five-carbon) sugar.

ribosome: The subcellular organelle on which the message of messenger RNA is translated into protein. The organelle on which protein synthesis occurs.

RMR: Resting metabolic rate.

RNI: Reference nutrient intake, a term introduced in the 1992 UK Tables of Dietary Reference Values. See RDA.

salt: The product of a reaction between an acid and an alkali. Ordinary table salt is sodium chloride.

satiety: The state of satisfaction of hunger or appetite.

saturated: An organic compound in which all carbon atoms are joined by single bonds, as opposed to unsaturated compounds with carbon–carbon double bonds. A saturated compound contains the maximum possible proportion of hydrogen.

soluble fiber: Nonstarch polysaccharides that are soluble in water; pectin and the plant gums and mucilages.

starch: A polymer of glucose units. Amylose is a straight-chain polymer with 1–4 glycoside links between the glucose units. In amylopectin there are also branch points, where chains are linked through a 1–6 glycoside bond.

steroids: Compounds derived from cholesterol (itself also a steroid), most of which are hormones.

substrate: The substance or substances upon which an enzyme acts.

sugar: Chemically, a monosaccharide or small oligosaccharide. Cane or beet sugar is sucrose, a disaccharide of glucose and fructose.

teratogen: A compound that can cause congenital defects in the developing fetus.

transcription: The process whereby a copy of the region of DNA containing the gene for a single protein is copied to give a strand of messenger RNA.

transcriptome: The mRNA present in an organism, showing which genes are being expressed. Hence, the science of transcriptomics.

translation: The process protein synthesis, whereby the message of messenger RNA is translated into the amino acid sequence.

triacylglycerol: The main type of dietary lipid and the storage lipid of adipose tissue. Glycerol esterified with three molecules of fatty acid; also known as triglycerides.

triglyceride: Alternative (and chemically incorrect) name for triacylglycerol.

unsaturated: An organic compound containing one or more carbon–carbon double bonds, and therefore less than the possible maximum proportion of hydrogen.

urea: The main excretory end product of amino acid metabolism.

valency: The number of bonds that an atom must form with other atoms to achieve a stable electron configuration.

van der Waals forces: Individually weak forces between molecules depending on transient charges due to transient inequalities in the sharing of electrons in covalent bonds.

Vegan: A strict vegetarian who will eat no foods of animal origin.

vegetarian: One who does not eat meat and meat products. An ovo-lactovegetarian will eat milk and eggs, but not meat or fish; a lactovegetarian milk but not eggs; a vegan will eat only foods of vegetable origin.

vitamin: An organic compound required in small amounts for the maintenance of normal growth, health, and metabolic integrity. Deficiency of a vitamin results in the development of a specific deficiency disease, which can be cured or prevented only by that vitamin.

zymogen: Inactive precursor of an enzyme (especially proteolytic enzymes) that is activated after secretion.

Subject index

A

B

C

N

O

P

Q

R

S

T

U

V

W

X

Z